Oral Cancer: Epidemiology, Diagnosis and Management

Oral Cancer: Epidemiology, Diagnosis and Management

Edited by **Kimball Cho**

hayle medical

New York

Published by Hayle Medical,
30 West, 37th Street, Suite 612,
New York, NY 10018, USA
www.haylemedical.com

Oral Cancer: Epidemiology, Diagnosis and Management
Edited by Kimball Cho

International Standard Book Number: 978-1-63241-305-5 (Hardback)

Printed in China.

Contents

Preface

This book brings about important researches in the field of oral cancer relating to its prognosis and treatment. Oral cancer is a crucial public health problem on a global scale and even though, the oral cavity is easily accessible, early diagnosis is still far behind the improved detection of cancers of the colon, melanoma, breast, and prostate. Consequently, death rate due to oral cancer for the last four decades has continued to be over 50% despite significant progresses in treatment modalities. This is contrasting against significant reduction in death rates due to cancers of colon, melanoma, prostate, and breast during the same period. The aim of this book is to serve as a useful source of reference on the etiologic/risk factors, management philosophies, progression indicators, present clinical diagnostic tools, and molecular biomarkers of oral cancer, thereby extensively elucidating this vast topic for interested readers.

Various studies have approached the subject by analyzing it with a single perspective, but the present book provides diverse methodologies and techniques to address this field. This book contains theories and applications needed for understanding the subject from different perspectives. The aim is to keep the readers informed about the progress in the field; therefore, the contributions were carefully examined to compile novel researches by specialists from across the globe.

Indeed, the job of the editor is the most crucial and challenging in compiling all chapters into a single book. In the end, I would extend my sincere thanks to the chapter authors for their profound work. I am also thankful for the support provided by my family and colleagues during the compilation of this book.

Editor

Part 1

Epidemiology and Risk Factors

1

Overview of Oral Cancer

Kalu U. E. Ogbureke[1,*] and Christopher Bingham[2]
[1]*Department of Oral Biology, College of Dental Medicine, Georgia Health Sciences University, Augusta, Georgia,*
[2]*Department of Periodontology, College of Dental Medicine, Georgia Health Sciences University, Augusta, Georgia, USA*

1. Introduction

Cancer is the second most common cause of death in the Western world, after cardiovascular diseases (Johnson, 1991; 2001). Worldwide, an estimated cancer incidence of about 10 million was reported for the year 2009 (Jemal et al., 2010), and 1 out of every 3 persons is estimated to suffer from cancer by the age of 75 years (Johnson, 1991; 2001). It is also estimated that about 7.9 million people world-wide will die from cancer this year (Jemal et al., 2010), accounting for nearly 12% of deaths worldwide (Jemal et al., 2010). In the United States alone, an estimated 569,490 deaths from cancer are projected for the 2010 (Jemal et al., 2010). Recent published estimates of worldwide frequency of the 16 major cancers indicate that in developing countries with a high prevalence of infectious and nutritional diseases, cancer remains a major cause of death (Parkin, Laara and Muir, 1988). This may account partly for the current statistics whereby more than half the global incidence of cancer is from the so-called developing countries, since an estimated 70-80% of the global population resides in these areas (Parkin et al., 1998). The estimated annual incidence of cancer ranges from 48 to 225 per 100,000 in developing countries (Parkin et al., 1998).

2. Oral cancer - Epidemiologic overview

"Oral cancer" encompasses all malignancies originating in the oral cavity. Oral cancer ranks sixth in the overall incidence for the 10 most common cancer sites worldwide and third in the developing countries (Johnson, 2001)). There is also a marked disparity in geographic incidence between the "high" and "low" prevalence areas of the world, suggesting major geographic differences in risk factors (Johnson, 1991; 2001). Most of these factors have been identified through epidemiologic studies.

For statistical purposes, oral cancer is often grouped together with cancers of the pharynx as "oropharyngeal" cancer (Daftary et al., 1992). In the Western world, oral cancer is relatively uncommon, and in the context of all malignant tumors, incidence in the United States and Great Britain ranges from 2 to 3% (Batsakis, 1979; Jemal et al., 2008). Relative incidence of

---

* Corresponding Author

up to 5% however has been reported for the United States (Batsakis, 1979), and higher rates have been reported for the so-called "high risk" areas of Europe with incidence equally varying with different socioeconomic groups within these areas (Johnson, 1991). Worldwide, it is estimated that about 300,000 people will be diagnosed with oral cancer in 2010 (Jemal et al., 2010). Of these, 126,000 will die from the disease (Jemal et al., 2010). In the United States alone, an estimated 35,000 new cases of oral cancer will be diagnosed in 2009 with an estimated 7,500 resultant deaths (Jemal et al. 2008). In the Asian subcontinent of Bangladesh, India, Pakistan, and Sri Lanka, oral cancer is the most common malignancy, accounting for about one-third of all malignancies within the subcontinent (Daftary et al., 1991; Jonson, 2001). About 100,000 new cases are estimated to occur annually in these regions that include Burma, Cambodia, Malaysia, Nepal, Singapore, Thailand, and Vietnam (Daftary et al., 1991).

The paradox in the foregoing gloomy statistics is that, although the oral cavity and oropharynx are easily accessible to dentist and physicians for routine examinations and the biopsy of suspicious lesions that often present with outstanding features, early diagnosis has been painfully slow when compared with the enhanced early detection of breast, colon, prostate cancers, and melanoma (Mashberg A, 2000). As a result, the mortality rate from oral cancer for the past three and a half decades has remained high (over 50%) in spite of new treatment modalities. In contrast, there has been a considerable decrease in mortality rates for cancers of the breast, colon, prostate, and melanoma during the same period (Mashberg A, 2000). Examination of the colonic mucosa, which requires endoscopic examination for evaluation of colon cancer, reveals 36% of localized colon cancers among the United States population (Mashberg A, 2000). An identical percentage of localized oral/oropharyngeal cancers are diagnosed without endoscopy among the same population (Mashberg A, 2000). This paradox was eloquently summed up in a four decades-old publication highlighting ". . . the poor prognosis of a form of cancer, which presents exceptionally good opportunity for early treatment" (Banoczy and Csiba, 1976; Wright 1994).

The impediment to early diagnosis of oral and oropharyngeal cancers, despite increased assiduousness on the part of dentists and oral physicians in their examination of patients at risk, stems from the persistence of archaic paradigms, and the lack of an easily available diagnostic adjunct. In order to increase the early detection of oral cancers, and by so doing increase the survival rates of oral cancer patients, there is therefore the need to identify diagnostic screening modalities that identify early oral malignant lesions with precision.

About 95% of oral cancers are classified histologically as oral squamous cell carcinoma (OSCC; Mashberg, 2000; Johnson, 2001, Sargeran et al., 2008). The remaining 5% include such histologic variants as oral verrucous carcinoma, adenosquamous carcinoma, adenoid squamous cell carcinoma, mucoepidermoid carcinoma, and basaloid squamous cell carcinoma. Mucoepidermoid carcinomas are malignancies of salivary gland origin and, within the oral cavity, arise from minor salivary glands, while adenosquamous carcinomas are currently believed to arise from the oral mucosa with subsequent glandular changes among the tumor cells. Basaloid squamous cell carcinoma, a relatively newly recognized entity, is a rare histologic variant of OSCC with marked predilection for the base of tongue in addition to the supraglottic larynx and hypopharynx. Often included in the remainders are metastatic carcinomas from regional sites distant to the oral cavity.

3. Etiologic risk factors for oral cancer

Oral cancer is a multifactorial disease. Exposure to one of three broad groups of carcinogenic stimuli, namely, chemical, physical, and viral, is known to induce cancer in genetically and systemically conditioned oral mucosa. Within the oral cavity, it appears that carcinomas are caused predominantly by chemical carcinogens, although evidence implicating viral and physical stimuli in the development of some oral cancers continues to mount (Syrjanen, 2005; Reddout et al., 2007). The pathogenesis of oral cancer is equally complex, and exposure to carcinogens does not inevitably result in the development of oral cancer. This is because a number of familial, dietary, hormonal, and sex-related factors are known to modulate neoplastic processes generally. Tobacco and alcohol have emerged as the most important culprits contributing to the etiology of oral cancers. Other factors frequently cited are ultraviolet light, nutritional and dietary factors, precancerous lesions, immunosuppression, genetic, and dental factors.

3.1 Tobacco and tobacco products

An association between the use of tobacco and oral cancer can be traced to the early 18th century, when lip cancer was observed with some frequency in tobacco users (Sawyer and Wood, 1992). The strong association of cancers of the oral cavity and oropharynx with tobacco use is well established (Johnson, 2001). Epidemiological studies show that the risk of developing oral cancer is five to nine times greater for smokers than for nonsmokers, and this risk may increase to as much as 17 times for heavy smokers of 80 or more cigarettes per day (Neville and Day, 2002). Approximately 80 percent of oral cancer patients are smokers, and this is two to three times greater than that of the general population (Silverman and Griffith, 1972; Blot et al., 1988; Mashberg et al., 1993; Jovanovic et al., 1993; Andre et al., 1995, Lewin et al., 1998). In addition, treated oral cancer patients who continue to smoke have a two- to six- times greater risk of developing a second malignancy of the upper aerodigestive tract than those who stop smoking (Silverman and Griffith, 1972; Silverman and Shillitoes, 1998).

Oral smokeless tobacco (snuff and chewing tobacco) have also been associated with an increased risk for oral cancer (Brown et al., 1965). In one study of women in the southern United States, chronic users of snuff were estimated to have a four times greater risk of developing oral cancer (Winn et al., 1981, Johnson, 2001). In addition, a significant number of oral cancers in smokeless tobacco users develop at the site of tobacco placement. However, the use of smokeless tobacco appears to be associated with a much lower cancer risk than that associated with smoked tobacco. For example, although the state of West Virginia has the highest consumption of chewing tobacco in the United States, the incidence of oral cancer in West Virginia is below the U.S. national average (Bouquot and Meckestroth, 1998). Recent studies from Scandinavia have suggested that the use of Swedish snuff (which is nonfermented and has lower nitrosamine levels) is not associated with an increased risk for oral cancer (Johnson, 2001; Neville, 2002).

The habit of oral smokeless tobacco use is evolving as "fashionable" amongst the youth in many Western countries, and may partly account for spikes in the rate of oral cancers and potentially malignant lesions observed in this age group in recent decades (Johnson, 1991). The importance of teenage use of smokeless tobacco lies in the considerable length of time that the oral mucosa of teenagers indulging in this habit are bathed in high concentrations of numerous carcinogens contained in smokeless tobacco (Sawyer and Wood, 1992). In addition to carcinogens usually associated with smoking, smokeless tobacco contains ^{210}polonium (originating from phosphate fertilizers used to grow tobacco), ^{226}radium, and ^{210}lead (Main and Lacavalier, 1988). Furthermore, tobacco-specific nitrosamines present in smokeless tobacco, and readily extracted in saliva and further enhanced in alkaline environments, often are of higher concentrations than in cigarette smoke (Sawyer and Wood, 1992).

In India and Southeast Asia, the chronic use of betel quid (*paan*) in the mouth has been strongly associated with an increased risk for oral cancer (Murti et al., 1985; Murti et al., 1995). The quid typically consists of a betel leaf that is wrapped around a mixture of areca nut and slaked lime, usually with tobacco and sometimes with sweeteners and condiments. The slaked lime results in the release of an alkaloid from the areca nut, which produces a feeling of euphoria and well-being in the user. Betel quid chewing often results in a progressive, scarring precancerous condition of the mouth known as oral submucous fibrosis. In India, one study showed a malignant transformation rate of 7.6 percent for oral submucous fibrosis (Murti et al., 1985).

Marijuana use is also considered to be a potential risk factor and may be partly responsible for the rise in oral cancers seen among young adults (Zhang et al., 1999; Silverman, 2001; Schantz and Yu, 2002). Marijuana smoke contains known carcinogens such as benzopyrene and benzanthracene (aromatic hydrocarbons), and the concentration of these carcinogens is postulated to be considerably higher than that in cigarette smoke (Sawyer and wood, 1992). However, further epidemiological studies are necessary to confirm the purported association of marijuana and oral cancer, particularly in younger patients.

3.2 Alcohol

The relationship between alcohol, particularly hard liquor, and squamous cell carcinoma has been recognized for a long time (Wynder, 1971), and has been identified as a major risk factor for cancers of the upper aerodigestive tract (Neville and Day, 2002). What presented as a significant challenge, until recently, was the assessment of the independent role of alcohol in oral cancers due to the difficulty in separating the effects of heavy alcohol consumption from those of smoking and other risk factors, including nutritional (Kato and Nomura, 1994). Most heavy consumers of alcohol beverages also are heavy smokers.

In studies controlled for smoking, moderate-to-heavy drinkers have been shown to have a three- to nine- times greater risk of developing oral cancer (Blot et al., 1988; Mashberg et al., 1993; Jovanovic et al., 1993; Andre et al., 1995; Lewin et al., 1998). One study from France showed that heavy drinkers, consuming more than 100 grams of alcohol per day (a typical serving of beer, wine, or liquor approximates 10 to 15 grams of alcohol), had a 30 times greater risk of developing oral and oropharyngeal cancer (Andre et al., 1995). Thus, it would appear that smoking is not a necessary prerequisite for alcohol induced cancers. Of greater significance however is the synergistic effect of alcohol and smoking; some subsets of patients who are both heavy smokers and heavy drinkers can have over one hundred times greater risk for developing a malignancy (Blot et al., 1988; Andre et al., 1995).

While the mechanism of alcohol-induced carcinogenesis remains unclear, it is apparent that alcohol acts primarily as a co-carcinogen or promoter. Carcinogenesis also may be related to nutritional deficiencies associated with alcoholism. Systemically, alcohol may lead to impaired absorption of nutrients and vitamins. It has been suggested that alcohol acts as a solvent facilitating the entry of carcinogens into exposed cells (Sawyer and Wood, 1992). In addition to creating a nutritional deficiency state (Harris et al., 1997; Johnson, 2001), alcohol may alter epithelial cell metabolism, or suppress immunity (Cotran, Kumar and Robbins, 1989). There is some evidence that carcinogenic contaminants rather than ethanol may be responsible for the increased incidence of alcohol-associated cancers (Bennie, 1976).

3.3 Human Papilloma Viruses (HPV)

The role of HPV as an etiologic agent in cancer was first recognized in the uterine cervix (where it is present in about 99.7% of cases), and the prognostic significance of HPV-associated cervical cancer is now well established (Clifford, Boyle and Franceschi S, 2003; Reddout, 2007). HPV-16 and -18 are the major high-risk types and predominate in invasive anogenital cancers (Clifford et al., 2003; Reddout, 2007). On the other hand there is as yet no clear evidence to support a causative role for HPV in OSCCs, and any potential pathogenic mechanism of HPV-associated OSCCs is still confounding. At best, an association between HPV infection and oral cancer is accepted by most investigators in this field.

In oral lesions, HPV-16 is by far the most common subtype associated with OSCCs and oral premalignant lesions (OPL) exhibiting epithelial dysplasias (Reddout, 2007). HPV-16 DNA has been identified in primary tumors of the tonsil, hypopharynx, oral cavity, tongue, and nasopharynx, as well as in cell-lines derived from these regions (Syrjanen, 2005; Reddout, 2007). Metastatic lymph nodes lesions have also been shown to contain DNA of the same HPV type as in the primary tumor in 76% of the cases, supporting the involvement of HPV in the development of OSCC (Clifford et al., 2003; Syrjanen, 2005; Reddout, 2007).

The prevalence of HPV-16 in OSCC is now considered to be as high as 50% if not more, making it likely that every alternate OSCC patient is HPV-16 positive (Syrjanen, 2005; Reddout, 2007). The association is strongest in the oropharynx, most notably in the tonsil and base of tongue, which present more frequent basaloid histomorphology and less frequent p53 mutations (Clifford et al., 2003). In addition, HPV-16 has been detected in extremely low copy numbers (compared to copy numbers in OSCC and dysplastic OPLs) in some human "normal" oral mucosa (NOM), suggesting that a threshold viral DNA copy number is required for the role of oncogenic HPVs in oral carcinogenesis. HPV-18 is far less commonly associated with oral cancers, and has been found in up to just 14 percent of cases (Kang and Park, 2001).

It is now established that the products of two early genomic regions of high-risk HPVs, E6 and E7, are capable of forming specific complexes with vital cell cycle regulators (Kang and Park, 2001). For example, E6 binds to p53 to induce p53 degradation, while E7 interacts with pRb resulting in blockage of the downstream activities of pRb (Kang and Park, 2001). Both p53 and pRb are oncosuppressors, and the overall outcome of their functional dysregulation is an uncontrolled DNA replication and impairment of apoptosis. The combined effects of apoptotic impairment and uncontrolled DNA replication are increased tendency towards cellular transformation and tumorigenesis.

3.4 Nutritional factors

The role of metabolic and dietary deficiencies in the etiology of OSCC was long suspected before concrete evidence began to emerge. Peterson (1919) and Kelly (1919) independently described the symptom complex of chronic dysphagia, mucosal atrophy of the hypopharynx, and chronic anemia in middle-aged women who also had cricoid carcinomas. The term sideropenic dysphagia was introduced, and used to describe the disease complex now referred to as Paterson-Kelly (or Plummer-Vinson; P-V) syndrome. P-K syndrome is marked by diminished iron stores and the absence of stainable bone marrow iron. Other components of the syndrome include riboflavin and other vitamin deficiencies. Subsequent studies by Ahlbom (1936) confirmed not only the importance of P-K syndrome in the development of pharyngeal cancers, but also showed that this applied to the buccal mucosa, tongue, and all levels of the esophagus.

There is a high incidence of oral cancer in parts of the world where iron deficiency is endemic (Prime, MacDonald and Rennie, 1982). Iron metabolism is essential for the overall integrity and health of epithelia of the digestive tract, and its importance may lie in its contribution to normal enzymes. Rennie and MacDonald (1982), and Rennie, MacDonald and Dagg (1982) demonstrated quantitative histologic changes in the oral epithelium in human iron deficiency anemia and in experimental iron deficiency in hamsters. The authors noted that the oral epithelium in iron deficiency is atrophic with reduced maturation compartment, but an increased keratinized compartment (Rennie et al., 1982). Subsequent cell kinetic studies by Rennie and MacDonald (1984) showed increased cell proliferation, indicating that, in spite of the atrophy, epithelial turnover is rapid. This observation suggested a possible increase in susceptibility to chemical carcinogens due to both an increase in the population of potentially vulnerable dividing cells and to a more permeable epithelium.

Increased cancer risks also are attributable to dietary factors, notably low intake of fruits and vegetables (Winn et al., 1984; Winn, 1995). Increased consumption of fruits and vegetables were said to be protective against oral cancer when controlled for demographic characteristics, tobacco and alcohol use, relative weight, and the intake of other food items (Winn et al., 1984). The reduction of risk is seen to be consistent with the hypothesis that Vitamin C and/or Vitamin A and ß-carotene intake is associated with a reduced risk of oral and pharyngeal cancers (Ibrahim, Jafarey and Zuberi, 1977). Interestingly, intervention trial studies with ß-carotene and Vitamin A in patients with oral precancer have been shown to result in substantial regression of the lesions (Stich et al., 1988a, 1988b).

Degenerative changes occur in riboflavin deficiency, a frequent finding in alcoholics. This may partly explain the relationship between alcoholism and oral cancer (Wynder and Klien, 1965). It also may be that alcohol increases the risk of oral cancer by lowering nutritional status via a substitution of non-nutritive calories for vitamins, minerals, and other elements; alternatively, that poor nutrition allows the deleterious effects of alcohol to be manifested.

3.5 Impaired immunity

Generally, patients with malignancies have some degree of immunosuppression that tends to worsen with the progression of their malignancy. Immunosuppression appears to predispose some individuals to an increased risk for oral cancer. Carcinomas of the lip have been reported in a number of kidney transplant patients receiving immunosuppressive medications, and oral carcinomas have been documented in young AIDS patients (van Zuuren, de Visscher JGAM, Bouwes Bavinck JN, 1988; Flaitz et. al., 1995; de Visscher, Bouwes Bavinck JN and van der Waal, 1997; Flaitz and Silverman, 1998). It is however still debated as to whether immunosuppression in malignant disease represents an effect or a cause of the malignancy. Some studies have suggested that immunosuppressive states may represent the effect rather than the cause of cancer (Johnson, 1991), while others have suggested that OSCC, despite its local manifestations, is most likely a "regional" disease process that becomes "clinically significant" only when the patient's immunologic status is altered (Mashberg and Samit, 1989).

It would appear however that a factor such as advanced age, which diminishes immune competence and immune cellular surveillance, increases the risks of oral cancer. Overt immune suppression induced by chemicals or drugs, or caused by specific viral infections such as the human immunodeficiency virus (HIV), or Epstein Barr virus (EBV), increases the risk of oral cancers. Barr et al. (1989); Bradford et al. (1990) variously suggested that HPV may play an etiologic role in squamous cell carcinoma in renal allograft recipients.

3.6 Oral Premalignant Lesions

Oral premalignant lesions (OPLs) are lesions, often presenting on the oral mucosa, which possess a higher than normal propensity for transformation to OSCC with time if untreated. The current model for oral carcinogenesis postulates a step-wise transformation from normal to pre-malignant to invasive carcinoma phenotype. Histologically, the transition process involves progression from benign epithelial hyperplasia to various degrees of epithelial dysplasia (mild, moderate, severe) to carcinoma in situ, and finally to invasive OSCC. With respect to transition to OSCC, oral leukoplakia, oral erythroplakia, and speckled leukoplakia are the most notable and most studied OPLs (Figure 1.1). The transition rate of oral leukoplakia to OSCC is estimated at between 4 and 18%, while that of OLP is to be between 1 and 4%.

Although erythroplakia is not nearly as common as leukoplakia, it is much more likely to show dysplasia or carcinoma histologically. In a study by Shafer and Waldron (1975) of biopsies of erythroplakic lesions from 65 patients, all cases showed some degree of epithelial dysplasia: 51 percent showed invasive squamous cell carcinoma; 40 percent were carcinoma in situ or severe epithelial dysplasia; and the remaining 9 percent demonstrated mild-to-moderate dysplasia (Shafer and Waldron, 1975). Thus, true clinical erythroplakia is a much more worrisome lesion than leukoplakia (Mashberg and Samit, 1995). Likewise, in a mixed leukoplakia-erythroplakia (erythroleukoplakia), the erythroplakic (red component) is more likely to demonstrate dysplastic changes than is the white component, making it imperative that that biopsy sites be selected to ensure that the specimen incorporates the red component. In addition, a number of studies have suggested that oral lichen planus (OLP), especially the erosive form, may be associated with an increased cancer risk, although other investigators have questioned the strength of this association (Silverman et al., 1991; Barnard et al., 1993; Eisenberg, 2000).

4. Site distribution in oral cancer

Symptomatic lesions present with symptoms and signs such as intraoral pain and/or dysfunction, extraoral swelling, and cervical lymphadenopathy. These signs and symptoms alert the clinician to the need to evaluate the oral cavity for obvious primary lesions. Site distribution in OSCC is usually described in relation to the symptomatic lesions, which are often amenable to classification under the "T" category of the TNM classification of malignant tumors (Neville and Day, 2002). The TNM classification allows for the clinical staging of oral malignant tumors on the basis of the size of the primary tumor, T, the absence or presence of corresponding regional node spread, and the absence or presence of distant site/organ metastases (Neville and Day, 2002). In OSCC, T1 lesions are 2cm or less in greatest dimension; T2 lesions are more than 2cm but not more than 4cm in greatest dimension; T3 lesions are more than 4cm in greatest dimension, and T4 lesions are those that have invaded adjacent contiguous structures such as the cortical bone, inferior alveolar nerve, deep extrinsic muscles of the tongue, maxillary sinus, or salivary glands regardless of their apparent visual dimension (Neville and Day, 2002).

Early asymptomatic lesions are relatively small (T1) and, not infrequently, elude clinical diagnosis by conventional systems (Mashberg and Meyers, 1976; Neville and Day, 2002). These early asymptomatic lesions, often presenting as erythroplastic lesions, were studied by Mashberg and Meyers (1976) who consequently provided guidance toward enhanced accurate designation of sites of origin of these early asymptomatic lesions (Mashberg and Meyers, 1976). In this respect, the authors further concluded thus: "The described locations in the literature may be points of termination or extension of the lesion rather than sites of origin, e.g., a symptomatic lesion (T2 or T3) in the floor of mouth may have extended to and invaded the alveolus; hence, based on clinical and x-ray evidence, it may have been reported as a gingival or alveolar lesion" (Mashberg and Meyers (1976).

There are geographic variations in the frequency of sites of involvement, probably related to such risk factors as occupation and lifestyle, oral habits, and certain socio-cultural practices, such as the mode of tobacco use (Paymaster, 1962; Brown et al., 1965). For example, presentation of intraoral cancers among the population of the high risk areas of Southeast Asia and the Southeast United States is slightly different. Consistent with the role of the risk factors alluded to above the most prone sites in the high risk areas of Southeast Asia are the buccal, retromloar, and commissural mucosa (Paymaster, 1962; Brown et al., 1965).

4.1 The lip

The World Health Organization (WHO) revision of the International Classification of Diseases (ICD) defines cancer of the lips as malignant lesions of the vermilion area of the upper and lower lips (Daftary et al., 1992). Cancers in these areas are not considered intraoral cancers (Daftary et al., 1992). Over 90% of lip cancers involve the lower lip (Neville and Day, 2002). Lip lesions are easily detectable partly because the lip is the most visible structure of the oral cavity complex. Lip squamous cell carcinomas usually arise in actinic cheilosis, a premalignant condition, which is a "cousin" to actinic keratosis of the skin. Actinic cheilosis is characterized by atrophy of the vermilion border, clinically visible as dry, scaly changes. Ulcerated foci alternating with partial healing may appear as the lesion progresses. Not infrequently, patients mistake these recurring ulcerated lesions for "fever blisters." Subsequently, the evolving cancer slowly becomes a crusted, non-tender, indurated ulcer or mass (Neville et al., 2009; Silverman, Dillon and Fischbein, 1998).

In Romania, Hungary, Yugoslavia, and parts of Canada and the United States, the vermilion area of the lips are the commonest sites of oral cancer (Johnson, 1991; 2001), and it has been reported that about half of all cases of oral cancer in the Nordic countries occur on the lips (Ringertz, 1971). The lateral aspect of the lower lip is more frequently involved than the mid-portion (Daftary et al., 1992). Race and ethnic variations in the incidence of lip cancer occur worldwide. Among most white population, the lip constitutes the most common site for oral cancer (Spitzer et al., 1975; Johnson, 1991; 2001). Considerable agreement over the association between lip cancer and occupation exists; the disease being common amongst white males who engage in outdoor occupations, such as farming and fishing, which expose them excessive sunlight (Spitzer et al., 1975; Johnson, 1991; 2001). On the other hand, lip cancer is relatively rare in black males, and females of both white and black races (Bernia, 1948; Spitzer et al., 1975; Johnson, 1991; 2001).

In a 1984 study reported by Douglass and Gammon there was variation in the incidence of lip cancer between the male non-Maori (1.7/ 100,000) and the Maori (0.2/100,000) population of New Zealand (Douglass and Gammon, 1984). The authors similarly highlighted ethnic differences in the incidence of lip cancer in Israel where males born in Israel had a higher rate of lip cancer (3.5/100,000) than male immigrants from Europe/America (2.9/100,000), or Africa/Asia (0.8/100,000).

4.2 The tongue and floor of mouth

The tongue is the most common site for intraoral carcinoma and accounts for about 40 percent of all cases in the oral cavity proper, with tumors occurring on the posterior lateral border and ventral surfaces of the tongue (Neville and Day, 2002). The incidence of floor-of-mouth squamous cell carcinoma closely approximates that of the tongue (Neville and Day, 2002). In the black population however the floor of mouth distinctly is the most common site for OSCC (Batsakis, 1979). Thus, anatomically, the lateral tongue and floor of mouth (extending to the lateral soft palate and tonsillar area) combine to form a horseshoe-shaped region of the oral mucosa, which is at greatest risk for cancer development (Neville and Day, 2002). Two major factors may explain the high-risk status of this composite region: first, carcinogens in saliva pool at the floor of the mouth with the tongue providing a lid; second, this complex is covered by a thinner, non-keratinized mucosa, thus providing limited barrier to carcinogen ingress (Jovanovic et al., 1993).

4.3 Buccal mucosa

The mucosal surface of the cheek extends from upper to lower vestibular sulci, where the mucosa reflects itself to cover the upper and lower alveolar ridges. The buccal mucosa also forms the commissure of the lip and covers the ramus of the mandible. A number of buccal squamous cell carcinomas originate in the commisural areas before spreading posteriorly to involve the mucosa along the occlusal plane of the teeth, or at the retromolar area (Batsakis, 1979). It has been suggested that, because commissural cancers have better prognoses than buccal mucosa cancers, the former ought to be separated from the latter for purposes of site designation (Daftary et al., 1992). However, this suggestion appears not to have gained wide acceptance. Buccal cancers usually arise on the mucosa lying against the wisdom teeth, and correspond to the common site of placement of tobacco-containing quid. The lesion then grows to obscures the site of origin (Singh and von Essen, 1966; Batsakis, 1979; Daftary et al.,

1992). Results of some studies indicate a consistent increase in the incidence of buccal cancers in relation to smokeless tobacco use (Brown et al., 1965; Winn et al., 1981). These findings underscore the importance of local etiologic factors in the site distribution of intraoral cancers.

4.4 The gingiva and alveolar ridge

Cancer of the gingivae and alveolar ridge are usually grouped together. Squamous cell carcinomas of the gingival and alveolar ridge generally are less common than those of the lip, tongue, and floor of mouth (McCarthy and Shklar, 1964). Similar to buccal and commissural cancers, Daftary et al., (1992) suggested that lesions of the gingivae and alveolar ridge be separated because of differences in prognosis. The incidence of carcinoma of the gingivae and alveolar ridge among the rural women of the Southeast United States is relatively high (Rosenfield and Callaway, 1963). The reported incidence of cancer of the gingival and alveolar ridge in three Indian populations ranged from 0.6/100,000 to 1.4/100,000 per annum among women (Daftary et al., 1992). Carcinoma of the gingivae generally arises in the premolar and molar regions and more frequently, on the lower than on the upper arch (Cady and Catlin, 1969). These correspond to the sites of retention of tobacco quid in those who practice the habit.

4.5 The palate

Squamous cell carcinomas of the palate are in the Western countries and the United States (Daftary et al., (1992). Again, incidence significantly reflects different habits. In India, for example where the habit of "reverse smoking" is prevalent among the population, the relative frequency of squamous cell carcinoma of the palate is high (Gupta et al., 1980; Daftary et al., 1992). The habit of reverse smoking is exemplified by the practice of placing the glowing end of a local form of cigar called "chuttas" inside the mouth. In areas where reverse smoking is practiced palatal cancer comprise 38 to 48 percent of all oral cancers (Gupta et al., 1980; Daftary et al., (1992). Lesions of the hard palate may arise in the midline or to one side close to the palatal gingivae (Batsakis, 1979).

Primary squamous cell carcinomas arising in the soft palate are uncommon, accounting for 2 percent of overall oral cancer in reverse-smoking areas (Ramulu et al., 1973), but only 0.4 percent in non-reverse smoking areas (Wahi et al., 1965). However, reports of later studies by Mashberg and Meyers (1976) indicated a greater frequency of lesions primarily arising from the soft palate than is ordinarily documented with the "late" symptomatic lesions. On analyzing the site distribution of 222 cases of early asymptomatic OSCCs, the authors found that 64 of these (28.8 percent) occurred in the "soft palate complex" comprising the soft palate, anterior pillar of fauces, and retromolar trigone. Thus, some of the lesions designated hard palate lesions at the time of diagnosis may have earlier arisen from the soft palate before spreading to the hard palate at a late symptomatic stage.

5. Diagnosis and management of oral cancer

Early diagnosis of oral cancer has emerged as a priority public health objective whereby oral health professional play leading role (Neville and Day, 2002). It is presumed that early diagnosis of cancer should lead to less damage from interventional treatment and to a better prognosis. Because most individual are seen more commonly by primary care physicians and general dentists than by specialists, it is imperative for these clinicians to perform screening examinations to identify potential oral and pharyngeal cancers. In addition to the need for improved early detection by clinicians, it is also important that the patient and general public are knowledgeable about the disease (Yellowitz and Goodman, 1995; CDC, 1998). Delays in identification and recognition of suspicious lesions contribute to advanced stage at diagnosis and lower survival statistics (Shafer, 1975; Hollows, McAndrew and Perini, 2000).

5.1 Diagnosis of oral cancer

A distinction has been made in the early detection of oral cancers between "screening" (test aimed at evaluating presence of the disease in asymptomatic individuals) and "detection of cases" (applying specific procedure to patients with a suspicious lesion; Lestón and Dios, 2010). Nevertheless, conventional visual examination accompanied by palpation of suspicious lesions remains the gold standard screening methodology for oral precancer and cancer, while biopsy and histopathologic examination remains the universal diagnostic confirmatory test of choice (Lestón and Dios, 2010). Thus, in spite of the availability of several techniques that have been advocated as aids to oral cancer diagnosis (summarized in Table; adapted from Lestón and Dios, 2010) suspected malignant lesions must be biopsied in order to establish a definitive diagnosis.

Toluidine blue
Light-based detection systems
Chemiluminescence (ViziLite Plus®; Microlux/DL®)
Tissue fluorescence imaging (VELscope®)
Tissue fluorescence spectroscopy
Cytology or brush biopsy (OralCDx®)
Specific analysis (, SCCAA, IAP, CYFRA, , and others)
Specific analysis (, , , CYFRA 21-1, TPS, IL-1B, DUSP 1, HA3, , , SAT, miRNA, and others)
Imaging (DPT, CT, CBCT, MRI)

Table 1. Some techniques advocated for the clinical diagnosis of OSCC supplementing conventional oral examination, and histopathologic examination of suspicious lesions *(adapted from Lestón and Dios, 2010)*.

In turn, the accurate diagnosis of potentially malignant and malignant oral lesions depends on the quality of the biopsy, selection of appropriate technique (e.g. incisional versus excisional), the applicability of the adequate clinical information, and competent interpretation of the biopsy results. Oral biopsy specimens can be affected by a number of artifacts resulting from crushing, fulguration, injection, or incorrect fixation and freezing (Trullenque-Eriksson et al., 2009). Results of cytologic examination of specimens obtained from non-invasive procedures such as brush biopsies or comparable techniques must not constitute the sole basis for a diagnosis of malignancy (or the absence) leading to definitive treatments. This is because these non-invasive techniques often are fraught with several pitfalls accounting for high rates of false-negative and false-positive results.

5.2 Management of oral cancer patients

While an exhaustive discussion on the management of oral cancer and precancerous lesions is not intended in this review, it is generally recommended that leukoplakias exhibiting degrees of epithelial dysplasia equal to, or worse than, moderate epithelial dysplasia be removed completely when possible (Epstein et al., 2007). On the other hand, the management guideline for mild dysplastic lesions is far less standardized with varied schools of thought ranging from those advocating a "wait-and-see" approach to those advocating total removal of all dysplastic lesions regardless of the degree of epithelial dysplasia. In addition, management decisions for mild epithelial dysplasia appear to be influenced by the size, location, and apparent etiologic factor accounting for the lesion. Some early dysplastic lesions where an etiologic agent (e.g. smoking) is identified have been known to regress and may reverse to normal on elimination of the etiologic factor responsible.

Patients with invasive oral cancer are best managed by a coordinated, multidisciplinary team of health care professionals, which may include a head and neck surgeon, oral and maxillofacial pathologist, general pathologist, radiation oncologist, neuroradiologist, reconstructive surgeon, medical oncologist, general dentist, oral and maxillofacial surgeon, maxillofacial prosthodontist, dental hygienist, nurse specialist, speech pathologist, nutritionist, and tobacco cessation counselor (Ord and Blanchaert, 2001).

Up to 15 percent of individuals with oral cancer harbor a second primary, making a complete head and neck examination that includes the larynx imperative (Lippman and Hong, 1989). Endoscopy of the larynx, esophagus, trachea, and lungs to rule out the possibility of other lesions in the high-risk patient is now performed routinely. For patients who present with a neck mass but no obvious primary site (or if the neck mass is more amenable to biopsy than the primary tumor), a fine needle aspiration remains the diagnostic method of choice rather than an open biopsy, because open biopsy has been reported to be related to a lower survival rate when not accompanied by a simultaneous neck dissection (Lefebvre et al., 1990; Kleid and Millar, 1993).

Also, imaging studies are now routines during the evaluation of primary oral tumors and neck disease. Both contrast-enhanced computed tomographic (CT) scans and magnetic resonance imaging (MRI) may be utilized in determining the extent of the primary tumor, invasion, regional node status, and distant metastasis, thereby providing important staging information (Som, Curtin and Mancuso, 1999, Robbins, 1999). Positron emission tomography (PET) scans are also becoming an increasingly popular tool for the identification of primary, recurrent, and metastatic diseases.

The treatment options for primary OSCCs are variable and depend on the size and location of the tumor, lymph node status, presence or absence of distant metastases, the patient's ability to tolerate treatment, and the patient's desires. Surgery and/or radiation therapy remain the gold standards for treatment of cancers of the lip and oral cavity. Oropharyngeal cancer may be treated with surgery and/or radiation therapy for early-stage disease. For advanced-stage disease, surgery with adjuvant radiation therapy may be indicated, although recent evidence suggests that the addition of chemotherapy to radiation therapy may provide a survival advantage over radiation therapy alone in this population (Forastiere, 1998; Calais et al., 1999). It is important to take into account disease status and prevalence of occult disease in the neck when evaluating primary cancers of the lip, oral cavity, and oropharynx (Robbins et al., 2001). Regardless of the treatment modality used, many patients will require consideration of problems related to airway protection, enteral feedings, xerostomia, mucositis, dysphagia, and voice change.

6. References

Ahlbom HE. Simple achlorhydric anaemia, Plummer-Vinson syndrome and carcinoma of the mouth, pharynx and oesophagus in women. Br Med J 1936; 2: 331-333.

Andre K, Schraub S, Mercier M, et al. Role of alcohol and tobacco in the aetiology of head and neck cancer: A case-control study in the Doubs region of France. Oral Oncol, Eur J Cancer 1995; 31B: 301-309.

Banoczy J, Csiba A. Occurrence of epithelial dysplasia in oral leukoplakia. Oral Surg 1976; 42:766-774

Barnard NA, Scully C, Eveson JW, et al. Oral cancer development in patients with oral lichen planus. J Oral Pathol Med 1993; 22: 421-424.

Barr BBB, Benton EC, McLaren K, Bunney MH et al. Human Papillomavirus infection and skin cancer in renal allograft recipients. Lancet 1989; I: 124-128.

Batsakis JG. Tumors of the Head and Neck, Clinical and pathologic Consideration,, 2nd Edition 1979. Ch. 6, pp144-146. Baltimore: Williams and Wilkins Co.

Bennie WH. A perspective of oral cancer: Epidemiology and aetiology of oral cancer in Britain. Proceedings of the Royal Society of Medicine 1976; 69: 737-740.

Bernia JL. Carcinoma of the lip: preliminary statistical analysis of eight hundred and twenty-seven cases. J Am Dent Assoc 1948; 36: 262-270.

Blot WJ, McLaughlin JK,Winn DM, et al. Smoking and drinking in relation to oral and pharyngeal cancer. Cancer Res 1988; 48: 3282-3287.

Bouquot JE, Meckstroth RL. Oral cancer in a tobacco-chewing U.S. population - no apparent increased incidence or mortality. Oral Surg Oral Med Oral Pathol Oral Radiol Endod 1998; 86:697-706

Bradford CR, Hoffman HT, Wolf GT, Carey TE, Baker SR, McClatchey KD. Squamous carcinoma of the head and neck in organ transplant recipient: possible role of oncogenic viruses. Laryngoscope 1990; 100: 190-194.

Brown RL, Suh JM, Scarborough JE, et al. Snuff dippers' intraoral cancer: Clinical characteristics and response to therapy. Cancer 1965; 18: 2-13.

Brown RL, Suh JM, Scarborough JE, Wilkins SA Jr., Smith RR. Snuff dipper's intraoral cancer: clinical characteristics and response to therapy. Cancer 1965; 18: 2-13.

Cady B, Catlin D. Epidermoid carcinoma of the gum: A 20-year survey. Cancer 1969; 23: 551-596.

Calais G, Alfonsi M, Bardet E, et al. Randomized trial of radiation therapy versus concomitant chemotherapy and radiation therapy for advanced-stage oropharynx carcinoma. J Natl Cancer Inst 1999; 91: 2081–2086.

Carpenter RD,Yellowitz JA, Goodman HS. Oral cancer mortality in Maryland. Maryland Med J 1993; 42: 1105-1109.

Centers for Disease Control and Prevention. Preventing and controlling oral and pharyngeal cancer. Recommendations from a national strategic planning conference. MMWR 1998; 47RR- 14.

Chaturvedi AK, Engels EA, Anderson WF, Gillison ML. Incidence trends for human papillomavirus-related and -unrelated oral squamous cell carcinomas in the United States. J Clin Oncol 2008; 26: 612-9.

Clifford GM, Boyle P, Franceschi S. Human papilloma virus types in invasive cervical cancer worldwide: a meta-analysis. Br J Cancer 2003; 189: 12-19.

Cotran R, Kumar V, Robbins S. Environmental Pathology. In Robbins' Pathologic Basis of Diseases 1989; Ch. 9. Philadelphia: W.B. Saunders.

Daftary DK, Murti PR, Bhonsle RB, Gupta PC, Mehta FS, Pindborg JJ. Oral squamous cell carcinoma, In Oral Diseases in the Tropics, eds Patbhu SR, Wilson DS, Daftary DK, Johnson NW 1992. Ch. 37, pp. 429-448. Oxford: Oxford University Press.

Daftary DK, Murti PR, Bhonsle RB, Gupta PC, Mehta FS, Pindborg JJ. Risk factors and risk markers for oral cancer in high incidence areas of the world. In Oral Cancer: Detection of Patients and Lesions at High Risk, ed Johnson NW, 1991. Ch. 2. Cambridge: Cambridge University Press.

de Visscher JG, Bouwes Bavinck JN, van der Waal I. Squamous cell carcinoma of the lip in renal-transplant recipients. Report of six cases. Int J Oral Maxillofac Surg 1997; 26: 120-123.

Eisenberg E. Oral lichen planus: A benign lesion. J Oral Maxillofac Surg 2000; 58: 1278-1285.

Epstein JB, Sciubba J, Silverman S, Sroussi HY. Utility of toluidine blue in oral premalignant lesion and squamous cell carcinoma: continuing research and implications for clinical practice, Head Neck 2007; 29: 948–958.

Flaitz CM and Silverman S Jr. Human immunodeficiency virus (HIV)-Associated Malignancies. In Silverman S Jr (ed) Oral Cancer, 4th ed. Hamilton, Ontario, Canada: BC Decker, Inc., 1998: 165-170.

Flaitz CM, Nichols CM, Adler-Storthz K, et al. Intraoral squamous cell carcinoma in human immunodeficiency syndrome virus infection. A clinicopathologic study. Oral Surg Oral Med Oral Pathol Oral radiol Endod 1995; 80: 55-62.

Forastiere A, Goepfert H, Goffinet D, et al. NCCN practice guidelines for head and neck cancer. National Comprehensive Cancer Network Proceedings. Oncology 1998; 12: 39–247.

Gillison ML, Koch WM, Capone RB, Spafford M, Westra WH, Wu L, Zahurak ML, Daniel RW, Viglione M, Symer DE, Shah KV, Sidransky D. Evidence for a causal association between human papillomavirus and a subset of head and neck cancers. J Natl Cancer Inst 2000; 92: 709-20.

Goldenberg D, Harden S, Masayesva BG, Ha P, Benoit N, Westra WH, Koch WM, Sidransky D, Califano JA. Intraoperative molecular margin analysis in head and neck cancer. Arch Otolaryngol Head Neck Surg 2004; 130: 39-44.

Gupta PC, Mehta FS, Daftary DK, et al., Incidence rates of oral cancer and natural history of oral precancerous lesions in a 10-year follow-up study of Indian villagers. Commun Dent Oral Epidemiol 1980; 8: 287-333.

Harris C, Warnakulasuriya KAAS, Gelbier S, Johnson NW, Peters TJ. Oral and dental health in alcohol misusing patients. Alcohol Clin Exp Res 1997; 21: 1707-9.

Hollows P, McAndrew PG, Perini MG. Delays in the referral and treatment of oral squamous cell carcinoma. Br Dent J 2000; 188: 262-265.

Ibrahim K, Jafarey NA, Zuberi SJ. Plasma vitamin "A" and carotene levels in squamous cell carcinoma of the oral cavity and oro-pharynx. Clin Oncol 1977; 3: 203-207.

Jemal A, Siegel R, Ward E et al. Cancer statistics, 2008. CA Cancer J Clin 2008; 58:71-96. Sargeran K, Murtomaa H, Safavi SM, Vehkalahti MM, Teronen O. Survival after diagnosis of cancer of the oral cavity. Br J Oral Maxillofac Surg. 2008; 46: 187-191.

Jemal A, Siegel R, Xu J, Ward E. Cancer statistics, 2010. CA Cancer J Clin 2010; 60:277-300.

Johnson NW. A global view of the epidemiology of cancer of oral cancer. In Oral Cancer: Detection of Patients and Lesions at Risk, ed. Johnson, N.W. 1991. Ch.1. Cambridge: Cambridge University Press.

Johnson NW. Tobacco use and oral Cancer: a global perspective. J Dent Educ 2001; 65: 328-339.

Joseph BK. Oral cancer: prevention and detection. Med Princ Pract 2002; 11(Suppl 1): 32-35,

Jovanovic A, Schulten EA, Kostense PJ, et al. Tobacco and alcohol related to the anatomical site of oral squamous cell carcinoma. J Oral Pathol Med 1993; 22:459-462.

Kato I, Nomura AM. Alcohol in the aetiology of upper aero-digestive tract cancer. Eur J Cancer Oral Oncol 1994; 30B: 75-81.

Kelly AB. Spasm at the entrance of the esophagus. Proc R Soc Med 1919; 12 (Laryngol Sect): 235.

Kleid S, Millar HS. The case against open neck biopsy. Aust N Z J Surg 1993; 63: 678–681.

Lee JJ, Hong WK, Hittelman WN, Mao L, Lotan R, Shin DM, Benner SE, Xu XC, Lee JS, Papadimitrakopoulou VM, Geyer C, Perez C, Martin JW, El Naggar AK, Lippman SM. Predicting cancer development in oral leukoplakia: ten years of translational research. Clin Cancer Res 2000; 6: 1702-1710.

Lefebvre JL, Coche-Dequeant B, Van JT, et al. Cervical lymph nodes from an unknown primary tumor in 190 patients. Am J Surg 1990; 160: 443–446.

Lestón JS, Dios PD. Diagnostic clinical aids in oral cancer. Oral Oncol 2010; 46: 418-422.

Lewin F, Norell SE, Johansson H, et al. Smoking tobacco, oral snuff, and alcohol in the etiology of squamous cell carcinoma of the head and neck. A population-based case-referent study in Sweden. Cancer 1998; 82:1367-1375.

Lippman SM, Hong WK. Second primary tumors in head and neck squamous cell carcinoma: The overshadowing threat for patients with early-stage disease. Int J Radiat Oncol Biol Phys 1989; 17: 691–694.

Main JHP, Lacavaliar DR. Smokeless tobacco and oral disease: a review. J Can Dent Assoc 1988; 54: 586-591.

Mashberg A, Boffetta P,Winkelman R, et al. Tobacco smoking, alcohol drinking, and cancer of the oral cavity and oropharynx among U.S. veterans. Cancer 1993; 72:1369-1375.

Mashberg A, Samit A. Early diagnosis of asymptomatic oral and oropharyngeal squamous cancers. CA Cancer J Clin 1995; 45: 328-351

Mashberg A, Samit AM. Early detection, diagnosis, and management of oral oropharyngeal cancer. J Cancer Clinicians 1989; 39: 67-88.

Mashberg A. Diagnosis of early oral and oropharyngeal squamous carcinoma: obstacles and their amelioration. Oral Oncol. 2000; 36: 253-255.

McCarthy PL, Shklar G. Diseases of the Oral Mucosa, Diagnosis, Management, Therapy 1964. Ch. 29, pp. 304-328. New York: McGraw-Hill Book Company.

Murti PR, Bhonsle RB, Gupta PC, et al. Etiology of oral submucous fibrosis with special reference to the role of areca nut chewing. J Oral Pathol Med 1995; 24: 145-152.

Murti PR, Bhonsle RB, Pindborg JJ, et al. Malignant transformation rate in oral submucous fibrosis over a 17-year period. Community Dent Oral Epidemiol 1985; 13: 340-341.

Neville BW, Damm DD, Allen CM, et al. Oral & Maxillofacial Pathology. 2nd ed. Phila., PA: Saunders; 2009; 337-369.

Neville BW, Day TA. Oral cancers and precancerous lesions. CA cancer J Clin 2002; 52: 195-215.

Ord RA, Blanchaert RH Jr. Current management of oral cancer. A multidisciplinary approach. J Am Dent Assoc 2001; 132: 19S–23S

Parkin SM, Laara E, Muir CS. Estimates of the worldwide frequency of sixteen major cancers in 1980. International Journal of Cancer 1988; 41: 184-197.

Paterson DR. A clinical type of dysphagia. Proc R Soc Med 1919; 12 (Laryngol Sect): 285-291.

Paymaster JC. Some observations on oral and pharyngeal carcinomas in the state of Bombay. Cancer 1962; 15: 578-583.

Prime SS, MacDonald DG, Rennie JS. The effects of iron deficiency on experimental oral carcinogenesis. Br J Cancer 1983; 47: 413-418.

Ramulu C, Raju MVS, Venkatarathnam G, Reddy CRRM. Nicotinic stomatitis and its relations to carcinoma of the hard palate in reverse smokers of chuttas. J Dent Res 1973; 52: 711-718.

Reddout N, Christensen T, Bunnell A et al. High risk HPV types 18 and 16 are potent modulators of oral squamous cell carcinoma phenotypes in vitro. Infectious Agents and Cancer 2007; doi: 101186/1750-9378-2-21.

Reddout N, Christensen T, Bunnell A et al. High risk HPV types 18 and 16 are potent modulators of oral squamous cell carcinoma phenotypes in vitro. Infectious Agents and Cancer 2007; doi: 101186/1750-9378-2-21.

Reibel J: Prognosis of oral pre-malignant lesions: significance of clinical, histopathological, and molecular biological characteristics. Crit Rev Oral Biol Med 2003; 14: 47-62.

Rennie JS, MacDonald DG, Dagg JH. Quantitative analysis of human buccal epithelium in iron deficiency anaemia. J Oral Pathol 1982; 11: 39-46.

Rennie JS, MacDonald DG. Quantitative histologic analysis of the epithelium of the ventral surface of the hamster tongue in experimental iron deficiency. Archives of oral Biology 1982; 27: 393-397.

Ringertz N (ed). Cancer incidence in Finland, Iceland, Norway and Sweden. A comparative study by the cancer registries. Acta Pathologica Microbiologica Scandinavia, Section A, Supplement 224, pp 105.

Robbins KT, Atkinson JL, Byers RM, et al. The use and misuse of neck dissection for head and neck cancer. J Am Coll Surg 2001; 193: 91–102.

Robbins KT. Integrating radiological criteria into the classification of cervical lymph node disease. Arch Otolaryngol Head Neck Surg 1999; 125: 385–387.

Rosenfield L, Callaway J. Snuff dipper's Cancer. Am J Surg 1963; 106: 840-844.

Sawyer DR, Wood NK. Oral cancer: Etiology, recognition and management. In The Dental Clinics of North America. Topics in Oral Dignosis I, eds. D'Ambrosia JA, Fotos PG. 1992; 36: 919-944.

Schantz SP,Yu GP. Head and neck cancer incidence trends in young Americans, 1973-1997, with a special analysis for tongue cancer. Arch Otolaryngol Head Neck Surg 2002; 128: 268-274.

Schwartz SR, Yueh B, McDougall JK, Daling JR, Schwartz SM. Human papillomavirus infection and survival in oral squamous cell cancer: a population based study. Otolaryngol Head Neck Surg 2001; 125: 1-9.

Scully C. Oncogenes, tumor suppressors and viruses in oral squamous carcinoma. J Oral Pathol Med 1993; 22: 337-347.

Seoane J, Varela-Centelles P, Ramirez J.R, Romero MA, De La Cruz A. Artefacts produced by suture traction during incisional biopsy of oral lesions, Clin Otolaryngol 2002; 27: 549–553.

Shafer WG. Initial mismanagement and delay in diagnosis of oral cancer. J Am Dent Assoc 1975; 90: 1262-1264.

Silverman S Jr, Dillon WP, Fischbein NJ. Diagnosis In: Silverman S Jr ed. Oral Cancer. 4th ed. Hamilton, Ontario, Canada: BC Decker Inc; 1998; 41-66.

Silverman S Jr, Gorsky M, Lozada-Nur F, et al. A prospective study of findings and management in 214 patients with oral lichen planus. Oral Surg Oral Med Oral Pathol 1991;72:665-670.

Silverman S Jr, Griffith M. Smoking characteristics of patients with oral carcinoma and the risk for second oral primary carcinoma. J Am Dent Assoc 1972; 85:637-640.

Silverman S Jr, Shillitoe EF. Etiology and Predisposing Factors. In: Silverman S Jr ed. Oral Cancer, 4th ed. Hamilton, Ontario, Canada: BC Decker Inc; 1998, 7-24.

Silverman S Jr. Demographics and occurrence of oral and pharyngeal cancers. The outcomes, the trends, the challenge. J Am Dent Assoc 2001; 132: 7S-11S.

Singh AD, von Essen CF. Buccal cancer in South India. Etiologic and clinical aspects. Am J Roentgenol 1966; 96: 6-14.

Som PM, Curtin HD, Mancuso AA. An imaging-based classification for the cervical nodes designed as an adjunct to recent clinically based nodal classifications. Arch Otolaryngol Head Neck Surg 1999; 125: 388–396.

Spitzer WO, Hill GB, Chambers LW, Helliwell BE, Murphy HB. The occupation of fishing as a risk factor in cancer of the lip. New Engl J Med 1975; 293: 419-424.

Stich HF, Rosen MP, Hornby AP, Mathew B, Sankaranarayan R, Nair MK. Remission of oral leukoplakias and micronuclei in tobacco/betel quid chewers treated with ß-carotene plus vitamin A. Int J Cancer 1988; 42: 195-199.

Stich HF, Rosen MP, Hornby AP, Mathew B, Sankaranarayan R, Nair MK. Response of oral leukoplakias to the administration of vitamin A. cancer letters 1988; 40: 93-101.

Syrjanen S. Human papilloma virus (HPV) in head and neck cancer. J Clin Virol 2005; 32: (suppl) 59-66.

Syrjanen S. Human papilloma virus (HPV) in head and neck cancer. J Clin Virol 2005; 32: (suppl) 59-Kang MK, Park N-H. Conversion of normal to malignant phenotype: telomere shortening, telomerase activation, and genomic instability during immortalization of human oral keratinocytes. Crit Rev Oral Biol Med 2001; 12: 38-54

Trullenque-Eriksson A, Muñoz-Corcuera M, Campo-Trapero J, Cano-Sanchez J, Bascones-Martinez A. Analysis of new diagnostic methods in suspicious lesions of the oral mucosa, Med Oral Patol Oral Cir Bucal 2009; 14: E210–E216.

van Zuuren EJ, de Visscher JGAM, Bouwes Bavinck JN. Carcinoma of the lip in kidney transplant recipients. J Amer Acad Dermatol 1988; 38: 497-499.

Wahi PN, Lahiri B, Kehar U, Arora S. Oral and oropharyngeal cancers in North America. Br J Cancer 1965; 19: 627-641.

Warnakulasuriya KA, Tavassoli M, Johnson NW. Relationship of p53 overexpression toβ other cell cycle regulatory proteins in oral squamous cell carcinoma. J Oral Pathol Med 1998; 27: 376-381.

Weinberger PM, Yu Z, Haffty BG, Kowalski D, Harigopal M, Brandsma J, Sasaki C, Joe J, Camp RL, Rimm DL, Psyrri A. Molecular classification identifies a subset of human papillomavirus--associated oropharyngeal cancers with favorable prognosis. J Clin Oncol 2006; 24: 736-47.

Winn DM, Blot WJ, Shy CM, et al. Snuff dipping and oral cancer among women in the southern United States. N Engl J Med 1981; 304:745-749.

Winn DM, Ziegler RG, Pickle LW, et al. Diet in the etiology of oral and pharyngeal cancer among women from the southern United States. Cancer Res 1984; 44: 1216-1222.

Winn DM. Diet and nutrition in the etiology of oral cancer. Am J Clin Nutr 1995;61:437S-445S.

Wright Jm. Oral Precanerous lesions and conditions. Semin Dermatol 1994; 13:125-131

Wynder EL, Klein VE. The possible role of riboflavin deficiency in epithelial neoplasm. 1. Epithelial changes of mice in simple deficiency. Cancer 1965; 18: 167-180.

Wynder EL. The etiology aspects of squamous cell cancers of the head and neck. J Am Med Assoc 1971; 215: 452-453.

Yellowitz JA, Goodman HS. Assessing physicians' and dentists' oral cancer knowledge, opinions and practices. J Am Dent Assoc 1995; 126:53-59.

Zhang ZF, Morgenstern H, Spitz MR, et al. Marijuana use and increased risk of squamous cell carcinoma of the head and neck. Cancer Epidemiol Biomarkers Prev 1999; 8: 1071-1078.

2

Oral Cancer – An Overview

Raghu Radhakrishnan, Bijayata Shrestha and Dipshikha Bajracharya
Department of Oral Pathology, Manipal College of Dental Sciences, Manipal University, India

1. Introduction

Neoplasms of diverse cellular origin arise in the oral cavity and among these oral squamous cell carcinoma (OSCC) arising from the mucosa of the oral cavity constitutes to over 90%[1, 2]. Oral cancer encompasses all the malignancies originating in the oral tissues, including cancers of the lip, tongue, gingiva, floor of the mouth, buccal mucosa, palate and the retromolar trigone. It is the 6th most common cancer worldwide[3]. Oral squamous cell carcinoma is described as an invasive epithelial neoplasm with varying degrees of squamous differentiation and a propensity to early and extensive lymph node metastases, occurring predominantly in alcohol and tobacco using adults generally in the 5th and 6th decades of life.

Globally about 5, 00,000 new cases of oral and oropharyngeal cancers are diagnosed and three quarters of these are from the developing world[7, 8, 9]. Approximately 3, 89,650 cases occurred in the year 2000 out of which 2, 66,672 were in the oral cavity (ICD - 9 140 - 5) and 1, 22,978 for the cancer of oropharynx (ICD - 9 146, 8-9). This represented about 5% of all cancers for men and 2% for women[10]. Oral and oropharyngeal cancers remain one of the more common cancers in the South and South East Asian countries, as opposed to Western society, where it accounts for only about 1 - 4% of the of reported cancers incidence [4]. For example, the incidence of oral cancer in India is high, constituting about 12% of all cancer in men and 8% in women[5]; mortality rate is equally high in this population, ranking number one in men and number three in women[6]. Oral and oropharyngeal cancers therefore qualify as major public health problem, not only in India, but also globally.

Worldwide, oral cancer incidence rates appear to have been stabilizing over the last decade[12], but the greater frequency of oral cancer in certain regions and among specific populations is a cause for concern since their overall 5-year survival rate is 53% and it has not changed in the last two decades[13]. With this heightened awareness, research to further investigate the detection, diagnosis and prevention or oral cancer has recently been included as one of the targeted priorities supported by the National Institute of Dental and Craniofacial Research (NIDR) in the United States[14].

The overall 5 - year survival rate for patients without clinically evident cervical lymph node metastases is 85% . However, patients with microscopic lymph node metastases have a survival rate of 54%. It has been estimated that 20-50% of patients without clinically evident cervical lymph node metastases do in fact have microscopic metastases and therefore poorer prognosis[87]. Among the Indian population, the overall 5- year observed and relative survival rates were 30.5% and 39.7%, respectively. Survival steadily declined with advancing age and advanced clinical stages. 5-year observed survival was 59.1% for localized cancer, 15.7% for cancers with regional extension and 1.6% for those with distant metastasis. Those with tongue, buccal mucosa and retromolar trigone cancers had poor survival rates[11].

2. Risk factors for oral cancer

The cancer epidemic in developed countries, and increasingly in developing countries, is due to the combined effect of the ageing of populations, and the high or increasing levels of prevalence of cancer risk factors[15]. About 95% of patients with oral cancer are over 40 years of age at diagnosis, and the mean age at diagnosis is 60 years. The association of oral cancer with increasing age is consistent with the disease process being related to environmental risk factors. Risk rises dramatically among males from about 7/1, 00,000 at the age of 30 to approximately 80/1, 00,000 for the 60 year old[15].

The development of oral cancer in many cases appears to be due to chronic exposure to topical carcinogens, notably tobacco and alcohol[16] proposed to interact synergistically to increase cancer. However, there is a distinct geographical variation among the risk factors contributing to oral cancer. In the Western population exposure to sunlight (lip cancer), cigarette-smoking, and alcohol consumption are the frontline etiologic culprits compared with the use of smokeless tobacco and combustible tobacco more prevalent in the South East Asian countries[17].

The concurrent use of tobacco and alcohol accounts for 75% of all oral cancers[18]. Other risk factors for oral cancers includes over exposure to sun rays, particularly the cancer of the lip, and malnutrition or poor dietary intake of essential minerals[19]. Currently the role of viruses such as human papillomavirus[20, 21, 22, 23] is also implicated as a major risk factor. They are believed to induce cancers by altering the DNA and the chromosomal structures of the cells and by inducing proliferative changes of the cells they infect.

An increased consumption of fruits and vegetables is associated with lower risk of oral cancers[24]. Thus, primary preventive measures in oral cancer includes, avoidance of tobacco and alcoholic intake, avoiding exposure to certain viruses and exposure to sunlight and consumption of fruits and vegetables.

Tobacco: Overwhelming majority of carcinomas is closely linked to tobacco usage in various forms. Tobacco may be consumed as smoking tobacco or smokeless tobacco. It is used in various forms such as chewing tobacco, oral use of snuff, smoking of cigars, cigarettes, bidis, pipes, among others (Table - 1.1).

The smoking of tobacco is a widespread habit practiced by people from most cultures and societies throughout the world. While the custom of tobacco smoking is almost universal in its occurrence, there is considerable variation with respect to the amount of tobacco smoked and the form in which it is smoked. Smokeless tobacco is tobacco that is not burnt when it is used and is usually placed in the oral or nasal cavities against the mucosal sites that permit the absorption of nicotine into the human body. The two main types are the chewing tobacco and snuff. It may be used alone or in combination with other substances such as lime.

Smoking Tobacco	
Cigarette	Finely cured tobacco treated with sugars, flavoring agents wrapped in paper.
Bidi	Small quantity of shredded sun cured tobacco which is hand rolled into a piece of tendu (temburni tree leaf - Diospyrous melanoxylon).
Cigars	Made of cigar tobaccos, wrapped in a tobacco leaf, paper or reconstituted tobacco.
Chutta	Hand made cigar containing cured tobacco in a dried tobacco leaf wrapping.
Pipe - Briar Pipe, Meerschaum Pipe (England), Chillum (India)	Pipe tobaccos are of variable composition usually consist of blended tobaccos to which sugars and flavoring agents such as liquorices are added.
Smokeless tobacco	
Chewing tobacco	Plug tobacco, loose leaf tobacco and twist (roll) tobacco (Western World).
	Khaini, Pattiwala tobacco, Mainpuri tobacco, Mishri, Zarda, Kiwam, Gudakhu, Shammah, Nass, Naswar.
Snuff	A moist type, consisting of very finely cut tobacco which is used in the mouth and a dry type, which is finely pulverized tobacco and which is used orally or nasally.

Table 1.1. Different forms of tobacco and usage

Among the different smoking habits, the cigarette or cigar increased the risk of cancer by 6 times, hookah and pipe by 16 times and bidi smoking by 36 times[25] as compared to non smokers. In the largest population-based case-control study of oral cancer yet conducted[16], strong positive trends in risk were observed according to amount and duration of each type of tobacco and amount of alcohol consumption. Relative to nonsmokers, heavy cigarette smokers (40+/day for 20+ years) experienced a four-fold risk (men) and ten-fold risk (women) after adjusting for alcohol intake. After controlling for smoking, moderate drinkers (15-29 alcoholic drinks/week) had a three-fold risk of oral cancer and heavy drinkers (> 30 drinks/week) experienced an eight- to nine-fold risk. Combined heavy smoking and drinking resulted in a greater than 35-fold excess risk.

The chewing of quid containing betel leaves, tobacco, and lime and the smoking of bidi contribute to the majority of cases in parts of India and Southeast Asia[26, 27]. Among users of snuff, cancerous lesions typically arise at the site where smokeless tobacco or quid, is held in contact with the buccal mucosa or gingiva. Although not as prevalent as cigarette smoking, habitual use of pipes, cigars, and smokeless tobacco is associated with relative risks for cancers of the mouth as great as that for cigarette smoking[28]. The site of origin of oral cancer usually corresponds to the placement of tobacco quid[29]. The patients who chewed and smoked tobacco together had a tenfold higher risk of cancer of the oral cavity relative to the non-chewing, non-smokers, whereas the patients who only chewed tobacco had a six fold higher risk of cancer and the patients who only smoked had a threefold increase in the same risk[30]. It has also been demonstrated that the relative risk of chewing betel quid without tobacco for oral cancer was lowered compared to chewing betel quid with tobacco[31]. The role of areca nut in oral carcinogenesis is a matter of debate, however, areca nut and lime when used has had a definite carcinogenic effect, even when chewed without tobacco[32].

Tobacco consumption is positively correlated with accumulation of DNA damage, and exposure to tobacco related chemical carcinogens could provide direct damaging effects on the cellular DNA in the human oral cavity[33, 34]. DNA damaging agents found in tobacco include benzi (a) pyrene (B (a) P) and tobacco specific N′-nitrosamines (TSNAs). Examples of TSNAs are N nitrosonornicotine (NNN) and 4- [methylnitrosoamino]-1-[3-pyridyl]-1-butanone (NNK) and these chemicals exhibit carcinogenicity in animals[33, 35]. In fact, damaged genomic DNA has been detected as DNA adducts in various tissues of cigarette smokers[36, 37]. Nitrosamines contain the organic functional group N-N=O, and are formed by the nitrosation (addition of an N=O group) of secondary and tertiary amines. Another chemical term for these tobacco amines is an "alkaloid", an organic base that contains nitrogen and is located in a seed plant. TSNA are created during fermentation, curing and burning of the tobacco leaf. These findings strongly suggest a causal role of tobacco use in oral carcinogenesis[38].

Alcohol: The independent risk of alcohol in oral cancer etiopathogenesis is uncertain as most of the alcohol users are smokers as well. Alcohol is thought to be associated with carcinogens through several mechanisms in that it may damage the oral mucosa through a direct effect on cell membranes, removing lipids and increasing the permeability of the oral mucosa to noxious carcinogenic substances. It also has systemic effects and alcohol related liver damage may potentiate the action of carcinogens in the oral mucosa by reducing the body's ability to detoxify harmful compounds. Alcohol also has immunosuppressive effect and this together with a degree of nutritional deficiency may also contribute to the carcinogenic process. In addition, acetaldehyde a direct metabolite of alcohol is a carcinogen and may be produced both systemically and by the oral micro flora.

Viruses: Both RNA-containing and DNA-containing viruses have been identified as carcinogenic. These viruses may incorporate one or more of the functional genes into the host DNA and secondly the persistent expression of this viral genome may maintain the host cell in the transformed state. Although Epstein - Barr virus (EBV), Herpes Simplex viruses (HSV), Retroviruses and Human papillomaviruses (HPVs) have all been implicated to play a role in the development of oral carcinoma, HPV is increasingly highlighted as a risk factor in oral carcinogenesis[39, 40, 41, 42].

HPVs, especially those genotypes of known high oncogenic potential in uterine cervix and skin such as HPV 16 and 18, are found in a variable but small proportion of oral cancers. This has lead to the speculation that HPV infection, perhaps arising from oral/ genital contact, might be important in some cases. Of interest is the observation that HPV containing cancers at these sites do not generally show TP53 mutations, contrary to HPV DNA negative cancers[43].

It is well known that E6 protein from "high risk" HPV interact with E6 associated protein (E6/E6-AP) complex, which binds to and induces degradation of p53 protein[44, 45]. "High risk" HPV infection, however, directly abrogates the innate check point mechanisms against such environmental challenge, resulting in the accumulation and propagations of mutations. Hence, the viral infection in combination with existing chemical carcinogens may be the paramount causative agents for the development of oral cancer[46].

Diet and deficiency states: Recent epidemiologic studies have indicated that diet may play an important role in the origin of these cancers. Findings have pointed to the protective effects of a diet consistently high in fresh fruits; vegetables; vitamins A, C, and E; and carotenoids, even with adjustment for alcohol intake and smoking[47, 48, 49, 50, 51]. A reduced risk of oral cancer associated with vitamin E supplementation has been shown in one study[52]. Certain deficiency states may cause epithelial atrophy, which renders the epithelium vulnerable to action of carcinogens. Vegetarianism versus non vegetarianism has failed to show any role in oral cancer development[53]. High levels of carotenoids have been shown to be strongly related to lower risk of oral cancer development. The possible role of micronutrient ingestion with an associated antioxidant effect has been emphasized. Natural carotenoid compounds, dietary selenium, folate and vitamin A, C and E have been stated to offer protective effects regarding cancer development[54]. Iron deficiency anemia, a relatively common disorder, may produce atrophic oral changes (as seen in patients with Plummer-Vinson syndrome) that may predispose to malignant transformation[55].

Oral cancer affects men more often than women because of heavier indulgence in both tobacco and alcohol habits in most countries[58, 59]. However, in India the oral cancers are also common among women due to tobacco chewing habits. The male to female ratios, globally, however, is lower for cancer of the oral cavity than for cancer of the oropharynx, perhaps suggesting that higher exposure to tobacco smoking and alcohol drinking are required to induce oropharyngeal than oral cancer[60]. An epidemiological review on oral cancer in India showed that the mean age was 57.1 years for males and 58.6 years for female patients with peak age frequency in the sixth decade for men and seventh decade for women[5].

Other factors: Carcinoma of the vermilion border of the lip is more often linked to working outdoors in fair skinned individuals regularly exposed to sun light. This has been attributable to the effect of UV radiation[26, 56]. Orodental factors like poor oral hygiene, faulty restorations, sharp teeth and ill-fitting dentures may also play a role in the etiology of oral cancers[57].

3. Clinical features

The clinical features of oral cancer differ considerably for different intraoral locations. Patients with small oral and oropharyngeal SCC are often asymptomatic or may present with vague symptoms and minimal physical findings. Hence, a high index of clinical suspicion is needed to diagnose small lesions, especially if the patients have tobacco and alcohol habits. Patients may present with red lesions, mixed red and white lesions or white plaques. Co existing white plaques may be observed adjacent to carcinomas and this implies an origin in a pre existing white lesion though the prevalence of this association varies considerably. However, most patients present with signs and symptoms of locally advanced disease. The clinical features may vary according to the affected intra oral site. Mucosal growth and ulceration, pain from the lesion, referred pain to the ear, malodor from the mouth, difficulty with speaking, discomfort while chewing, pain with swallowing, weight loss, swelling in the neck are the common presenting symptoms of locally advanced oral cancers. Occasionally patients present with enlarged neck nodes without any symptoms from oral or oropharyngeal lesions. Extremely advanced cancers present as ulceroproliferative growths with areas of necrosis and extension into the surrounding structures. In the advanced stages patients may present with orocutaneous fistula, intractable bleeding, severe anaemia and cachexia.

Tumors may arise in any part of the oral cavity and its preferential occurrence varies with the geographical domain reflecting different risk factors. Within the oral cavity, oral cancer may be localized to buccal mucosa, upper and lower gingiva, hard palate, anterior two thirds of the tongue, including the dorsal, ventral and lateral surfaces, and floor of the mouth. The most common oropharyngeal site of involvement for SCC is the base of tongue.

Oral cancers have a varied clinical presentation in that they may be exophytic or endophytic. Exophytic lesions typically have surfaces that are irregular, fungating, papillary or verruciform and its color may vary from normal to red to white, depending on the degree of vascularity and the amount of surface keratin. The surface is often ulcerated, and the tumor feels indurated on palpation. The endophytic growth pattern is characterized by a depressed, irregularly shaped, ulcerated central area with a surrounding "rolled" border of normal, red or white mucosa. The rolled border results from invasion of the tumor downward and laterally under adjacent epithelium.

Carcinoma of the lip is typically found in light skinned persons with either long term exposure to ultraviolet radiation from sunlight or a history of sunburn early in life. It also may arise at the site where a cigarette, cigar or pipe stem is held by the patient. Almost 90% of lesions are located on the lower lip. The typical vermilion carcinoma is a crusted, oozing, non tender, indurated ulceration that is usually less than 1cm in its greatest diameter. The tumor is characterized by a slow growth rate and metastasis is a late event[61, 62].

The most common intraoral carcinoma is the tongue, usually the posterior-lateral and ventral surfaces. Cancer of the tongue may appear as a red area interspersed with nodules or as an ulcer infiltrating deeply, leading to reduced mobility of the tongue. These tumors are painful. Advanced stages are associated with drooling. Lesions near the base of the tongue are particularly insidious, since they may be asymptomatic until they attain advanced stage. Even then the only manifestation may be a sore throat and dysphagia. The specific site of development of these tumors is of great significance, since the lesions on the posterior portion of the tongue are usually of a higher grade of malignancy, metastasize earlier and offer a poorer prognosis, especially because of their inaccessibility for early diagnosis and treatment. Metastasis occurs with greater frequency in cases of tongue cancer. In India, the cancers over the anterior 2/3 of tongue are related to the tobacco chewing habit and posterior 1/3 lesions are related to bidi smoking[63, 64].

Carcinoma of the floor represents 15 – 30% of all intra oral cancers. Cancers of the floor of the mouth may arise as a red area, a small ulcer or as a papillary lesion. Most patients present with discomfort or irritation at the site of the tumor. This type of cancer affecting predominantly the males of the higher age group has shown to be associated with tobacco usage and alcohol drinking[65]. The typical carcinoma in the floor of the mouth is an indurated ulcer of varying size situated on one side of the midline. Because of its location, early extension into the lingual mucosa of the mandible and into the mandible proper as well as into the tongue occurs with considerable frequency. Of all intra oral carcinomas, oral floor lesions are the most likely to arise from a preexisting leukoplakia or erythroplakia. It is also the oral cancer site most often associated with the development of a second primary malignancy of another aerodigestive tract location or a distant organ. Metastasis from the floor of the mouth are found most commonly in the submandibular group of lymph nodes and since the primary lesion frequently occurs near the midline where a lymphatic drainage occurs contra lateral metastases are often present[66].

Cancer of the buccal mucosa may present as an ulcer with indurated raised margin, exophytic or verrucous on the side with the placement of betel quid. In advanced stages these lesions infiltrate into the adjacent bone and overlying skin. Leukoplakia is a common predecessor of carcinoma of buccal mucosa and they originate in the commissural areas and spreads posteriorly. The most common sites of metastases are the sub maxillary lymphnodes[67, 68].

Carcinomas from gingiva and alveolar ridge are usually painless and most frequently arise from keratinized mucosa. It is generally agreed that carcinoma of the mandibular gingiva is more common that the involvement of maxillary gingiva. Carcinoma of the gingiva usually manifested initially as an area of ulceration which may be purely erosive or may exhibit an exophytic granular or verrucous type of growth. The tumor arises more commonly in edentulous areas, although it may develop in a site in which teeth are present. The attached gingiva is more frequently involved than the free gingiva. The proximity of the underlying periosteum and bone usually invites early invasion of these structures. In maxilla, gingiva carcinomas often invade into the maxillary sinus, or it may extend onto the palate or into the tonsillar pillar. In the mandible, extension into the floor of the mouth or laterally into the cheek as well as deep into the bone is rather common. Of all the intra oral carcinomas, this one is least associated with tobacco smoking and has the greatest predilection for females[69].

Tumors of the alveolar ridge may occasionally present difficulty in wearing dentures or may present loose teeth associated with pain and bleeding during brushing of teeth. Tumors of the hard palate are not particularly common lesions and palatal carcinomas usually manifests itself as a poorly defined, ulcerated, painful lesion on one side of the midline. It crosses the midline, and may extend laterally to include the lingual gingiva or may posteriorly extend to involve the tonsillar pillar or uvula. Tumors of the hard palate often presents as papillary or exophytic growths, rather than a flat or ulcerated lesion.

Cancers of the soft palate and oropharyngeal mucosa has the same basic clinical appearance as more anterior carcinomas, except that in this posterior location the patient often is unaware of its presence and the diagnosis may be delayed. The tumor site is greater than that of more anterior carcinomas and the proportion of cases with cervical and distant metastasis at diagnosis is higher[70].

4. Relevant diagnostic procedures

Early detection of cancer is the most effective means of reducing mortality. Accurately identifiable biomarkers for early detection may provide newer avenues and constitute potential targets of cancer and its risk assessment. Screening for oral cancer should include a thorough history and physical examination. The clinician should visually inspect and palpate the head, neck, oral and pharyngeal regions. This procedure involves digital palpation of neck node regions, bimanual palpation of the floor of mouth and tongue. Protraction of the tongue with gauze is necessary to visualize fully the posterior lateral tongue and tongue base. The clinician should review the social, familial and medical history and should document risk habits, a history of head and neck radiotherapy, familial history of head and neck cancer and a personal history of cancer.

The diagnosis is confirmed by biopsy. The specimen is taken from the clinically most suspicious area, avoiding necrotic or grossly ulcerated areas and biopsy specimens from more than one biopsy site may need. In patients with enlarged cervical lymph nodes and an obvious primary in the oral cavity, the biopsy is always taken from the primary site and not from the lymph node. In such situations, fine needle aspiration cytology may be carried out to verify the involvement of the node. If no obvious primary site is found in patients presenting with neck nodes, fine needle aspiration of the lymph node can be performed to help establish the diagnosis. In patients for whom fine needle aspiration is non diagnostic, excisional lymph node biopsy is required. Patients with SCC of the oral cavity or oropharynx have a risk of multiple primary tumors in the pharynx or larynx, as well as in the tracheobronchial region and oesophagus so routine panendoscopy is often performed to evaluate these sites.

Imaging: Intra oral and dental radiographs, in combination with orthopantomography, may help in identifying involvement of the underlying bone. Three dimensional imaging with computed tomography (CT) and magnetic resonance imaging (MRI) is frequently used to supplement the clinical evaluation and staging of the primary tumor and regional lymph nodes. CT scan or MRI gives more information about the local extent of the disease and also help to identify lymph node metastases. MRI is more informative when evaluating the extent of soft tissue and neurovascular bundle involvement. The combination of soft tissue characterization and anatomical localization afforded by CT and MRI make them valuable tools in the preoperative assessment of patients. Distant metastasis from oral cancer is uncommon at presentation. At minimum, a routine radiograph of the chest is performed to rule out lung metastases.

5. Tumor spread

Local spread of oral SCC, in the early stages, is relatively predictable in tissues that have not been previously irradiated. It is influenced by local anatomical features. Lip SCC spreads superficially and then into deeper tissues. Floor of mouth SCC spreads superficially rather than in depth, invading into the myelohyoid muscle or the sublingual gland only at late stage. Tumor involving the lateral margin of tongue, whether arising there directly or by superficial spread from the floor of mouth, tends to spread deep within the tissue. The intrinsic muscles of tongue run in small bundles in all directions such that invading tumor encounters some muscle running at right angles to the surface. Tumors of palate spread superficially rather than deep and this is also true for more posterior tumors of the oropharynx.

Spread of SCC into bone is a frequent problem. The mandible is involved much more frequently than the maxilla. Tumors in the mandible can involve the inferior alveolar nerve with a particular likelihood of spread posteriorly along the nerve. Cancers arising in gingiva or alveolus and those involving these sites by extension from adjacent sites are unlikely to invade into the mandible[71].

Tumor spread in previously irradiated soft tissues tends to be more extensive and less predictable than in normal tissues and as a consequence requires more extensive surgery if excision is attempted. Spread to local lymph nodes worsens the prognosis in oral and oropharyngeal cancer. The mechanism of spread from primary site to lymph nodes is almost always by dissemination. The lymph nodes in the neck are divided into levels. The lymphatic drainage from the head and neck sites is relatively predictable[72].

Levels at high risk for metastasis from OSCC are level I, II and III and to a lesser extent level IV. Although Level II is the most frequently involved, some tumors spread to Level III or IV, with or without involvement of Level I. This has given rise to the concept of skip metastasis. Bilateral spread to the neck is likely to occur from tumors involving the midline, especially tumors of the posterior tongue or soft palate. Extra capsular spread of tumor involving lymph nodes is associated with a poor prognosis. There have been many studies attempting to predict the presence of lymphatic spread from features of the primary tumor[66, 73].While the implementation of multi-modality neoadjuvant therapy for the treatment of head and neck cancer has resulted in an improvement in local regional control, there has been a resultant increase in the reported incidence of distant metastasis. This shift in the pattern of patient treatment failure highlights the importance of identifying patients at high risk of developing metastasis, accurately detecting metastasis, and improving treatment strategies for advanced disease. Currently, metastatic lesions from head and neck primaries portend a poor prognosis[73].

Pattern of the invasive front is a useful predictor in that a non cohesive front is associated with increased likelihood of metastases. Other factors associated with increased risk of metastases are perineural spread at the invasive front, lymphovascular invasion and tumor thickness. For diagnostic purposes, a thickness of 5mm or greater is used as indicating increased risk of nodal spread[74]. Until recently hematogeneous spread of oral cancer had been regarded as less important than local and lymphatic spread. However, its importance is increasing as loco-regional control improves. Blood borne spread most often involves lung[75, 76]. The best predictor of the likelihood of spread is involvement of the neck at multiple levels. This suggests that the route of entry of tumors into the circulation is most often via the large veins in the neck and that haematogenous spread is in effect tertiary spread following extracapsular spread from neck nodes.

6. Staging

Clinical staging refers to an assessment of the extent of the disease before undertaking treatment. The purpose of staging is for the selection of the most appropriate treatment plan, for meaningful comparison of the end results reported from different sources and for determining tumor size, extent of metastasis, and other indicators of patient prognosis.

TNM clinical classification if carcinomas of the lip and oral cavity[77, 78]

T - Primary tumor
TX - Primary tumor cannot be assessed
T0 - No evidence of primary tumor

Tis - Carcinoma in situ
T1 - Tumor 2cm or less in its greatest dimension
T2 - Tumor more than 2cm but not more than 4cm in greatest dimension
T3 - Tumor more than 4cm in greatest dimension
T4a (Lip)
- Tumor invades through cortical bone, inferior alveolar nerve, floor of mouth or skin (Chin or nose)
T4b (Oral cavity)
- Tumor invades through cortical bone, into deep / extrinsic muscles of the tongue (genioglossus, hyoglossus, palatoglossus and styloglossus), maxillary sinus or skin of face
T4b (Lip and oral cavity)
- Tumor invades through masticator space, pterygoid plates, or skull base or encases internal carotid artery
NOTE - Superficial erosion alone of bone/ tooth socket by gingival primary is not sufficient to classify tumor as T4
N - Regional Lymph nodes (Cervical nodes)
NX - Regional lymph nodes cannot be assessed
N0 - No regional lymph node metastasis
N1 - Metastasis in a single ipsilateral lymph node, 3cm or less in greatest dimension.
N2 -
N2a - Metastasis in a single ipsilateral lymph node, more than 3cm but not more than 6 cm or less in greatest dimension.
N2b - Metastasis in multiple ipsilateral lymph nodes, none more than 6 cm in greatest dimension.
N2c - Metastasis in bilateral or contralateral lymph nodes, none more than 6 cm in greatest dimension
N3 - Metastasis in a lymph node more than 6 cm in greatest dimension
Note - Midline nodes are considered ipsilateral nodes.
(M) - Distant metastasis
MX - Distant metastasis cannot assessed
M0 - No evidence of distant metastasis
M1 - Distant metastasis is present

7. Stage grouping

Stage 0	Tis	N0	M0
Stage I	T1	N0	M0
Stage II	T2	N0	M0
Stage III	T1,2,3	N1	M0
Stage IVA	T1,2,3	N2	M0
	T4a	N0,N1,N2	M0
Stage IVB	Any T	N3	M0
	T4b	Any N	M0
Stage IVC	Any T	Any N	M1

8. Grading

Squamous differentiation, often seen as keratinization with variable "pearl" formation and invasive growth are the prerequisite features of SCC. Invasion is manifested by the disruption of basement membrane and extension into the underlying tissue, often accompanied by stromal reaction. Angiolymphatic and perineural invasion are additional signs of malignancy.

The tumors are traditionally graded into well - moderately - , and poorly differentiated SCC. Well differentiated SCC resembles closely normal squamous epithelium. Moderately differentiated SC contains distinct nuclear pleomorphism and mitotic activity, including abnormal mitoses; there is usually less keratinization. In poorly differentiated SCC, immature cells predominate, with numerous typical and atypical mitoses and minimal keratinization. Most SCC is moderately differentiated, so grading by differentiation is really of limited prognostic value, as compared to pattern of invasion. Broder's[82] grading was the first of the systems which initiated quantitative grading of cancer. This classification system was based on the estimated ratio of differentiated to undifferentiated elements in the tumor. The author suggested a grading system in which a grade I lesion was highly differentiated (its cells were producing much keratin), while grade IV were poorly differentiated (cells were anaplastic and showed no keratin formation) (Tab 1.2).

Grade I:	• Numerous epithelial pearls, considerable cellular keratinization with inter cellular bridges; • Less than 2 mitoses per high power field, • Atypical mitosis and multinucleated giant cells rarely present, minimal nuclear and cellular pleomorphism.
Grade II:	• Epithelial pearls infrequent or even absent; neither keratinization of individual cells nor the presence of intercellular bridges; • 2-4 mitoses per high power field with occasional atypical mitosis; • Moderate pleomorphism of cells and nuclei.
Grade III:	• Epithelial pearls rarely seen; negligible cellular keratinization and no inter cellular bridges; • More than 4 mitoses per high power field with frequent atypical mitoses, cellular and nuclear pleomorphism marked.
Grade IV:	• Highly anaplastic, practically no keratin formation

Table 1.2. Histologic Grading of Oral Cancer[82]

Later Anneroth et al developed a much better classification system in 1987[79] (Tab 1.3)

Morphologic parameters	1	2	3	4
Degree of keratinization	Highly keratinized (50% of cells)	Moderately keratinized (20-50% of cells)	Minimal keratinization (5-20% of cells)	No Keratinization (0-5% of cells)
Nuclear Polymorphism	Little nuclear polymorphis m (>75% mature cells)	Moderate to abundant nuclear polymorphism (50-70% mature cells)	Abundant nuclear polymorphism (25-50% mature cells)	Extreme polymorphism (0-25% mature cells)
Number of mitosis/high power field	0-1	2-3	4-5	>5
Pattern of invasion	Pushing, well delineated infiltrating border	Infiltrating solid cords, bands of strands	Small groups of cords of infiltrating cells	Marked and wide spread cellular dissociation in small groups
Stage of invasion	Carcinoma in situ or questionable invasion	Direct invasion but involving lamina propria only	Invasion below lamina propria adjacent to muscle, salivary gland and periosteum	Extension and deep invasion replacing most of the stromal tissue and infiltrating jaw bones
Lympho-plasmocytic invasion	Marked	Moderate	Slight	None

Table 1.3. Histologic Grading of Malignancy of tumor cell population (points)

All the above features are graded in the most poorly differentiated parts of the tumors. Each morphologic feature is graded from 1 to 4, and a total malignancy score is the sum of scores. A high total score indicates a poor prognosis. However this system had a few drawbacks as it was complicated and time consuming. Besides which the evaluations of features were dependent on a large and representative biopsy.

Invasive front

Tumor growth at the invasive front can show an expansive pattern, an infiltrative pattern or both. Expansive growth pattern is characterized by large tumor islands with well defined pushing margins and is associated with a better prognosis. Infiltrative growth pattern is characterized by scattered small irregular cords or single tumor cells, with poorly defined infiltrating margins and is associated with a more aggressive course[80].

Bryne et al[81] modified this system as they found that deep, invasive cells of the tumor appears to be histologically less differentiated than cells in the more superficial parts. They included a new parameter "invasive cell grading" into the system proposed by Anneroth et al.[79] The grading system described by Bryne et al[81] consists of five morphological features namely degree of keratinization, nuclear polymorphism, number of mitoses, mode of invasion and plasma-lymphocytic infiltration. Each of these features was scored from 1 to 4 according to the definitions given by Anneroth et al[79]. Only the cells at the deep, invasive margins of the tumor were graded. The scores for each morphological feature were summed into a total malignancy score.

9. Prognosis and predictive factors

Tumor size and nodal status are the most significant prognostic factors. Histological grade correlates poorly with patient outcome. The value of grading improves when only the deeply invasive margins of the tumor are evaluated. Tumors invading with pushing borders are less aggressive than tumors showing a non cohesive front showing diffuse spread with tiny strands or single cells. Major risk factors that adversely influence prognosis are two or more positive regional nodes, extra capsular extension of nodal disease or positive margins of resection. The other important histologic features associated with poor prognosis are tumor thickness and vascular invasion[83, 84, 85, 86, 87].

Second Primary Tumors: It has been recognized that patients with oral cancer are at a risk of second tumors in the upper aero digestive tract. This has been reported to occur in 10 - 35% of cases[88, 89]. These may be synchronous with the index tumor or, if occurring after intervals of longer than months are described as metachronous. Recurrence of the index tumor after treatment can be diagnosed by the pathologist where the tumor is in deeper tissue and not associated with epithelial surface. However, the most frequent situation of the second tumors is when they arise from surface epithelium adjacent to the treated index tumor. On morphological grounds these are diagnosed as second primary tumors. The increasing use of molecular biological techniques has allowed distinction to be made between molecularly distinct second primary tumors and second field tumors derived from the same genetically altered field as the index tumor.

10. Glossary

Oral cancer: Cancer of the lip, tongue, salivary glands, and other sites in the mouth
Oral Leukoplakia: A predominantly white lesion of the oral mucosa that cannot be characterized as any other definable lesion; some oral leukoplakias will transform into cancer.
Precancerous lesion: A morphologically altered tissue in which cancer is more likely to occur than its apparently normal counter part.

Quid: Defined as "a substance or mixture of substances placed in the mouth or chewed and remaining in contact with the mucosa, in raw or any manufactured or processed form." Clear delineation on contents of the quid (areca quid, tobacco quid and areca and tobacco quid) are recommended as absolute criteria for finer sub divisions to be added if necessary.
Betel quid: The betel quid refers to any quid wrapped in betel leaf and is therefore a specific variety of quid
Nass - a preparation of local tobacco, ash and cotton or sesame oil
Naswar - a mixture of powdered tobacco, slaked lime, cardamom oil
Betel quid - fresh betel leaf, fresh areca nut, slaked lime, catechu and tobacco
Pan masala - areaca nut, slaked lime, catechu, condiments and tobacco
Mainpuri - Tobacco, slaked lime, arecanut, camphor and cloves
Mawa - Areca nut, tobacco and slaked lime
Khainin - Tobacco and slaked lime
Gutka - An industrially manufactured tobacco and areca product

11. References

[1] Johnson NW. A global view of the epidemiology of oral cancer. In: N. W. Johnson (eds.), Oral Cancer: The Detection of Patients and Lesions at Risk, pp. 3–26. Cambridge, United Kingdom: Cambridge University Press, 1991.
[2] Boyle P, Macfarlane, GJ, Zheng T, Maisonneuve P, Evstifeeva T and Scully C. Recent advances in epidemiology of head and neck cancer. Curr Opin Oncol. 1992; 4: 471–477.
[3] Parkin DM, Stjernsward J and Muir CS. Estimates of the worldwide frequency of twelve major cancers. Bull WHO. 1984; 62:163 - 182.
[4] Silverman S. Oral cancer. Hamilton, London: BC Decker, 1998.
[5] Sankaranarayanan R. Oral Cancer in India; An epidemiologic and Clinical review. Oral Surg Oral Med Oral Pathol. 1990; 69: 325 - 330.
[6] Indian Council of Medical Research (ICMR): Annual reports of National cancer Registry Project of India. New Delhi: ICMR, 1982, 1984.
[7] Parkin DM, Pisani P and Ferlay J. Estimates of the worldwide incidence of eighteen major cancers in 1985. Int J Cancer. 1993; 19, 54: 594 - 606
[8] Stewart BW and Kleihues P (eds). World Cancer Report. Lyon: WHO International Agency for Research on Cancer; 2003.
[9] Petersen PE. The World Oral Health Report 2003: Continuous improvement of oral health in the 21st century - the approach of the WHO Global Oral Health Programme. Community Dent Oral Epidemiol. 2003; 31: 3–24.
[10] World Health Organization Classification of Tumors. International Agency for Research on Cancer. Pathology and Genetics of Head and Neck Tumors, IARC Press, Lyon, 2005.
[11] Yeole BB, Ramanakumar AV and Sankaranarayanan R. Survival from oral cancer in Mumbai (Bombay), India. Cancer Causes Control. 2003; 14: 945-52.
[12] Parkin DM, Whelan SL, Ferlay J, Raymond L and Young J (editors). Cancer Incidence in five continents. IARC Scientific Publication No. 143, VI. Lyon, France: International Agency for Research on Cancer; 1997.
[13] Swango PA. Cancers of the oral cavity and pharynx in the United States: an epidemiologic overview. J Public Health Dent. 1996; 56: 309-18.
[14] National Institute of Dental and Craniofacial Research (NIDR). Prevention and Early detection: Keys to Oral Cancer. JADA. 1993; 124: 81-82.

[15] Fearlay J, Bray F, Pisani P and Parkin DM, GLOBOCAN 2000: Cancer incidence, mortality and prevalence worldwide, version 1.0. IARC Cancer Base No.5.Lyon: IARC Press; 2001.

[16] Blot WJ, McLaughlin JK, Winn DM, Austin DF, Greenberg RS, Preston-Martin S, et al. Smoking and drinking in relation to oral and pharyngeal cancer. Cancer Res. 1988; 48: 3282-7.

[17] Graham S: Dentition, diet, tobacco and alcohol in the epidemiology of oral cancer. J Natl Cancer Inst. 1977; 59: 1611 - 1618.

[18] Wynder EL, Mushinski MH and Spivak JC. Tobacco and alcohol consumption in relation to the development of multiple primary cancers. Cancer. 1977; 40: 1872-8.

[19] Devise SS, Blot WJ and Fraumeni JF. Changing patterns in the incidence of esophageal and gastric carcinoma in the United States. Epidemiology. 1990; 1: 116-21.

[20] Gillison ML, Koch WM and Shah KV. Human papillomavirus in head and neck squamous cell carcinoma: are some head and neck cancers a sexually transmitted disease? Curr Opin Oncol. 1999; 11: 191-9.

[21] Koch WM, Lango M, Sewell D, Zahurak M and Sidransky D. Head and neck cancer in nonsmokers: a distinct clinical and molecular entity. Laryngoscope. 1999; 109: 1544-51.

[22] D'Costa J, Saranath D, Sanghvi V and Mehta AR. Epstein-Barr virus in tobacco-induced oral cancers and oral lesions in patients from India. J Oral Pathol Med. 1998; 27: 78-82.

[23] Shimakage M, Horii K, Tempaku A, Kakudo K, Shirasaka T and Sasagawa T. Association of Epstein-Barr virus with oral cancers. Hum Pathol. 2002; 33: 608-14.

[24] Winn DM. Diet and nutrition in the etiology of oral cancer. Am J Clin Nutr. 1995; 61: 437S-445S.

[25] Hirayama T. An epidemiological study of oral and pharyngeal cancer in Central and South-East Asia. Bull World Health Organ. 1966; 34: 41-69.

[26] Mahboubi E and Sayed GM: Oral Cavity and Pharynx. pp. 583-595. In Cancer Epidemiology and Prevention (Schottenfeld D, Fraumeni JF Jr, Eds.). Philadelphia: W.B. Saunders, 1982.

[27] Jayant K and Deo MG: Oral cancer and culture practices in relation to betel quid and tobacco chewing and smoking. Cancer Detect Prev. 1986; 9: 207-213.

[28] Winn DM, Blot WJ, Shy CM, Pickle LW, Toledo A and Fraumeni JF. Snuff dipping and oral cancer among women in the southern United States. N Engl J Med. 1981; 305: 745-749.

[29] Gupta PC. Betel quid and oral cancer: prospects for prevention. IARC Sci Publ. 1991; 105: 466-70.

[30] Jayant K. Statistical appraisal of the association of smoking habits to the oral and pharyngeal cancers. Ind J Cancer. 1977; 14:293-299.

[31] Gupta PC, Pindborg JJ and Mehta S. Comparison of carcinogenicity of betel quid with and without tobacco: an epidemiologic review. Ecology of Disease. 1982; 1:213-219.

[32] Atkinson L, Purohit R, Reay-Young P and Scott GC. Cancer reporting in Papua, New Guinea. National Cancer Institute Monographs 1982; 62: 65-71.

[33] Preston-Martin S and Correa P. Epidemiological evidence for the role of nitroso compounds in human cancer. Cancer Surv. 1989; 8: 459-73.

[34] Stich HF, Parida BB and Brunnemann KD. Localized formation of micronuclei in the oral mucosa and tobacco-specific nitrosamines in the saliva of "reverse" smokers, Khaini-tobacco chewers and gudakhu users. Int J Cancer. 1992; 50: 172-6.

[35] Hoffmann D, Djordjevic MV and Brunnenmann KD. New brands of oral snuff. Food and Chemical Toxicology. 1991; 29: 65 – 68.

[36] Baan RA, van den Berg PT, Steenwinkel MJ and van der Wulp CJ. Detection of benzo[a]pyrene-DNA adducts in cultured cells treated with benzo[a]pyrene diol-epoxide by quantitative immunofluorescence microscopy and 32P-postlabelling; immunofluorescence analysis of benzo[a]pyrene-DNA adducts in bronchial cells from smoking individuals. IARC Sci Publ. 1988; 89: 146-54.

[37] Pulera N, Petruzzelli S, Celi A, Puntoni R, Fornai E, Sawe Uet al. Presence and persistence of serum anti-benzo[a]pyrene diolepoxide-DNA adduct antibodies in smokers: effects of smoking reduction and cessation. Int J Cancer. 1997 17; 70: 145-9.

[38] Hecht SS and Hoffmann D. Tobacco-specific nitrosamines, an important group of carcinogens in tobacco and tobacco smoke. Carcinogenesis 1988; 9: 875-884.

[39] Vasudevan DM and Vijayakumar T. Viruses in human oral cancers. J Exp Clin Cancer Res. 1998; 17: 27-31.

[40] Park NH, Li SL, Xie JF and Cherrick HM. In vitro and animal studies of the role of viruses in oral carcinogenesis. Eur J Cancer B Oral Oncol. 1992; 28B: 145-52.

[41] Flaitz CM, Nichols CM, Adler-Storthz K and Hicks MJ. Intraoral squamous cell carcinoma in human immunodeficiency virus infection. A clinicopathologic study. Oral Surg Oral Med Oral Pathol Oral Radiol Endod. 1995; 80: 55-62.

[42] Hille JJ, Webster-Cyriaque J, Palefski JM and Raab-Traub N.Mechanisms of expression of HHV8, EBV and HPV in selected HIV-associated oral lesions. Oral Dis. 2002; 8: 161-8.

[43] Herrero R, Castellsague X, Pawlita M, Lissowska J, Kee F, Balaram P, et al. IARC Multicenter Oral Cancer Study Group. Human papillomavirus and oral cancer: J Natl Cancer Inst. 2003; 95:1772-83

[44] Huibregtse JM, Scheffner M and Howley PM. Cloning and expression of the cDNA for E6-AP, a protein that mediates the interaction of the human papillomavirus E6 oncoprotein with p53. Mol Cell Biol. 1993; 13: 775-84.

[45] Scheffner M, Huibregtse JM, Vierstra RD and Howley PM. The HPV-16 E6 and E6-AP complex functions as an ubiquitin-protein ligase in the ubiquitination of p53. Cell. 1993; 75: 495-505.

[46] Kim HJ, Guo W and Park NH. HPV-16 E6 oncoprotein induces mutations via p53-dependent and -independent pathways. Oncol Rep. 2000; 7: 707-12.

[47] McLaughlin JK, Gridley G, Block G, Winn DM, Preston-Martin S, Schoenberg JB, et al. Dietary factors in oral and pharyngeal cancer. J Natl Cancer Inst. 1988; 80: 1237-43.

[48] Franceschi S, Bidoli E, Baron AE, Barra S, Talamini R, Serraino D, et al. Nutrition and cancer of the oral cavity and pharynx in north-east Italy. Int J Cancer. 1991; 47: 20-5.

[49] Franco EL, Kowalski LP, Oliveira BV, Curado MP, Pereira RN, Silva ME, et al. Risk factors for oral cancer in Brazil: a case-control study. Int J Cancer 1989; 43: 992-1000.

[50] Gridley G, McLaughlin JK, Block G, Blot WJ, Winn DM, Greenberg RS, et al. Diet and oral and pharyngeal cancer among blacks. Nutr Cancer. 1990; 14: 219-225.

[51] La Vecchia C, Negri E, D'Avanzo B, Boyle P and Franceschi S. Dietary indicators of oral and pharyngeal cancer. Int J Epidemiol. 1991; 20: 39-44.

[52] Gridley G, McLaughlin JK, Block G, Blot WJ, Gluch M and Fraumeni JF Jr. Vitamin supplements use and reduced risk of oral and pharyngeal cancer. Am J Epidemiol 1992; 135: 1083-1092.

[53] Shanta V and Krishnamurthy S. A study of etiological factors in oral squamous cell carcinoma. Br J Cancer. 1959; 13: 382 - 388.

[54] Zheng W, Blot WJ, Diamond EL, Norkus EP, Spate V, Morris JS, et al. Serum micronutrients and the subsequent risk of oral and pharyngeal cancer. Cancer Res. 1993; 53: 795-8.

[55] Larsson LG, Sandström A and Westling P. Relationship of Plummer-Vinson disease to cancer of the upper alimentary tract in Sweden. Cancer Res. 1975; 35: 3308-16

[56] Lundeen RC, Langlais RP and Terezhalmy GT. Sunscreen protection for lip mucosa: a review and update. J Am Dent Assoc. 1985; 111: 617-21.

[57] Wahi PN, Kehar U and Lahiri B. Factors influencing oral and oropharyngeal cancers in India.Br J Cancer. 1965; 19: 642-60.

[58] Graham S, Dayal H, Rohrer T, Swanson M, Sultz H, Shedd D, et al. Dentition, diet, tobacco, and alcohol in the epidemiology of oral cancer. J Natl Cancer Inst. 1977; 59: 1611-8.

[59] Mehta FS, Pindborg JJ, Gupta PC and Daftary DK. Epidemiologic and histologic study of oral cancer and leukoplakia among 50,915 villagers in India. Cancer. 1969; 24: 832-49.

[60] Franeschi S, Bidoli E, Herrero R and Munoz N. Comparison of cancers of the oral cavity and pharynx worldwide: etiological clues. Oral Oncol. 1990; 36: 106 - 115.

[61] Baker SR and Krause CJ. Carcinoma of the lip. Laryngoscope. 1980; 90: 19-27.

[62] Hjortdal O, Naess A and Berner A. Squamous cell carcinomas of the lower lip. J Craniomaxillofac Surg. 1995; 23: 34-7.

[63] Rao DN and Desai PB. Risk assessment of tobacco, alcohol and diet in cancers of base tongue and oral tongue--a case control study. Indian J Cancer. 1998; 35: 65-72.

[64] Prince S and Bailey BM. Squamous cell carcinoma of the tongue; review. J Oral Maxilofac Surg. 1999; 37: 164-174.

[65] Sankaranarayanan R, Duffy SW, Day NE, Nair MK and Padmakumary G. A case-control investigation of cancer of the oral tongue and the floor of the mouth in southern India. Int J Cancer. 1989; 44: 617-21.

[66] Woolgar JA and Scott J. Prediction of cervical lymph node metastasis in squamous cell carcinoma of the tongue/floor of mouth. Head Neck. 1995; 17: 463-72.

[67] Hirayama T. An epidemiological study of oral and pharyngeal cancer in central and South East Asia. Bulletin of WHO. 1966; 34: 41 - 69

[68] Dhawan IK, Verma K, Khazanchi RK, Madan NC, Shukla NK and Saxena R. Carcinoma of buccal mucosa: incidence of regional lymph node involvement. Indian J Cancer. 1993; 30: 176-80.

[69] Sankaranarayanan R, Duffy SW, Padmakumary G, Day NE and Padmanabhan TK. Tobacco chewing, alcohol and nasal snuff in cancer of the gingiva in Kerala, India. Br J Cancer. 1989; 60: 638-43.

[70] Brennan CT, Sessions DG, Spitznagel EL Jr and Harvey JE. Surgical pathology of cancer of the oral cavity and oropharynx. Laryngoscope. 1991; 101: 1175-97.

[71] McGregor AD and MacDonald DG. Routes of entry of squamous cell carcinoma to the mandible. Head Neck Surg. 1988; 10: 294 - 301.

[72] Mukherji SK, Armao D and Joshi VM. Cervical nodal metastases in squamous cell carcinoma of the head and neck: what to expect. Head Neck. 2001; 23: 995 - 1005.
[73] Genden EM, Ferlito A, Bradley PJ, Rinaldo A and Scully C. Neck Disease and distant metastases Oral Oncol. 2003; 39: 207 - 212.
[74] Charoenrat P, Pillai G, Patel S, Fisher C, Archer D, Eccles S, et al. Tumor thickness predicts cervical nodal metastases and survival in early oral tongue cancer. Oral Oncol. 2003; 39: 386 - 390.
[75] Ferlito A, Shaha AR, Silver CE, Rinaldo A and Mondin V. Incidence and site of distant metastases from head and neck cancer. ORL J Otorhinolarygol Relat Spec. 2001; 63: 202 - 207.
[76] Osaki T, Yoneda K, Yamamoto T, Kimura T, Matuoka H, Sakai J, et al. Clinical investigation on pulmonary metastasis of head and neck carcinomas. Oncology. 2000; 59: 196 - 203.
[77] Greene FL, Page DL, Fleming ID, Fritz AG, Balch CM, Haller DG et al. (2002) American Joint Committee on Cancer. Cancer Staging Manual. Springer: New York.
[78] Sobin LH and Wittekind C (2002). TNM Classification of Malignant Tumors. 6th ed. John Wiley and Sons: New York.
[79] Anneroth G, Batsakis J and Luna M. Review of the literature and a recommended system of malignancy grading in oral squamous cell carcinomas. Scand J Dent Res. 1987; 95: 229-49.
[80] Bryne M, Jenssen N and Boysen M. Histological grading in the deep invasive front of T1 and T2 glottic squamous cell carcinomas has high prognostic value. Virchows Arch. 1995; 427: 277 - 281.
[81] Bryne M, Koppang HS, Lilleng R, Stene T, Bang G and Dabelsteen E. New malignancy grading is a better prognostic indicator than Broders' grading in oral squamous cell carcinomas. J Oral Pathol Med. 1989; 18: 432-7.
[82] Goyanna R, Torres Et and Broders AC. [Histological grading of malignant tumors; Broder's method.] Hospital (Rio J). 1951; 39: 791-818.
[83] Platz H, Fries R and Hudec M. Retrospective DOSAK Study on carcinomas of the oral cavity: results and consequences. J Maxillofac Surg. 1995; 13: 147 - 153.
[84] Kearsley JH and Thomas S. Prognostic markers in cancers of the head and neck region. Anticancer Drugs. 1993; 4: 419 - 429.
[85] Roland NJ, Caslin AW, Nash J and Stell PM. Value of grading squamous cell carcinoma of the head and neck. Head Neck. 1992; 1: 224 - 229.
[86] Bryne M, Koppang HS, Lilleng R and Kjaerheim A. Malignancy grading of the deep invasive margins of oral squamous cell carcinomas as high prognostic value. J Pathol. 1992; 166: 375 - 381.
[87] Hiratsuka H, Miyakawa A, Nakamari K, Kido Y, Sunakawa H and Kohama GG. Multivariate analysis of occult lymph node metastasis as a prognostic indicator for patient with squamous cell carcinoma of the oral cavity. Cancer. 1997; 80: 351-356.
[88] van Oijen MG, Leppers Vd Straat FG, Tilanus MG and Slootweg PJ. The origins of multiple squamous cell carcinomas in the aero digestive tract. Cancer. 2000; 88: 884-93.
[89] van Oijen MG and Slootweg PJ. Oral field cancerization: carcinogen-induced independent events or micrometastatic deposits? Cancer Epidemiology Biomarkers Prep. 2000; 9: 249-56.

3

Oral Squamous Cell Carcinoma Clinical Aspects

Nicolás Bolesina, Fabián L. Femopase,
Silvia A. López de Blanc, Rosana A. Morelatto and María Alicia Olmos
Universidad Nacional de Córdoba, Córdoba
Argentina

1. Introduction

Oral cancer (OC) is considered a serious public health problem that causes great morbidity and mortality in the population. While OC has a lower incidence than other malignant tumors, it is known to produce high mortality and serious disturbances or discomfort in the patient as a consequence of either the tumor itself or of the treatment. The Oral Squamous Cell Carcinoma is the most common malignant tumor of the lip, oral cavity and oropharynx (90% of the cases) while the remaining 10% of the cases are mainly melanomas, sarcomas, minor salivary gland carcinomas and metastatic cancers (Scully et al., 2006).

In this chapter the attention is focused on the clinical characteristics of **OSCCs**.

Topics: Clinical presentation, Symptoms, Diagnosis, Prognosis, Oral and Dental Management and Psychological aspects of patient care.

2. Clinical presentation. Symptoms

Oral Squamous Cell Carcinoma (**OSCC**) presents different clinical aspects which are related with the location of the tumor, evolution time, precancerous lesions and risk factors. The most frequent clinical aspects are: tumor, ulcer, vegetans, verrucous and mixed forms such as ulcerous-vegetans or verrucose- ulcers (Boring et al., 1994).

The diagnosis of early lesions such as in-situ or microinvasive carcinoma, represents a real challenge for health professionals. Leukoplakia, erythroplakia or erythroleukoplakia are the most frequent clinical aspects, which may present superficially eroded areas. Chorion infiltration may be suspected when increased consistency on palpation is observed. The abovementioned lesions are asymptomatic, tend to keep their size, may show changes in the surface and do not respond to local treatments. The lesion can progress and develop as an exophytic, irregular lobulated lesion or adopt an endophytic growth pattern characterized by a depressed ulcer with grayish-white edges, elevated, everted and indurate borders and an infiltrated base. In most cases, lesions are asymptomatic; pain appears only when muscles or nerves are invaded at advanced stages of the disease. (Neville et al., 2002; Silverman et al., 1998)

According to different authors, the lip is the most common location of **OSCCs**. In such cases, patients are likely to consult a physician or a dermatologist while in cases of tongue tumors, consultation to the dentist is more frequent. The paramedial area of the inferior lip is the most often region affected by lip cancer whereas the most prevalent precancerous lesions are actinic chronic cheilitis. **OSCCs** most common clinic manifestations are the loss of superficial tissue, erosion, ulcers (Fig.1) and occasionally exophytic shaped lesions: keratotic, verrucous or vegetant, with tumorous or "skin horn" aspect (Neville et al., 2002; Silverman et al., 1998). Chronic exposure to the sun produces in affected patients an alteration of the shape of the lip called lip everted or "lip on balcony".

A significant atrophy of the vermillion area with scales that do not tend to shed and therefore accumulate to form keratosis can often be observed. This type of lesions alternate with white lesions and erythro-leukoplakia areas that are prone to cracking, erosion or ulceration which are called actinic cheilitis. Lip cancer develops slowly and in advanced stages it can extend to the corner of the mouth or to the gingiva. It can also develop metastatic lymph nodes in submental and submandibular areas (Grinspan, 1983).

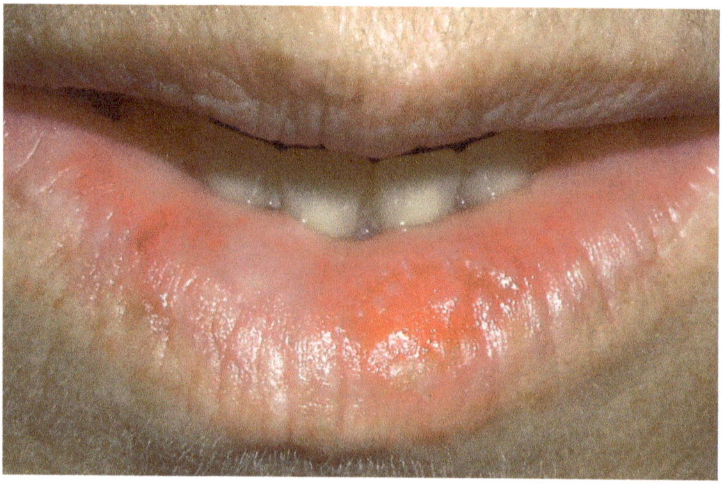

Fig. 1. In-situ carcinoma of the lower lip vermillion

Tongue carcinoma is the most commonly observed OC into the oral cavity; traumatic lesions, leukoplakia and lichen planus are predominant precancerous conditions. Tongue carcinoma represents 30-40% of OCs, the lateral tongue being the most frequent situation (80%), followed by ventral and dorsum (Brandizzi et al., 2008).

Lateral border of the tongue and ventral surface OCs are usually preceded by traumatic lesions caused by sharp cusps or sharp edged teeth, by badly positioned teeth or by maladjusted dentures that chronically rub the mentioned areas. Ulcerated forms are the most frequently observed, see Fig 2, followed by exophitic tumor, which generally produce pain irradiating to the ear. In the ventral area, ulcer-vegetant or mixed forms predominate. Tumors on the dorsum are generally associated to lichen planus or to leukoplakia lesions. They are clinically observable as ulcerated forms tend to expand on the surface rather than go deeper into it. The lateral border of the tongue and the floor of the mouth (with extensions to the back lateral soft palate and tonsillar areas) combine to form a horse shoe-shaped region in the oral mucosa that was described by Jovanovic et al., (1993) as highly risky for cancer development and also as a bad prognostic area.

These tumors tend to evolve towards the ventral side and to the floor of the mouth. In the first consultation, 40% of the patients have lymph nodes. When the lesion has more than 4 cm, lymph nodes are present in 90% of the cases (Grinspan et al., 1983). Tumors located in the anterior half of the tongue usually lead to lymphadenopathy in the suprahyoid region while those located in the posterior half lead to submaxillary, carotid and lateropharyngeal nodes. Contralateral nodes are more frequent from tumors in the ventral surface and floor of the mouth (Shah et al., 1990; Grinspan, 1983).

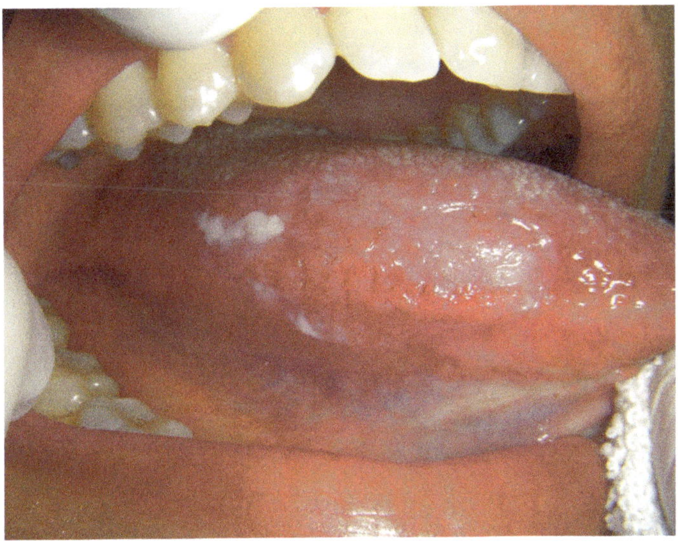

Fig. 2. Tongue infiltrant SCC, T2 N1 Mo

According to our experience in Argentina, **OSCCs** in gum and alveolar ridge are the 2nd most frequent locations (Brandizzi et al., 2008.) which is not the case in other countries (Boudewijn et al., 2009, Chandu et al., 2005). It is difficult to detect previous lesions when the carcinoma is located in the gingival or alveolar ridge. In such locations, however, it is common to associate them with periodontal disease.

Chronic inflammatory processes would release genotoxic mediators that would stimulate the accumulation of genetic defects leading to the appearance of malignant cells. In its initial stage, gingival carcinoma looks like a red or/and white spot slightly vegetant, extending on the surface due to the resistance offered by the periosteum (**Fig 3**). As **OSCC** advances, it adopts a tumoral shape, it may invade the bones, produce loosening of teeth and cause pain or trismus. Its progress through the lymph affects the submental, submandibular and carotid regions, these ones becoming the most common bilateral metastases. The antero inferior lesions progress towards the floor of the mouth and to the ventral side of the tongue. If the tumor is located in the posterior zone, it invades the floor of the mouth as well as the masticatory muscles.

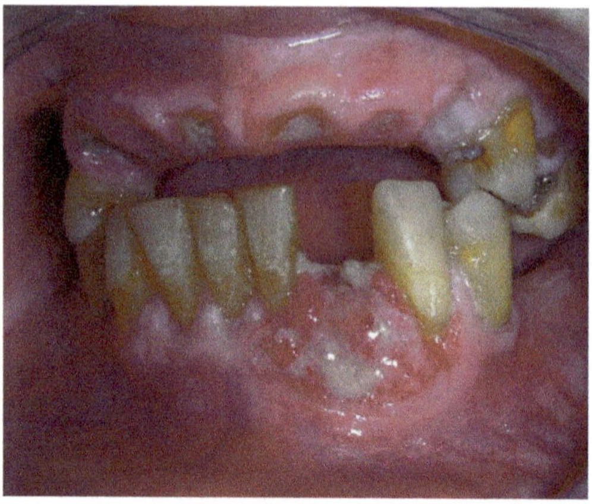

Fig. 3. Gum carcinoma, the tooth was lost due to bone tumor invasion

The floor of the mouth **OSCC** starts mainly in the anterior area as red and/or white spots, plaque or nodular, ulcerated lesions, later indurated at palpation (**Fig. 4**). It is not painful at an early stage although the tongue´s mobility can eventually be impaired. It advances from the surface to the depths of the tissues, invading the floor of the mouth muscles, the submental, submaxillary and cervical nodes.

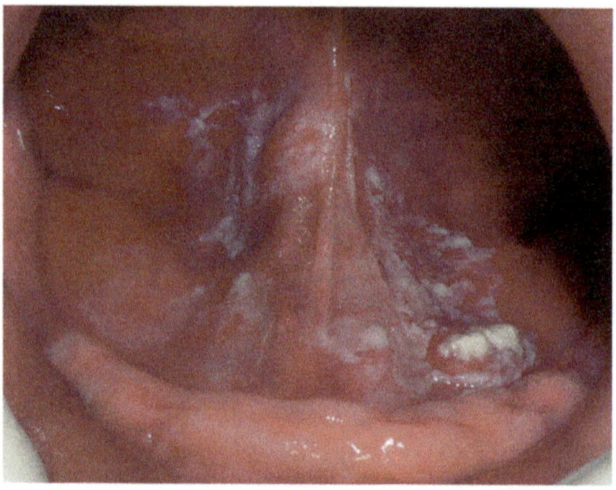

Fig. 4. Floor of the mouth, infiltrant SCC, two foci born in a leukoplakia

Most buccal mucosa SCC is characterized by developing on previous lesions. The leukoplasiform and erythroplastic forms are commonly observed in the anterior part of the buccal mucosa while in the posterior one it is more often secondary to traumatic lesions or lichen planus. One of the first signs of the transformation is the induration of erythoplastic lesions that tend to develop an exophytic aspect as they grow (Fig. 5). This type of SCC rarely presents ulcers whereas differentiated histopathologic forms are predominant. When SCC appears in the posterior third of the buccal mucosa, it usually presents itself as endophytic or ulcers; undifferentiated histological types is the most frequent that have a worse prognosis than in the anterior third. The affected nodes are generally situated in the submaxillary area and less frequently in the cervical or facial ones (Grinspan, 1983; Jovanovic et al., 1993).

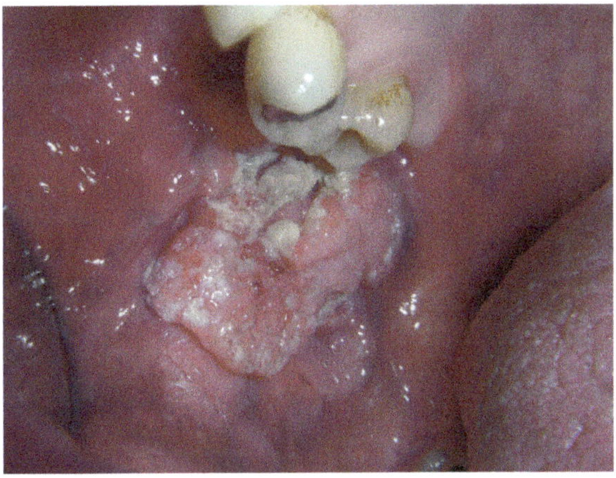

Fig. 5. OSCC of the buccal mucosa, an exophytic aspect.

When we analized the habits associated to **OSCC** location, we observed that 85%-90% of the patients affected with floor of the mouth and oropharygeal carcinoma were smokers and drinkers. Fewer than 40% of those with gum and tongue carcinoma had both habits (Fig. 6).

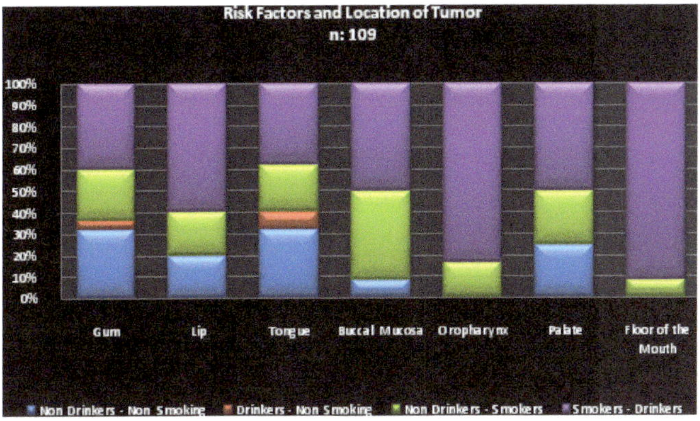

Fig. 6. Risk factors and location of the tumor

To highlight: It is essential for everyone to undergo a proper oral examination. Pain in itself is not a reliable indicator of malignancy; in many of the studied cases, early lesions were associated with only minor discomfort.

2.1 Lymph nodes

According to the natural history of **OSCCs**, invasive lesions would lead to their spreading through the lymph nodes. Mobile, painless nodes whose volumes increase in course of time, and fix to surrounding tissue in the advanced stages, are those clinically suggestive of malignancy.

Union for International Cancer Control (**UICC**) recommended to classify the location of lymph nodes in the following levels:

Level I: submandibular and submaxillary nodes.
Level II: upper jugular nodes.
Level III: jugular media.
Level IV: lower jugular.
Level V: nodes in the posterior triangle, bounded at the back by the anterior border of the trapezius muscle, anteriorly by the posterior border of the sternocleidomastoid and below by the clavicle. Descriptive purposes can be divided into high, medium and low by two horizontal planes: the superior plane is situated below the hyoid bone and the inferior one in the lower edge of the cricoid cartilage.
Level VI: lymph nodes in the central compartment, which extends from the suprasternal notch to the hyoid bone. Lateral boundaries are formed on each side by the body´s internal carotid sheath.
Level VII: lymph nodes located in the upper mediastinum, below the suprasternal notch.

2.2 TNM system and staging

According to the literature, the first classification of malignant tumors is Pierre Denoix´s (1944) Tumor Node Metastasis (**TNM**), based on the extent of primary tumor (**T**), involvement of regional lymph nodes (**N**) and metastasis at distance (**M**). Such classification also applies to **OSCCs** of the mouth. Proper classification and staging allows the physician to determine treatment more appropriately, evaluate results of management more reliably and compare worldwide statistics reported from various institutions.

Currently, the American Joint Committee on Cancer (**AJCC**) and the **UICC** periodically update cancer staging, which is used by physicians and health care professionals throughout the world to facilitate the uniform description of neoplastic diseases. **UICC** rules to classify tumors are:

- The classification applies only to carcinomas in the lip vermilion, in the oral cavity, pharynx, larynx, sinuses mucous including minor salivary gland tumors.
- There should be histological confirmation. When the histology comes from another institution, it is recommended to have it reviewed by the pathologist in the working team.
- The extent of the disease should be evaluated by clinical examination, endoscopy and imaging.

In patients with advanced **OSCC** plus a history of heavy smoking, chest Computer Tomography (**CT**) is recommended before deciding on treatment because of the considerable possibility of undetected metastases in previous X-Ray tests.

The staging of each case must be determined before treatment and should not be changed whatever findings emerge after starting it. You can add such findings but you cannot change the staging. If doubts arise concerning it, assigning the patient the lowest category is the most convenient procedure.

Tables 1 shows the **TNM** classification and **Table 2** describes the staging.

T **Tumor**	N **Nodule**	M **Metastasis**
Tis: in situ Carcinoma	N0: nonpalpable regional lymph node	M0: No distant metastasis
T1: < 2 cm. diameter	N1: ipsilateral single ≤3 cm palpable nodes	M1: clinical or radiographic evidence of metastasis
T2: 2 to 4 cm. diameter	N2: ipsilateral or contralateral palpable lymph nodes 3 to 6 cm. subdivided into: N2a: an ipsilateral single node 3 to 6 cm. N2b: ipsilateral multiple ≤6 cm. N2c: contralateral or bilateral ≤6 cm.	
T3: Tumor >4 cm. diameter	N3: >6 cm.	
T4: invaded adjacent tissues T4a: moderately advanced local disease T4b: very advanced local disease		

Table 1. **TNM** Classification of malignant Tumors

Stage	Tumor	Node *	Metastasis
Stage 0	Tis	N0	M0
Stage I	T1	N0	M0
Stage II	T2	N0	M0
Stage III	T1 T2 T3 T3	N1 N1 N0 N1	M0 M0 M0 M0
Stage IVA moderately advanced local/ regional disease	T4a T4a T1 T2 T3 T4a	N0 N1 N2 N2 N2 N2	M0 M0 M0 M0 M0 M0
Stage IVB very advanced local/regional disease	T4b	Any N	M0
Stage IVC distant metastatic disease	Any T Any T	N3 Any N	M0 M1

* Extracapsular spread (ECS) of disease is added as ECS + or ECS – as a descriptor.
These descriptors will not influence nodal staging.

Table 2. Stage grouping for oral cavity, oropharyngeal, hypopharyngeal and laryngeal cancers from **UICC**: **TNM** Classification of Malignant Tumours

3. Variables that influence diagnosis

3.1 Diagnostic delay

Oral cancer is a global health problem of increasing incidence and mortality rates; more than 500,000 patients worldwide are estimated to have oral cancer (Parkin et al., 2005). The International Association for Cancer Research (IARC) and the World Health Organization (WHO) latest records show an incidence of 263,020 cases (3.8 rate) with high mortality 127,654 (1.9 rate), (Ferlay et al., 2010).

Unfortunately, the 5-year survival rate has not changed during the last half of the century, still being around 50–55% in spite of the advances in diagnosis and treatment (Neville and Day, 2002). Early diagnosis is a foremost step for reducing cancer mortality (Boyle et al., 2003), since the identification of smaller lesions allows less aggressive and debilitating treatments. However, almost half of intraoral cancers have late diagnosis (stages III or IV).

Diagnostic delay is, therefore, the main reason why most patients´ OSCCs are discovered in advanced stages when their diagnoses are finally made. Late diagnosis is the result of either patient or professional delay (Kerdpon & Sriplung, 2001, Rogers et al., 2007).

There is a vast literature about the results of research on this interesting topic carried out in populations from all over the world (Table 5).

We investigated OSCC diagnosis delay in Córdoba in a retrospective study of clinical records of OSCC patients, examined in the Stomatology B service (a referral clinic for oral soft-tissue lesions) and in the Oncohematology Unit of Hospital Nacional de Clínicas (Morelatto et al., 2007). We included in that study patients diagnosed with OSCC as their first cancer between 1992 and 2004. Oral exams and diagnosis at both centers were made by the same trained professionals and supervised by the same head professor. Age, sex and location of the OSCC, first signs or symptoms, and first consultation with a health professional (HP) were studied. Stage at the moment of the diagnosis was classified according to the 1997 version of the UICC, AJCC. The symptoms were classified as pain, swelling, ulceration, white lesions, poor denture fit and others. Stages III and IV (S III and S IV) were defined as advanced tumors and S I and S II as early ones (Brohua et al., 2005).

In order to study the OSCC diagnostic delay, the authors described the following categories:

A- Patient delay: considers the time elapsed between the first sign or symptom noticed by the patient and the first consultation with a HP. B- Professional delay: considers the period of time between the first consultation with a HP and the referral to the specialist who performed the biopsy (Kerdpon & Sriplung, 2001). C- Patient and professional delay: considers the period of time between the final diagnosis and the beginning of treatment (Kowalski & Carvalho, 2001).

A lapse of more than 30 days in any category (A, B or C) was regarded as delay (Shah & Lydiatt, 1995). The data aforementioned were statistically analyzed.

In our study, 68% of the patients in the early stage and 54% in the advanced stage evidenced patient delay (see Table 3). On the other hand, 72% of the patients in the early stage and 61%

in the advanced stage had a professional delay of more than 30 days (Table 4). In both cases, the delay was more pronounced in early stages.

Delay A	<30 days n (%)	30-60 days n (%)	60-120 days n (%)	>120 days n (%)	Total delay n (%)
S I and II	6 (32)	2 (10)	3 (16)	8 (42)	13 (68)
S III and IV	23 (46)	12 (24)	8 (16)	7 (14)	27 (54)*
Total	29 (42)	14 (20)	11(16)	15(21)	40 (58)

*In one patient, delay A was unknown.

Table 3. Patient delay (A) related to the stage of the tumor.

Delay B	<30 days n (%)	30-60 days n (%)	60-120 days n (%)	>120 days n (%)	Total delay n (%)
S I y II*	5 (28)	4 (22)	-	9 (50)	13 (72)*
S III y IV	20 (39)	6 (12)	18 (35)	7 (14)	31 (61)
Total	25 (36)	10 (14)	18 (26)	16 (23)	44 (64)

* In one patient, delay B was unknown.

Table 4. Professional delay (B) related to the stage of the tumor

A similar finding was reported in Greece and in the Netherlands with 52% of patients with more than 3 weeks (Pitiphat et al., 2002) and 46 days of delay, respectively (Jovanovic et al.,1992). A median time of 3 months or more until diagnosis was described for Canada (Elwood & Gallagher, 1985), Italy (Mashberg et al., 1989), Finland (Soderholm, 1990), Denmark (Wildt et al., 1995) and Israel (Gorsky &Dayan, 1995). Although the results obtained in Argentina were more optimistic than in those of some other populations, the proportion of patients who had delayed diagnosis was still considerably high. The mean time between the first symptom and the consultation with a HP (delay A) was 2.5 months in females and 2.3 in males. The percentage of delay A of more than 1 month (68%) in Córdoba is similar to the value found by Jovanovic et al., 1992 (53.7%) and lower than results obtained by Pinholt et al., 1997, (92%).

It should be considered that there are some limitations in the present research namely, that many patients did not exactly recall the onset of their symptoms (Wildt et al., 1995). Pain was the most common first symptom, but more than half of the patients did not visit a medical facility to receive treatment before one month following that occurrence. Onizawa et al., 2003 consider that the symptom may not be bothersome or severe enough to seek professional help.

The time elapsed between the first symptom and its diagnosis was longer for women than for men in our population (77.5 and 67.8 days respectively); Wildt et al., 1995, reported similar results. In our research, we observed that 100% of lip cancers and 38% of tongue lesions were staged as early cancers at the time of diagnosis, while Gorsky & Dayan, 1995 in Israel found 82% in lip and 58% of tongue tumors in that stage. According to our research professional delay (B) was the most related variable to the stage of the tumor at the time of diagnosis. As shown in Table 4, B was more important in early stages; this observation is relevant because treatment delay worsens the prognosis.

Country	Author / Year	N	Delay
The Netherlands	Jovanovic et al., 1992	50	patient
Australia	Dimitroulis et al., 1992	51	patient
Brazil	Kowalski et al.,1994	336	professional
Israel	Gorsky et al., 1995	543	professional
Denmark	Wildt et al., 1995	167	patient
Malaysia	Khoo et al., 1998	65	Patient and professional
Canada	Allison et al., 1998	188	professional
Thailand	Kerdpon et al., 2001	161	patient and professional
Japan	Onizawa et al., 2003	152	professional
The Netherlands	Tromp et al., 2005	306	patient
Ireland	O´Sullivan et al., 2005	370	patient
Netherlands	Brouha et al., 2007	173	professional

Table 5. Responsibility of diagnostic delay in oral cancer in different countries according to several authors

OSCC diagnostic delay has been thoroughly studied and its causes seem to be always the same: (i) unawareness of most of the population regarding the potential malignancy of oral lesions (patients' delay), (ii) inaccurate diagnosis on the part of the HP and (iii) delay in referral for treatment (Allison et al., 1998; Dimitroulis et al., 1992), see Table 5.

Medical practitioners usually prescribe various medications; it is more common, however, that dentists adopt a more mechanical approach such as extracting teeth or adjusting dentures (Kerdpon & Sriplung, 2001). Both tend to be slow in suspecting malignancy.

The findings of the present study also indicate that patients are partially responsible for delay in OSCC diagnosis.

3.2 Awareness

Due to the apparent lack of awareness of patients suffering from **OSCC** assisted by different services in various countries, we studied the general public in Cordoba City to assess levels of awareness and knowledge of oral cancer, risk factors, suspicious clinical signs and parameters related to early consultation to **HP** (Robledo et al., 2008). Anonymous surveys were carried out, obtaining a systematic sampling from the 2004-2005 telephone directory of Cordoba City. Four hundred effective surveys were made to Argentine citizens older than 18. Results: 41 % of the participants did not know of the existence of **OC**, the highest percentage of poor or no information was found among people younger than 30 years of age. Only 60% of those who knew about **OC** were able to name a risk factor, being tobacco the most easily associated. It is surprising that only 3% of the questioned people associated alcohol, related tobacco-alcohol consumption or unadjusted dentures as risk factors. Only 45% had some knowledge about clinical manifestations, pain and ulcers being the most frequently mentioned. Though most of the surveyed population had consulted a dentist one or several times a year, only 32% could recall if they had had a comprehensive oral exam. Evidently, the population badly needs to be informed about risk factors and first clinical manifestations of OC and about the importance of early consultation.

In a study of Humphris et al. (2004), a randomized controlled trial found that patients attending primary care who had read an information leaflet about head and neck cancer had increased awareness of risk compared to patients who had not seen the leaflet. A questionnaire of awareness of signs and symptoms and risks of oral cancer showed that all those who received the leaflet (smokers, non-smokers and past smokers) reported greater knowledge ($p < 0.001$). Smokers were 16 times more likely to perceive that they were at greater risk.

It would also be highly necessary to have access to professionals with further training in the detection of precancerous lesions and OC early signs.

4. Prognosis. Survival rate

Cancers of the oral cavity have a high mortality rate and, despite the current progress in treatments, the situation has not improved. A five-year survival rate ranging from 30% to 80% has been reported from several parts of the world. Survival rates are lower in developing countries (Sargeran et al. 2008). We made a research on that subject in Córdoba in an retrospective study of 89 clinical records of **OSCC** patients, followed in the Stomatology B Service and in the Oncology Unit of Hospital Nacional de Clínicas between 1989-2005, (Bolesina et al., 2007). Survival rates were related to age, gender, location, stage, risk factors and treatment; 74% of the patients were male, age range was 23-93, median age 60 years. The lowest survival rate was found between 61 and 70 years of age. After five years of **OSCC** diagnosis, the general survival rate reached 35—40 %. The most frequent cancer location was in the tongue (26%), followed by gum (23%) and floor of the mouth (11%). The highest mortality rate was due to tumors situated in the base of the tongue, gum and floor of the mouth, 100%, 88% and 85%, respectively. It was noted that 100% base of the tongue tumors , 90% gingiva and floor of the mouth tumors were discovered in advanced stages while 100% of lip tumors were diagnosed in early stages.

The observed survival rate in **OSCC** stage I was 75% whereas only 23% patients survived in stage IV. When all the variables were analysed and related to survival rates, a value of $p = 0.001$ was obtained for tumor stages (Fig. 7).

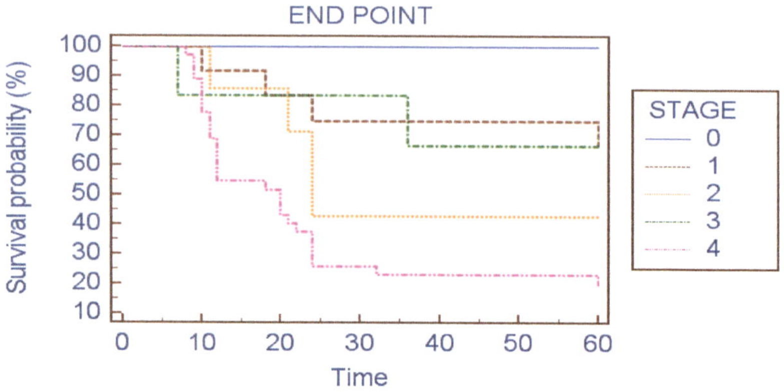

Fig. 7. Five year survival rates, according to **OSCC** stage at the moment of diagnosis

When surgery was the only treatment indicated, patient survival rate was 55%. When radiotherapy complemented surgery, the rate decreased to 33%, which is in good agreement with the literature (Sargeran et al., 2008).

As far as risk factors are concerned, it has to be pointed out that 49% of the patients were smokers and heavy drinkers; higher mortality rates were found specially in male patients having these habits compared to those with only one or none of them. The p value obtained for alcohol consumers and tobacco smokers was 0.04, see Fig 8.

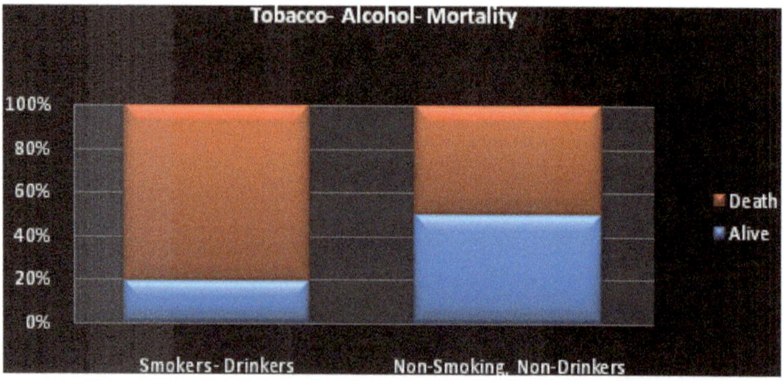

Fig. 8. Percentaje of patients who died before 5 years, related to risk factors

In our study, we did not have a significant enough sample of young patients to reach definitive conclusions. However, previous studies show that younger people have a considerably better five-year survival. Age is therefore a determining factor to good outcomes for OSCC patients (Warnakulasurilya et al. 2007). Although it is well known that tobacco smoking and alcohol consumption are the strongest risk factors for the development of head and neck cancer, little information is available concerning both the prognostic value of these habits and that of quitting them after diagnosis.

Non-smokers with early stage OSCC have a better prognosis than former or current smokers at the same stage (Vora et al., 2003), which agrees with the results obtained in our study.

Smoking cessation after diagnosis or starting OC therapy can improve survival rates. It is reported that head and neck cancer patients who admitted to continuing smoking during their radiotherapy treatment had a lower response and survival prospects than those who claimed to quit smoking prior to starting the treatment, with 2.5 RR (95% CI 1.4–4.4) (Browman et al., 1993). RR of recurrence of the disease among smokers (non drinkers) was 2.9 compared to non/ex-smokers and 3.8 for those smoking >2 packets a day (Stevens et al., 1983). In a retrospective study in Southern England, RR for multiple primary cancers was higher in those patients who continued smoking and drinking after therapy (Warnakulasuriya et al., 2003).

To sum up, these studies provide clear evidence that smoking cessation even after an oral cancer diagnosis improves prognostic outcomes. Oral cancer patients who were current drinkers showed higher mortality rates than former or non drinkers (Kowalski et al., 1994). Quitting drinking after diagnosis was also associated with improved survival outcomes, but the hazard ratios did not reach statistical significance.

The findings suggest that rising alcohol consumption since the 1950s is more closely related to increasing intra-oral cancer incidence and mortality than smoking, a fact that is more evident among younger males since the early 1970s (Hindle et al., 2000).

There are a myriad of risk factors that lead to OC, among them Human Papilloma Virus and other infections, chronic inflammations and social and environmental carcinogen conditions. These issues are the subject of continuous studies being carried on at present by several scientific teams.

5. Patient management

The decision about the adequate treatment for each patient should be made by an interdisciplinary committee of specialists in head and neck tumors. The choice of treatment largely depends on the site and stage of the disease and on the overall health status of the patient. Early stages of intraoral cancers are likely to be cured by surgery or radiation therapy. The election of the type of treatment is determined by the anticipated functional and cosmetic results and by the availability of the particular expertise required from the surgeon or radiation therapist for each patient. Advanced tumors (stages III and IV) are generally treated by surgery, followed by radiation therapy.

The treatment for head and neck cancers, especially those involving the oral cavity, has changed in the last 10–20 years. It is now widely accepted that for advanced OC tumors, surgery combined with radiation therapy has a better outcome than if only one of those modalities is used. Although the impact of neo-adjuvant chemoradiation may increase survival, it may also increase morbidity considerably.

It is worth mentioning that current advent of state-of-the-art technology applied to cancer treatments has significantly improved the quality of life of OC patients. However, there are only few data as to the length of survival in relation to new devices such as gamma rays, electrons, protons and atomic nuclei, tridimensional (3DR), stereotactic, Modulated Intensity Radiotherapy (MIR) and Image-Guided Radiation Therapy (IGRT). The new technology allows the professional to better adjust radiation to the tumor, thus diminishing the damage inflicted to the surrounding healthy tissues, especially major salivary glands and maxillaries. Brachytheraphy is a still used resource; it requires the isolation of the radiated patient and it should be carried out by highly experienced professionals.

In spite of all the above mentioned innovations, the occurrence of complications is high, which would inevitably delay the standard therapeutic protocols. This fact, in turn, would make patients prone to recurrence or to metastases.

5.1 More frequent oral complications

All treatments usually applied to deal with **OSCC** and also with head and neck cancers have a negative impact on the patients, especially on their oral cavity; several complications can arise due to direct damage to oral tissues or to indirect regional or systemic toxicity. What is more, dental care is regarded by many patients as a low priority in their treatment. Surprisingly, 90% of the treated patients were found to have dental diseases such as caries, periodontal diseases or sepsis (Toljanic et al., 2002). The factors that influence intensity and duration of oral damage are: the medical and nutritional status of the patient, tobacco and alcohol use, oral hygiene and dental status, previous surgical interventions, and the indicated radiation treatment.

5.1.1 Surgical risks and complications

Surgical management of intraoral lesions typically includes both the primary lesion and cervical lymph nodes. Ideally, surgery is selected when permanent control of the tumor is sought. The tumour staging is essential to determine whether only surgery is indicated or whether radiation or chemotherapy may be needed later.

The risks and sequels of surgery primarily depend on or develop from the extent of the tumor and its relationship to contiguous oral structures. Sequels may include disorders in speech and swallowing, pain, limitations in oral motor function; infections, enteral nutrition (e.g. tube feedings), facial, neck and shoulder malfunction, disturbances in mental health, fibrosis, cosmetic deficits and bone lesions.

During resection of oral cancers, teeth and their supporting bone are often removed. In order to achieve functional rehabilitation, it is necessary to replace missing elements. Some patients may require an intraoral prosthesis for obturation of a velopharyngeal deficit or to reshape and augment the contours of a resected hard palate. The work of a speech therapist is crucial in this venture (Vendrell & Ranking, 1999).

5.1.2 Potential oral manifestations of radiation therapy

Patients that receive radiation therapy in the oropharyngeal area for malignant tumors may undergo radiation therapy for 7 weeks with a dose going up to 7000cGy, depending on tumor type and location. Radiotherapy is associated with side effects that vary in intensity and duration and are dependent on several factors. Not all patients will experience all possible complications but they should be aware of the potential risks.

Acute and chronic complications in the short and long term have been studied by different authors; some complications are described below. Hyposalivation during the 1st week of radiation treatment amounts to 50-60% of the usual saliva flow. After a 7- week conventional treatment, it decreases to 20%.

Hyposalivation subjective symptom xerostomy implies several other symptoms like dysphagia, dysgeusia, dysosmia and speach difficulties (Jansma et al., 1989).

Xerostomy brings about a change in oral microflora and, as a result, cariogenic microorganisms *streptococos mutans y lactobacilos* prevail in the saliva, causing caries and periodontal diseases. The oral mucosa becomes soft, irritable and susceptible of fungal infections (candidiasis) and inflammations (Daly & Drane,1972; Hinds,1971).

Recently, preventive measures to decrease the effects of radiation induced xerostomy have been widely studied. To begin with, patients should give up tobacco, alcohol and spicy, too hot, too cold or too hard foods and replace them by soft and moist nutrients. Secondly, they should be advised to be well hydratated and to use saliva substitutes.

Salivary gland tissue does not recover from high doses of radiation. The quality and quantity of saliva is permanently changed. Taste loss and alterations may begin with the first 200-400 cGy. After three weeks of therapy, it takes 500-8,000 times normal concentrations of taste stimulant to elicit a normal taste response. Taste acuity levels usually return to normal within 2-12 months following completion of therapy, if adequate saliva is available (Jasma et al., 1989). Both mucositis and decreased salivary flow may contribute to taste alteration.

Mucositis: Oral mucositis is the inflammation that takes place in the oral epithelium as a result of antineoplastic treatments such as radiotherapy, chemotherapy or bone marrow transplant which are very frequent in these treatments for oncohematologic disease. Not only do the consequences of the inflammation affect the quality of life of the patient but it can also mean a limitation in the application of the treatment, as well as an increase in hospital length of stay and therapeutic costs.

Radiation-induced mucositis depends on the absorbed radiation dose, fractioning, delivery modality and soft tissue status. Other influential patient-related variables are age, sex, nutritional condition, oral microbiota, salivary flow and inflammation among others.

The study of the degrees of severity of oral mucositis has yielded different results coming from diverse research centers. This constitutes a major obstacle for the study of mucositis. The lack of a uniform systematic approach adopted for its evaluation by means of oral examination makes it difficult to assess its consequences.

The various existing scales to measure mucositis were analyzed by López Castaño et al., 2005; Stone et al., 2007; Sonis et al., 1999; World Health Organization, 1979 (see **Table 6**).

1	burning sensation and eritema
2	eritema, ulcers and possibility of solid food intake
3	ulcers, liquid diet
4	impossible feeding

Table 6. Mucositis WHO Classification

Oral Infections: Health care providers should be concerned about preventing oral local and systemic infections in addition to managing their symptoms. Treating infections as soon as they are detected will help to reduce pain, as well as control the spread of infection. A fungal, bacterial or viral culture is recommended if infection is suspected.

In patients undergoing head and neck radiotherapy, *Candida* colonization tends to increase during the course of the treatment and remains increased if xerostomia occurs (Epstein et al., 1998; Ramirez-Amador et al., 1997). Candidiasis can cause a burning or scalding sensation, can distort taste and may interfere with swallowing. Its spread to the esophagus or systemic dissemination is a serious consequence (Rankin & Jones, 1999). Other opportunistic fungal infection is Histoplasmosis.

Bacterial and viral infections are more common in neutropenic patients than in those affected by oral cancers. The detection and treatment of those infections represent a challenge to health professionals and should be the subject of a more extensive study.

Nutritional deficiency: It is caused by the effects of mucositis, xerostomy, hypogeusia, and loss of appetite that can make eating an unpleasant painful chore, quite apart from the psychological implications that such discomforts may have on the eating function. Symptoms may include rapid weight loss, dehydration, nutritional stomatitis, and secondary oral infection, specifically candidiasis (Rankin & Jones, 1999).

Caries: Even patients that have not suffered from dental caries for some time can develop them when submitted to radiotherapy. Those caries differ considerably in clinical appearance, development, and progression from dental caries in non-irradiated patients. Radiation has a pernicious effect on the teeth since it makes them prone to decalcification. Post-radiation lesions develop in a distinct manner with initial sheer fracture of enamel followed by rapid decay of the exposed underlying dentin (Jansma et al.,1993; Jongebloed et al., 1988). Such lesions are mainly developed when the flow of saliva diminishes or when its properties are altered (Brown et al., 1975; Carl & Schaff, 1974). Furthermore, post- radiation lesions tend to occur at gingival margins, cusp tips, and incisal surfaces in contrast to typical caries, which develop in pits, fissures and proximal areas.

There are three kinds of radiation- related carious lesions:

First type: the lesion superficially covers the cervical tooth area, slowly progressing inwards until it often provokes the crown total destruction. This is less frequent in the molars, although the caries tend to appear on the surfaces of the whole molar area.

The second type of lesion is a generalized superficial defect that first affects the buccal and later the lingual or palatal surfaces of the tooth crowns. The proximal surfaces are less affected.This lesion often begins as a diffuse, punctate defect and then progresses to generalized, irregular erosion of the tooth surfaces. In this type of lesion, decay localized at the incisal or occlusal edges is often observed. The result is a destruction of the coronal enamel and dentin, especially on the buccal and palatal surfaces.

Third type: the lesion extends as a heavy brown-black discoloration over the whole set of tooth crown together with a marked wear of the oclusal and incisal sides (Vissink et al., 2003).The areas just below the contact points seem to be the last areas to be affected by radiation caries.

Trismus and / or fibrosis: Spasms and/or fibrosis of the masticatory muscles and temporomandibular joint (TMJ) capsule, usually occurs 3-6 months after radiation therapy, with unpredictable frequency and severity. It is worsened by some surgical resections (Rankin & Jones, 1999).

Limited opening may interfere with oral hygiene, dietary intake, use of prostheses and restricted access to dental care and general anesthesia (Barker et al., 1996).

It is often observed that floor of the mouth and neck fibrosis bears a relation with individual predisposing factors, among which peripheric circulatory disorders can be mentioned.

Soft tissue necrosis/osteoradionecrosis (ORN): Soft tissue and bone necrosis may develop because tissues within the field of radiation become hypovascular, hypoxic and hypocellular. The threat of this sequel persists indefinitely, although the risk is minimal when the total dose of radiation is < 5000 cGy.

The effects of radiation on bone, periosteum, connective tissue, and vascular epithelium generally develop over time and include suppressed osteoblastic activity, decreased cell numbers, disorganization of bone remodelling, hypovascularity and increased fibrosis. Smaller blood vessels are more sensitive than large vessels. Initially, there is a periarteritis and endarteritis that progress to fibrosis and loss of endothelium. This results in the narrowing and possible obliteration of the lumen, reducing the blood supply to all tissues within the radiation field.

Factors that may contribute to an increased risk of necrosis include compromised vascularity from previous surgery, poor nutritional or health status, uncontrolled diabetes and heavy tobacco or alcohol use. Trauma may result from tooth extraction, invasive periodontal procedures and intraoral prosthetic appliances. The necrosis process may take place spontaneously or result from trauma, leading to non-healing soft tissue, bone lesions, and necrosis. The mandible is much more susceptible to ORN than the maxilla. The incidence of ORN is twice as high in dentate patients as it is among edentulous patients.

Clinical manifestations of ORN may include pain, orofacial fistulas, exposed necrotic bone, pathologic fracture and suppuration (Barker et al., 1996).

The management of patients with ORN depends on the severity of the necrosis which may be controlled by local irrigation, antibiotic treatment, local sequestrectomy or wide segmental excision with or without reconstruction. Hyperbaric oxygen therapy is considered an adjunctive treatment for ORN, often used in conjunction with surgery, and has been associated with better success rates than surgery alone (Aitasalo et al., 1995; McKenzie et al., 1993).

5.2 Oral and dental management

5.2.1 Pre oncologic treatment oral preparation

With the increasing trend in outpatient management, including cancer therapies, every health care professional is a potential and integral part of the cancer treatment team that once existed solely within the hospital environment. To provide optimal therapy, a functional, communicative, interactive team is critical to the successful management and outcome of the cancer patient. This includes the evaluation and treatment planning considering the overall patient health, tumor site, stage and tumor biologic status and patient´s cultural/socioeconomic status. Dentists, as part of a multidisciplinary team, have an active role before, during and after the treatment (Shaw, 1997).

The aims of oral care programs for **OC** patients are:

- to improve oral function and quality of life.
- to improve and keep oral hygiene so as to reduce risk and severity of oral complications.
- to eliminate oral infections and avoid tooth originated systemic ones.
- to prevent, eliminate or control oropharyngeal pain.
- to prevent or control salivary gland dysfunctions and tooth destruction.
- to prevent or reduce the incidence of bone necrosis.

The first step of the treatment should be a panoramic X-Ray in order to have a global vision. If tooth extractions are necessary for non-restorable or doubtful prognosis teeth (see criteria in Table 7), they should be made 15-20 days before radiation treatment and 5-10 days before chemotherapy.

Caries (nonrestorable).
Active periapical disease (symptomatic teeth).
Moderate to severe periodontal disease (with mobility grade 2 and 3).
Furcation lesions of grade II and III, periodontal pocket $\leq$ 4 mm).
Endo-periodontal processes.
Lack of opposing teeth, compromised hygiene.
Extensive periapical lesions (if not chronic or well localized).
Partial impaction or incomplete eruption.

Table 7. Criteria for pre-radiotherapy extractions

Before starting radiotherapy, tissues must be healthy without tearing or leaks either in the oral mucosa or in the alveolar bones. Besides, endodontic treatment of deeply decayed teeth must be carried out, glass ionomer and resins must be used for cavity obturation, metallic reconstructions must be avoided, planing and polishing of the dental and prosthetic sharp cusps must be performed. There must be a tight control of microflora and of oral hygiene techniques. Fluoride tooth paste and adequate prothesis disinfection are highly advisable.

5.2.2 During radiotherapy treatment

A weekly check up by the interdisciplinary team will allow the professionals involved to detect early lesions and to make sure that the patient follows all preventive indications.

Good results were obtained when a preventive program including mechanical and chemical biofilm control was put into practice.

5.2.3 After a radiotherapy treatment

Very strict oral hygiene as well as frequent visits to the dentist are mandatory to prevent infections and caries formation since extractions are highly unadvisable due to impending ORN risk.

It has become essential to implement specific training courses dealing with OC patient care, which should be progressively included in the grade curricula.

6. Psychological aspects of patient care

Oral cancer is a complex health problem that deeply affects the life of the patient since it involves vital body areas related to communication and emotions. Comparatively, it is even more disturbing than general cancer since head and neck cancer is clearly related to functional speech and swallowing problems; therefore, OC patients are among the most distressed sufferers.

We will point out here some of the characteristics of the patients given the painful experience they have to go through.

6.1 Patient´s previous history

6.1.1 Alexithymia

It refers to a specific disturbance in psychic functioning characterized by difficulties in the capacity to verbalize affections and to elaborate fantasies. **OSCC** leads the patient to a forced mutism sometimes preceded by poor verbal communication. Although initially described in the context of psychosomatic illnesses, alexithymic characteristics may be observed in patients with a wide range of medical and psychiatric disorders (Sifneos, Nemiah, 1973, cited by Marty, 1995).

6.1.2 Traumatic episodes

The existence of events that greatly disturbed the patients' emotional lives may be interpreted as cumulative trauma. The clinical records of such patients reveal episodes of labour dissatisfaction, overadjustment to extreme labour conditions, submission, unquestioned acceptance of social position, tragic loss of close relatives, change of roles or loss of working status.

6.1.3 Vulnerability

OSCC patients are vulnerable since the lesion is associated with unhealthy habits like alcoholism and tobacco addiction. Such habits are sometimes disruptive behaviours that appear as a consequence of unresolved affective problems. Bodily vulnerability (Zukerfeld, R. 1999, 2005) is defined as the possibility of either dysfunctional somatic behaviours and reactions to adverse, stressing factors or to cumulative trauma.

6.2 Emotional state during treatment

Treatment shocks the **OC** patients in a global way, affecting their quality of life. They have to process a great deal of endogenous and exogenous stimuli. When the treatment is indicated, the first struggle is required: the patients have to adapt to a new routine, thus altering their usual habits; they have to accept new schedules and new premises even when they are far removed from their usual places of residence. The newly established routine increases the patients´ dependence since they need the care and attention of other persons as well as having to take care of themselves. Side effects produced by irradiation in the oral cavity make tasting, chewing and swallowing difficult. These impairments lead to loss of appetite and loss of weight, all of which tend to unbalance their emotional state. Gaining weight becomes a major worry for the patients and their families. In some cases, the restrained, underlying anguish that has dominated the patient´s life finds a way out in the disease itself. That chronic state of dejection has been described in systemic patients as hidden depression, devoid of complaints or whining (Marty, 1966).

6.3 Interdisciplinary approach

In 2010, a partly structured, written survey was carried out. It was addressed to individual patients and to those acting as their companions who attended the Oncology Service at Hospital Nacional de Clínicas with the aim of finding out their opinion about the interdisciplinary care they were receiving. They were questioned about: Overall service performance (favourable or unfavourable), presence of several health professionals during consultation, patient´s suggestions to improve the service, optional therapies they would like to receive. The interviewed patients had been in contact with the service for a minimum of 3 months and a maximum of 6 years. Results: 53% of interviewed were male; 59% were smokers, 41% drank alcohol, 42% consumed both alcohol and tobacco. The 88% were satisfied, using the option "favourable" to describe their opinion about the service. They regarded the presence of dentists and psychologists in the team as very valuable; 71% declared they ignored the profession of the people present at consultation and 59 % stated they preferred to be seen by several professionals. Concerning the medical services they would like to be offered, their preference rates were: social work (25%), physiotheraphy and language theraphy (18% each one) and personalized psychotherapy 12%. The following conclusions were drawn from the aforementioned results: the interdisciplinary team appears as a recommended approach for **OC** patients, not only because it focuses the disease comprehensively but also because the patients themselves expressed a positive point of view in its regard. Although the interdisciplinary approach to cancer patients is established in health systems, it is important to know how good this model works from the patient´s viewpoint.

- The dynamics of consultation is mainly based on a unilateral information medical request, being the patient´s role fairly secondary. Most patients did not know the specialty of the professionals present at consultation.

The patient plays a leading role both in defining and privileging his health problems and in accepting or refusing the possible solutions. Helping the patient to become active and to regain control of his own life is a desirable aim in every medical case. However, when dealing with **OC** patients, this goal acquires a special dimension.

6.4 The role of the psychologist

Psycho oncology conceives cancer as a symptom of an illness comprising myriads of factors both at its starting point, during its course and in its recovery stage (Middleton, 2002). As a field of knowledge, psycho oncology goes beyond the limits of disciplinary knowledge. The role of the psychologist in the **OC** team may be summarized as follows:

- Pave the way for a more interactive consultation by stimulating the patient´s participation in such a way that communication can flow more easily among patient, relatives and medical team.
- Ask for and provide information.
- Bring into consultation aspects related with the patient´s lifestyle : food, sleeping habits, leisure time, side effects of the treatment.
- Lower the patient´s depersonalization caused by their illness and its demanding attention.
- Propose the patient to make a critical reflection about the association between his lifestyle and his illness.
- Assign due importance to the role of their companions and to their supporting net of relations. Encourage, support, challenge the patient and their family.
- Contribute to install the idea that the illness should be perceived as a meaningful experience, as a chance for reflection and change.
- Understand the incidence of psycho social factors during the course of the illness.

As a member of the medical team dealing with OC patients, the psycho oncologist acts as a catalyst. His presence helps the patients´ psychological state, which may contribute to a better understanding of their reality.

7. Conclusion

OSCC has a bad prognosis and survival time is short in spite of the technological advances applied to treatments.

Most patients, disregarding the initial symptoms, go to consultation at advanced **OSCC** stages. Pre-malignant lesions may appear 10 years before the initial **OSCC** manifestations. Although the carcinoma may be preventable through treatment of pre-cancerous lesions, many dentists and family physicians are not performing the opportunistic oral cavity exams. Oral cavity cancers can be detected easily with a simple oral examination, but compared to cancers that involve more elaborate screening tests (i.e., breast, prostate and colon), the rate of early diagnosis has not improved over time.

OSCC is related to preventable risk factors. Therefore, we strongly advocate that doctors should discourage all their patients from smoking and drinking excessively. Furthermore, intensive public promotion and educational campaigns are imperative to increase patient awareness.

Dental professionals have an important role both in primary prevention of oral cancer -by inducing healthy life styles- and in secondary prevention by detecting oral cancer or its precursor lesions at early stages.

8. Acknowledgment

We want to express our gratitude to our teachers Dr Hector Lanfranchi, Dr Julio Diaz and Dr David Grinspan, and to all B Stomatology Service members for their unfailing support and cooperation.

Our thanks to Julia for her work as translator and proof-reader.

We thank the Science and Technology Secretary (SeCyT) and the National University of Cordoba (UNC) for their financial support.

9. References

Aitasalo, K., Grenman, R., Virolaine, E., Niinikoski, J. & Klossner, J. (1995). A modified protocol to treat early osteoradionecrosis of the mandible. *Undersea Hyperb Med,* Vol 22, No2, pp.(161–70), ISSN: 1066-2936

Allison, P., Franco, E. & Feine, J. (1998). Predictors of professional diagnostic delay for upper aerodigestive tract carcinoma. *Oral Oncol,* Vol 34, pp. (127–32). ISSN: 1368-8375

Barker, G., Barker, B. & Gier, R. (1996). Oral management of the cancer patient: A guide for the health professional. Kansas City, MO: University of Missouri - Kansas City.

Bellm, L., Epstein J., Rose-Ped, A., Aitasalo, K., Grenman, R., Virolaine, E., Niinikoski, J. & Klossner, J. (1995). A modified protocol to treat early osteoradionecrosis of the mandible. *Undersea Hyperb Med* 1995; Vol 22, No2, pp. (161–70). ISSN: 1066-2936

Bolesina, N., Morelatto, R., Belardinelli, P., Fernández, E., Herrera, G., López de Blanc, S. (2007) http://iadr.confex.com/iadr/arg07/preliminaryprogram/abstract_114584.htm, ISSN: 0022-0345

Boring, C., Squires, T. & Tong, T. (1994). Cancer Statistics. *Cancer J Clin,* Vol 44, pp. (7-26). ISSN: 1432-1335

Boyle, P., Autier, P. & Bartelink, H. et al. (2003). European code against cancer and scientific justification: third version. *Ann Oncol,* Vol. 14, No7, pp. (973–1005). ISSN: 0923-7534

Boudewijn, J., Braakhuis, A., Otto Visser, C. & René Leemans, A. (2009). Oral and oropharyngeal cancer in The Netherlands between 1989 and 2006: Increasing incidence, but not in young adults. *Oral Oncol,* Vol 45, No e85, pp. (89-87). ISSN: 1368-8375

Brandizzi, D., Gandolfo, M., Velazco, M., Cabrini, R. & Lanfranchi, H. (2008). Clinical features and evolution of oral cancer: A study of 274 cases in Buenos Aires, Argentina. *Med Oral Patol Oral Cir Bucal,* Vol Sep1, No13 (9), pp.(E544-8), ISSN 1698-6946.

Brohua, X., Tromp, D., Horijk, G., Winnubst, J. & De Leew, R. (2005). Role of alcohol and smoking in diagnostic delay of head and neck cancer patients. *Acta Otolaryngol ,* Vol. 125, No. 5, (May), pp. (552-556). ISSN: 0001-6489

Brohua, X., Tromp, D., Koole, R., Hordijk, G., Winnbust, J. & De Leeuw, J. (2007). Professional delay in head and neck cancer patients: analysis of the diagnostic pathway. *Oral Oncol,* Vol.43, pp. (551-556). ISSN: 1368-8375

Browman, G., Wong, G., Hodson, I., Sathya J., Russell, R. & McAlpine, L., et al. (1993) Influence of cigarette smoking on the efficacy of radiation therapy in head and neck cancer. *New Eng J Med.* Vol.328, pp. (159–163). ISSN: 0028-4793

Brown, L., Dreizen, S. & Handler, S., et al. (1975). The Effects of Radiation Induced Xerostomia on Human Oral Microflora. *J Dent Res,*Vol. 54, No. 4, pp. (740-750). ISSN: 0022-0345

Carl W. & Schaff N. (1974). Dental Care for the Cancer Patient. *J Surg Oncol,* Vol. 6, No. 4, pp. (293-310). ISSN: 1096-9098

Chandu A., G. Adams, A. C. H. Smith. (2005). Factors affecting survival in patients with oral cancer: an Australian perspective. *Int. J. Oral Maxillofac. Surg.*, Vol. 34, pp. (514–520). ISSN: 0901-5027

Daly, T. & Drane, J. (1972). Management of Dental Problems in Irradiated Patients. University of Texas Press, Houston, Texas.

Dimitroulis, G., Reade, P. & Wiesenfeld, D. (1992). Referral patterns of patients with oral squamous cell carcinoma, Australia. *Eur J Cancer B Oral Oncol*, Vol 28B, pp. (23–7). ISSN: 0964-1955

Elwood, J. & Gallagher, R. (1985). Factors influencing early diagnosis of cancer of the oral cavity. *CMAJ*, Vol 133, pp. (651–6). ISSN: 1488-2329

Epstein, J., Chin, E., Jacobson, J., Rishiraj, B. & Le N. (1998). The relationship among fluoride, cariogenic oral flora, and salivary flow rate during radiation therapy. *Oral Surg Oral Med Oral Pathol Oral Radiol Endod;* Vol. 86, No. 3, pp. (286–292). ISSN: 1079-2104

Ferlay, J., Shin, H., Bray, F., Forman, D., Mathers, C. & Parkin, D. (2010). Estimates of worldwide burden of cancer in 2008: GLOBOCAN 2008. *International Journal of Cancer*, 127, 12, 15 (Dec 2010), pp. (2893–2917). ISSN: 1097-0215

Gao, W. & Guo, C. (2009). Factors related to delay in diagnosis of oral squamous cell carcinoma. *J Oral Maxillofac Surg*, Vol 67, pp. (1015-1020). ISSN 0278-2391

Gorsky, M. & Dayan, D. (1995). Referral delay in diagnosis of oro/oropharyngeal cancer in Israel. *Eur J Cancer B Oral Oncol*, Vol 31B, pp. (166–8). ISSN: 0964-1955

Grinspan, D. (1983). Enfermedades de la Boca. Tomo V. Editorial Mundi S.A.I.C.y F., ISBN: 950-545-010-9, Buenos Aires Argentina.

Hindle, M., Downer, D., Moles D. & Speight P. (2000). Is alcohol responsible for more intra-oral cancer? *Oral Oncol* Vol 36, pp. (328-333). ISSN: 1368-8375

Hinds E. (1971). Dental Care and Oral Hygiene Before and After Treatment. Radiation Caries. *J Am. Med Assoc*, Vol 215, pp. (964-6). ISSN: 1538-3598.

Humphris, G., Freeman R. & Clarke H. (2004). Risk perception of oral cancer in smokers attending primary care: a randomized controlled trial. *Oral Oncol.* Vol. 40, No. 9, pp. (916-924). ISSN: 1368-8375

Jansma, J., Vissink, A., Gravenmade, E., Visch L., Fidler V. & Retief D. (1989). In vivo study on the prevention of post-radiation caries. *Caries Res*, Vol 23, pp. (172-178). ISSN: 0008-6568

Jansma, J., Vissink, A. & Jongebloed, W., Retief, D., Johannes's-Gravenmade, E. (1993). Natural and induced radiation caries: a SEM study. *Am J Dent*, No. 6, pp. 130–136. ISSN: 0894-8275

Jongebloed, W., Gravenmade, E. & Retief, D. (1988). Radiation caries. A review and SEM study. *Am J Dent* Vol. 1, pp. (139–146).ISSN: 0894-8275

Jovanovic, A., Kostense, P., Schulten, E., Snow G. & Van Der Waal, I. (1992). Delay in diagnosis of oral squamous cell carcinoma; a report from the Netherlands. *Eur J Cancer B Oral Oncol*, 28B, pp. (37–8). ISSN: 0964-1955

Jovanovic, A., Schulten, E. & Kostense, P. et al. (1993). Tobacco and alcohol related to the anatomical site of oral squamous cell carcinoma. *J Oral Pathol Med*, Vol 22, pp. (459-462). ISSN: 0904-2512

Kerdpon, D. & Sriplung, H. (2001).Factors related to delay in delay in diagnosis of oral squamous cell carcinoma in southern Thailand. *Oral Oncol*, Vol. 37, No. 2, (Feb), pp. (127-31). ISSN: 1368-8375

Khoo, S., Shanmuhasuntharam, P., Mahadzir, W., Tay, K., Latif, A. & Nair, S. (1998). Factors involved in the diagnosis of oral squamous cell carcinoma in Malaysia. *Asia Pac J Public Health*, Vol 10, pp. (49–51). ISSN: 1010-5395 .

Kowalski, L., Franco, E. & Torloni, H., et al. (1994). Lateness of diagnosis of oral and oropharyngeal carcinoma: factors related to the tumour, the patient and health professionals. *Eur J Cancer B Oral Oncol.*; No. 30B, pp: (167-173). ISSN: 0964-1955

Kowalski, L. & Carvalho, A. (2001). Influence of time delay and clinical upstaging in the prognosis of head and neck cancer. *Oral Oncol* , Vol. 37, No. 1, pp. (94-98). ISSN: 1368-8375

Liu, L., Kumar S., Sedghizadeh P., Jayacar A., & Shuler C. (2008). Oral squamous cell carcinoma incidence by subsite among diverse racial and ethnic populations in California. *Oral Surg Oral Med Oral Pathol Oral Radiol Endod*, Vol 105, pp.470-80. ISSN:1079-2104

López Castaño, F., Oñate Sánchez, R., Roldán Chicano, R. & Cabrerizo Merino, M. (2005). Revisión Measurement of secondary mucositis to oncohematologic treatment by means of different scale. *Med Oral Patol Oral Cir Bucal*, Vol.10, pp. (412-21). ISSN: 1698-4447.

Marty, P. (1995). *La psicosomática del adulto,* 2do Edición, Amorrortu, ISBN: 950-518-523-5, Buenos Aires.

Mashberg, A., Merletti, F., Boffetta, P., Gandolfo, S., Ozzello, F., Fracchia, F. & Terracini, B. (1989). Appearance, site of occurrence, and physical and clinical characteristics of oral carcinoma in Torino, Italy. *Cancer*, Vol 63, pp. (2522–7). ISSN: 1097-0142.

McKenzie, M., Wong, F., Epstein, J. & Lepawsky, M. (1993). Hyperbaric oxygen and postradiation osteonecrosis of the mandible. *Eur J Cancer B Oral Oncol*, Vol 29B, No 3, pp. (201–7). ISSN: 0964-1955.

Middleton, J. (2002). Psico-oncología en el siglo XXI, en *Revista Actualidad Psicológica N° 298, Clínica de Pacientes con cáncer,* pp. (30-32). ISSN 0325-2590

Morelatto, R., Herrera, M., Fernández, E., Corball A., López de Blanc S. (2007). Diagnostic delay of oral squamous cell carcinoma in two diagnosis centers in Córdoba Argentina. *J Oral Pathol* , 36 (7) pp (405-08). ISSN: 0904-2512.

Neville, B., Damm, D. & Allen, C. et al. (2002). *Oral & Maxillofacial Pathology*. 2nd ed. Phila., PA: Saunders, pp. (337-369).

Neville, B. & Day, T. (2002). Oral cancer and precancerous lesions. *CA – A Cancer J Clin*, No 52, pp. (195–215). ISSN: 1542-4863

Olmos, M. 2010, Evaluación de un servicio público de atención de cáncer de cabeza y cuello. 5to Congreso Multidisciplinario de Salud Comunitaria del Mercosur, San Luis, Argentina, set. 2010.

Onizawa, K., Nishihara, K., Yamagata, K., Yusa, H., Yanagawa, T. & Yoshida, H. (2003). Factors associated with diagnostic delay of oral squamous cell carcinoma. *Oral Oncol*, Vol 39, pp. (781–8). ISSN: 1368-8375

O'Sullivan E. (2001). Some insights into the potential for the earlier detection of oral cancer: A population-based study. In: Seventh International Congress on Oral Cancer, April 2001, The Hague, Netherlands. *Oral Oncol*, Vol 37, pp. (553). ISSN: 1368-8375

Parkin, D., Bray, F., Ferlay, J. & Pisani, P. (2005). Global cancer statistics, 2002. *CA-A Cancer J Clin*, Vol.55, pp. (74–108). ISSN: 1542-4863

Pinholt, E., Rindum, J. & Pindborg, J. (1997). Oral cancer: a retrospective study of 100 Danish cases. *Br J Oral Maxillofac Surg*, Vol. 35, pp. (77–80). ISSN: 0266-4356

Pitiphat, W., Diehl, S., Laskaris, G., Carstsos, V., Douglass, C. & Zavras, A. (2002). Factors associated with delay in the diagnosis of oral cancer. *J Dent Res*, Vol. 81, pp. (192–197). ISSN: 0022-0345

Ramirez-Amador, V., Silverman, S. Jr, Mayer, P., Tyler, M. & Quivey, J. (1997). Candidal colonization and oral candidiasis in patients undergoing oral and pharyngeal radiation therapy. *Oral Surg Oral Med Oral Path Oral Radiol Endod;* Vol. 84, No. 2, pp. (149–153). ISSN: 1079-2104.

Robledo, G., Belardinelli, P., Herrera, C., Criscuolo, I., López de Blanc, S. (2008). Level of Public Awareness about Oral Cancer in Cordoba, Argentina. *Rev Claves en Odontología 2008*, Vol. 15, N° 61: pp. (23-30). ISSN: 1666-0706.

Rogers, S., Pabla, R., Mc Sorley, A. Lowe, D., Brown, J. & Vaughan, E. (2007). An assessment of deprivation as a factor in the delay presentation, diagnosis and treatment in patients with oral and oropharyngeal squamous cell carcinoma. *Oral Oncol*, Vol. 43, pp. (649). ISSN: 1368-8375

Sargeran, K., Murtomaa, H., Safavi, SM., Vehkalahti, MM., Teronen, O. (2008). Survival after diagnosis of cancer of the oral cavity. *Br J Oral Maxillofac Surg*, Vol. 46, 3, pp. (187–191). ISSN:0266-4356.

Scully C. and Felix D. (2006). Oral Medicine —Update for the dental practitioner Oral cáncer. *Br Dent J*, Vol. 200, N 1, pp 13-17. ISSN: 007-0610

Schávelszon, J. 2002. La psico-oncología en el tratamiento del cáncer, en *Revista Actualidad Psicológica. N° 298*, Clínica de Pacientes con cáncer, 9-11. ISSN: 0325-2590, Buenos Aires.

Shah, J., Candela, F. & Poddar, A. (1990). The patterns of cervical lymph node metastasis from squamous carcinoma of the oral cavity. *Cancer,* Vol 66, pp. (109-113). ISSN: 1097-0142

Shah, J. & Lydiatt, W. (1995). Treatment of cancer of the head and neck. *CA Cancer J Clin*, No. 45, pp. (352–368). ISSN: 1542-4863

Shaw H. (1997). The British Association of Head and Neck Oncologists within the wider perspectives of the USA and Europe. *Ann R Coll Surg Engl*, Vol May, No 79 (3 Suppl), pp. (111-4). ISSN: 0035-8843

Silverman, S. Jr, Dillon, W. & Fischbein, N. (1998). Diagnosis In: Silverman S. Jr ed. Oral Cancer. 4th ed. Hamilton, Ontario, Canada: BC Decker Inc, pp. (41-66).

Soderholm A. (1990). Oral carcinoma of the mandibular region. *Br J Oral Maxillofac Surg*, Vol 28, pp. (383–9). ISSN: 0266-4356

Sonis, S., Eilers, J., Epstein J., LeVeque, F., Liggett, W. Jr. & Mulagha, M.T., et al. (1999). Validation of a new scoring system for the assessment of clinical trial research of oral mucositis induced by radiation or chemotherapy. *Mucositis Study Group. Cancer* No. 85, pp. 2103-2113.

Stevens M.H., Gardner J.W., Parkin J.L. & Johnson L.P. (1983). Head and neck cancer survival and life-style change. *Arch Otolaryngol.* No.109, pp. 476–479. ISSN: 0886-4470

Stone R., Potting C.M.J., Clare S., Uhlenhopp M., Davies M., Mank A. & Quinn B. (2007). Management of oral mucositis at European transplantation centers. *European Journal of Oncology Nursing*, Vol 11, pp. S3-S9. ISSN: 1462-3889

Stone, R., Potting, C., Clare, S., Uhlenhopp, M., Davies, M., Mank, A. & Quinn, B. (2007). Management of oral mucositis at European transplantation centres. *European Journal of Oncology Nursing*, Vol 11, pp. (S3-S9). ISSN: *1462-3889*

Sznajder, A., 2006 *Posgrado en Salud Social y Comunitaria- Programa Médicos Comunitarios- Módulo 8 Trabajo en Equipo en Salud-* Plan Federal de Salud- Ministerio de Salud y Ambiente de la Nación Argentina, ISBN 950-38-0035-8. Buenos Aires.

Toljanic J., Heshmati R. & Bedard J. (2002). Dental follow-up compliance in a population of irradiated head and neck cancer patients. *Oral Surg Oral Med Oral Pathol Oral Radiol & Endod*, Vol 93, No 1, pp. 35-8. ISSN: 1079-2104.

Tromp D., Brouha X., Hordijk G., Winnubst J. & De Leeuw R. (2005). Patient and tumor factors associated with advanced carcinomas of the head and neck. *Oral Oncol*, Vol 41, pp. 313–9. ISSN: 1368-8375

Vendrell Rankin K. & Daniel L. (1999). Oral Health in cancer Therapy. A guide for health care professionals, Texas Cancer Council.

Vissink A., Jansma J., Spijkervet F., Burlage F. & Coppes R. (2003). Oral sequelae of head and neck radiotherapy. *Crit Rev Oral Biol Med,*Vol 14, pp. 199–212. ISSN: 1045-4411

Vora H., Shah N., Patel D., Trivedi T. & Chikhlikar P. (2003). Prognostic significance of biomarkers in squamous cell carcinoma of the tongue: multivariate analysis. *J Surg Oncol.* No. 82, pp. 34–50. ISSN: 1096-9098.

Walker, M., Williams K. & Wichman B. (2008). Post-radiation dental index: development and reliability. *Support Care Cancer* No. 16, pp. 525–530. ISSN: 1433-7339

Warnakulasuriya, K., Robinson, D. & Evans, H. (2003). Multiple primary tumours following head and neck cancer in southern England during 1961–1998. *J Oral Pathol Med.* No. 32, pp. 443–449. ISSN: 0904-2512

Warnakulasuriya, S., Mak, V, Moller, H. (2007) Oral cancer survival in young people in South East England. *Oral Oncol,* 43 pp982-986. *ISSN: 1368-8375*

West, R., Alkhatib, M., McNeill, A. & Bedi, R. (2006). Awareness of mouth cancer in Great Britain. *Br Dent J* No.,200, pp. 167–169. ISSN: 0007-0610.

Wildt, J., Bundgaard, T. & Bentzen, S. (1995). Delay in the diagnosis of oral squamous cell carcinoma. *Clin Otolaryngol Allied Sci*, Vol 20, pp. 21–5. ISSN: 0307-7772

World Health Organization. (1979). Handbook for reporting results of cancer treatment. WHO Offset Publications. Vol. 48. World Health Organization, Geneva, Switzerland, pp. 15-22.

Zukerfeld, R.-Zukerfeld, R. (1999). *Psicoanálisis tercera tópica y vulnerabilidad somática,* Lugar Editorial, ISBN 959-892-077-7, Buenos Aires.

Zukerfeld, R.-Zukerfeld, R. (2005). *Procesos Terciarios, de la vulnerabilidad a la resiliencia,* Lugar Editorial, ISBN 950-892-245-1, Buenos Aires.

4

Oral Cancer and Potentially Cancerous Lesions – Early Detection and Diagnosis

C. S. Farah[1,2], P. J. Ford[1,2], K. Allen[1,2], A. Vu[1,2] and M. J. McCullough[3]
[1]*The University of Queensland, School of Dentistry, Brisbane*
[2]*The University of Queensland, UQ Centre for Clinical Research, Herston*
[3]*The University of Melbourne, Melbourne Dental School, Melbourne*
Australia

1. Introduction

Cancer of the oral cavity, also known as "oral cavity cancer" or more simply "oral cancer", affects the tongue, gingiva, floor of mouth, palate, tonsils and oropharynx.[1, 2] However, the most common form of oral cancer, oral squamous cell carcinoma (OSCC), can affect any tissue lined with oral mucosal epithelium.[2, 3] Oral cancer is one of the most common malignancies in the world, ranking eighth and thirteenth for males and females respectively.[1] Typically, patients with this cancer are over 40 years of age, although younger patients with regular exposure to risk factors associated with oral cancer can also present with potentially malignant and malignant oral mucosal lesions.[1, 3] Known aetiological risk factors include tobacco, betel quid, alcohol, and micronutrient deficiency.[1, 3, 4] Avoidance of these will reduce the probability of normal cells transforming to malignant cells.[4] In some cases though - namely, oral cancer in women under 45 years of age, tobacco use and alcohol consumption do not appear to play a role.[1] Instead, recent studies have suggested human papillomavirus (HPV) as a possible causative factor in cancers of the base of tongue, tonsils and oropharynx.[1, 2, 4]

Early detection of potentially malignant oral lesions (PMOLs) is important for improving the probability of complete recovery, since the stage of malignancy at the time of diagnosis influences morbidity and mortality.[1, 3, 5, 6] In most countries, the five-year survival rate is about 50% but can be as low as 15% if the cancer has spread to the lymphatic circulation.[1, 6] Unfortunately, more than 60% of patients present with stage III and IV oral cancer.[5] It is therefore important for all clinicians to recognize potentially malignant changes in oral mucosa and early-stage oral cancer in a visual and tactile examination, even though PMOLs may not become malignant.[1] In fact, only a small percentage of dysplastic lesions, and even fewer non-dysplastic lesions, undergo malignant transformation.[1, 3] PMOLs can be asymptomatic patches of white, red or speckled red-white,[1-3] with sharp or distinct borders and surface irregularity.[2] When these patches cannot clinically be characterised as any other condition, they are termed leukoplakia, erythroplakia and erythro-leukoplakia (speckled erythroplakia) respectively.[1] The most common PMOL is leukoplakia, although erythroplakia and erythro-leukoplakia have a higher likelihood of becoming malignant.[1-3] If undetected, they may turn into invasive cancer by growing or enlarging, causing tissue destruction, induration, and fixation to deeper structures.[2, 3] Pain, dysesthesia, paraesthesia, loss of function, dysphagia, dysarthria, odynophagia, tooth mobility and cervical lymphadenopathy may also be present in invasive oral cancer.[2, 3] Hence, it is clearly important to detect potentially malignant oral mucosal lesions early.

Although many new technologies exist for helping clinicians detect lesions at an earlier stage, delay in detection still occurs, and this can be both patient and practitioner mediated, with patient delay contributing to the greatest proportion of total delay time. By targeting this delay, there is potential to detect lesions at an earlier stage, thus improving survival rates.

Screening programs serve to detect disease and allow for early intervention. In the case of oral cancer, early recognition and subsequent treatment of potentially malignant and malignant lesions is the key to improving 5 year survival rates.[7] Despite the fact that early detection and treatment increase survival rates and decrease morbidity, over the past few decades the 5-year survival rate has not significantly improved.[8] Despite the oral cavity being accessible to visual inspection, most cancers are diagnosed at a late stage of disease which can negatively impact prognosis.[9-12] Not only is survival compromised, but there is greater possibility for disfigurement and functional disturbances that can adversely affect the patient's quality of life post treatment.[13, 14] Diagnosis of oral cancer at an early asymptomatic stage is rare, with most patients seeking help only after the onset of symptoms.[9]

Delay in detection can be attributed to both the patient and practitioner and the key to improving survival rates is reduction of this delay. Patient delay is defined as the time between the patient's recognition of symptoms and their first consultation with a healthcare provider.[8] It is commonly recognized that patient delay constitutes the largest proportion of total delay time, although the amount varies between studies.[8, 10, 12, 15-20] Reasons for patient delay have been hypothesized and explored, however findings have been inconsistent. This may be in part due to differences in the population under study, study design or recall bias. Professional delay has been described as the time between a patient's initial consultation with a healthcare worker to the time of definitive diagnosis.[8] It has been proposed that only about 1 in every 63,000 patient visits will yield a positive tumour screen. This inherent rarity of detection may place the practitioner at a decreased vigil.[21] Although we rely partially on the patient to notice and present with symptoms, there is a professional and legal expectation on the dental practitioner to be able to identify a lesion and appropriately refer.[21] It is expected of general dental practitioners that upon patient presentation, oral cancer screening will occur.[22, 23]

Current literature has attempted to identify reasons for delay, however these appear to be diverse and dependent on the context of the study. Patient socioeconomic factors such as age or gender are usually not found to relate to duration of delay; neither are lesion factors such as size or location. Self medication has often been associated with longer delay. So while the knowledge base of this area of research is growing, more work is clearly needed. Further qualitative studies are required to explore factors which influence both patient and practitioner behaviors surrounding oral cancer detection and diagnosis. Qualitative methods are capable of eliciting contextually rich information to provide greater insights into factors associated with delay. Screening for oral lesions is not occurring consistently, with practitioners often citing a lack of time, financial incentives or training as barriers. Dental and medical practitioners are often unaware of where their duty lies in terms of screening for oral cancer, however both disciplines express the need for education on both oral cancer detection and referral pathways. Further research is required in this field to inform effective interventions.

2. Screening

Oral cancer screening is 'the process by which a practitioner evaluates an asymptomatic patient to determine if he or she is likely or unlikely to have a potentially-malignant or malignant lesion'.[2] This definition implies more than a visual and tactile examination of the oral mucosa and includes assessment of the patient's risk profile - at a minimum a consideration of their age, tobacco and alcohol use. The aim of screening is to enhance the early detection of oral cancer and pre-cancer, and thereby enhance patient survival and outcomes. Due to the relatively low prevalence of oral cancer, population based screening is not currently justified.[24] Opportunistic screening (conducting an oral mucosal examination when the patient presents for periodic examination or other treatment), or targeting of groups known to be at higher risk for oral cancer is likely to be more cost-effective.[25] The profile of a high risk individual is that of an older male with a heavy use of tobacco and alcohol, poor diet and of low socioeconomic status.[9, 26] Emerging knowledge of the role of human papillomavirus (HPV) in the pathogenesis of oral cancer however is challenging the relevance of this profile. HPV positive oral cancer is associated with younger age and does not appear to be linked with gender, alcohol or tobacco use.[27, 28]

While the purpose of screening is to detect oral lesions, it also provides an excellent opportunity for the practitioner to engage the patient in a discussion about oral cancer. This serves to raise patient awareness about oral cancer generally, its risk factors and the importance of the screening examination that has just been performed. Patients may also examine themselves for early signs of oral cancer, however evidence for the usefulness of this approach is currently limited.[29, 30] The effectiveness of any screening program will be influenced by a number of factors. These factors include those relating to the patient, the practitioner, the availability and demonstrated efficacy of diagnostic aids, and those factors relating to the health system. These will be discussed in detail in the following sections.

3. Patient factors

Patient delay is defined as the time it takes for patients to seek help following self discovery of symptoms.[8] This term is widely accepted however it should be interpreted cautiously so as not to infer blame on the part of the patient. The mean patient delay varies between studies, with anywhere from 11 weeks to 6 months cited.[12, 17] Mean patient delay can be affected by large outliers in studies and for this reason it is useful to also include median delay, however not all studies report both.[31] Some studies collect data on a categorical basis, reporting the percentage of patients that present within a given time frame. It is difficult to define what excessive patient delay is, however a reduction in mean and median values would improve survival rates.

3.1 Public awareness of oral cancer

The public know little about the clinical presentation of oral cancer, although most are aware it is usually detected in late stages of disease.[32] Most people are able to identify tobacco and previous experience of oral cancer as risk factors, but less people are aware of other risk factors such as alcohol, older age and poor diet.[32] Flyers and brochures in dental clinics may increase awareness of oral cancer. They may not only prompt patients to request a mucosal screening, but also motivate them to be more aware of self screening opportunities.[33] Leaflets have been shown to render patients more open to mucosal screening, with educational self screening pamphlets also resulting in high compliance.[33, 34] Not all practices however will promote awareness of oral cancer, as they believe it will create patient anxiety.[6, 35] This worry was unfounded in a study of dental professionals who attempted to integrate screening into their practices, finding patients had a positive disposition towards screening for oral cancer.[35] Although most patients were aware of oral cancer, some reported being totally unaware of the potential for it to occur.[16] Most patients who were aware of oral cancer had minimal knowledge.[16] Lack of awareness and knowledge of oral cancer has been reported to increase patient delay, thus making information available to patients may be a vital part in improving survival rates.[21] Although surgeries can make pamphlets available in the waiting room, it has been shown in numerous studies that those patients most at risk of developing oral cancer do not regularly attend a dentist.[21, 36-38] Television has the potential to reach a wider audience and educate about the importance of self screening and prompt presentation to a practitioner. Following an oral cancer campaign in Scotland, two thirds of those surveyed remembered hearing about oral cancer six months prior.[39] The majority of those patients saw it on television.[39] Around half of the patients felt encouraged to seek help because of the campaign.[39] In another study, several patients diagnosed with oral cancer remember having seen a television commercial, with two patients presenting to a health care professional as a result of these commercials.[16] Although television has the potential to reach a wide audience, oral cancer has a relatively low prevalence. For this reason it has been suggested a more cost effective mechanism is to target those most at risk of the condition.[40]

3.2 Self medication contributing to delay

Scott *et al.* performed a systematic literature review of articles published between 1975 and 2005 to identify known factors associated with patient delay.[20] The majority of factors investigated in studies reviewed were not shown to be related to the duration of patient delay. This may be because studies regarding patient delay are few in number and not all are considered rigorous in terms of study design.[20] In Thailand, it was reported that patients who had used traditional herbal medicine had a longer duration of delay.[20, 41] Self medication being associated with longer duration of patient delay has since been demonstrated in other studies. Patients may attempt to treat symptoms with over the counter products, with some seeking advice from pharmacists who commonly advise gels, creams or mouthrinses.[16, 42] These patients then wait to see whether their oral condition resolves following self medication, increasing duration of delay.[18] This highlights the importance of the pharmacist's awareness of oral cancer as they may be an initial point of call for a patient developing oral symptoms.[37, 42] One study showed that after pharmacies were given an educational package on oral cancer, more staff advised a mystery shopper querying a 4 week old non healing ulcer to present to a healthcare practitioner.[43] Although the shopper could be advised to visit either their doctor or dentist, most staff advised the shopper to visit a doctor.[43] Following the intervention only 45% of staff advised help seeking behavior, however this was higher than prior to the intervention.[43] A limitation of this study was that only one staff member was approached at each pharmacy, and this may not have been representative of the overall impact of the educational material provided. Not only are patients self medicating symptoms before diagnosis, one study has demonstrated that patients often trial alternative therapies before undergoing conventional cancer treatment.[44]

3.3 Socio demographic factors contributing to delay

Studies consistently report no correlation between age and delay, however, whether other factors such as gender, financial status, location or size of lesion play a role in patient delay has not yet been substantiated, with studies often generating conflicting results.[8, 15-17, 41, 45-50] Gender is not usually demonstrated to influence duration of delay[8, 15-17, 41, 47-49, 51]. Only one study contradicted this, with women taking longer to present to a practitioner following self discovery of symptoms.[12] However in this study there was a male/female ratio of 5.4/1, with only a small number of females.[12] Two studies noted unmarried patients exhibit longer delay, both suggesting this is because married patients have more support.[17, 52] As other studies did not show marital status influenced delay, the differences may be a result of cultural factors. Two studies found longer delay in non smokers.[17, 45] Patients who do not smoke may feel that since they are at lesser risk of developing oral cancer, their lesion is not of concern.[17] This being said, patients who smoke and drink alcohol are more likely to present with concurrent illness and they often have poorer prognosis partly due to increased delay.[53] Heavy drinkers have been shown to display an increased duration of delay, and in the same study only light smokers demonstrated excessive delay.[54] Difficulty obtaining access to a practitioner is often shown to influence delay.[19, 55] A study comparing the waiting time for patients to see a dentist established that those with potentially malignant lesions (ulceration) were seen much faster than those requesting prosthetic treatment, showing dental surgeries will prioritise cases.[56] Eleven percent of appointments in this study were made because of symptoms similar to oral cancer. Unfortunately however a comparison of waiting times for other symptoms such as prolonged pain or numbness was not incorporated.[57] Patients afflicted with oral cancer are often of low socioeconomic background and financial barriers may play an important role in patient delay.[55] Practitioners agreed that patients of low socioeconomic background exhibited greater delay.[58] This is exemplified by the high patient delay experienced in the USA compared to Canada.[10] The USA has a healthcare system whereby individuals pay for their own health expenses, whereas in Canada some healthcare is provided by the government. One study did however report that most individuals in the USA diagnosed with oral cancer had health insurance coverage, and those that had no coverage did not exhibit excessive delay.[46] A study performed in the UK reported that an oral cancer patient waited to see a free NHS dentist rather than be seen immediately by a private dentist, for which a fee would be charged. [8] Only three out of 44 patients interviewed in England identified costs of a dental check up to be a large barrier.[42] Financial barriers are dependent on the health care system utilised in the country where the research is performed, further complicating study comparisons.

3.4 Lesion factors contributing to delay

Most studies have found tumour factors such as site, symptoms, size and stage did not have an association with duration of delay.[8, 18, 41, 47] One study indicated that patients with oral cancer located in more commonly found sites such as the tongue, floor of mouth and retromolar pads presented faster than those with cancer located in uncommon sites such as on the hard palate and gingivae.[12] However the small number of individuals with cancer in uncommon sites in this study means that the results should be interpreted with caution.[12] Another study also showed that lesion site was associated with delay, but again a small sample size of uncommon cancer sites meant they were also unable to draw strong conclusions.[15] Those with cancer in more visible sites such as the lip or tongue have been shown to be diagnosed at earlier stages than others.[49] A lesion's maximal diameter was shown to be inversely proportional to delay by one study.[15] The patient's interpretation of symptoms has commonly been shown to influence duration of delay. The most common oral symptoms noticed by a patient are a non healing ulcer or sore, persistent lumps or swellings, sore tongue or mouth and sore throat, abscess or boil.[42, 49] Patients sometimes attribute these symptoms to an infection, dental problem or problem with a prosthesis.[51] Those that believe their lesion to be innocuous will often wait longer to be seen by a health care practitioner.[8, 18, 42, 51, 59] Some patients are aware there is a chance their symptoms are cancerous, but do not believe they are.[59] This highlights the need for both awareness of oral cancer presentation and the understanding that anyone may be afflicted. One study revealed patients also require guidance on how to interpret oral symptoms.[40] Of patients diagnosed with oral cancer, most can retrospectively pinpoint symptoms attributable to cancer and the majority of patients diagnosed with oral cancer report presenting as a result of their symptoms.[16, 46] This being said, symptom recognition is not a reliable method of detecting tumours at an early stage since about 25% of oral cancers remain silent until they reach an advanced size.[21] Although tumours may not necessarily be detected at an early stage, attribution of symptoms to cancer can at least lead to earlier detection.

3.5 Barriers and triggers to help seeking

Understanding the barriers and triggers to help seeking is crucial to institute effective mechanisms to decrease patient delay. Patient delay should not be influenced by whether the patient actually has a malignant lesion, since both benign and malignant lesions can exhibit similar symptoms. Despite this, most studies only include patients with a diagnosis of oral cancer. A more recent study took this into account and included patients who had potentially malignant lesions.[19] As was the case with patients diagnosed with oral cancer, patients delayed seeking help as they believed their symptoms were minor and some attempted self care prior to seeking help.[19] One study hypothesized that patients who had previously experienced benign lesions may have longer delay time, since they are less inclined to believe their condition needs attention.[15] Some patients had a negative attitude towards dental practitioners due to a previous negative experience or apprehension, with others not wanting to waste practitioners' time.[19, 51] Only about half of the patients interviewed in the USA had a regular dentist.[46] Often patients were found to have competing responsibilities or priorities such as work commitments or comorbidities.[19] Most previous studies have only looked at the barriers to help seeking. In order to institute effective public awareness however, triggers should also be identified. One study which queried patients about the triggers, found patients presented following either a change in symptoms, if they had another reason to visit a practitioner, had a fear of worsening symptoms, excessive worry, dislike of symptoms or were advised by significant others.[19] Attribution of symptoms to something sinister will not always inspire help seeking behaviour, with a fear of diagnosis sometimes leading to delay.[55] Another study also investigated triggers to presentation, finding the dominant triggers to be anxiety and worry, need to resolve uncertainty, avoidance of problems getting worse and being advised by others to seek help.[42] Being advised by others to seek help has been shown to trigger help seeking behavior in subsequent studies, as well as receipt of new information from sources such as media or medical literature.[59] Development of a neck mass usually inspires a patient to visit a healthcare practitioner, however by this stage it is well advanced.[51] Most studies are conducted retrospectively, meaning they are subject to significant recall bias. Gao *et al.* instituted a system whereby family members were requested to confirm descriptions in order to decrease recall bias.[15] It was however found by Rogers *et al.* that the majority of patients will wait up to a month before telling anyone about their symptoms.[42] It is not apparent whether family members will be subject to the same recall bias, or simply tend to agree with the patient.

4. Practitioner factors

As with patient delay, a wide variance of mean and median professional delay time has been cited. This can be attributed to differing definitions of delay, recall bias or incomplete records. Although professional delay does not tend to contribute greatly to total delay, it is arguably the easiest part of delay to target. Professional delay has been proposed to occur as a result of lack of rigour in screening, lack of confidence in detection, low prevalence rates, inadequate knowledge and lack of incentives for screening.

4.1 Mucosal examination

A dentist's attitude to screening is an important factor in detecting early malignancy, as unless patients present with a complaint there is complete reliance on the dentist to identify mucosal lesions.[60, 61] It has been shown that patients who develop an oral cancer and who regularly attend a dentist are more likely to have their cancer diagnosed in its early stages.[46] Often, asymptomatic lesions are discovered incidentally during dental examination.[47, 62, 63] However, even following a routine dental examination malignant lesions are sometimes missed. This was demonstrated in a study where oral and maxillofacial surgeons detected oral cancer in patients referred for extraction of teeth.[47] The majority of dentists claim to perform mucosal screening for every patient, and in some cases they target screening to individuals over the age of 40.[14, 64] Of dentists working in nursing homes in Ohio, 83% reported performing mucosal exams for each patient, although only half actually identified increasing age as a risk factor for oral cancer.[65] Screening practices are found to be inconsistent between studies; only a third of dentists in Germany reported performing routine oral cancer examinations.[66] In the same study, only 66% of dentists questioned felt adequately trained to examine patients for oral cancer, despite the majority agreeing that dentists are qualified to perform these examinations.[66] In this study, questionnaires were sent out with a dental association journal and there was a response rate of only 14%, resulting in biased data, so the real picture is likely to be even worse.[66] Similar results were found in a separate study when questionnaires were sent to dental and medical professionals.[67] Although some practitioners cited a lack of time as a barrier to screening, the reality is that it takes less than 2 minutes to perform a thorough head and neck exam.[35, 38] Lack of financial incentives to perform mucosal screening may therefore be impeding on motivation to do so.[35] Almost all dentists surveyed in a study in Ohio felt oral cancer screening should be a separate reimbursable procedure, with all agreeing mucosal examinations should occur for all patients over 40 annually.[65] Lack of rigour regarding screening may be the result of the relatively low incidence of oral cancer; the average dentist only encounters about 2 tumour cases during a lifetime.[21, 61] Clinicians should however be performing mucosal examinations not only to pick up cancer, but also other lesions, including potentially malignant lesions. What motivates a clinician to undertake a mucosal exam is yet to be determined, however if practitioners are only undertaking a mucosal exam to detect oral cancer the low prevalence rates may indeed play a role.

4.2 Risk assessment

Alcohol and smoking are prominent risk factors for of oral cancer.[7] Some practitioners will take this into account and perform a more thorough mucosal exam for smokers while others do not consider this a factor influencing their screening behaviour.[61, 68] One study demonstrated that dentists will often take into account risk factors when deciding whether to refer.[22] Dentists are in a position to provide smoking cessation advice. It has been shown however that some dentists don't believe there is any benefit providing this advice due to lack of financial incentives, a belief that people do not want the advice or the belief that patients do not want to quit.[6, 37, 69] The belief that patients don't want smoking cessation advice has been contradicted since, with about half the dental patients surveyed suggesting they would try to quit if advice was offered.[69] Almost two thirds of dentists questioned in Germany agreed dentists should be trained to provide smoking cessation, but only about a quarter felt they were able to provide advice.[66] Although a number of dentists claimed to provide smoking cessation advice, only a small number follow up with the patient and help them to quit.[64] The number of dentists requesting information about and providing advice on a patient's drinking habits has consistently been even lower.[37, 64, 66] This may be a result of less awareness of the role of alcohol in oral cancer.[37] About two thirds of dentists surveyed in Germany believed dentists should be trained to provide smoking cessation advice, and more than 50% felt training in alcohol cessation was important.[66] It has been suggested that compulsory continuing education should be implemented to educate practitioners about the effects of tobacco and alcohol on the oral mucosa and how to provide cessation advice.[64] Although practitioners may be aware of the risk that alcohol and smoking pose to the patient, there is still a lack of readiness to provide support to patients in modifying their risk behaviors. Patients diagnosed with oral cancer don't always link their smoking habits as a causative factor, highlighting the importance of public awareness of risk factors.[16] Targeting high risk groups for screening has been proposed as a feasible screening plan.[21] Practitioners involved could be trained to assist patients with reducing their risk from lifestyle factors such as tobacco and alcohol. They would therefore not only detect lesions earlier but also work with their patients to help them reduce their risk. Diagnostic delay has been associated with increased co-morbidities, which is concerning as over 25% of head and neck cancer patients also have illness in more than one body part.[53] These co-morbidities are often tobacco associated.[53]

4.3 Practitioner knowledge of oral cancer

It has been shown in some studies that practitioners lacked confidence in detecting cancer; however this has been contradicted in other studies.[14, 61] Dentists are often looking for cancer as opposed to potentially malignant lesions. Changing this philosophy is important in ensuring lesions are identified at an early stage where treatment is less radical.[61] Dentists should be able to determine whether a lesion has malignant potential or is already malignant, with non homogenous lesions being referred straight away.[7] Non homogenous leukoplakia is often shown to have a marked increase in malignant change when compared with homogeneous leukoplakia.[7, 70] Erythroplakia exhibits higher malignant potential, with about half these lesions showing invasive carcinoma.[7] Alarmingly, health care providers surveyed in Scotland were more concerned about leukoplakia than erythroplakia.[37] This study included general medical practitioners as well as general dental practitioners with no distinction between groups in terms of oral cancer knowledge. Another study suggested that dentists do give due concern to erythroplakia.[61] A study comparing oral cancer knowledge between doctors and dentists found that dentists could identify more risk factors and oral changes associated with oral cancer.[68] It was shown that dentists are more confident in detecting oral cancer than doctors, despite most patients presenting to their doctor regarding oral lesions.[11, 21, 37, 42, 47] Patients may present to a doctor rather than a dentist because they do not view their oral lesion as a problem with their dentition or dentures, thus there is a need for the public to be made aware that it is appropriate to go to their dentist if they become aware of a mucosal lesion.[47] Doctors perceive lack of training and time to be barriers to oral cancer screening, similar to the dentist's disposition.[37] Doctors could be advised that if there is an oral condition they are unsure of, patients can be advised to seek the opinion of a dentist. It could be argued that this referral could contribute to delay, however Macpherson *et al.* found most doctors will refer if a lesion persists for 4-5 weeks compared to most dentists who wait only the recommended 2 weeks.[37] Although Jovanovic *et al.* found no significant difference in delay between doctors and dentists, their study analysed the records of 41 patients whereas Macpherson *et al.* sent questionnaires to 357 doctors and 331 dentists.[37, 47] Using questionnaires to record behavior introduces bias in itself, making interpretation difficult.

4.4 Need for continuing education

When practitioners are interviewed, they often exhibit the belief that there should be compulsory continuing education courses in oral cancer.[35, 58] Participants in one study wanted to know more about referral pathways, biopsy procedure and guidelines for screening.[35] Courses have been shown to be effective in promoting screening methods, with practitioners reporting better screening habits following attendance.[35, 58] A lack of confidence in detection has been made apparent as some dentists did not feel that they should deal with diseases such as cancer as they are "not medical doctors".[35] This lack of confidence also extends to doctors, as both doctors and dentists felt that they had inadequate training and were not confident in detecting oral lesions.[37] If that is the case, further compulsory continuing education courses on oral cancer could help to shift this belief and make practitioners more aware of their responsibility. Practitioners who have undertaken more recent continuing education courses in oral cancer have had greater knowledge in the area.[14] Despite the benefit of such courses, about one third of dentists from a Western US multistate dental practice group reported having never attended a continuing education course on oral cancer.[14] An association has been demonstrated between knowledge of risk factors and diagnosis, and number of lesions referred or biopsied by a practitioner.[71]

4.5 Referral and patient mediated professional delay

Some studies have found dentists will wait 2 weeks to review a lesion prior to referral. This is recommended since oral cancer can mimic traumatic lesions which resolve in 2 weeks.[6, 37,

[50] A difficulty in implementing the two week rule is that patients may delay in presentation for the second appointment, for reasons similar to initial delay.[72] In some cases, patients can also delay in effecting a referral.[58, 72] For this reason practitioners should convey urgency to the patient if a suspicious lesion is referred.[50] Not only should practitioners convey urgency to the patient, but also to the specialist, since mentioning malignancy or possibility of a tumour in the referral letter, or accompanying a referral letter with a phone call can categorise a referral as urgent.[50] Specialists will prioritise a patient if malignancy is suspected. Dentists have been shown to display difficulty in conveying their suspicions in referral letters, especially when compared to their medical counterparts.[73] Practitioners should also follow up referred patients to ensure they are utilising their referral, effectively decreasing this proportion of professional delay.[72] Patient anxiety has been shown to modify the decision to refer.[6, 61] Although it is important to allay the concerns of an anxious patient, a suspicious lesion should be referred regardless of whether the patient is concerned. Cues for frank malignancy are more likely to prompt a referral when compared with premalignancy and it has been demonstrated in numerous studies that if a practitioner is in doubt, they will refer. [22, 61] Again, greater emphasis needs to be placed on the detection of potentially malignant and premalignant lesions if a decrease in delay is sought.

Not only does referral involve the practitioner identifying and referring a patient for examination, there is a distinct need to communicate to the patient why they are being referred. A part of professional delay that is difficult to control for in studies is patient mediated professional delay, that is when patients do not attend a specialist appointment for a prolonged period of time following referral.[10] The need for a patient to promptly attend a specialist appointment should be communicated to the patient without causing undue distress. Rogers *et al.* found 1 in 6 patients were not satisfied with advice received upon their first medical consultation, however whether patients were dissatisfied with either advice given from a doctor or dentist was not represented and the reasons they weren't happy was also not explored.[42] The practitioner should be able gauge the patient's emotional and social well being and deliver medical information that the patient is able to comprehend.[36] Upon issuing a referral, practitioners will often tell the patient they have seen something suspicious and would like a second opinion.[6] Dentists worry about using language to avoid anxiety, tending to refrain from using words associated with malignancy and some believe this helps calm the patient.[6] Following questioning from the patient regarding possibility of oral cancer, dentists tend to say they do not think the lesion is malignant.[6] Although this may help decrease patient anxiety, there is also a need to ensure that the patient also sees the issue of obtaining a definitive diagnosis as urgent. Both medical and dental practitioners believe more training in detection and referral pathways are necessary.[37]

4.6 Delays between diagnosis and treatment

Once a diagnosis of oral cancer has been made, delay can occur in obtaining treatment for these patients. Not only does this delay cause stress to the patient, tumour size may increase during this time period.[74] Alarmingly, a study in Denmark showed the amount of delay increased from 1992 to 2002. This was attributed to a shortage of radiotherapy capacity.[75] They also observed that more imaging procedures were carried out, but could not prove a cause and effect relationship.[75] In one study factors such as ethnicity, primary site and insurance correlated with delay between diagnosis and treatment.[76] It has been suggested that longer planning time is needed for complex cases, thus some delay in this instance appears warranted.[76]

5. Health system factors

The structure and organisation of a country's health system is a critically important yet poorly recognised factor influencing the early detection of oral cancer and pre-cancer. It can contribute to both patient and professional delay. Low socioeconomic status has been previously discussed in this chapter as a barrier to accessing health care for the symptoms of oral cancer. Financial barriers to health care depend on the funding model of the health system. If health care is funded by the government then theoretically this barrier is removed. However, real access to public health care also depends on the available resources. Inadequately resourced public health care results in waiting lists. This forces patients to seek care in the private sector, or to neglect health care. In addition, health systems that ensure culturally safe practice enhance access for groups at high risk, Indigenous and recent immigrant populations.[77] Whether the health system values and supports prevention and early detection will influence practitioner behaviour in performing a thorough screen including a risk assessment and providing support for patients in modifying their health behaviours. If the practitioner is reimbursed for these activities or in the case of the public sector, if this contributes to productivity targets, then these behaviours are likely to be valued by the patient and occur more frequently.

Health systems globally are stretched ever further dealing with the challenges of an ageing population and the increased burden of complex chronic diseases. Dental health systems are often prioritised lower than general health systems and so public funding for oral health care may suffer a significant shortfall. Oral cancer, similarly to other oral disease, is almost entirely preventable. If it can be detected early, the outcomes are substantially better. Putting aside the gains in human health and quality of life, from a purely cost perspective, it makes sense to invest in programs which focus on the prevention and early detection of all oral diseases, including oral cancer. The health care team paradigm is now well accepted as a necessity for providing optimal patient care. In a number of countries, including Australia and New Zealand, oral health therapists are tertiary trained practitioners who work in the dental team. They have expertise in recognition of oral abnormalities, risk assessment and health promotion.[78] Novel models of care, in which oral health therapists are used to screen, risk assess, provide support for health behaviour modification and refer for treatments outside their scope of practice, are currently being trialled. Continuing education programs, and the establishment of clear clinical guidelines and criteria for referral[79] are agreed to be necessary to support primary care clinicians in confidently and effectively performing oral cancer screening for their patients.

6. Diagnostic aids

The quest for reduction in professional delay of detection, and a desire to improve early detection of oral cancer has driven the development of diagnostic aids designed to improve visualisation of malignant and potentially malignant oral lesions. Methods for visualising and detecting PMOLs include conventional oral examination (COE), vital tissue staining, light based detection systems which rely on tissue reflectance (ViziLite, Microlux/DL), and autofluorescence (VELscope, Identafi). Several key issues are considered when assessing a particular diagnostic aid. These include the effectiveness of the visualisation method in detecting oral cancer and precancer; whether or not the method can distinguish premalignant or malignant lesions from other benign conditions; and if an accepted "gold standard" comparison such as scalpel biopsy and histopathological assessment was used in assessing the efficacy of the diagnostic aid. Where possible, sensitivity, specificity, positive predictive value (PPV) and negative predictive value (NPV) are used to determine the effectiveness and accuracy of each aid. Sensitivity is the proportion of people who have the disease and test positive, while specificity refers to the proportion of people who do not have the disease and test negative. PPV is the proportion of people with positive test results who have the disease, whereas NPV is the proportion of people with negative results and do not have the disease.

6.1 Conventional oral examination

Conventional oral examination under normal incandescent or halogen light illumination is the standard method for screening for oral cancer.[5] It typically involves visual inspection of the oral cavity and palpation of the lymph nodes for clinical signs of abnormalities such as changes in colour, texture, ulceration, persistent swelling and enlarged lymph nodes.[1] Several studies have reported relatively high sensitivity and specificity values for COE. In a prospective study involving two oral cancer screening programs, over 2,300 people underwent a thorough oral examination by a dentist.[80] An oral medicine specialist then examined participants to give a definitive 'true' clinical diagnosis, thus providing a "soft" gold standard. The combined sensitivity and specificity of these two screening programs was 0.74 and 0.99 respectively,[80] which is consistent with sensitivity and specificity values of other screening programs.[81-83] The results from this study, along with six other prospective studies with calculated sensitivity and specificity, were included in a meta-analysis by Downer *et al.*[84] These studies reported a range of sensitivity and specificity values, from 0.60 to 0.97 and 0.74 to 0.99 respectively. When pooled together, the overall sensitivity for COE was 0.848 while the overall specificity was 0.965.[84] This indicates that COE has relatively few false negatives, and even less false positives. However, the ability of a clinician to screen for potentially malignant and malignant lesions will vary, depending on their knowledge and clinical judgement. Nonetheless, Downer *et al.*'s heterogeneity analysis of the eight studies found that dentists and specifically trained basic health workers can screen with similar degrees of accuracy.[84]

Despite the relatively high sensitivity and specificity, there is still some controversy about the use of COE as clinicians often cannot purely use this method to discriminate progressive from non-progressive lesions, and benign from malignant lesions.[85] For definitive diagnosis, an incisional biopsy with histopathological analysis is required.[1, 3] Furthermore, not all early lesions are easily seen under a dental operating light.[2, 5, 85, 86] In a pilot study by Thomson, 26 untreated patients with either a PMOL or unilateral OSCC had a biopsy of clinically normal-looking mucosa taken from the corresponding, contralateral anatomical site.[87] After histological assessment, 6 (23%) samples had reactive changes, 7 (27%) had some form of dysplasia (mild, moderate or severe), 1 (0.04%) had carcinoma in situ (CIS) and 1 (0.04%) had microinvasive squamous cell carcinoma.[87] Sites with a high proliferation rate such as the ventral tongue and floor of mouth, and were exposed to carcinogens, were also found to be more susceptible to dysplastic changes.[87] It is therefore particularly important to identify high-risk patients so that an even higher level of suspicion is maintained when examining these patients, especially since a randomised controlled trial (RCT) reported a significant decrease in mortality in males who used alcohol or tobacco, or both, when they were screened for oral cancer.[88] However, a recent Cochrane review assessed this RCT and cautioned the interpretation of this statement, as the study had several methodological problems which may have introduced bias.[24] Furthermore, since this study was conducted in India where the prevalence of oral cancer is higher, results from this study may not be applicable to low-prevalence populations.[24] More RCTs are required as there currently is insufficient evidence to support oral cancer screening with COE in the general population. Nonetheless, it is clear that COE alone is not perfect. Therefore, the use of an adjunctive technique that has high specificity and sensitivity for highlighting PMOLs and OSCC should aid a clinician in detecting and diagnosing these lesions at an early stage, and consequently improve prognosis.[85]

6.2 Vital tissue staining

Tolonium chloride, more commonly known as toluidine blue (TB), is an acidophilic metachromatic dye of the thiazine group that preferentially stains nucleic acids and abnormal tissues.[5, 89] The increased nuclear density and the loss of intracellular adherence in dysplastic and malignant tissues allows TB dye to penetrate through the epithelium and be retained in these tissues, thereby staining these areas of abnormality blue.[89, 90] Although TB has primarily been marketed as an adjunct for detecting potentially malignant and malignant oral lesions not identified by COE, it has also been recommended for determining the risk of potentially malignant oral lesions progressing to cancer, monitoring suspicious lesions, determining the optimal biopsy site, assessing the extent and margins of potentially malignant and malignant oral lesions, and for assessing the outcome after treatment for dysplasia and cancer in follow-up appointments.[90, 91] Until recently, TB was commercially available as kits under the trade names 'OraScan' (Germiphene), 'OraScreen' (Stafford-Miller Ltd.) and 'OraTest' (Zila Pharmaceuticals). However, TB is now available as part of ViziLite Plus under the name, TBlue[630] (Zila Tolonium Chloride) Oral Lesion Marking System, and may be used at the discretion of the clinician for demarcating any lesion that requires further study or biopsy.[92]

Whilst there is extensive literature on TB, many only provided background information, expert opinion and/or described a technique but did not provide additional data.[90] An early meta-analysis by Rosenberg *et al.* of 12 studies conducted between 1964 and 1984 reported 93.5 to 97.8% sensitivity and 73.3 to 92.9% specificity for the detection of oral cancers.[93] A later systematic review by Grey *et al.* of 14 studies conducted between 1970 to 1999, half of which were also included in Rosenberg *et al.*'s paper, reported sensitivity varying from 40 to 100% and specificity from 31 to 92%.[90] Another recent systematic review of adjuncts to oral examination assessed 15 studies from 1967 to 2005.[94] In this review, sensitivity and specificity of TB as a diagnostic adjunct ranged from 38 to 98% (median 85%) and 9 to 93% (median 67%) respectively. PPV varied from 33 to 93% (median 85%) and NPV from 22 to 92% (median 83%).[94] Although there are discrepancies in the sensitivity and specificity ranges due to the different inclusion and exclusion criteria of these reviews, the median values suggest that TB has high sensitivity but relatively lower specificity.

Findings from an observational study of 45 oral mucosal lesions by Allegra *et al.* are consistent with this idea.[95] Allegra *et al.* reported 96.2% sensitivity and 77.2% specificity for TB staining, with a PPV of 86.6% and a NPV of 93.3%. In comparison, sensitivity and specificity for clinical examination were 53% and 80% respectively, whereas the PPV was 84.2% and NPV was 46.1%. There was a statistically significant difference in both sensitivity and NPV between TB and clinical examination. Therefore, TB was better at identifying suspected lesions than COE, and had a very low probability of a positive histological result coming from a negatively stained lesion.[95] These results are consistent with previous studies.[96, 97] In contrast, a recently published paper of case series by Cancela-Rodriguez *et al.* reported higher specificity than sensitivity.[89] Whilst the sensitivity of 65.5% was lower than previous reports, the specificity of 73.3% was consistent with other studies. The PPV of 35.2% was also lower, which the authors attributed to the lower prevalence of dysplastic and malignant lesions in their study when compared with others, whereas the NPV of 90.6% was again consistent with other papers.[89]

On the whole, the relatively lower specificity values were a result of relatively high numbers of false positive findings. In several studies, TB stained normal variations of anatomy, and benign inflammatory and traumatic lesions due to their increased cell activity.[89, 96-100] To reduce the number of unnecessary biopsies and to exclude inflammatory and traumatic lesions, Mashberg suggested restaining any TB-stained lesion after 10 to 14 days.[98] Any lesion that still stained after this period should be evaluated for cancer by biopsy,[98] as OSCC, CIS and high-grade dysplasia retained TB fairly consistently.[5, 97, 101] Furthermore, a prospective longitudinal study by Zhang *et al.* reported that lesions - including benign lesions with high-risk clinical and molecular characteristics - which stained with TB had an increased risk of malignant transformation.[101] However, staining of all early-stage dysplasias does not always occur,[5] probably because these lesions do not have the molecular changes associated with OSCC progression.[102] Conversely, TB has been shown to stain lesions that were undetected by COE.[90, 103]

Current literature suggests that the use of TB by trained and experienced practitioners may be useful in high-risk patients in a specialist setting, as most TB studies have been conducted in specialist clinics on higher-risk patients or patients who already have a known lesion.[5, 94] With only one published community-based randomised controlled trial (RCT),[104] there is insufficient data to support the use of TB as an adjunct to COE in general practice on the general population. In this RCT, 7,975 participants were randomly allocated to either the experimental group (TB) or the control group (placebo dye), and were visually examined by experienced dentists who were trained by an oral pathologist to detect oral lesions. It was found that the use of TB did not significantly improve the detection rate of PMOLs; however, significantly more oral submucous fibrosis and slightly more leukoplakia were detected when TB was used as an adjunct than with visual screening alone. In addition, there was no significant difference between the two groups in reducing the incidence of oral cancer after five years. Further RCTs in the general population with longer follow-up periods are needed to confirm these results, particularly since the malignant transformation of PMOLs has a long natural history.[104]

Problems with experimental design and analysis of results are the main reasons contributing to the poor quality of many studies on TB. Care must be taken when interpreting and comparing results as methods and definitions are inconsistent. Common issues that need to be considered include whether or not a non-pharmaceutical grade (laboratory) TB solution or a higher standard, pharmaceutical grade TB solution was used, the method of applying TB (rinse versus local swab), if a two rinse procedure was used instead of one rinse to rule out inflammatory lesions, and the definition of a positive stain. Staining intensity is a contentious issue, with some studies defining a positive result if there is an intense blue stain, while in other studies a positive result is if there is any blue staining.[5, 91] Further complicating this matter is the inclusion of equivocal results in some studies, and whether or not they should be considered as positive or negative in statistical analysis. Grey *et al.* showed that equivocal results can significantly affect statistical values in individual studies,[90] which may mean that accuracy results are underestimated.[94] Interpretation of TB stains can therefore be difficult and its use should be limited to trained and experienced clinicians, otherwise there may be more unnecessary biopsies taken and higher numbers of false positive and negative results.

6.3 Tissue reflectance (ViziLite, Microlux/DL)

There are several screening devices marketed as adjuncts to COE that enhance tissue reflectance to aid clinicians to detect PMOLs and OSCCs. These devices include ViziLite Plus (Zila Pharmaceuticals, Phoenix, Arizona, USA), Microlux/DL (AdDent, Danbury, CT, USA) and Orascoptic DK (Orascoptic, a Kerr Company, Middleton, WI, USA).[1, 2, 85, 105] ViziLite Plus utilises a disposable chemiluminescent light packet to provide diffuse blue-white light between 490 to 510 nm in wavelength.[92, 106] Chemiluminescence occurs when a chemical reaction produces light which can vary in intensity, lifetime and colour depending on the type of reaction.[107] In contrast, Microlux/DL and Orascoptic DK use a diffuse white light from a battery-powered light-emitting diode (LED).[108] Regardless of the type of light, these devices claim to enhance tissue reflectance of oral tissues after the mouth has been rinsed with 1% acetic acid for 60 seconds.[92, 108, 109] According to the manufacturers, a cytoplasmic dehydration agent such as acetic acid can alter the refractile properties of oral mucosal abnormalities with atypical non-keratinized squamous epithelium, as these cells have an increased nuclear:cytoplasmic ratio.[92, 108, 109] Consequently, dysplastic lesions become more visible as they appear white (hence termed an 'acetowhite lesion') against the light blue appearance of normal tissue.[85, 92, 105, 108-110]

Several studies have evaluated the efficacy of tissue reflectance as a technique for visualising and detecting oral mucosal lesions; however, the number of publications available is still quite limited. The majority of these are on ViziLite, with only one study on Microlux/DL and none on Orascoptic DK.[5] Although several studies have been published regarding the efficacy of ViziLite, there appears to be conflicting results. In a pilot study involving 150 patients, a variety of hard and soft oral lesions were examined using ViziLite.[110] All benign lesions without hyperkeratinisation, hyperparakeratinisation, chronic inflammatory infiltrate and/or an altered nuclear:cytoplasmic ratio did not appear acetowhite. However, all lesions with a clinical diagnosis of leukoedema and two out of fourteen frictional keratoses were ViziLite positive. In addition, three leukoplakic lesions appeared acetowhite. Two of these, including the one that was not detected by COE, had signs of cellular atypia, while the third was later diagnosed as a non-specific ulcer.[110] This finding is consistent with two other papers that reported positive results with a non-specific ulcer,[105] and four cases of traumatic ulcers.[111] These results suggest that ViziLite has fairly high sensitivity but low specificity and PPV,[5] and this idea is supported by several studies.[105, 107, 112] In a study by Ram and Siar involving 40 patients with a PMOL, primary squamous cell carcinoma, or a history of either condition, sensitivity and specificity was 100% and 14.2% respectively.[107] In another study by Farah and McCullough involving 55 patients with an oral white mucosal lesion, sensitivity was again 100% while specificity was 0%.[105] Unlike Ram and Siar who reported an accuracy of 80.6%, Farah reported an accuracy of only 18.2%.[105, 107] This considerable difference in accuracy is most likely attributed to the different sample population.[105] A recent study by Awan *et al.* also reported high sensitivity and low specificity, with the values being 77.3% and 27.8% respectively.[112] The lower sensitivity has been attributed to the sample population, which included a wider range of oral lesions than the two previous studies.[112] In contrast, a recent study reported a sensitivity of 0% and specificity of 75.5%.[113] In this study by Mehrotra *et al.*, there were three dysplastic lesions and one cancerous lesion out of 102 patients examined with ViziLite - none of which had a positive ViziLite result. Consequently, the NPV was very high, at 94.8%, while PPV was 0%.[113] Although not specified by the authors, the dysplastic and cancerous lesions may have been red, which is reportedly less preferentially highlighted by chemiluminescence than lesions with a white component.[111, 112, 114] This may be due to the fact that erythroplakia has either atrophied epithelium or epithelium that has had no change in thickness, and that acetic acid does not enhance the refractile properties of erythroplakia.[111]

Clearly, the ability to differentiate between keratotic, inflammatory, potentially malignant and malignant lesions is poor with ViziLite.[105, 107, 111] Nevertheless, there are reports that ViziLite improves visualisation of lesions - particularly leukoplakias, although there are conflicting results. Epstein *et al.* found a significant improvement in the brightness, sharpness and texture of lesions using ViziLite,[114] while Kerr *et al.* noticed a significant improvement in only sharpness, a trend towards enhanced brightness, and no significant improvement in texture.[111] Two other studies also noticed improved brightness and sharpness of oral lesions with chemiluminescence.[112, 115] Visualisation of intraoral lesions was reportedly enhanced in Farah's paper, however this was not statistically significant.[105] In contrast, visualisation can be more difficult due to an increase in mucosal surface reflectivity as a result of stimulated salivary flow following an acetic acid rinse.[106, 111, 112] Most studies have also found at least one new lesion that was not seen by COE;[105, 106, 110, 111, 114] however, the general consensus is that ViziLite does not provide any additional benefit to COE.[105, 106, 113]

Although there have been several studies on ViziLite, the only published study assessing the efficacy of Microlux/DL as a diagnostic aid in visualising oral mucosal lesions is a prospective study by McIntosh *et al.*[85] In this study, 50 patients referred to an oral medicine specialist unit because of an oral mucosal white lesion were examined by an oral medicine specialist. Lesions were assessed clinically and were given a provisional diagnosis before undergoing incisional biopsy and histopathological analysis. With a gold standard diagnostic test to compare to, sensitivity, specificity, PPV and NPV could be accurately assessed. Results from this study found a sensitivity of 77.8%, a specificity of 70.7%, a PPV of 36.8% and a NPV of 93.5%. These results indicate that while Microlux/DL is fairly good for highlighting potentially malignant oral mucosal lesions and the presence of no disease, the ability to differentiate between benign and malignant lesions is poor. Furthermore, the system did not find any new lesions, modify the provisional diagnosis, or change the biopsy site, although it did improve lesion visibility and border distinctness of the majority of lesions when compared to COE. Furthermore, the emitted light from Microlux/DL was found to be very similar to a standard LED headlight.[85] From these results alone, Microlux/DL does not appear to be a great benefit to COE, particularly since the sensitivity and specificity scores in this study are lower than Downer *et al.*'s calculated overall sensitivity and specificity for COE.[84, 108] A limitation of the study was that a specialist performed the examinations rather than a general dental practitioner, and more trials are required to validate these findings in a general population.[85] A significant finding however, was that examination of PMOLs with white light is more useful than standard incandescent or halogen light.

More research is needed to support the use of chemiluminescence and tissue reflectance as an adjunct to COE. The published papers on both ViziLite and Microlux/DL have flaws in their experimental design; the most common being the lack of a definitive diagnostic gold standard comparison (incisional biopsy and histopathology) for all lesions.[106, 107, 110, 111, 114] To compensate, several studies used results from brush cytology as their main diagnostic comparison,[106, 110, 114] but this does not provide a definitive diagnosis.[5] Other weaknesses in studies include small sample size,[85, 105, 107] recruiting patients from specialist clinics instead of from the general population,[85, 105, 107, 111] and the use of specialists instead of general dental practitioners.[85, 105, 111] As a consequence, results should be interpreted with caution as they cannot be generalised to general practitioners, nor to the general population where the prevalence of oral cancer and precancer is much lower.[115] In addition, there was a potential for conflicts in interest in two studies.[114, 115] Larger, well-designed clinical trials are required to determine the ability of these devices in improving the visualisation of potentially malignant lesions that cannot be identified by COE.[5]

6.4 Tissue autofluorescence imaging (VELscope, Identafi)

Another light-based adjunct to COE is a handheld device called a Visually Enhancing Lesion Scope (VELscope; LED Dental Inc., Burnaby, BC, Canada). Using the idea that cellular fluorophores are excited by high intensity light of particular wavelengths, this device utilizes blue light 400 to 460 nm in wavelength to cause tissue autofluorescence.[5] This technology is based on the fact that both the superficial epithelium and underlying stroma of developing premalignant lesions have changes in their optical properties.[116] Normal oral epithelium appears pale green when directly viewed through a narrow-band filter, as green-red fluorescence is excited from fluorophores in the oral tissues.[1, 2, 5, 117] In contrast, dysplastic cells or potentially early tumours appear dark green to black due to the cellular and structural changes which occur in neoplastic tissue.[1, 5, 117, 118] Cellular alterations such as decreased flavin adenine dinucleotide concentration and collagen matrix breakdown have been associated with loss of fluorescence visualisation (FV).[117, 118] Furthermore, decreased fluorescence as a result of increased absorption and scattering of light occurs when there are structural changes in both the epithelium and lamina propria such as hypertrophy, hyperchromatism, cellular/nuclear pleomorphism and increased microvascularity.[117, 118]

Being relatively new, the number of published literature about the efficacy of VELscope for visualising and detecting potentially malignant lesions is limited. While the general consensus is that VELscope has very high sensitivity, the specificity has ranged quite considerably depending on the study. In three observational (cross-sectional) studies, the reported values for sensitivity ranged from 97% to 100% and for sensitivity, 80% to 100%.[117-119] In contrast, while Awan *et al.* had fairly high sensitivity, specificity was significantly lower.[112] The reported sensitivity for dysplasia and leukoplakia/erythroplakia was 84.1% and 87.1% respectively, while the specificity was 15.3% and 21.4% respectively.[112] Two recent studies have noted both low specificity and sensitivity with VELscope.[113, 120] A cross-sectional study by Mehrotra *et al.* found 50% sensitivity and 38.9% specificity after examining 156 patients seeking dental care with VELscope.[113] More recently, a prospective study by Farah *et al.* reported a sensitivity of 30%, a specificity of 63% and an accuracy of 55% when VELscope was used alone to examine 118 lesions from 112 patients.[120] The large discrepancy for specificity in these studies is most likely attributed to the sample population. Lane *et al.* and Poh *et al.* recruited patients with biopsy-confirmed oral dysplasia or SCC and Scheer *et al.* included patients with an increased risk of mucosal abnormalities.[117-119] In contrast, Mehrotra *et al.* enrolled patients with lesions deemed clinically innocuous according to COE,[113] while Farah *et al.* recruited patients with white or mixed white or red oral mucosal lesions,[120] and in the study conducted by Awan *et al.*, the only inclusion criteria was the presence of white, red and mixed white and red oral lesions.[112] Only one study used VELscope in a private general dentistry practice.[121] In this retrospective observational study, 905 patients were examined with VELscope. The authors reported a 1.3% prevalence of mucosal abnormalities, with 83% of these lesions being potentially premalignant.[121] When compared with results from incisional biopsies, studies demonstrated that VELscope could reveal high-risk lesions such as severe dysplasia and CIS; however, milder forms of dysplasia were not always detected.[113, 117-119] Despite this, there are several published case studies of new lesions being uncovered with VELscope in patients with a history of epithelial dysplasia or CIS.[122, 123] Furthermore, Farah *et al.* reported that VELscope revealed five lesions not found during COE, enhanced visualisation of 34.74% of cases, changed the clinical provisional diagnosis of 22 lesions, and changed the biopsy site of four lesions.[120] Border distinctness and visibility of benign and dysplastic lesions, however, were not different.[120] VELscope may also play a role with reducing the risk of tumour recurrence as it can be used before the excision of lesions to delineate malignant and premalignant subclinical extensions.[118]

A high number of false positives with VELscope resulted in low specificity and PPV values, with reported PPV ranging from 6.4% to 54.5%, while NPV ranged from 97.5% to 100%.[113, 119, 120] Inflammatory and traumatic lesions such as oral lichen planus, granulation tissue, chronic inflammation, ulcerations and hyperkeratosis had loss of FV and were therefore false positive results.[119] These tissues displayed less autofluorescence as they also had increased submucosal blood flow, altered metabolic activity and structural changes.[113, 119] To discriminate inflammatory lesions from dysplastic lesions, soft pressure should be applied to reduce blood flow to the area.[120] Blanched inflammatory lesions will have normal autofluorescence whereas potentially malignant and malignant lesions remain unchanged.[113, 119-122] However, applied pressure to dysplastic and OSCC lesions can still cause blanching, even though these lesions had loss of fluorescence.[120] Interestingly, one study found a gain of autofluorescence in verrucous leukoplakias that had no dysplasia.[119] From this, the authors proposed that invasive carcinomas will also have a gain in autofluorescence and therefore, loss of fluorescence would not be an applicable indicator for malignancy in verrucous lesions.[119] Nonetheless, Balevi calculated, using Bayes' theorem and the sensitivity and specificity values from existing literature, a PPV of 1.27% and a false positive rate of 98.63% if VELscope was used to routinely screen the total population for oral cancer.[124] The author concluded that as VELscope has such a high misdiagnosis rate in the general population, the use of VELscope should be limited to oral cancer specialist clinics where the prevalence of oral cancer is most likely greater than 10%.[124]

It is clear that there is currently an insufficient body of evidence to support the use of VELscope as an adjunct to COE for oral cancer screening in general practice. While VELscope does show promise, it cannot differentiate inflammatory and traumatic lesions from premalignant and malignant lesions. Therefore, use of the device requires skill and training in order to interpret results.[113, 119, 120] With low specificity, the clinician still needs to conduct a thorough examination and use their clinical judgement as well as the patient's history to determine the need for further investigation,[120] otherwise, there will be an increased risk of overtreatment and a higher number of unnecessary referrals.[112] Most published studies on VELscope have a small sample population that is not representative of the general population - namely, they were patients with a history of potentially malignant and malignant oral lesions.[117-120, 122, 123] In addition, a major limitation of VELscope is that the difference between loss of fluorescence and diminished fluorescence is subjective and depends on the experience of the user.[112, 119] When this is compounded with specialists who were not blinded,[117, 118] it is possible that results may have been overestimated. Consequently, the results from current literature cannot be applied to the general population and general practitioners. Until larger, blinded, randomized-controlled clinical trials can evaluate the performance of VELscope in populations where the prevalence for oral cancer is low, the use of this device should be restricted to specialist oral cancer clinics.

It is possible that the newest oral cancer screening system on the market, Identafi (previously marketed as Identafi 3000 ultra; DentalEZ Group, Malvern, PA, USA), may show more potential than its light-based screening predecessors. Identafi utilizes both optical autofluorescence and reflectance spectroscopy, in addition to traditional white light, to screen for PMOLs and OSCC.[86] According to the manufacturer, areas with biochemical and morphological changes in cells can be visually identified by exciting oral tissues using a combination of multi-spectral light.[86] Although highly concentrated white light may be considered slightly better for visualising oral lesions than incandescent operatory lights,[85] it cannot be used alone as it is still difficult to differentiate premalignant lesions with inflammation, oral lichen planus/lichenoid reactions and other benign conditions which clinically appear similar to precancer.[125] Consequently, the device also employs violet and green-amber light for detecting changes in fluorescence and reflectance respectively, thereby making it possible to locate areas of diseased tissue.[86]

Unlike VELscope which uses blue light, Identafi uses violet light to excite tissues and induce fluorescence.[86] As dysplastic and cancerous tissues have lower blue-green fluorescence intensity than normal tissues when they are excited by light with wavelengths between 330 to 470 nm,[116] abnormal tissues should appear dark brown or black when exposed to the 405 nm violet light emitted by Identafi.[86] A study by Roblyer *et al.* found that the optimal excitation wavelength of light for discriminating normal tissue from dysplasia and invasive cancer is 405 nm.[125] At this wavelength, the authors reported a sensitivity of 95.9% to 100% and a specificity of 91.4% to 96.2% for differentiating dysplasia and cancer from normal tissue.[125] Based on these results, it can be expected that Identafi may have similar values for sensitivity and specificity. A recent case report illustrated how autofluorescence tissue imaging with Identafi aided in diagnosing a metastatic tumour that was clinically innocuous.[126] Furthermore, an unpublished study by Zuluaga *et al.* involving 120 patients from four clinical centres found that the violet light had 100% NPV and a PPV nearing 60% for differentiating between normal and dysplastic or malignant tissue in one cohort.[127] The other cohorts had similar findings, and the authors expect that the overall PPV will be improved in the entire cohort with the addition of green-amber light.[127]

Tissue reflectance can be enhanced with the addition of green-amber light (dominant 545 nm).[86, 127] Although the haemoglobin absorption is strongest at 420 nm,[128] this light can delineate the vasculature of lesions from surrounding normal tissues as its wavelength is close to one of the two primary bands of haemoglobin absorption (*Q*-band peak of 542 nm).[86, 128] Premalignant and malignant tissues will appear diffuse due to their disorganised growth of blood vessels.[86] Therefore, as abnormal signs of morphologic changes can be highlighted, the addition of this light is expected to reduce the rate of false positives.[86, 127] However, further research is required to determine the efficacy of a multispectral system like Identafi.

7. Conclusions

Morbidity and mortality rates for oral cancer can be improved if potentially malignant oral mucosal lesions are found before they reach an advanced stage. Investigation of socio demographic factors in relation to patient delay is an important area deserving of further attention. Themes have emerged through the use of qualitative studies regarding barriers and triggers to patient presentation. Drawing upon the triggers associated with help seeking behavior and creating awareness of the symptoms of oral cancer may allow patients to attribute their signs to something more serious. Educational interventions and self screening promotion aimed at the population have the potential to create awareness of oral cancer. Patients have stated that if they were more aware of oral cancer, they would have presented sooner regarding their signs and symptoms. As it has been shown that patients often tell a family member or friend about their symptoms, increased knowledge among the public may ensure that the patient is advised to seek help by their loved ones. Educational interventions should also be targeted at pharmacists, as their advice has the potential to decrease patient delay should a patient seek advice from a pharmacy.

Dentists should be performing opportunistic screening on patients at dental appointments; however this is not happening consistently. Lack of confidence signals the need for further training, which can be done at both the undergraduate level and following graduation in the form of continuing professional development. As patients will commonly present to their doctor regarding an oral lesion, continuing education courses should also be made available for doctors. Identification of risk factors and effective patient counseling has the potential to decrease the incidence of oral cancer and there is need for improvement in this area. Risk factor analysis and effective communication could be integrated into continuing education courses. Practitioners should be more involved in creating awareness of oral cancer and this may be as simple as making pamphlets available at their surgeries.

Problems exist with interpreting data from many studies performed in this area. Often studies are performed retrospectively, thus incorporating memory bias or relying on records which may be incomplete. The low incidence of oral cancer renders sample sizes small, making it difficult to generalize the results. Continued investigation of the barriers and triggers to help seeking behavior and identification of factors involved in professional delay is required in order to inform effective interventions.

Although many new diagnostic aids are available to help clinicians detect oral mucosal lesions earlier, the current screening devices and methods are limited by their inability to detect and discriminate between benign and malignant lesions, and thus cannot be used alone as an alternative to COE - they must be used as an adjunct. As skill and training are required in order to interpret results, the use of these devices and methods should be limited to specialist centres and experienced and trained clinicians, if they are to be recommended for use at all. Currently, there is still insufficient evidence to support the use of vital tissue staining and technology based on tissue reflectance and autofluorescence, particularly since none have consistently shown that they are more effective than COE.

8. References

[1] McCullough MJ, Prasad G, Farah CS. Oral mucosal malignancy and potentially malignant lesions: an update on the epidemiology, risk factors, diagnosis and management. *Aust Dent J.* Jun 2010;55 Suppl 1:61-65.

[2] Rethman MP, Carpenter W, Cohen EE, et al. Evidence-based clinical recommendations regarding screening for oral squamous cell carcinomas. *J Am Dent Assoc.* 2010;141(5):509-520.

[3] Neville BW, Day TA. Oral cancer and precancerous lesions. *CA Cancer J Clin.* Jul-Aug 2002;52(4):195-215.

[4] Warnakulasuriya S. Causes of oral cancer--an appraisal of controversies. *Br Dent J.* Nov 28 2009;207(10):471-475.

[5] Lingen MW, Kalmar JR, Karrison T, Speight PM. Critical evaluation of diagnostic aids for the detection of oral cancer. *Oral Oncol.* Jan 2008;44(1):10-22.

[6] Brocklehurst PR, Baker SR, Speight PM. A qualitative study examining the experience of primary care dentists in the detection and management of potentially malignant lesions. 2. Mechanics of the referral and patient communication. *Br Dent J.* 2010;208(2):E4; discussion 74-75.

[7] Farah CS, McCullough MJ. Oral cancer awareness for the general practitioner: new approaches to patient care. *Aust Dent J.* 2008;53(1):2-10.

[8] Scott SE, Grunfeld EA, Main J, McGurk M. Patient delay in oral cancer: a qualitative study of patients' experiences. *Psychooncology.* 2006;15(6):474-485.

[9] van der Waal I, de Bree R, Brakenhoff R, Coebergh JW. Early diagnosis in primary oral cancer: is it possible? *Med Oral Patol Oral Cir Bucal.* 2011;1(16):e300-305.

[10] Peacock ZS, Pogrel MA, Schmidt BL. Exploring the reasons for delay in treatment of oral cancer. *J Am Dent Assoc.* 2008;139(10):1346-1352.

[11] McLeod NM, Saeed NR, Ali EA. Oral cancer: delays in referral and diagnosis persist. *Br Dent J.* 2005;198(11):681-684.

[12] Abdo EN, Garrocho Ade A, Barbosa AA, et al. Time elapsed between the first symptoms, diagnosis and treatment of oral cancer patients in Belo Horizonte, Brazil. *Med Oral Patol Oral Cir Bucal.* 2007;12(7):E469-473.

[13] Rogers SN. Quality of life perspectives in patients with oral cancer. *Oral Oncol.* 2010;46(6):445-447.

[14] LeHew CW, Epstein JB, Kaste LM, Choi YK. Assessing oral cancer early detection: clarifying dentists' practices. *J Public Health Dent.* 2010;70(2):93-100.

[15] Gao W, Guo CB. Factors related to delay in diagnosis of oral squamous cell carcinoma. *J Oral Maxillofac Surg.* 2009;67(5):1015-1020.

[16] Grant E, Silver K, Bauld L, Day R, Warnakulasuriya S. The experiences of young oral cancer patients in Scotland: symptom recognition and delays in seeking professional help. *Br Dent J.* 2010;208(10):465-471.

[17] Pitiphat W, Diehl SR, Laskaris G, Cartsos V, Douglass CW, Zavras AI. Factors associated with delay in the diagnosis of oral cancer. *J Dent Res.* 2002;81(3):192-197.

[18] Scott S, McGurk M, Grunfeld E. Patient delay for potentially malignant oral symptoms. *Eur J Oral Sci.* 2008;116(2):141-147.

[19] Scott SE, Grunfeld EA, Auyeung V, McGurk M. Barriers and triggers to seeking help for potentially malignant oral symptoms: implications for interventions. *J Public Health Dent.* 2009;69(1):34-40.

[20] Scott SE, Grunfeld EA, McGurk M. Patient's delay in oral cancer: A systematic review. *Community Dent Oral Epidemiol.* 2006;34(5):337-343.

[21] McGurk M, Scott SE. The reality of identifying early oral cancer in the general dental practice. *Br Dent J.* 2010;208(8):347-351.

[22] Brocklehurst PR, Baker SR, Speight PM. Factors which determine the referral of potentially malignant disorders by primary care dentists. *J Dent.* 2010;38(7):569-578.

[23] Wade J, Smith H, Hankins M, Llewellyn C. Conducting oral examinations for cancer in general practice: what are the barriers? *Fam Pract.* 2010;27(1):77-84.

[24] Brocklehurst P, Kujan O, Glenny AM, et al. Screening programmes for the early detection and prevention of oral cancer. *Cochrane Database Syst Rev.* 2010(11):CD004150.

[25] Speight PM, Palmer S, Moles DR, et al. The cost-effectiveness of screening for oral cancer in primary care. *Health Technol Assess.* Apr 2006;10(14):1-144, iii-iv.

[26] Conway DI, Petticrew M, Marlborough H, Berthiller J, Hashibe M, Macpherson LM. Socioeconomic inequalities and oral cancer risk: a systematic review and meta-analysis of case-control studies. *Int J Cancer.* Jun 15 2008;122(12):2811-2819.

[27] Fakhry C, Gillison ML. Clinical implications of human papillomavirus in head and neck cancers. *J Clin Oncol.* Jun 10 2006;24(17):2606-2611.

[28] Gillison ML, D'Souza G, Westra W, et al. Distinct risk factor profiles for human papillomavirus type 16-positive and human papillomavirus type 16-negative head and neck cancers. *J Natl Cancer Inst.* Mar 19 2008;100(6):407-420.

[29] Scott SE, Rizvi K, Grunfeld EA, McGurk M. Pilot study to estimate the accuracy of mouth self-examination in an at-risk group. *Head Neck.* Oct 2010;32(10):1393-1401.

[30] Elango KJ, Anandkrishnan N, Suresh A, Iyer SK, Ramaiyer SK, Kuriakose MA. Mouth self-examination to improve oral cancer awareness and early detection in a high-risk population. *Oral Oncol.* Jul 2011;47(7):620-624.

[31] Gomez I, Warnakulasuriya S, Varela-Centelles PI, et al. Is early diagnosis of oral cancer a feasible objective? Who is to blame for diagnostic delay? *Oral Dis.* 2010;16(4):333-342.

[32] Hertrampf K, Wenz HJ, Koller M, Wiltfang J. Public awareness about prevention and early detection of oral cancer: A population-based study in Northern Germany. *J Craniomaxillofac Surg.* May 16 2011;[Epub ahead of print].
[33] Elango KJ, Anandkrishnan N, Suresh A, Iyer SK, Ramaiyer SK, Kuriakose MA. Mouth self-examination to improve oral cancer awareness and early detection in a high-risk population. *Oral Oncol.* 2011;47(7):620-624.
[34] Humphris GM, Field EA. The immediate effect on knowledge, attitudes and intentions in primary care attenders of a patient information leaflet: a randomized control trial replication and extension. *Br Dent J.* 2003;194(12):683-688.
[35] Laronde DM, Bottorff JL, Hislop TG, et al. Voices from the community--experiences from the dental office: initiating oral cancer screening. *J Can Dent Assoc.* 2008;74(3):239-241.
[36] Newton JT. Reactions to cancer: communicating with patients, family and carers. *Oral Oncol.* 2010;46(6):442-444.
[37] Macpherson LM, McCann MF, Gibson J, Binnie VI, Stephen KW. The role of primary healthcare professionals in oral cancer prevention and detection. *Br Dent J.* 2003;195(5):277-281.
[38] Kao SY, Chu YW, Chen YW, Chang KW, Liu TY. Detection and screening of oral cancer and pre-cancerous lesions. *J Chin Med Assoc.* 2009;72(5):227-233.
[39] Rodgers J, Macpherson LM. General dental practitioners' perceptions of the West of Scotland Cancer Awareness Programme oral cancer campaign. *Br Dent J.* 2006;200(12):693-697.
[40] Scott SE, Weinman J, Grunfeld EA. Developing ways to encourage early detection and presentation of oral cancer: What do high-risk individuals think? *Psychol Health.* Jan 1 2011;[Epub ahead of print]:1-14.
[41] Kerdpon D, Sriplung H. Factors related to delay in diagnosis of oral squamous cell carcinoma in southern Thailand. *Oral Oncol.* 2001;37(2):127-131.
[42] Rogers SN, Vedpathak SV, Lowe D. Reasons for delayed presentation in oral and oropharyngeal cancer: the patients perspective. *Br J Oral Maxillofac Surg.* Jul 29 2010;[Epub ahead of print].
[43] Rogers SN, Lowe D, Catleugh M, Edwards D. An oral cancer awareness intervention in community pharmacy. *Br J Oral Maxillofac Surg.* 2010;48(7):498-502.
[44] Kato I, Neale AV. Does use of alternative medicine delay treatment of head and neck cancer? A surveillance, epidemiology, and end results (SEER) cancer registry study. *Head Neck.* 2008;30(4):446-454.
[45] Rogers SN, Pabla R, McSorley A, Lowe D, Brown JS, Vaughan ED. An assessment of deprivation as a factor in the delays in presentation, diagnosis and treatment in patients with oral and oropharyngeal squamous cell carcinoma. *Oral Oncol.* 2007;43(7):648-655.
[46] Watson JM, Logan HL, Tomar SL, Sandow P. Factors associated with early-stage diagnosis of oral and pharyngeal cancer. *Community Dent Oral Epidemiol.* 2009;37(4):333-341.
[47] Jovanovic A, Kostense PJ, Schulten EA, Snow GB, van der Waal I. Delay in diagnosis of oral squamous cell carcinoma; a report from The Netherlands. *Eur J Cancer B Oral Oncol.* 1992;28B(1):37-38.

[48] Wildt J, Bundgaard T, Bentzen SM. Delay in the diagnosis of oral squamous cell carcinoma. *Clin Otolaryngol Allied Sci.* 1995;20(1):21-25.
[49] Morelatto RA, Herrera MC, Fernandez EN, Corball AG, Lopez de Blanc SA. Diagnostic delay of oral squamous cell carcinoma in two diagnosis centers in Cordoba Argentina. *J Oral Pathol Med.* 2007;36(7):405-408.
[50] Hollows P, McAndrew PG, Perini MG. Delays in the referral and treatment of oral squamous cell carcinoma. *Br Dent J.* 2000;188(5):262-265.
[51] Brouha XDR, Tromp DM, Hordijk GJ, Winnubst JAM, de Leeuw JRJ. Oral and pharyngeal cancer: Analysis of patient delay at different tumor stages. *Head Neck-J Sci Spec.* 2005;27(11):939-945.
[52] Sargeran K, Murtomaa H, Safavi SM, Teronen O. Delayed diagnosis of oral cancer in Iran: challenge for prevention. *Oral Health Prev Dent.* 2009;7(1):69-76.
[53] Paleri V, Wight RG, Silver CE, et al. Comorbidity in head and neck cancer: a critical appraisal and recommendations for practice. *Oral Oncol.* 2010;46(10):712-719.
[54] Brouha X, Tromp D, Hordijk GJ, Winnubst J, De Leeuw R. Role of alcohol and smoking in diagnostic delay of head and neck cancer patients. *Acta Otolaryngol Orient.* 2005;125(5):552-556.
[55] Santos LC, Batista Ode M, Cangussu MC. Characterization of oral cancer diagnostic delay in the state of Alagoas. *Braz J Otorhinolaryngol.* 2010;76(4):416-422.
[56] Lopez-Jornet P, Camacho-Alonso F. New barriers in oral cancer. Patient accessibility to dental examination--A pilot study. *Oral Oncol.* 2006;42(10):1022-1025.
[57] Alho OP, Teppo H, Mantyselka P, Kantola S. Head and neck cancer in primary care: presenting symptoms and the effect of delayed diagnosis of cancer cases. *CMAJ.* 2006;174(6):779-784.
[58] Morse DE, Velez Vega CM, Psoter WJ, et al. Perspectives of San Juan healthcare practitioners on the detection deficit in oral premalignant and early cancers in Puerto Rico: a qualitative research study. *BMC Public Health.* 2011;11(1):391.
[59] Scott SE, McGurk M, Grunfeld EA. The process of symptom appraisal: cognitive and emotional responses to detecting potentially malignant oral symptoms. *J Psychosom Res.* 2007;62(6):621-630.
[60] Kujan O, Duxbury AJ, Glenny AM, Thakker NS, Sloan P. Opinions and attitudes of the UK's GDPs and specialists in oral surgery, oral medicine and surgical dentistry on oral cancer screening. *Oral Dis.* 2006;12(2):194-199.
[61] Brocklehurst PR, Baker SR, Speight PM. A qualitative study examining the experience of primary care dentists in the detection and management of potentially malignant lesions. 1. Factors influencing detection and the decision to refer. *Br Dent J.* 2010;208(2):E3; discussion 72-73.
[62] Scott SE, Grunfeld EA, McGurk M. The idiosyncratic relationship between diagnostic delay and stage of oral squamous cell carcinoma. *Oral Oncol.* 2005;41(4):396-403.
[63] Guggenheimer J, Verbin RS, Johnson JT, Horkowitz CA, Myers EN. Factors delaying the diagnosis of oral and oropharyngeal carcinomas. *Cancer.* 1989;64(4):932-935.
[64] Cruz GD, Ostroff JS, Kumar JV, Gajendra S. Preventing and detecting oral cancer. Oral health care providers' readiness to provide health behavior counseling and oral cancer examinations. *J Am Dent Assoc.* 2005;136(5):594-601.

[65] Mahalaha SA, Cheruvu VK, Smyth KA. Oral cancer screening: practices, knowledge, and opinions of dentists working in Ohio nursing homes. *Spec Care Dentist.* 2009;29(6):237-243.
[66] Klosa K, Wiltfang J, Wenz HJ, Koller M, Hertrampf K. Dentists' opinions and practices in oral cancer prevention and early detection in Northern Germany. *Eur J Cancer Prev.* 2011;20(4):313-319.
[67] Jaber L, Shaban S, Hariri D, Smith S. Perceptions of healthcare practitioners in Saudi Arabia regarding their training in oral cancer prevention, and early detection. *Int J Health Care Qual Assur.* 2011;24(1):8-18.
[68] Carter LM, Ogden GR. Oral cancer awareness of general medical and general dental practitioners. *Br Dent J.* 2007;203(5):E10; discussion 248-249.
[69] Afifah R, Schwarz E. Patient demand for smoking cessation advice in dentist offices after introduction of graphic health warnings in Australia. *Aust Dent J.* 2008;53(3):208-216.
[70] Amagasa T, Yamashiro M, Uzawa N. Oral premalignant lesions: from a clinical perspective. *Int J Clin Oncol.* 2011;16(1):5-14.
[71] Patton LL, Elter JR, Southerland JH, Strauss RP. Knowledge of oral cancer risk factors and diagnostic concepts among North Carolina dentists. Implications for diagnosis and referral. *J Am Dent Assoc.* 2005;136(5):602-610.
[72] Tromp DM, Brouha XD, Hordijk GJ, Winnubst JA, de Leeuw JR. Patient factors associated with delay in primary care among patients with head and neck carcinoma: a case-series analysis. *Fam Pract.* 2005;22(5):554-559.
[73] Dimitroulis G, Reade P, Wiesenfeld D. Referral patterns of patients with oral squamous cell carcinoma, Australia. *Eur J Cancer B Oral Oncol.* 1992;28B(1):23-27.
[74] Jensen AR, Nellemann HM, Overgaard J. Tumor progression in waiting time for radiotherapy in head and neck cancer. *Radiother Oncol.* 2007;84(1):5-10.
[75] Primdahl H, Nielsen AL, Larsen S, et al. Changes from 1992 to 2002 in the pretreatment delay for patients with squamous cell carcinoma of larynx or pharynx: a Danish nationwide survey from DAHANCA. *Acta Oncol.* 2006;45(2):156-161.
[76] Caudell JJ, Locher JL, Bonner JA. Diagnosis-to-treatment interval and control of locoregionally advanced head and neck cancer. *Arch Otolaryngol Head Neck Surg.* 2011;137(3):282-285.
[77] Anderson LM, Scrimshaw SC, Fullilove MT, Fielding JE, Normand J. Culturally competent healthcare systems. A systematic review. *Am J Prev Med.* Apr 2003;24(3 Suppl):68-79.
[78] Tsang A. *Oral Health Therapy Programs in Australia and New Zealand.* 1 ed: Robert T Watts; 2010.
[79] Brocklehurst PR, Baker SR, Speight PM. Oral cancer screening: what have we learnt and what is there still to achieve? *Future Oncol.* Feb 2010;6(2):299-304.
[80] Jullien JA, Downer MC, Zakrzewska JM, Speight PM. Evaluation of a screening test for the early detection of oral cancer and precancer. *Community Dent Health.* Mar 1995;12(1):3-7.
[81] Downer MC, Evans AW, Hughes Hallet CM, Jullien JA, Speight PM, Zakrzewska JM. Evaluation of screening for oral cancer and precancer in a company headquarters. *Community Dent Oral Epidemiol.* Apr 1995;23(2):84-88.

[82] Ikeda N, Downer MC, Ishii T, Fukano H, Nagao T, Inoue K. Annual screening for oral cancer and precancer by invitation to 60-year-old residents of a city in Japan. *Community Dent Health.* Sep 1995;12(3):133-137.

[83] Mathew B, Sankaranarayanan R, Sunilkumar KB, Kuruvila B, Pisani P, Nair MK. Reproducibility and validity of oral visual inspection by trained health workers in the detection of oral precancer and cancer. *Br J Cancer.* 1997;76(3):390-394.

[84] Downer MC, Moles DR, Palmer S, Speight PM. A systematic review of test performance in screening for oral cancer and precancer. *Oral Oncol.* Mar 2004;40(3):264-273.

[85] McIntosh L, McCullough MJ, Farah CS. The assessment of diffused light illumination and acetic acid rinse (Microlux/DL) in the visualisation of oral mucosal lesions. *Oral Oncol.* Dec 2009;45(12):e227-231.

[86] Identafi: How it works. 2010; http://www.identafi.net/identafi. Accessed 16 April, 2011.

[87] Thomson PJ. Field change and oral cancer: new evidence for widespread carcinogenesis? *Int J Oral Maxillofac Surg.* Jun 2002;31(3):262-266.

[88] Sankaranarayanan R, Ramadas K, Thomas G, et al. Effect of screening on oral cancer mortality in Kerala, India: a cluster-randomised controlled trial. *Lancet.* Jun 4-10 2005;365(9475):1927-1933.

[89] Cancela-Rodriguez P, Cerero-Lapiedra R, Esparza-Gomez G, Llamas-Martinez S, Warnakulasuriya S. The use of toluidine blue in the detection of pre-malignant and malignant oral lesions. *J Oral Pathol Med.* Apr 2011;40(4):300-304.

[90] Gray M, Gold L, Burls A, Elley K. *The clinical effectiveness of toluidine blue dye as an adjunct to oral cancer screening in general dental practice*2000.

[91] Epstein JB, Guneri P. The adjunctive role of toluidine blue in detection of oral premalignant and malignant lesions. *Curr Opin Otolaryngol Head Neck Surg.* Apr 2009;17(2):79-87.

[92] ViziLite Plus. http://www.zila.com/assets/file/ViziliteBlueTBlue630_0507.pdf. Accessed 16 April, 2011.

[93] Rosenberg D, Cretin S. Use of meta-analysis to evaluate tolonium chloride in oral cancer screening. *Oral Surg Oral Med Oral Pathol.* May 1989;67(5):621-627.

[94] Patton LL, Epstein JB, Kerr AR. Adjunctive techniques for oral cancer examination and lesion diagnosis: a systematic review of the literature. *J Am Dent Assoc.* Jul 2008;139(7):896-905; quiz 993-894.

[95] Allegra E, Lombardo N, Puzzo L, Garozzo A. The usefulness of toluidine staining as a diagnostic tool for precancerous and cancerous oropharyngeal and oral cavity lesions. *Acta Otorhinolaryngol Ital.* Aug 2009;29(4):187-190.

[96] Epstein JB, Feldman R, Dolor RJ, Porter SR. The utility of tolonium chloride rinse in the diagnosis of recurrent or second primary cancers in patients with prior upper aerodigestive tract cancer. *Head Neck.* Nov 2003;25(11):911-921.

[97] Epstein JB, Oakley C, Millner A, Emerton S, van der Meij E, Le N. The utility of toluidine blue application as a diagnostic aid in patients previously treated for upper oropharyngeal carcinoma. *Oral Surg Oral Med Oral Pathol Oral Radiol Endod.* May 1997;83(5):537-547.

[98] Mashberg A. Tolonium (toluidine blue) rinse--a screening method for recognition of squamous carcinoma. Continuing study of oral cancer IV. *JAMA.* Jun 19 1981;245(23):2408-2410.

[99] Onofre MA, Sposto MR, Navarro CM. Reliability of toluidine blue application in the detection of oral epithelial dysplasia and in situ and invasive squamous cell carcinomas. *Oral Surg Oral Med Oral Pathol Oral Radiol Endod.* May 2001;91(5):535-540.

[100] Warnakulasuriya KA, Johnson NW. Sensitivity and specificity of OraScan (R) toluidine blue mouthrinse in the detection of oral cancer and precancer. *J Oral Pathol Med.* Mar 1996;25(3):97-103.

[101] Zhang L, Williams M, Poh CF, et al. Toluidine blue staining identifies high-risk primary oral premalignant lesions with poor outcome. *Cancer Res.* Sep 1 2005;65(17):8017-8021.

[102] Guo Z, Yamaguchi K, Sanchez-Cespedes M, Westra WH, Koch WM, Sidransky D. Allelic losses in OraTest-directed biopsies of patients with prior upper aerodigestive tract malignancy. *Clin Cancer Res.* Jul 2001;7(7):1963-1968.

[103] Mashberg A. Reevaluation of toluidine blue application as a diagnostic adjunct in the detection of asymptomatic oral squamous carcinoma: a continuing prospective study of oral cancer III. *Cancer.* Aug 15 1980;46(4):758-763.

[104] Su WW, Yen AM, Chiu SY, Chen TH. A community-based RCT for oral cancer screening with toluidine blue. *J Dent Res.* Sep 2010;89(9):933-937.

[105] Farah CS, McCullough MJ. A pilot case control study on the efficacy of acetic acid wash and chemiluminescent illumination (ViziLite) in the visualisation of oral mucosal white lesions. *Oral Oncol.* Sep 2007;43(8):820-824.

[106] Oh ES, Laskin DM. Efficacy of the ViziLite system in the identification of oral lesions. *J Oral Maxillofac Surg.* Mar 2007;65(3):424-426.

[107] Ram S, Siar CH. Chemiluminescence as a diagnostic aid in the detection of oral cancer and potentially malignant epithelial lesions. *Int J Oral Maxillofac Surg.* Jul 2005;34(5):521-527.

[108] Microlux/DL. 2007; http://www.addent.com/docs/instructions/microlux-dl_english.pdf. Accessed 16 April, 2011.

[109] Orascoptic DK User Manual. http://www.orascoptic.com/cms-filesystem-action/manuals/um_ordk_old.pdf. Accessed 16 April, 2011.

[110] Huber MA, Bsoul SA, Terezhalmy GT. Acetic acid wash and chemiluminescent illumination as an adjunct to conventional oral soft tissue examination for the detection of dysplasia: a pilot study. *Quintessence Int.* May 2004;35(5):378-384.

[111] Kerr AR, Sirois DA, Epstein JB. Clinical evaluation of chemiluminescent lighting: an adjunct for oral mucosal examinations. *J Clin Dent.* 2006;17(3):59-63.

[112] Awan KH, Morgan PR, Warnakulasuriya S. Evaluation of an autofluorescence based imaging system (VELscope) in the detection of oral potentially malignant disorders and benign keratoses. *Oral Oncol.* Apr 2011;47(4):274-277.

[113] Mehrotra R, Singh M, Thomas S, et al. A cross-sectional study evaluating chemiluminescence and autofluorescence in the detection of clinically innocuous precancerous and cancerous oral lesions. *J Am Dent Assoc.* Feb 2010;141(2):151-156.

[114] Epstein JB, Gorsky M, Lonky S, Silverman S, Jr., Epstein JD, Bride M. The efficacy of oral lumenoscopy (ViziLite) in visualizing oral mucosal lesions. *Spec Care Dentist.* Jul-Aug 2006;26(4):171-174.

[115] Epstein JB, Silverman S, Jr., Epstein JD, Lonky SA, Bride MA. Analysis of oral lesion biopsies identified and evaluated by visual examination, chemiluminescence and toluidine blue. *Oral Oncol.* Jun 2008;44(6):538-544.

[116] Schwarz RA, Gao W, Daye D, Williams MD, Richards-Kortum R, Gillenwater AM. Autofluorescence and diffuse reflectance spectroscopy of oral epithelial tissue using a depth-sensitive fiber-optic probe. *Appl Opt.* Feb 20 2008;47(6):825-834.

[117] Lane PM, Gilhuly T, Whitehead P, et al. Simple device for the direct visualization of oral-cavity tissue fluorescence. *J Biomed Opt.* Mar-Apr 2006;11(2):024006.

[118] Poh CF, Zhang L, Anderson DW, et al. Fluorescence visualization detection of field alterations in tumor margins of oral cancer patients. *Clin Cancer Res.* Nov 15 2006;12(22):6716-6722.

[119] Scheer M, Neugebauer J, Derman A, Fuss J, Drebber U, Zoeller JE. Autofluorescence imaging of potentially malignant mucosa lesions. *Oral Surg Oral Med Oral Pathol Oral Radiol Endod.* May 2011;111(5):568-577.

[120] Farah CS, McIntosh L, Georgiou A, McCullough MJ. The efficacy of tissue autofluorescence imaging (VELScope) in the visualization of oral mucosal lesions. *Head Neck* 2011.

[121] Huff K, Stark PC, Solomon LW. Sensitivity of direct tissue fluorescence visualization in screening for oral premalignant lesions in general practice. *Gen Dent.* Jan-Feb 2009;57(1):34-38.

[122] Kois JC, Truelove E. Detecting oral cancer: a new technique and case reports. *Dent Today.* Oct 2006;25(10):94, 96-97.

[123] Poh CF, Ng SP, Williams PM, et al. Direct fluorescence visualization of clinically occult high-risk oral premalignant disease using a simple hand-held device. *Head Neck.* Jan 2007;29(1):71-76.

[124] Balevi B. Assessing the usefulness of three adjunctive diagnostic devices for oral cancer screening: a probabilistic approach. *Community Dent Oral Epidemiol.* Apr 2011;39(2):171-176.

[125] Roblyer D, Kurachi C, Stepanek V, et al. Objective detection and delineation of oral neoplasia using autofluorescence imaging. *Cancer Prev Res (Phila Pa).* May 2009;2(5):423-431.

[126] Vigneswaran N, Koh S, Gillenwater A. Incidental detection of an occult oral malignancy with autofluorescence imaging: a case report. *Head Neck Oncol.* 2009;1:37.

[127] Zuluaga AF, Vigneswaran N, Bradley RK, Gillenwater A, Nichols CM, Poh CF. Identafi®3000 ultra A multispectral tool for improved oral lesion evaluation. *Biomedical Optics.* Vol paper BSuD105. Miami, Florida: OSA Technical Digest (Optical Society of America); 2010.

[128] Rajaram N, Gopal A, Zhang X, Tunnell JW. Experimental validation of the effects of microvasculature pigment packaging on in vivo diffuse reflectance spectroscopy. *Lasers Surg Med.* Sep 2010;42(7):680-688.

5

A Literature Analysis of the Risk Factors for Oral Cancer

Shih-An Liu
National Yang-Ming University, Taichung Veterans General Hospital
Taiwan, R.O.C.

1. Introduction

Oral cancer is one of the top ten most common cancers in men. It is estimated that 190,000 new oral cavity cancer cases were diagnosed in 2008 worldwide with 83,000 deaths (Ferlay et al., 2010). In Taiwan, oral cancer has been one of the top 10 causes of death from cancer since 1991. According to the annual report from the Department of Health of the Executive Yuan, the death toll for oral cancer in males has been increasing at a surprising rate (Liu et al., 2006). Although advances in the treatment of oral cancers have been made in the last four decades, benefits have not been reflected in mortality figures. Therefore, primary prevention such as cessation of tobacco smoking and alcohol consumption along with early detection are necessary control procedures to improve the prognosis for oral cancer (Ramadas et al., 2003). However, it is crucial to identify relevant risk factors for contracting oral cancer before implementation of prevention programs. Here, we review the relevant literature and critically appraise the risk factors for contracting oral cancer.

2. Materials and methods

Web-based exploration of electronic resources was carried out to screen published literature. We searched for relevant articles (published up to May 2011) in the Medline/PubMed database. These searches included the use of free text and index terms, such as "risk factor", "oral cancer" and "head/neck cancer", in order to expand the number of potentially pertinent studies retrieved. Furthermore, we checked the relevant references cited in the retrieved articles for further studies to review. The levels of evidence and grades of recommendation of the cited studies are listed in Table 1. The process of article selection is summarized in Figure 1.

3. Risk factors for contracting oral cancer

All relevant risk factors in the literature are listed in Table 1. Further description of risk factors for oral cancer are discussed below.

3.1 Lifestyle factors

The etiology of oral cancer involves multiple factors and the most important are life style factors, such as cigarette smoking, alcohol consumption and betel quid chewing.

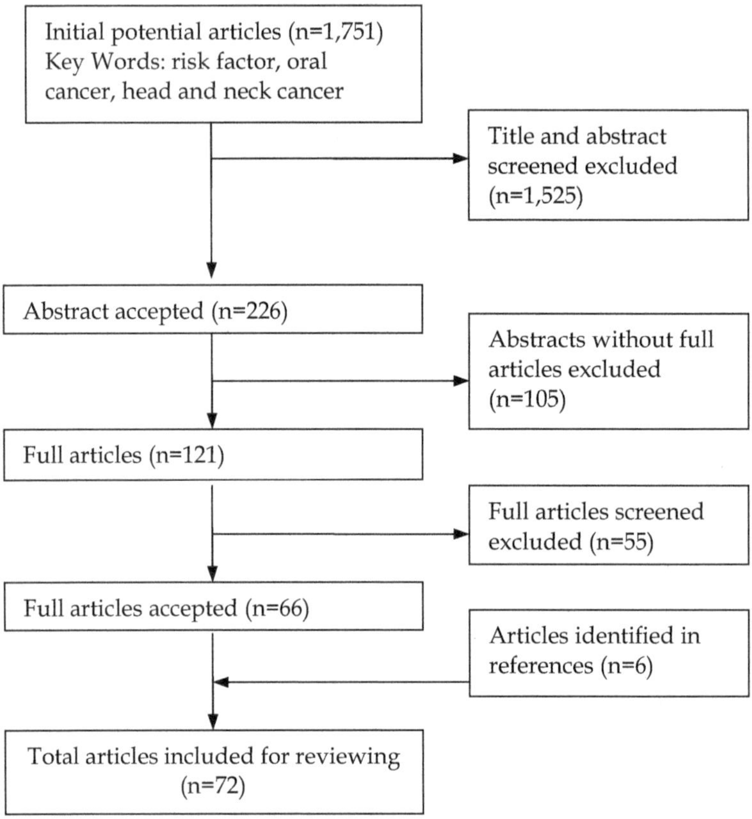

Fig. 1. Results of literatures search. The figure illustrates the whole process of searching for articles for inclusion in this review.

3.1.1 Tobacco smoking

Data from the National Cancer Institute's Surveillance, Epidemiology, and End Results (SEER) program revealed state-specific increases in oral cancer in United States. Further analysis indicated such states had comparatively higher percentages of smokers currently, as well as historically (Bunnell et al., 2010). It was estimated that a betel quid-chewing patient consumes 310,000 pieces of betel quid and a smoking patient consumes 14,000 packs of cigarettes before the diagnosis of oral cavity cancer on average. Besides, betel quid chewer and cigarette smoker were more prone to be diagnosed with oral cavity cancer at a younger age than abstainers (Tsai et al., 2009). Furthermore, heavy smoker were not only more likely to be diagnosed at a younger age but also at an advanced stage. Apart from active smoking, patients who were exposed to passive smoke were also found to have higher odds ratios (1.62 ~ 2.46) for contracting oral cavity and oropharynx cancers in a hospital-based case control study (Lee et al., 2009). The odds ratios or relative risks for contracting oral cancer among cigarette smoker, alcohol drinkers, or betel quid chewers are summarized in Table 2.

Risk factors	Grade of recommendation	Level of evidence
Lifestyle factors		
Cigarette smoking	A ~ B	1c ~ 3b
Alcoholic consumption	B	2b ~ 3b
Betel quid chewing	B	2b ~ 3b
Genetic factors	B	2b ~ 3b
Infectious factors	B	3a ~ 3b
Environmental factors	B	2b ~ 3b
Dietary factors	B	2b ~ 3b
Socio-economic factors	B	3a ~ 3b
Ethnicity and race	B	2b ~ 3b
Others	B	2b ~ 3a

Table 1. Relevant risk factors for contracting oral cancer in the literature

Variable	Odds ratios or Relative risk (95% CI[a])	Study design	Reference
Smoking			
Cigarette smoking	8.4 (3.5 ~ 20.4)	Case-control	Ko et al., 1995
Current smoker	6.41 (3.32 ~ 12.37)	Case-control	Castellsagué et al., 2004
Habitual smoker	4.65 (2.74 ~ 7.89)	Cohort	Yen et al., 2008
> 30 pack-years	2.9 (1.8 ~ 4.5)	Case-control	Smith et al., 2010
Smoker	1.68 (1.00 ~ 2.81)	Case-control	Ihsan et al., 2011
Bidi smoking	2.6 (1.4 ~ 4.9)	Cohort	Jayalekshmi et al., 2011
> 40 pack-years[b]	8.46 (6.22 ~ 11.50)	Case-control	Lee et al., 2011
>= 60 pack-years	10.1 (6.1 ~ 16.7)	Case-control	Lubin et al., 2010
Former smoker[b]	5.49 (4.06 ~ 7.41)	Case-control	Szymanska et al., 2011
Alcohol			
Alcohol drinking	3.2 (1.8 ~ 5.6)	Case-control	Ko et al., 1995
Current drinker	3.46 (1.88 ~ 6.35)	Case-control	Castellsagué et al., 2004
Habitual drinker	0.95 (0.29 ~ 3.11)	Cohort	Yen et al., 2008
>= 30 grams per day[c]	1.92 (1.08 ~ 3.40)	Cohort	Shanmugham et al., 2010
> 21 drinks per week[d]	4.8 (2.8 ~ 8.3)	Case-control	Smith et al., 2010
Alcohol consumption	1.71 (1.20 ~ 2.44)	Case-control	Li et al., 2011
Alcohol drinker[b]	4.62 (3.39 ~ 6.28)	Case-control	Szymanska et al., 2011
Betel quid			
Betel chewing	8.5 (4.4 ~ 16.2)	Case-control	Ko et al., 1995
Habitual chewer	10.97 (3.22 ~ 37.34)	Cohort	Yen et al., 2008
Chewer	12.52 (5.45 ~ 28.77)	Cohort	Wen et al., 2010
Chewer	1.85 (1.02 ~ 3.33)	Case-control	Ihsan et al., 2011

All use abstainers as reference group

[a] CI: confidence interval

[b] Including oral cavity and oropharynx patients

[c] Women only

[d] One drink was equivalent to a 12-oz can or a bottle of beer, 4 oz glass of wine, or 1.5 oz shot of hard liquor

Table 2. The association of smoking, alcoholic consumption and betel quid chewing and the risk of contracting oral cavity cancer

Tobacco contains N-nitroso compounds which are well-known carcinogens. In addition, cigarette smoke condensate has the capacity to activate nuclear factor kappa-B in squamous cell lines. Nuclear factor kappa-B is a transcription factor and has been implicated in the regulation of many proinflammatory pathways, which might be one mechanism leading to carcinogenesis (Rohrer et al., 2010). Other tobacco-generated carcinogens include tobacco-specific nitrosamines (TSNAs, e.g. NNN, NNK, NAT and NAB), and free radicals that can inhibit antioxidant enzymes (such as, glutathione-S-transferase, glutathione reductase, superoxide dismutase, catalase, and glutathione peroxidase) (Scully, 2011). This specific antioxidant enzyme activity loss renders the oral epithelial cells more vulnerable to the harmful effects of both thiocyanate ions and hydroxyl free radicals produced by residual H_2O_2 in the presence of salivary redox-active metal ions. It has been demonstrated that thiocyanate ions and free radicals may adversely react with DNA, thus paving the way for progression of oral cancer (Reznick et al., 2003).

3.1.2 Alcohol consumption

Although alcoholic consumption is often cited as a known risk factor of oral cavity cancer (Altieri et al., 2004; Scully, 2011; Szymańska et al., 2011), some studies did find alcohol was not associated with an elevated risk of oral cavity cancer (Takács et al., 2011; Yen et al., 2008). One possible explanation for the seeming contradiction may be that different studies defined alcohol consumption differently. Also, not all studies collected quantitative data on alcoholic consumption. Furthermore, the different alcohol-drinking profiles of various regions made the comparisons among studies more complicated. On the other hand, a previous case control study found a lower risk of oral cavity cancer in postmenopausal women with moderate alcoholic consumption (Takács et al., 2011). The beneficial systemic changes, namely the increased insulin sensitivity and elevated estrogen levels may explain the protective effects in these latter groups of cases.

Ethanol may work as a carcinogenic initiator or as a promoter that enhances permeability of cells to other environmental carcinogens, such as cigarette smoke. Ethanol is oxidized to acetaldehyde mostly through alcohol dehydrogenase and, to a lesser extent, cytochrome P450 enzymes in chronic drinkers (Lubin et al., 2009). Acetaldehyde is classified as "carcinogenic to humans" (IARC Group 1) by the International Agency for Research on Cancer (IARC) (Lachenmeier et al., 2011). Acetaldehyde not only induces DNA-protein cross-linking and DNA interstrand cross-linking, but also interferes with DNA repair mechanism by inhibiting repair enzyme. Apart from alcoholic consumption, acetaldehyde may also be produced by oral bacterial flora in patients with poor dentition or poor oral hygiene (Homann et al., 2000). A previous study found that short-term salivary acetaldehyde increased due to direct exposure to alcoholic beverages (Lachenmeier et al., 2011). This may suggest a possible mechanism to explain the greater risk for oral cavity cancer associated with alcoholic consumption.

3.1.3 Betel quid chewing

Betel quid is one of the most commonly used psychoactive substances. It has been estimated that there are 600 million betel quid chewers worldwide (Wen et al., 2010). People who chew betel quid but do not smoke cigarettes or consume alcohol were reported to have an odds ratio of 10.97 (95% confidence interval: 3.22-37.34) for contracting oral cancer (Yen et al.,

2008). Another case-control study found betel quid chewer had an odds ratio of 6.9 (95% confidence interval: 3.1-15.2) for developing oral cancer after adjustment for smoking and drinking alcohol (Ko et al., 1995).

Arecoline, the major alkaloid of areca nut, has been known to induce cytotoxicity and genotoxicity in various systems (Lin et al., 2011). It is also mutagenic in both bacteria and mammalian cells (Chang et al., 2001). Arecoline was found to inhibit P53, repress DNA repair, and trigger DNA damage response in human epithelial cells via an *in-vitro* study (Tsai et al., 2008). Chewing betel quid induces local irritation and trauma in the oral mucosa, leading to chronic inflammation, oxidative stress, and cytokine production, and the traumatic wound offers easier access to the system for carcinogens contained in betel quid (Wen et al., 2010). Betel quid chewing not only causes genomic instability, but also has a close relationship with cell-mediated immunity, which could play a role in the malignant transformation of oral mucosa (Yen et al., 2008).

3.1.4 Synergistic effect

Many studies have found that there is a synergic effect of cigarette smoking, alcoholic consumption, and betel quid chewing in carcinogenesis of oral cavity mucosa (Castellsagué et al., 2004; Chang et al., 2001; Ko et al., 1995; Szymańska et al., 2011; Wen et al., 2010; Yen et al., 2008). Patients who smoked and also consumed alcohol had an odds ratio of 9.03 for contracting oral cavity cancers, whereas patients who only smoke or only consumed alcohol had odds ratios of 4.65 and 0.95, respectively when compared with abstainers (Yen et al., 2008). *In vitro*, the addition of extracellular nicotine worked synergistically on the arecoline-induced cytotoxicity and this may partially explain why those who chew betel quid and smoke cigarette are at great risk of contracting oral cancer (Chang et al., 2001).

3.2 Genetic factors

Genetic instability, either spontaneous or mutagen induced, has been regarded as a predisposing factor for neoplastic transformation (Patel et al., 2010). Cancer is the result of DNA mutations occurring spontaneously and from the action of different mutagens. A sequence of genetic changes leads finally to loss of growth control and immortality (Scully, 2011). Together with these changes are mechanisms that metabolise carcinogens, repair DNA damage, control growth, and defend the human body against cancer. The development from an ordinary healthy cell to a pre-malignant or a potentially malignant cell is called oncogenesis (carcinogenesis). The level of chromatin breaks induced by a mutagen challenge may serve as an indicator of an individual's capacity to repair damaged DNA. A previous study showed that mean level of chromosomal aberrations was higher in oral cancer patients when compared with that of healthy controls (Patel et al., 2010). A dose relationship between lifetime tobacco exposure and chromosomal aberrations was also found in aforementioned study. Apart from healthy tissues, genomic imbalances in premalignant lesion tissues also had a strong association with malignant transformation (Garnis et al., 2009).

3.2.1 Epidermal growth factor receptor

The epidermal growth factor receptor (EGFR) is the cell-surface receptor for members of the epidermal growth factor family (EGF-family) of extracellular protein ligands. Increased or aberrant expression of the EGFR or its ligands may lead to many processes important for tumor growth, including cell proliferation, survival, angiogenesis, invasion, and metastasis (Janmaat & Giaccone, 2003). A pervious study investigating EGFR gene in oral premalignant lesion specimens found that increased EGFR gene copy number was associated with higher risk of oral cancer (Taoudi Benchekroun et al., 2010). Other studies found significant increases in EGFR copy number and EGFR immuno-reactivity in oral squamous cell carcinoma patients when compared with long-term betel quid chewers, or compared with matched adjacent oral mucosa (Chiang et al., 2008).

3.2.2 P53

P53 is one of the most important tumor suppressor genes. Tumor suppressor genes work normally in cellular growth control by regulating the cell cycle, apoptosis, cell adhesion, and DNA repair. Silencing of tumor suppressor genes occurs in carcinogenesis. P53 mutation was also found to have an association with tobacco smoking and alcohol drinking. Inactivation of P53 by mutations is a critical molecular event in the upper aero-digestive tract carcinogenesis (Szymańska et al., 2010). Alteration of P53 expression is related to increased genomic instability in oral intraepithelial neoplasia and may accelerate the genetic modifications during oral tumorigenesis (Lippman et al., 2005). P53 codon72 polymorphism was found to be associated with a higher risk for contracting oral cancer (Kuroda et al., 2007).

3.2.3 Gene polymorphisms

Single nucleotide polymorphisms (SNPs) are genes areas that have altered DNA sequences which may not induce an aminoacid modification, or misrepresented DNA sequences that do not seem to have the potential for any unfavorable consequence in healthy people but may be markers for tendency to contract diseases (Scully & Petti, 2010). Certain genetic polymorphisms associated with enzymes for alcohol metabolism, such as, alcohol dehydrogenase genes and cytochrome P450 genes, are related to a greater risk of contracting oral squamous cell carcinoma. Besides, this risk is proportional to the amount of alcohol consumption (Marichalar-Mendia et al., 2010). Previous studies found hypoxia inducible factor-1 alpha gene polymorphisms C1722T and G1790A were associated with an increased risk of contracting oral cancer (Chen et al., 2009; Shieh et al., 2010). SNPs of the vascular endothelial growth factor gene were reported to have an association with development of oral cancer. The +936 T allele and the -2578 C/A SNP were expressed significantly more often in peripheral blood samples from oral squamous cell carcinoma patients when compared with those from healthy controls (Kämmerer et al., 2010). In a meta-analysis of case-control study, Arg194Trp polymorphism in the X-ray repair cross-complementing group 1 gene was significantly associated with oral cancer in an Asian population (Zhou et al., 2009).

3.2.4 Others

Promoter methylation of human MutL homolog1 (hMLH1) was found in 76% of oral squamous cell carcinoma patients but in none of the healthy control samples. The hMLH1 gene belongs to the human DNA mismatch repair system and is essential in reducing the accumulation of mutations and maintaining genomic stability (González-Ramírez et al., 2011).

3.3 Infectious factors

Infection can be induced by bacteria, fungus, and virus. Periodontal disease has been shown to increase the risk of oral cancer. This chronic infection and resultant low-grade systemic inflammatory response along with oxidative stress may be one possible pathway of carcinogenesis (Gasche et al., 2011). Also, the oral ecological shifts accompanying periodontal disease are characterized by proliferation of ketone-producing and nitrate-reducing microorganisms, which may contribute to increases in carcinogen concentrations (Divaris et al., 2010). Furthermore, several oral microorganisms can produce carcinogenic acetaldehyde from alcohol (Homann et al., 2000). This may explain why poor oral hygiene is associated with oral cancer. A case-control study conducted in Japan found that frequent toothbrushing could reduce the risk of upper aerodigestive tract cancer, especially in those who are heavy smokers and drinkers (Sato et al., 2011).

Candida albicans is the yeast most commonly isolated from the oral cavity. *Candida* may invade oral epithelium and may be causally involved in dysplastic change. Nitrosamines produced by *Candida* may activate specific proto-oncogens. *Candida* can also efficiently convert ethanol into carcinogenic acetaldehyde (Scully, 2011).

Presently, more than 100 types of human papilloma viruses (HPV) have been identified. HPV-16 and HPV-18 are the most common virus types identified in oral carcinoma. Two meta-analyses found HPV is an independent risk factor for oral and oropharyngeal carcinoma (Dayyani et al., 2010; Hobbs et al., 2006). Two proteins of HPV, E6 and E7, are thought to be involved in the carcinogenesis of oral cancer. The E6 protein can bind to the cellular P53 protein and this leads to the breakdown and reduction in concentration of P53 in the cancer cell. As a consequence, the damaged cancer cells lose their ability to repair DNA and cannot undergo apoptosis. The E7 protein has the ability to bind the cellular RB protein, releasing transcription factors, which are then free to transactivate the expression of other cellular proteins (Shillitoe, 2009). A previous study has showed a combination of herpes simplex virus seropositivity and a history of smoking was associated with a higher risk of oral cancer than would be expected from a purely additive effect (Starr et al., 2001), However, the nature of the herpes simplex virus genome makes it difficult to generate specific probes and the possible sequences that were detected have not been identified (Shillitoe, 2009).

3.4 Environmental factors

3.4.1 Sunlight

In Denmark, a population-based case-control study found that individuals who were employed in outdoor work for more than 10 years had a 1.67-fold (95% confidence interval 1.38 ~ 2.03) increased risk of contracting lip cancer (Kenborg et al., 2010). The lower lip receives more direct sunlight than the upper lip. Therefore, lip cancer tends to develop in lower lip. However, it is interesting to note that the basal cell cancer and cutaneous malignant melanoma were less prevalent in outdoor workers in aforementioned study.

3.4.2 Heavy metals

Heavy metals are extremely persistent in the environment and can induce unfavorable consequences on human body. Heavy metals are incorporated into food crops grown in the soils, and subsequently find their way into the human body following the consumption of such contaminated food items. The IARC classifies many heavy metals, such as arsenic (As), chromium (Cr), and nickel (Ni), as human carcinogens (Chiang et al., 2010). In an observational study conducted in Taiwan, the incidence of oral cancer was geographically associated with the concentrations of As and Ni in the patients' residential areas (Su et al., 2010). Blood levels of Ni and Cr in oral cancer patients were 1.6 and 1.4 times higher, respectively, than those of healthy controls in a case-control study. Individuals with high Ni blood level had a 16-fold higher relative risk of contracting oral cancer than those with low Ni blood level. Also, people with high Cr blood level had a 7-fold higher relative risk of contracting oral cancer than those with low Cr blood level (Yuan et al., 2011). The role of heavy metals in the mechanism of development of oral cancer warrants further investigation.

3.5 Dietary factors

It is interesting to find that caffeinated coffee drinking was inversely related with the risk of oral cavity cancer (odds ratio: 0.96, 95% confidence interval: 0.94 ~ 0.98) in a pooled case-control study (Galeone et al., 2010). In addition, people who had a dietary pattern of animal product consumption had a greater risk of developing oral cancer (odds ratio: 1.56, 95% confidence interval: 1.13-2.15) (Edefonti et al., 2010). Moreover, women with low folate intake had a higher risk of developing oral cancer if they also consumed a high amount of alcohol (Shanmugham et al., 2010). On the other hand, a traditional Mediterranean diet was found to reduce the risk of upper aerodigestive tract cancers in a case-control study conducted in Greece (Samoli et al., 2010). Intake of citrus fruit was also reported to lower the risk of developing oral cancer (Foschi et al., 2010). Although some studies showed that the Mediterranean-type diet and vegetable rich diet could reduce the risk of oral cancer, the evidence is still weak. The effect of individual food components and trace elements on carcinogenesis remains unclear (Meurman, 2010).

3.6 Socio-economic factors

There was a significant increase in the incidence of head and neck cancer including oral cancer in people with low level of education (odds ratios: 1.85 ~ 5.3) and lower income patients (odds ratios: 1.7 ~ 2.41) (Boing et al., 2011; Conway et al., 2008; Johnson et al., 2010; Madani et al., 2010; Swaminathan et al., 2009). Although there was a strong association between smoking/alcohol consumption and socioeconomic status, individuals with lower education level, lower income, lower occupational status/social class, and those performing manual labor still had a higher risk of contracting head and neck cancer including oral cancer after adjusting for smoking and alcohol consumption (Boing et al., 2011; Conway et al., 2008). Possible explanations includes, limited access to health care and health information, exposure to harmful physical environments and agents, and stresses caused by job insecurity or unemployment, and so on (Conway et al., 2008).

3.7 Ethnicity and race

The incidence rates of oral cancer vary considerably across racial/ethnic groups worldwide (Warnakulasuriya, 2009a). South Asians have higher incidence rates of oral cancer than people from most other countries. Black males in the United States have higher rates of oropharyngeal cancer than white males (Warnakulasuriya, 2009b). However, such results could be confounded by nutritional difference, smoking pattern, differences in the amounts of cigarettes smoked or alcohol consumed, and interaction among smoking, alcohol consumption, and betel quid chewing.

3.8 Others

A previous study about the development of secondary solid tumors after allogeneic hematopoietic bone marrow transplant in Japan found that the risk for developing oral cavity cancer among those who had received such a transplant was 35.25-fold (95% confidence interval: 17.59 ~ 63.06) higher than that of the age- and sex-adjusted general population (Yokota et al., 2011). Body mass index gain was inversely associated with upper aero-digestive tract cancers including oral cancer in a large scale, prospective, multi-center study in European countries. It was speculated that this phenomenon might be due to other confounding factors, including interactions of body fat distribution with smoking and/or drinking, biological mechanisms, indication of early tumor development or other related carcinogenic mechanisms (Lubin et al., 2010; Park et al., 2011). A retrospective study found a significant association between chronic trauma of oral mucosa and oral cancer after adjusting for confounding factors, such as smoking and alcohol consumption (Piemonte et al., 2010). Sexual behaviors, such as more frequent sexual partners and oral sex were also reported to be associated with increased risk of oral cancer (Heck et al., 2010). However, such results may be confounded by HPV infection status.

3.9 Controversial risk factors

Although some studies found that heredity/familial risk, marijuana (cannabis) smoking, khat (qat) chewing, nicotine replacement therapy, human immunodeficiency virus infection, and alcohol in mouthwashes were linked with higher risk of developing oral cancer, these results are controversial and further investigation is still needed to elucidate the relationship between aforementioned factors and oral cancer (Warnakulasuriya, 2009b).

4. Prevention of oral cancer

A majority of people are at greater risks of developing oral cancer as a result of exposure to tobacco and/or alcohol or betel quid. It is estimated that a billion men and 250 million women smoke cigarettes, 2 billion people consume alcohol, and 600-1,200 million people chew betel quid worldwide (Scully, 2011). Therefore, oral cancer is largely preventable by lifestyle modification. A previous study found at least three-quarters of oral cancers could be avoided by the elimination of unsafe lifestyles such as cigarette smoking and alcoholic consumption. Smoking cessation contributes to decreased risk of oral cancers, with 35% decrease in risk within 1-4 years and 80% decrease of risk by 20 years, reaching the level of those who have never smoked lifelong non-smokers (Marron et al., 2010).

The most frequently used screening method for oral cancer is visual and physical examination of oral mucosa. Many studies have demonstrated that such screening programs could detect potentially malignant and malignant lesions at very early stages. However, there is still not enough concrete evidence to conclude if screening alters disease-specific mortality in asymptomatic person seeking dental care (Rethman, et al., 2010).

Although the use of non-steroid anti-inflammatory drugs (NSAID) has been associated with a reduced risk of developing several types of cancer, no definite conclusion or consensus has been reached on the effect of NSAIDs on head and neck cancer risk. Further large-scale studies are mandatory to elucidate possible relationships between NSAIDs and head and neck cancer (Wilson et al., 2011).

5. Conclusion

Recognition of relevant risk factors for oral cancer can help physician to identify those patients at greater risk of developing oral cancer. Besides, it can help health authorities to implement effective programs to prevent oral cancer. Furthermore, it is important to educate the public about the relevant risk factors of contracting oral cancer so that those with unhealthy habits can modify their lifestyles.

6. References

Altieri, A. et al. (2004). Wine, beer and spirits and risk of oral and pharyngeal cancer: a case-control study from Italy and Switzerland. *Oral Oncology*, Vol.40, No.9, pp. 904-909, ISSN 1368-8375

Boing, AF. et al. (2011). How much do smoking and alcohol consumption explain socioeconomic inequalities in head and neck cancer risk? *Journal of Epidemiology and Community Health*, Vol.65, No.8, pp. 709-714, ISSN 0143-005X

Bunnell, A. et al. (2010). Analysis of primary risk factors for oral cancer from select US states with increasing rates. *Tobacco Induced Diseases*, Vol. 8, No. 1, pp. 5, ISSN 2070-7266

Castellsagué, X. et al. (2004). The role of type of tobacco and type of alcoholic beverage in oral carcinogenesis. *International Journal of Cancer*, Vol.108, No.5, pp. 741-749, ISSN 0020-7136

Chang, YC. et al. (2001). Synergistic effects of nicotine on arecoline-induced cytotoxicity in human buccal mucosal fibroblasts. *Journal of Oral Pathology & Medicine*, Vol. 30, No. 8, pp. 458-464, ISSN 0904-2512

Chen, MK. et al. (2009). The association between hypoxia inducible factor-1alpha gene polymorphisms and increased susceptibility to oral cancer. *Oral Oncology*, Vol.45, No.12, pp. e222-e226, ISSN 1368-8375

Chiang, CT. et al. (2010). Spatiotemporal trends in oral cancer mortality and potential risks associated with heavy metal content in Taiwan soil. *International Journal of Environmental Research and Public Health*, Vol.7, No.11, pp. 3916-3928, ISSN 1661-7827

Chiang, WF. et al. (2008). Association of epidermal growth factor receptor (EGFR) gene copy number amplification with neck lymph node metastasis in areca-associated oral carcinomas. *Oral Oncology*, Vol.44, No.3, pp. 270-276, ISSN 1368-8375

Conway, DI. et al. (2008). Socioeconomic inequalities and oral cancer risk: a systematic review and meta-analysis of case-control studies. International Journal of Cancer, Vol.122, No.12, pp. 2811-2819, ISSN 0020-7136

Dayyani, F. et al. (2010). Meta-analysis of the impact of human papillomavirus (HPV) on cancer risk and overall survival in head and neck squamous cell carcinomas (HNSCC). *Head & Neck Oncology*, Vol.2, pp.15, ISSN 1758-3284

Divaris, K. et al. (2010). Oral health and risk for head and neck squamous cell carcinoma: the Carolina Head and Neck Cancer Study. *Cancer Causes Control*, Vol.21, No.4, pp. 567-575, ISSN 0957-5243

Edefonti, V. et al. (2010). Nutrient-based dietary patterns and the risk of oral and pharyngeal cancer. Oral Oncology, Vol.46, No.5, pp. 343-348, ISSN 1368-8375

Ferlay, J. et al. (2010). Estimates of worldwide burden of cancer in 2008: GLOBOCAN 2008. *International Journal of Cancer*, Vol.127, No.12, pp. 2893–2917, ISSN 0020-7136

Foschi, R. et al. (2010). Citrus fruit and cancer risk in a network of case-control studies. *Cancer Causes Control*, Vol.21, No.2, pp. 237-242, ISSN 0957-5243

Galeone, C. et al. (2010). Coffee and tea intake and risk of head and neck cancer: pooled analysis in the international head and neck cancer epidemiology consortium. *Cancer Epidemiology, Biomarkers & Prevention*, Vol.19, No.7, pp. 1723-1736, ISSN 1055-9965

Garnis, C. et al. (2009). Genomic imbalances in precancerous tissues signal oral cancer risk. *Molecular cancer*, Vol.8, pp. 50, doi: 10.1186/1476-4598-8-50, ISSN 1476-4598

Gasche, JA. et al. (2011). Interleukin-6 promotes tumorigenesis by altering DNA methylation in oral cancer cells. *International Journal of Cancer*, Vol.129, No.5, pp. 1053-1063, ISSN 0020-7136

González-Ramírez, I. et al. (2011). hMLH1 promoter methylation is an early event in oral cancer. *Oral Oncology*, Vol.47, No.1, pp. 22-26, ISSN 1368-8375

Heck, JE. et al. (2010). Sexual behaviours and the risk of head and neck cancers: a pooled analysis in the International Head and Neck Cancer Epidemiology (INHANCE) consortium. *International Journal of Epidemiology*, Vol.39, No.1, pp. 166-181, ISSN 0300-5771

Hobbs, CG. et al. (2006). Human papillomavirus and head and neck cancer: a systematic review and meta-analysis. *Clinical Otolaryngology*, Vol.31, No.4, pp. 259-266, ISSN 1749-4478

Homann, N. et al. (2000). Increased salivary acetaldehyde levels in heavy drinkers and smokers: a microbiological approach to oral cavity cancer. *Carcinogenesis*, Vol.21, No.4, pp. 663-668, ISSN 0143-3334

Ihsan, R. et al. (2011). Investigation on the role of p53 codon 72 polymorphism and interactions with tobacco, betel quid, and alcohol in susceptibility to cancers in a high-risk population from North East India. *DNA and Cell Biology*, Vol.30, No.3, pp. 163-171, ISSN 1044-5498

Janmaat ML. & Giaccone G. (2003). Small-molecule epidermal growth factor receptor tyrosine kinase inhibitors. *The Oncologist*, Vol.8, No.6, pp. 576-86, ISSN 1083-7159

Jayalekshmi, PA. et al. (2011). Oral cavity cancer risk in relation to tobacco chewing and bidi smoking among men in Karunagappally, Kerala, India: Karunagappally cohort study. *Cancer Science*, Vol.102, No.2, pp. 460-467, ISSN 1347-9032

Johnson, S. et al. (2010). Socio-economic status and head and neck cancer incidence in Canada: a case-control study. *Oral Oncology*, Vol.46, No.3, pp. 200-203, ISSN 1368-8375

Kämmerer, PW. et al. (2010). Single nucleotide polymorphisms of the vascular endothelial growth factor gene associated with incidence of oral squamous cell carcinoma. *Journal of Oral Pathology & Medicine*, Vol.39, No.10, pp. 786-792, ISSN 0904-2512

Kenborg, L. et al. (2010). Occupational exposure to the sun and risk of skin and lip cancer among male wage earners in Denmark: a population-based case-control study. *Cancer Causes & Control,* Vol.21, No.8, pp. 1347-1355, ISSN 0957-5243

Ko, YC. et al. (1995). Betel quid chewing, cigarette smoking and alcohol consumption related to oral cancer in Taiwan. *Journal of Oral Pathology & Medicine,* Vol.24, No.10, pp. 450-453, ISSN 0904-2512

Kuroda, Y. et al. (2007). Association between the TP53 codon72 polymorphism and oral cancer risk and prognosis. *Oral Oncology,* Vol.43, No.10, pp. 1043-1048, ISSN 1368-8375

Lachenmeier, DW. & Monakhova, YB. (2011). Short-term salivary acetaldehyde increase due to direct exposure to alcoholic beverages as an additional cancer risk factor beyond ethanol metabolism. *Journal of experimental & clinical cancer research,* Vol.30, No.1, pp. 3, ISSN 0392-9078

Lee, YC. et al. (2009). Active and involuntary tobacco smoking and upper aerodigestive tract cancer risks in a multicenter case-control study. *Cancer epidemiology, biomarkers & prevention,* Vol.18, No.12, pp. 3353-3361, ISSN 1055-9965

Li, Y.; Yang, H. & Cao, J. (2011). Association between alcohol consumption and cancers in the Chinese population – A systematic review and meta-analysis. *PloS ONE,* Vol.6, No.4, pp. e18776, ISSN 1932-6203

Lippman, SM.; Sudbo, J. & Hong, WK. (2005) Oral cancer prevention and the evolution of molecular-targeted drug development. *Journal of Clinical Oncology,* Vol.23, No.2, pp. 346-356, ISSN 0732-183X

Liu, SA. et al. (2006). Nutritional factors and survival of oral cancer patients. *Head & Neck,* Vol.28, No.11, pp. 998-1007, ISSN 1043-3074

Lubin, JH. et al. (2009). Total exposure and exposure rate effects for alcohol and smoking and risk of head and neck cancer: a pooled analysis of case-control studies. *American Journal of Epidemiology,* Vol.170, No.8, pp. 937-947, ISSN 0002-9262

Lubin, JH. et al. (2010). Body mass index, cigarette smoking, and alcohol consumption and cancers of the oral cavity, pharynx, and larynx: modeling odds ratios in pooled case-control data. American Journal of Epidemiology, Vol.171, N0.12, pp. 1250-1261, ISSN 0002-9262

Madani, AH. et al. (2010). Relationship between Selected Socio-Demographic Factors and Cancer of Oral Cavity - A Case Control Study. *Cancer Informatics,* Vol.11, No.9, pp. 163-168, ISSN 1176-9351

Marichalar-Mendia, X. et al. (2010). Oral cancer and polymorphism of ethanol metabolising genes. *Oral Oncology,* Vol.46, No.1, pp. 9-13, ISSN 1368-8375

Marron, M. et al. (2010). Cessation of alcohol drinking, tobacco smoking and the reversal of head and neck cancer risk. *International Journal of Epidemiology,* Vol.39, No.1, pp. 182-196, ISSN 0300-5771

Meurman, JH. (2010). Infectious and dietary risk factors of oral cancer. Oral Oncology, Vol.46, No.6, pp. 411-413, ISSN 1368-8375

Park, SL. et al. (2011). The association between change in body mass index and upper aerodigestive tract cancers in the ARCAGE project: multicenter case-control study. *International Journal of Cancer,* Vol.128, No.6, pp. 1449-1461, ISSN 0020-7136

Patel, BP. et al. (2010). Mutagen sensitivity in oral cancer patients, healthy tobacco chewers and controls. *Acta cytologica,* Vol.54, No.2, pp. 169-174, ISSN 0001-5547

Piemonte, ED.; Lazos, JP. & Brunotto, M. (2010). Relationship between chronic trauma of the oral mucosa, oral potentially malignant disorders and oral cancer. *Journal of Oral Pathology & Medicine,* Vol.39, No.7, pp. 513-517, ISSN 0904-2512

Ramadas, K. et al. (2003) Interim results from a cluster-randomized, controlled oral cancer screening trial in Kerala, India. *Oral Oncology,* Vol.39, No.6, pp. 580-588, ISSN 1368-8375

Rethman, MP. et al. (2010). Evidence-based clinical recommendations regarding screening for oral squamous cell carcinomas. *Journal of American Dental Association,* Vol.141, No.5, pp. 509-520, ISSN 0002-8177

Reznick, AZ. et al. (2003). Inhibition of oral peroxidase activity by cigarette smoke: in vivo and in vitro studies. *Free Radical Biology & Medicine,* Vol. 34, No.3, pp. 377-384, ISSN 0891-5849

Rohrer, J.; Wuertz, BR. & Ondrey, F. (2010). Cigarette smoke condensate induces nuclear factor kappa-b activity and proangiogenic growth factors in aerodigestive cells. *Laryngoscope,* Vol. 120, No.8, pp. 1609-1613, ISSN 0023-852X

Samoli, E. et al. (2010). Mediterranean diet and upper aerodigestive tract cancer: the Greek segment of the Alcohol-Related Cancers and Genetic Susceptibility in Europe study. *The British Journal of Nutrition,* Vol.104, No.9, pp. 1369-1374, ISSN 0007-1145

Sato, F. et al. (2011). Inverse association between toothbrushing and upper aerodigestive tract cancer risk in a japanese population. *Head & Neck,* Jan 21. doi: 10.1002/hed.21649. (Epub ahead of print), ISSN 1043-3074

Scully C. Oral cancer aetiopathogenesis; past, present and future aspects. (2011). *Medicina Oral, Patología Oral y Cirugía Bucal,* Vol.16, No.3, pp. e306-11 ISSN 1698-4447

Scully, C. & Petti, S. (2010) Overview of cancer for the healthcare team: Aetiopathogenesis and early diagnosis. Oral Oncology, Vol.46, No.6, pp.402-406, ISSN 1368-8375

Shanmugham, JR. et al. (2010). Alcohol-folate interactions in the risk of oral cancer in women: a prospective cohort study. *Cancer Epidemiology, Biomarkers & Prevention,* Vol.19, No.10, pp. 2516-2524, ISSN 1055-9965

Shieh, TM. et al. (2010). Association between the polymorphisms in exon 12 of hypoxia-inducible factor-1alpha and the clinicopathological features of oral squamous cell carcinoma. *Oral Oncology,* Vol.46, No.9, pp. e47-e53, ISSN 1368-8375

Shillitoe, EJ. (2009). The role of viruses in squamous cell carcinoma of the oropharyngeal mucosa. *Oral Oncology,* Vol.45, No.4-5, pp. 351-355, ISSN 1368-8375

Smith, EM. et al. (2010). Tobacco and alcohol use increases the risk of both HPV-associated and HPV-independent head and neck cancers. *Cancer Causes & Control,* Vol.21, No.9, pp. 1369-1378, ISSN 0957-5243

Starr, JR. et al. (2001). Serologic evidence of herpes simplex virus 1 infection and oropharyngeal cancer risk. *Cancer Research,* Vol.61, No.23, pp. 8459-8464, ISSN 0008-5472

Su, CC. et al. (2010). Incidence of oral cancer in relation to nickel and arsenic concentrations in farm soils of patients' residential areas in Taiwan. *BMC public health,* Vol.10, pp. 67, ISSN 1471-2458

Swaminathan, R. et al. (2009). Education and cancer incidence in a rural population in south India. *Cancer Epidemiology,* Vol.33, N0.2, pp. 89-93, ISSN 1877-7821

Szymańska, K. et al. (2010). TP53 and EGFR mutations in combination with lifestyle risk factors in tumours of the upper aerodigestive tract from South America. *Carcinogenesis*, Vol.31, No.6, pp. 1054-1059, ISSN 0143-3334

Szymańska, K. et al. (2011). Alcohol and tobacco, and the risk of cancers of the upper aerodigestive tract in Latin America: a case-control study. *Cancer Causes & Control*, Vol.22, No.7, pp. 1037-1046, ISSN 0957-5243

Takács, D. et al. (2011). Decreased oral cancer risk by moderate alcohol consumption in non-smoker postmenopausal women. *Oral Oncology*, Vol.47, No.6, pp. 537-540, ISSN 1368-8375

Taoudi Benchekroun, M. et al. (2010). Epidermal growth factor receptor expression and gene copy number in the risk of oral cancer. *Cancer prevention research (Philadelphia, Pa.)*, Vol.3, No.7, pp. 800-809, ISSN 1940-6207

Tsai, KY. et al. (2009) Quantification of betel quid chewing and cigarette smoking in oral cancer patients. *Community Dentistry and Oral Epidemiology*, Vol.37, No.6, pp. 555-561, ISSN 0301-5661

Tsai, YS. et al. (2008). Arecoline, a major alkaloid of areca nut, inhibits p53, represses DNA repair, and triggers DNA damage response in human epithelial cells. *Toxicology*, Vol.249, No.2-3, pp. 230-237, ISSN 0300-483X

Warnakulasuriya, S. (2009a). Global epidemiology of oral and oropharyngeal cancer. *Oral Oncology*, Vol.45, No.4-5, pp. 309-316, ISSN 1368-8375

Warnakulasuriya, S. (2009b). Causes of oral cancer - an appraisal of controversies. *British Dental Journal*, Vol.207, No.10, pp. 471-475, ISSN 0007-0610

Wen, CP. et al. (2010). Cancer risks from betel quid chewing beyond oral cancer: a multiple-site carcinogen when acting with smoking. *Cancer Causes & Control*, Vol.21, No.9, pp. 1427-1435, ISSN 0957-5243

Wilson, JC. et al. (2011). Non-steroidal anti-inflammatory drug and aspirin use and the risk of head and neck cancer: a systemic review. *Cancer Causes & Control*, Vol.22, No.5, pp. 803-810, ISSN 0957-5243

Yen, TT. et al. (2008). The association of smoking, alcoholic consumption, betel quid chewing and oral cavity cancer: a cohort study. *European Archives of Otorhinolaryngology*, Vol.265, No.11, pp. 1403-1407, ISSN 0937-4477

Yokota, A. et al. (2011). Secondary solid tumors after allegeneic hematopoietic SCT in Japan. *Bone Marrow Transplantation*, Feb 28. (Epub ahead of print) doi:10.1038/bmt.2011.23, ISSN 0268-3369

Yuan, TH. et al. (2011). Possible association between nickel and chromium and oral cancer: a case-control study in central Taiwan. *Science of the Total Environment*, Vol.409, No.6, pp. 1046-1052, ISSN 0048-9697

Zhou, C. et al. (2009). The Arg194Trp polymorphism in the X-ray repair cross-complementing group 1 gene as a potential risk factor of oral cancer: a meta-analysis. *The Tohoku Journal of Experimental Medicine*, Vol.219, No.1, pp. 43-51, ISSN 0040-8727

6

Environmental Factors Identified in the Etiology of Oral Cancers in Taiwan

Chi-Ting Chiang[1,*], Tsun-Kuo Chang[2], Ie-Bin Lian[3], Che-Chun Su[4], Kuo-Yang Tsai[5] and Yaw-Huei Hwang[6]
[1]*Green Energy and Environment Research Laboratories, Industrial Technology Research Institute,*
[2]*Department of Bioenvironmental Systems Engineering, National Taiwan University,*
[3]*Graduate Institute of Statistics and Information Science, National Changhua University of Education,*
[4]*Department of Internal Medicine, Changhua Christian Hospital,*
[5]*Department of Oral and Maxillofacial Surgery, Changhua Christian Hospital,*
[6]*Department of Public Health, National Taiwan University*
Taiwan

1. Introduction

There is an extensive variation in the incidence and mortality rates of oral cancer in different regions and countries of the world. While oral cancer is predominantly prevalent in South Asia and Southeast Asia, countries such as India, Pakistan, Bangladesh and Taiwan also have persistently increasing trends in incidence rates (Reichart & Way, 2006). Oral cancer is much more predominant in Taiwanese males than in females and the prevalence in male peaks at age between 45 and 65 years old. A review of the Taiwan Cancer Registry Database (TCRD) shows that the mortality rate for oral cancer ranked the fourth among the top 10 leading causes of cancer death in Taiwan since 2003 (Bureau of Health Promotion [BHP], 2011a). In Taiwan, the oral cancer incidence rate in male grew by nearly 22.1% in 2008, with comparative figures for 1995 (BHP, 2011a). Between 1997 and 2007, the number of oral cancer cases per year grew from 2,795 to 5,458, representing an increase of 119%; the number of deaths due to oral cancer jumped from 1,163 cases to 2,312 cases per year, representing an increase of 99% (BHP, 2011b). In addition, according to the statistical report from the Department of Health of the Executive Yuan, young and middle-aged Taiwanese males (between the ages of 25 and 44) are most likely to develop oral cancer. It is even more worrisome to note that the trend in the age of oral cancer has tended towards decreased age-groups in Taiwan on a yearly basis in recent years. Oral cancer has recently become a notable public health concern in Taiwan. Therefore, from a public health perspective, it is important and imperative to study the clinical and epidemiologic characteristics of oral cancer in Taiwan.

The development of various types of cancer is very complex and is influenced by many risk factors including hereditary, socio-demographics (such as age, gender, ethnicity, level of education, etc.), lifestyle, and environmental factors. The International Agency for Research

---

* Corresponding Author

on Cancer (IARC) has identified intake of alcoholic beverages (AB), betel quid chewing (BQC) with tobacco, and cigarette smoking (CS) as human carcinogens, with the target organs including the oral cavity, pharynx, larynx and oesophagus (IARC, 1988, 2003). So far, results of numerous studies have demonstrated that BQC, CS, and AB clearly relate to the development of oral cancer, and are therefore the major etiological factors for oral cancer, (Blot et al., 1988; Cancela et al., 2009; Choi & Kahyo, 1991; Merletti et al., 1989; Ogden, 2005; Petti & Scully, 2005). In a case-control study carried out in Taiwan, the probability of oral cancer in patients who consumed tobacco, alcohol and betel quid was 123-fold higher than that of abstainers, indicating that these three activities act synergistically (Ko et al., 1995). In Taiwan, BQC is much strongly correlated to oral cancer among these three factors; however, as BQC and CS normally coexist, the effects of BQC on human health in Taiwan can hardly be distinguished from the integrated effects of both (Wen et al., 2005). Oral cancer is a male dominant disease amongst the Taiwanese; a finding consistent with the prevalence rate of BQC is much higher in males than in females in that population. Among Taiwanese aborigines, betel quid is frequently used in traditional festivals, ceremonial rituals as well as daily life in line with custom. In consequence, the aboriginal population in Taiwan has a relatively higher risk for oral cancer than the Han Chinese.

Annual age-standardized incidence rate (ASIR) for oral cancer for the 22 counties in Taiwan Island indicated that two regions in the eastern (Taitung and Hualien Counties) and in the middle (Changhua and Yunlin Counties) Taiwan have very high incidence than the other regions. Table 1 shows that from 1995 to 2008, the 14-year average incidence rates of oral cancer in males in Taitung, Hualien, Changhua, and Yunlin Counties were 43.6, 36.0, 42.6, and 41.5 cases per 100,000 person-years, respectively, which were higher than that for the rest of the 18 counties (24.0 cases per 100,000 person-years). Thus, these four counties are "hot spots" of oral cancer in Taiwan. Although the prevalence of BQC use in Taiwan has declined in the middle (18.3% to 9.3%) and the eastern (44.0% to 36.6%) parts of Taiwan (44.0% to 36.6%) between 1996 and 2002 (Yang et al., 2002), oral cancer incidence rates have been rising rapidly in the past several decades (Su et al., 2007). However, a dramatically distinct difference in male-to-female ratio for oral cancer incidence appears between these two areas, i.e. the middle and eastern Taiwan (Table 1). As shown in Table 2, a large proportion of the aboriginal population residing in both Hualien and Taitung Counties, the home of the aboriginal people, have a high incidence of oral cancer, and the prevalence rates for the use of BQC and CS in males and females are equally high(Table 3). In contrast, Changhua and Yunlin Counties have only a small proportion of aboriginal population living in them (Table 2). As can be seen in Table 1~3, Changhua County in particular belongs to a high-risk oral cancer area and has the abnormally high male-to-female ratio of oral cancer incidence in spite of the fact that that its BQC and CS activities are only moderately high among the 22 county regions. Based on the above discussion, these known major risk factors for oral cancer (BQC/CS prevalence and ethnicity) do not fully explain the geographical occurrence of oral cancer "hot spots" in Taiwan. Therefore, there may be other potential risk factors such as genetics, lifestyle, and environmental, yet unknown that influence the development of oral cancer among these population.

It is estimated that as many as two-thirds of all cancer cases are linked to environmental causes (National Cancer Institute & National Institute of Environmental Health Sciences [NCI & NIEHS], 2003). Industrialization and urbanization in Taiwan over the past two decades have chronically polluted a huge amount of farm soil due to the discharge of industrial wastewater into the irrigation systems. Moreover, according to the nationwide systematic survey of farm soil conducted by the Environmental Protection Administration (EPA) in Taiwan, Changhua County is known as the granary of Taiwan, where farm soil has been seriously polluted by heavy metals. Environmental factor is suspected to play a critical role in the process of developing oral cancer in Taiwan.

Year	Middle Taiwan				Eastern Taiwan				Others	
	Changhua		Yunlin		Taitung		Hualien			
	Male	Female	Male	Female	Male	Female	Male	Female	Male	Female
1995	28.4	2.5	22.6	1.7	25.6	7.9	13.7	4.3	13.3	1.6
1996	30.1	2.5	25.6	1.1	30.6	9.9	29.0	4.2	14.3	2.0
1997	31.2	2.0	36.3	1.7	32.5	13.9	23.1	7.1	16.7	2.0
1998	36.9	1.8	29.9	4.0	34.0	4.6	28.4	5.6	19.4	2.1
1999	40.7	1.8	37.9	3.7	41.2	7.2	35.0	5.7	20.7	2.3
2000	40.7	2.5	37.0	3.2	39.5	5.9	36.1	5.1	22.9	2.1
2001	41.4	2.2	38.4	2.8	37.6	14.5	24.6	6.7	23.3	2.5
2002	40.7	3.6	36.7	1.9	42.8	8.0	34.7	3.6	23.7	2.7
2003	46.5	3.3	55.8	4.1	61.0	14.5	41.2	6.0	27.3	2.6
2004	51.9	3.1	54.0	3.5	52.2	11.8	46.9	6.4	28.9	3.0
2005	48.0	2.9	51.4	2.6	50.5	12.2	42.1	7.5	29.2	2.8
2006	52.7	3.6	60.1	3.3	62.6	12.9	51.8	9.1	31.5	2.9
2007	52.4	3.0	47.8	4.1	44.6	8.7	48.8	5.5	31.9	2.7
2008	55.1	1.8	47.9	1.3	56.3	13.9	48.6	8.4	33.0	2.6
Average	42.6	2.6	41.5	2.8	43.6	10.4	36.0	6.1	24.0	2.4
Ratio	17.1		16.8		4.5		6.1		9.8	

Table 1. Annual age-standardized incidence rate (ASIR) of oral cancer and average male-to-female ratios of oral cancer incidence in middle and eastern Taiwan and the rest of the counties, 1995-2008.

Heavy metals are extremely persistent in the environment and can cause adverse effects on human health. Many metals, including arsenic (As), chromium (Cr[VI]), and nickel (Ni[II]), have been classified as human carcinogens (International Agency for Research on Cancer [IARC], 1987, 1990). Consequently, long-term exposure to heavy metals in the air, water, and soil may increase the risk of a certain type of human cancer. Previous studies have also found that the high content of soil heavy metals in the region had high incidence or mortality rates of several types of cancers, such as stomach, prostate, bladder, esophageal, and gastrointestinal cancers (Rheeder et al., 1994; Stocks & Davies, 1964; Türkdoğan et al., 2003). These findings indirectly suggested a possible link between local residents' exposure to heavy metals in soil and the incidence of cancer. Soil and the human body both intake environmental heavy metals, which can be absorbed through various ways. That is to say, soil and the human body are both recipients of environmental pollutants. Thus, the content of heavy metals in soil is an index of possible environmental exposure to heavy metal, and it can also slightly reflect the extent of the potential exposure on the human body in the living environment. In addition to socio-demographic factor (i.e. the ethnic distribution) and lifestyle factors (i.e. the prevalence of BQC and CS), the content of soil heavy metals as a environmental factor is to explore the association between oral cancer occurrence and heavy metal pollution in the environment in Taiwan.

The development of geographic information systems (GIS) has offered a more powerful and efficient ability to visually inspect the spatial patterns and processes over the last twenty years. On the other hand, many recent epidemiological studies have widely used spatial analyses to identify possible causes related to the occurrence or outbreak of various diseases. A wide variety of statistical techniques to detect and describe spatial and temporal clustering have been applied in a range of disciplines, including geography, ecology, econometrics, biostatistics and medicine (Ward & Carpenter, 2000). Investigation of potential clustering of disease occurrence is a foundation of epidemiology, which provides valuable information on possible causes of the disease of interest and methods that may be used for disease control and prevention (Ward & Carpenter, 2000). Constructing disease-specific maps to depict geo-referencing health data cartographically can facilitate the identification of possible causes of disease as well as provide an additional perspective on clinical medicine, epidemiological studies and health improvement (Chiang et al., 2010). In this way, GIS, when combined with spatial analytical methods, may be assisted in the study of healthcare issues. Kitron & Kazmierczak (1997) indicated that counties with most human cases and tick were clustered in parts of western Wisconsin by using a measure of spatial autocorrelation. Pfeiffer et al. (2007) used a spatial clustering method to identify a sequence of three epidemic waves of highly pathogenic avian influenza (HPAI) occurred in Vietnam during the time period 2004–2006. Additionally, spatial regression analysis quantifies the spatial pattern through creating a specific-contiguity weight and examining the relationship between the attributes of interest and latent explanatory variables that can interpret the observed spatial pattern (Zeng et al., 2008). Green et al. (2003) identified the geographical location of Diabetes Mellitus (DM) clusters in the City of Winnipeg in Canada, and indicated high rates of DM prevalence are strongly correlated with some risk factor indicators by the combination of both spatial clustering and spatial regression methods.

In this chapter, we used GIS and Moran-based spatial statistics to associate the township-level oral cancer mortality rates with the prevalence of BQC and CS, the distribution of aboriginal population, and the content of soil heavy metals. The purpose was to identify the geographical locations of "hot spots" of various surveillance variables over the entire township of Taiwan, and then to determine and explain the magnitude of spatial association among these surveillance variables.

County regions	2000	2001	2002	2003	2004	2005	2006	2007	2008	2009	Average
Hualien	20.6	20.2	20.0	19.7	19.5	19.1	18.8	18.5	18.2	18.0	19.3
Taitung	18.8	18.4	18.1	17.7	17.3	17.0	16.7	16.3	16.0	15.9	17.2
Pingtung	12.5	12.5	12.3	12.1	11.9	11.8	11.7	11.5	11.4	11.3	11.9
Taoyuan	9.2	9.3	9.5	9.8	10.1	10.4	10.8	11.1	11.3	11.4	10.3
Taipei	7.6	7.8	7.9	8.1	8.4	8.6	8.8	9.1	9.3	9.4	8.5
Nantou	6.0	6.0	6.0	5.9	5.9	5.8	5.7	5.7	5.6	5.6	5.8
Hsinchu	3.9	3.9	3.9	3.8	3.8	3.8	3.8	3.8	3.8	3.8	3.8
Taichung	3.3	3.4	3.4	3.5	3.6	3.7	3.7	3.8	3.9	3.9	3.6
Kaohsiung	3.3	3.4	3.3	3.4	3.3	3.4	3.4	3.4	3.4	3.4	3.4
Ilan	3.0	3.0	3.0	3.0	3.0	3.0	3.0	3.0	3.0	3.0	3.0
Taipei City	2.1	2.2	2.4	2.4	2.4	2.5	2.5	2.6	2.6	2.6	2.4
Miaoli	2.1	2.1	2.0	2.0	2.0	2.0	2.0	2.0	2.1	2.1	2.1
Kaohsiung City	1.8	1.8	1.9	2.0	2.1	2.1	2.1	2.2	2.2	2.3	2.0
Keelung City	1.6	1.6	1.6	1.6	1.6	1.7	1.7	1.7	1.7	1.7	1.7
Taichung City	1.0	1.1	1.1	1.2	1.2	1.3	1.3	1.4	1.4	1.4	1.2
Chiayi	1.1	1.1	1.1	1.1	1.1	1.1	1.1	1.1	1.1	1.1	1.1
Changhua*	0.7	0.7	0.7	0.8	0.9	0.9	0.9	0.9	0.9	0.9	0.8
Tainan	0.5	0.5	0.5	0.6	0.6	0.6	0.7	0.7	0.7	0.7	0.6
Hsinchu City	0.4	0.4	0.4	0.4	0.4	0.5	0.5	0.5	0.5	0.6	0.5
Tainan City	0.2	0.2	0.3	0.3	0.3	0.3	0.3	0.4	0.4	0.4	0.3
Yunlin*	0.2	0.2	0.2	0.3	0.3	0.3	0.3	0.3	0.3	0.3	0.3
Chiayi City	0.1	0.1	0.1	0.1	0.2	0.2	0.2	0.2	0.2	0.2	0.2

Table 2. The proportion of the aboriginal population in each county region throughout the Taiwan Island, 2000-2009.

The proportion is equal to the number of aboriginal population in county divided by the total number of aboriginal population throughout Taiwan Island.

County regions	BQC prevalence (%)			CS prevalence (%)		
	All	Male	Female	All	Male	Female
Taitung	24.4 (1)	30.0 (2)	18.0 (1)	14.4 (1)	47.4 (2)	14.4 (1)
Hualien	21.6 (2)	32.6 (1)	9.6 (2)	13.4 (2)	46.0 (5)	13.4 (2)
Pingtung	16.0 (3)	26.1 (3)	5.1 (3)	4.2 (15)	48.1 (1)	4.2 (15)
Yunlin	13.4 (4)	24.8 (4)	0.5 (10)	5.1 (9)	43.4 (7)	5.1 (9)
Chiayi	13.0 (5)	24.0 (5)	0.6 (7)	5.1 (9)	42.4 (10)	5.1 (9)
Nantou	12.9 (6)	23.7 (6)	1.2 (4)	6.3 (6)	46.3 (4)	6.3 (6)
Tainan	9.5 (7)	18.1 (7)	0.4 (12)	4.1 (16)	43.6 (6)	4.1 (16)
Miaoli	9.2 (8)	17.3 (8)	0.0 (20)	3.1 (20)	42.3 (11)	3.1 (20)
Taichung	8.4 (9)	15.9 (9)	0.6 (7)	4.4 (14)	41.6 (13)	4.4 (14)
Kaohsiung	8.4 (10)	15.7 (10)	0.7 (6)	5.0 (12)	42.8 (9)	5.0 (12)
Ilan	8.1 (11)	15.2 (11)	0.5 (10)	4.5 (13)	42.9 (8)	4.5 (13)
Taoyuan	7.7 (12)	14.7 (12)	0.6 (7)	6.6 (5)	41.5 (14)	6.6 (5)
Changhua*	7.3 (13)	14.1 (13)	0.1 (18)	2.9 (21)	36.3 (20)	2.9 (21)
Chiayi City	7.1 (14)	14.0 (14)	0.2 (17)	3.7 (18)	39.8 (16)	3.7 (18)
Tainan City	6.3 (15)	12.6 (15)	0.0 (20)	2.0 (22)	36.2 (21)	2.0 (22)
Keelung	6.2 (16)	12.0 (16)	0.3 (15)	6.7 (4)	46.5 (3)	6.7 (4)
Hsinchu	5.8 (17)	10.4 (20)	0.8 (5)	4.1 (16)	39.8 (16)	4.1 (16)
Hsinchu City	5.4 (18)	10.7 (17)	0.0 (20)	5.2 (8)	40.4 (15)	5.2 (8)
Taipei	5.4 (18)	10.6 (18)	0.3 (15)	5.3 (7)	41.9 (12)	5.3 (7)
Taichung City	5.3 (20)	10.5 (19)	0.4 (12)	6.8 (3)	39.0 (18)	6.8 (3)
Kaohsiung City	5.0 (21)	9.5 (21)	0.4 (12)	3.6 (19)	36.9 (19)	3.6 (19)
Taipei City	2.6 (22)	5.4 (22)	0.0 (20)	5.1 (9)	32.1 (22)	5.1 (9)

Numbers in parentheses indicate the ranks of the prevalence rates among the 22 county regions.

Table 3. The prevalence rates of BQC and CS in each county region throughout the Taiwan Island in 2005 (BHP, 2011c).

2. Materials and methods

2.1 Study area

This study was conducted mainly in Taiwan Island. Taiwan locates in the heart of the Festoon Islands at the west coast of Pacific Ocean, and it plays a vital and indispensable role as a key transport hub in the East Asian region. The political geography of Taiwan can be divided into four major regions as follows: the north, middle, south, and east regions, as shown in Fig. 1. The total area of Taiwan Island is about 36,000 square kilometres with a population of about 23 million, and a population density of 640 persons per square kilometres. Taiwan's population has grown very rapidly in a very short time. Taiwan is also becoming an increasingly dominating urban society with its population almost concentrated on the northern and southern of Taiwan Island, in two metropolitan cities of Taipei and Kaohsiung. The majority of ethnic groups in Taiwan are Han Chinese and aboriginal, whose proportions are 97.8% and 2.2% respectively. The latter live primarily in the eastern valleys and central mountainous areas (Lin et al., 2008). Over the past three decades, Taiwan's industry has transformed from early agriculture to manufacture (industrialization), and then from manufacture to high-tech innovation (knowledge work). In 1995, the compulsory health care delivery system in Taiwan, called the National Health Insurance (NHI), was implemented with an emphasis on equal access to health care, regardless of socioeconomic status.

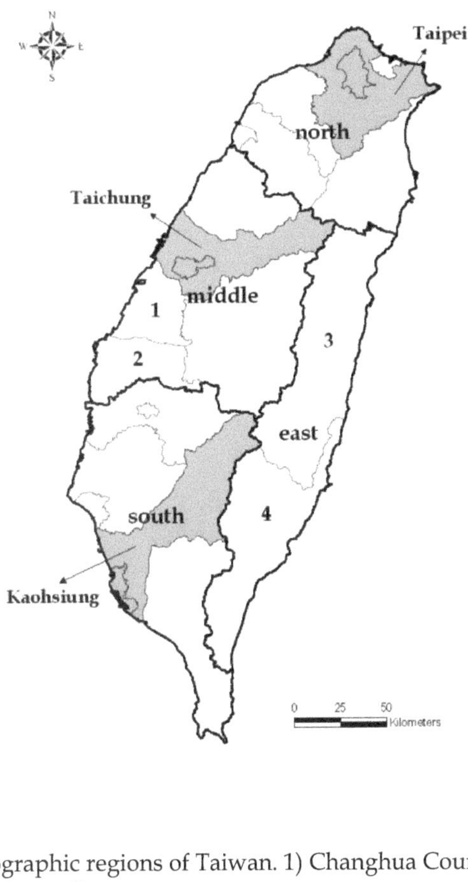

Fig. 1. Four major geographic regions of Taiwan. 1) Changhua County, 2) Yunlin County, 3) Hualien County, 4) Taitung County.

2.2 Data on oral cancer mortality rates

Taiwan established its comprehensive national cancer registry and database in 1979. Data on oral cancer mortality rates were obtained from the Atlas of Cancer Mortality in Taiwan constructed in 2003 by Taiwan's Department of Health (DOH), which contains age-standardized mortality rates (ASMR) in both genders of each township for each decade from 1972 to 2001. Additionally, data on ASMR of oral cancer in male and all gender (i.e. male plus female) for each township from 2001 to 2009 were obtained from the statistical reports on the leading cause of cancer death, which were also provided by Taiwan's DOH. Each township was treated as a unit in the analysis in this study.

2.3 Data on aboriginal population

In this study, a principal source of demographic data for the aboriginal population is the census. There are several culturally and ethno-linguistically distinct aboriginal tribes in Taiwan, who live mainly in the eastern plains and central mountains. In total, the Taiwanese aboriginal tribes consist of about 500,000 people. Data on aboriginal population of each township across Taiwan Island from 1998 to 2010 were retrieved from the Department of Household Registration Affairs.

2.4 Data on known risk habits of oral cancer

The prevalence rates of BQC and CS were estimated from the National Health Interview Survey (NHIS) data in 2002, which was conducted cooperatively by the National Health Research Institutes (NHRI) and Taiwan's DOH. The survey subjects included 1,086 males and 1,473 females from all over Taiwan Island. However, only data from males and all gender were considered in calculation due to the low rates of BQC and CS among females. Similarly, data on the prevalence rates of BQC and CS were studied based on the township level.

2.5 Data on the content of soil heavy metals

Soil data in this study were derived from a progressive, nationwide survey that determined the concentration in agricultural topsoil (0-15 cm) of arsenic (As), cadmium (Cd), chromium (Cr), copper (Cu), mercury (Hg), nickel (Ni), lead (Pb) and zinc (Zn), conducted by the Environmental Protection Administration (EPA) in Taiwan from 1986 to 1990 (Environmental Protection Administration, R.O.C. (Taiwan) [ROCEPA], 1985). The total concentration of extractable As and Hg in the soil was determined by the aqua regia method, as well as the other six heavy metals by the 0.1 N HCl extraction method. A grid cell size of 1,600 ha was used as sampling unit and 936 soil samples were collected across Taiwan Island. The area-weighted mean value represented the soil heavy metal content in each township.

2.6 Principal component analysis

Principal component analysis (PCA) is an exploratory data analysis tool introduced in 1901 by Karl Pearson (Pearson, 1901), and later on extended in 1933 by Harold Hotelling

(Hotelling, 1933). PCA is a linear eigenvector-based dimensionality reduction technique, which is based on orthogonal transforming a large set of potentially correlated variables into a new and smaller subset of uncorrelated variables with maximum variance. These new variables, called principal components (PCs), are obtained as linear combinations of the original variables. The number of PC is less than or equal to the number of original variables ($q \leqq p$). Eigenvalues quantify the amount of variability explained by each PC, and an eigenvalue greater than one is commonly used as a cut-off point for which PCs are retained. The first PC explains the maximum amount of total variability in the data, the second PC the next largest amount, and so on. For each observation, PC scores are the derived composite scores computed based on the eigenvectors for each PC. PC loadings are correlation coefficients between the PC scores and the original variables, which ranges from -1 to 1. Therefore, the result of a PCA can eliminate multi-collinearity existed among original variables in multiple regression analysis, and these PC scores can be used in subsequent analyses. The basic model structure for PCA is shown in equation (1).

$$\begin{cases} PC_1 = \ell_{11}X_1 + \ell_{12}X_2 + \cdots + \ell_{1p}X_p \\ PC_2 = \ell_{21}X_1 + \ell_{22}X_2 + \cdots + \ell_{2p}X_p \\ \vdots \quad \vdots \quad \vdots \quad \vdots \\ PC_q = \ell_{q1}X_1 + \ell_{q2}X_2 + \cdots + \ell_{qp}X_p \\ \vdots \quad \vdots \quad \vdots \quad \vdots \\ PC_p = \ell_{p1}X_1 + \ell_{p2}X_2 + \cdots + \ell_{pp}X_p \end{cases} \tag{1}$$

where $X_1, X_2, \cdots, X_p$ are the original variables; $PC_1, PC_2, \cdots, PC_p$ are new variables, namely the principal components; ℓ_{ij} is the correlation coefficient between the original variable j (X_j) and principal component i (PC_i), namely the PC loading. In this study, PC loadings greater than 0.75 in absolute value as strong correlation, were used to make decisions regarding significant loadings (Liu et al., 2003).

2.7 Moran-based autocorrelation statistics

The spatial autocorrelation exists when a value observed in one geographic location depends on the values at neighbouring locations. The spatial autocorrelation coefficient for one geographic location is similar to the traditional Pearson correlation coefficient. In this study, two different scales were applied in spatial autocorrelation analysis. The Moran index (Moran's I), a measure of spatial autocorrelation at global scale, which is used to estimate the magnitude of spatial association among all locations within the study area. The Moran's I statistic, the most common, is defined as following equation (2) (Moran, 1950). The global Moran's I only identify whether an overall spatial clustering propensity exists in a study area. Therefore, Anseline (1995) developed measure of spatial autocorrelation at local scale. The local Moran index (Moran's I_i), which provide the possible contribution of each location to the global Moran's I, is so called as local indicator of spatial association (LISA) (Anselin, 1995). The equation (3) is used to calculate the local Moran's I_i statistic. The LISA statistic is a spatial clustering method, which is used to identify significant local homogeneous (hot spots) or heterogeneous (cold spots) regions. The global Moran's I is the weighted average of local Moran's I_i. The null hypothesis (H_0) of the spatial autocorrelation test is that a variable value of interest is not associated with among neighbouring locations, while the alternative hypothesis (H_a) is that the neighbouring locations have similar variable values of interest. The null hypothesis is rejected if the significance test means there is spatial autocorrelation.

$$I = \frac{n}{\sum_{i=1}^{n}(x_i - \bar{x})^2} \times \frac{\sum_{i=1}^{n}\sum_{j=1}^{n} w_{ij}(x_i - \bar{x})(x_j - \bar{x})}{\sum_{i=1}^{n}\sum_{j=1}^{n} w_{ij}}, \quad i \neq j \qquad (2)$$

$$I_i = \frac{x_i - \bar{x}}{\sum_{i=1}^{n}(x_i - \bar{x})^2} \times \sum_{j=1}^{n} w_{ij}(x_i - \bar{x})(x_j - \bar{x}), \quad i \neq j \qquad (3)$$

where n is the number of regions in the study; x_i and x_j are the values of the variable of interest at regions i and j, respectively; w_{ij} is an element of an $(n \times n)$ binary spatial weight matrix, $\mathbf{W}$, defining the connection between regions i and j (e.g. 1 represents these two regions are adjacent and 0 for otherwise); $\mathbf{W}$ often is a row-standardized weight means that each row of the weight matrix must sum to one. Moran's ***I*** statistic ranges from -1 to 1, and it equals 0 when there is no spatial autocorrelation. Positive values of Moran's ***I*** statistics suggest spatial clustering, while negative values suggest dispersion, that is, high values are frequently found in the vicinity of low values.

In addition, the Moran scatter-plot and a local version of the Moran's ***I*** statistic for each region, which are valuable for gaining insights into the extent and nature of spatial clustering in a dataset (Anselin, 1996). The Moran scatter-plot is divided into four quadrants which all denote different levels of spatial association for each individual observation. The upper right quadrant of the Moran scatter-plot indicates regions with above average value share boundaries with neighbouring regions (High-High), i.e. hot spots. The lower left quadrant indicates regions with below average value on the variable of interest share boundaries with neighbouring regions (Low-Low), i.e. cold spots. The lower right quadrant indicates regions with above average values surrounded by regions with below average values (High-Low), and the upper right quadrant is opposite to the front (Low-High). The Moran scatter-plot values can be easily mapped and then further to explore where and how the spatial autocorrelation is located.

2.8 Spatial regression analysis

Many studies frequently focus on determining the correlation between potential environmental risk factors and diseases of concern through using multivariate linear regression analyses (Ashley, 1969; Dyomin et al., 1994). However, for analysis of observational data with spatial dependence, the classical linear regression model with spatial auto-correlated residuals violates the independence assumption for error. Spatial dependence effects must be incorporated into the specification of regression model and then the regression model must be estimated using appropriate estimation methods, such as maximum likelihood estimation method. The spatial lag model (SLM) regression can incorporate spatial dependence into the classical regression model (Anselin, 1988). Under

SLM specification, spatial autocorrelation in the dependent variable derives from exogenous influences. The SLM thus adds an additional predictor in the form of a spatially lagged exogenous variable to explain spatial dependence. A SLM commonly is expressed as equation (4) (Anselin, 1994):

$$y = \rho \mathbf{W} y + \mathbf{X}\beta + \varepsilon \tag{4}$$

where y is a $(n \times 1)$ vector of observation on the dependent variable; $\mathbf{X}$ is a $(n \times k)$ matrix representing the $(k-1)$ explanatory variables and 1s column to accommodate the constant term; β is a $(k \times 1)$ vector of regression coefficient to be estimated; ρ is a spatial autoregressive coefficient of spatial lag term; $\mathbf{W}$ is a spatial weight matrix defining the adjacent relation; ε is a $(n \times 1)$ vector of random error term. The SLM parameters are estimated using the maximum likelihood method.

The exploratory spatial data analyses and spatial regression were carried out using a cluster-detection software programme of GeoDa version 0.9.5-I, developed by Luc Anselin. For statistical inference, the significance was tested using a Monte Carlo test with 999 permutations at a significance level of 0.05.

3. Results and discussion

3.1 Principal component analysis for heavy metal in soil

This study conducted PCA to determine the major PCs influencing the pattern of soil heavy metal pollution in Taiwan.

Variables	PC1	PC2	PC3
As	-0.26	0.26	**0.89**
Cd	0.22	**0.85**	-0.05
Cr	**0.88**	-0.12	-0.01
Cu	**0.86**	-0.17	-0.04
Hg	0.53	0.04	0.27
Ni	**0.83**	-0.18	0.25
Pb	0.49	0.63	-0.06
Zn	**0.93**	-0.05	-0.08
Eigenvalue	3.71	1.26	1.01
% Total variance	46.42	15.80	12.63
Cumulative % variance	46.42	62.22	74.85[a]

[a] Total cumulative variance. The loading whose absolute value is greater than 0.75 of the total variance were in bold.

Table 4. Results from the principal component analysis (PCA) for heavy metals in soil.

Three PCs were extracted based on eigenvalues greater than one. These three PCs accounted for 74.85% of the total variance. Table 4 gives the results of PC loadings, eigenvalues, and cumulative percentage of variation explained by each of these retained three PCs after rotation. In practice, only PC loadings with absolute values greater than 0.75 were selected for the PC interpretation. Using this criterion, the first principal component (PC1) explained 46.42% of total variance with strong positive loadings on heavy metals Cr, Cu, Ni and Zn. The association of Cr, Cu, Ni and Zn in PC1 reflects the maximum influence of electroplating and other metal treatment plants on soil pollution Taiwan (Chang et al., 1997). The second principal component (PC2) included heavy metal Cd, which accounted for 15.80% of the total variance. Heavy metal Cd was dominated by PC2, which reflects the influence of pigments and plastic factories on soil pollution. The third principal component (PC3) included As, which accounted for 12.63% of the total variance. In Taiwan, according to previous studies, the As content in soil is closely related to the geologic parent materials (Chang et al., 1999). These three PCs were used to replace the original variables (i.e. eight kinds of heavy metals) to represent overall soil pollution by heavy metals in Taiwan. Additionally, PC scores were the derived composite scores computed for each township based on the eigenvectors for each PC, and they were used in subsequent analyses.

3.2 Correlation analysis of the explored variables

Correlation analysis is used as preliminary data analysis before applying more sophisticated techniques. A Pearson's correlation matrix is often used to explore for pairs of variables more likely to be associated. The Pearson's correlation matrix among male oral cancer mortality in different periods, male prevalence rates of BQC and CS, proportion of male aboriginal population as well as principle components PC1, PC2 and PC3 is constructed in Table 5.

Variables	Mortality (1972-1981)	Mortality (1982-1991)	Mortality (1992-2001)	Mortality (2001-2009)	Aborigines
BQC	**0.17	**0.16	**0.21	**0.30	*0.12
CS	-0.07	-0.03	-0.03	0.00	**0.15
Aborigines	-0.01	0.00	-0.01	0.01	
PC1	**0.22	**0.29	**0.26	**0.18	
PC2	0.06	0.05	0.03	-0.05	
PC3	**0.24	**0.19	**0.31	**0.38	

"Mortality (1)-(4)" indicate oral cancer mortality rates in males. "BQC and CS" indicate the male prevalence rate of betel quid chewing and cigarette smoking, respectively (n=301). "Aborigines" is used to denote the average proportion of the male aboriginal population (n=349). Three extractable principal components of PC1, PC2 and PC3 were determined by principal component analysis applied to eight heavy metals data (n=274).

* denotes significance at 0.05; ** denotes significance at 0.01.

Table 5. Pearson's correlation matrix among oral cancer mortality in male and related potential factors.

There was a positive and statistically significant correlation between proportion of aboriginal population and prevalence rates of BQC and CS, which implied BQC is actually a common habit in Taiwanese aborigines. As to the correlations among male oral cancer mortality and these other explored variables, prevalence rate of BQC, proportion of aboriginal population, and principle components PC1 and PC3 were found to be positively correlated with male oral cancer mortality (p-values < 0.05). These findings further validated the correlation between oral cancer and BQC, and indicated that soil heavy metal pollution is possibly related to oral cancer. Conversely, prevalence rate of CS, proportion of aboriginal population, and principle components PC2 had no statistically significant correlation with male oral cancer mortality (p-values > 0.05). Although CS is highly prevalent for Taiwanese, there is no apparent difference in geographical distribution of CS prevalence.

3.3 Global spatial autocorrelation of the explored variables

This study constructed a contiguity-based spatial weight for each township by queen contiguity relationships, which defines spatial neighbours as areas with a shared border and vertexes (Lai et al., 2009). The results of the global Moran's *I* analyses are summarized in Table 6. Table 6 shows the positive and statistically significant spatial autocorrelation for male oral cancer mortality in each period. In addition, there was a gradually increasing trend in the degree of spatial autocorrelation for oral cancer mortality, with ranges of global Moran's *I* values varying from 0.3701 to 0.6201 in the period of nearly forty years. The geographical distribution of aborigines across Taiwan exhibited a significantly positive spatial autocorrelation. There were also positive spatial autocorrelations in the geographical distributions of BQC and CS prevalence rates, and the Moran's *I* value in prevalence rate of BQC was greater than that of CS. Additionally, the geographical distributions of all these three PCs representing soil pollution by heavy metals in Taiwan had spatial autocorrelation. Among these three PCs, PC3 with the greatest positive Moran's *I* value displayed the strongest degree of spatial distribution.

Variables	Moran's *I*
Mortality (1972-1981)	**0.3701
Mortality (1982-1991)	**0.4134
Mortality (1992-2001)	**0.5906
Mortality (2001-2009)	**0.6201
Aborigines	**0.5729
BQC	**0.5726
CS	**0.3752
PC1	**0.5859
PC2	**0.1865
PC3	**0.7782

** denotes significance at 0.01.

Table 6. Global Moran's *I* of oral cancer mortality in male and related potential factors.

3.4 Local spatial clustering

The use of local indicator of spatial association (LISA) was to identify and explore the patterns of spatial clustering for each selected variable.

3.4.1 Spatial clusters of oral cancer mortality

Fig. 2 displays a map showing the distribution of high and low oral cancer mortality rates for male in the three 10-year periods from 1972 to 2001 and during the period of 2001 to 2009. Over the period of 1972 to 1981, a small number of clusters with high oral cancer mortality rate (i.e. hot spots) were observed, mainly located in the central and southernmost regions of Taiwan; the low-mortality clusters of male oral cancer (i.e. cold spots) were discovered in northern part of Taiwan. There was only an unusually apparent high-mortality cluster of male oral cancer centred on Changhua and Yunlin Counties of central Taiwan during 1982–1991; however, the high-mortality cluster located in southernmost Taiwan as in the previous time period of was disappeared. From 1992 to 2001, two distinctly large-ranges of high-mortality clusters were identified; one cluster was located in Taitung County of eastern Taiwan besides the previous cluster in central Taiwan. Over the past thirty years, the location and size of high-mortality cluster of male oral cancer in central Taiwan gradually expanded to include the entire Changhua County since 1972. As shown in the lower right figure of Fig. 2, the spatial clustering of male oral cancer mortality from 2001 to 2009 is identified. Although the main high-mortality clusters of male oral cancer in this period of time was slightly different from that in the last period of time, the main two hot spots were also exhibited in central and eastern regions of Taiwan, and cold spots were predominantly located in northern Taiwan.

3.4.2 Spatial clusters of related potential factors

The spatial clusters of high proportion of aborigines and high prevalence rates of BQC and CS for male are indentified are sequentially shown in the Fig. 3 above. The aboriginal population mostly resided in the eastern part of Taiwan, similarly, where one continuous and large-scale cluster with high proportion of aborigines was located. On the contrary, a cold spot of low proportion of aborigines distributed throughout the southwest and midwest Taiwan. For maps of prevalence rates of BQC and CS, an obvious cluster of high BQC prevalence rates was mainly in Taitung and Hualien Counties in eastern Taiwan, while the cluster position of high prevalence rates for CS extended from the northwest to the east.

The spatial clusters of each PC representing soil pollution by heavy metal are presented as Fig. 3 below. Clustering map for PC1, the spatial clusters of high PC1 scores mainly concentrated in the adjacent areas of Taichung and Changhua Counties in central Taiwan. There were five small and fragmented clusters of high PC2 scores spread from north to south throughout Taiwan except for the east. Three more apparent clusters of high PC3 scores were primarily focused on the southwest.

From the above results, the aggregation size of high-mortality rates of male oral cancer not only expanded with time, but also much more strongly clustered. However, the main gathering locations of aboriginal people and high BQC and CS prevalence rates for male were not totally consistent with that of high-mortality rates of oral cancer. Eastern Taiwan of

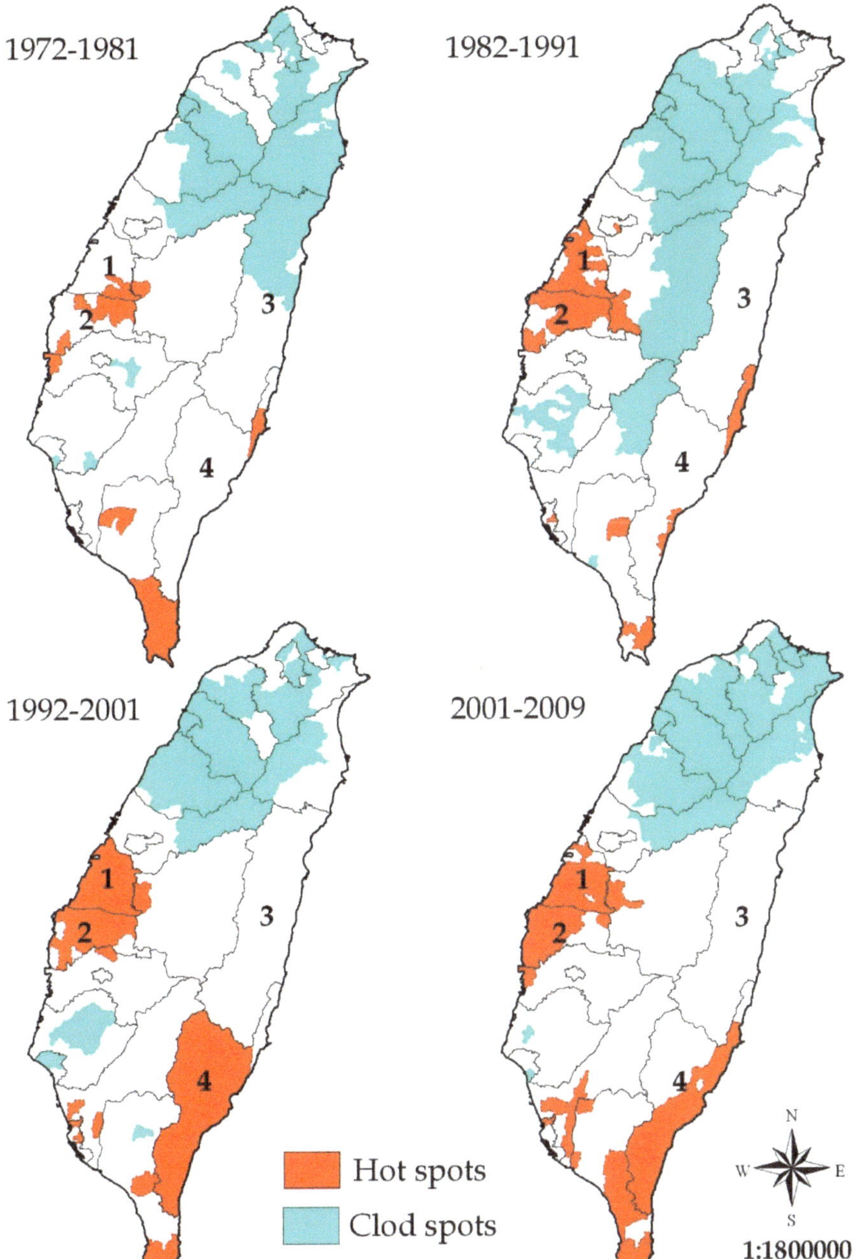

Fig. 2. Cluster locations of oral cancer mortality in males identified by local indicator of spatial association (LISA). 1) Changhua County, 2) Yunlin County, 3) Hualien County, 4) Taitung County.

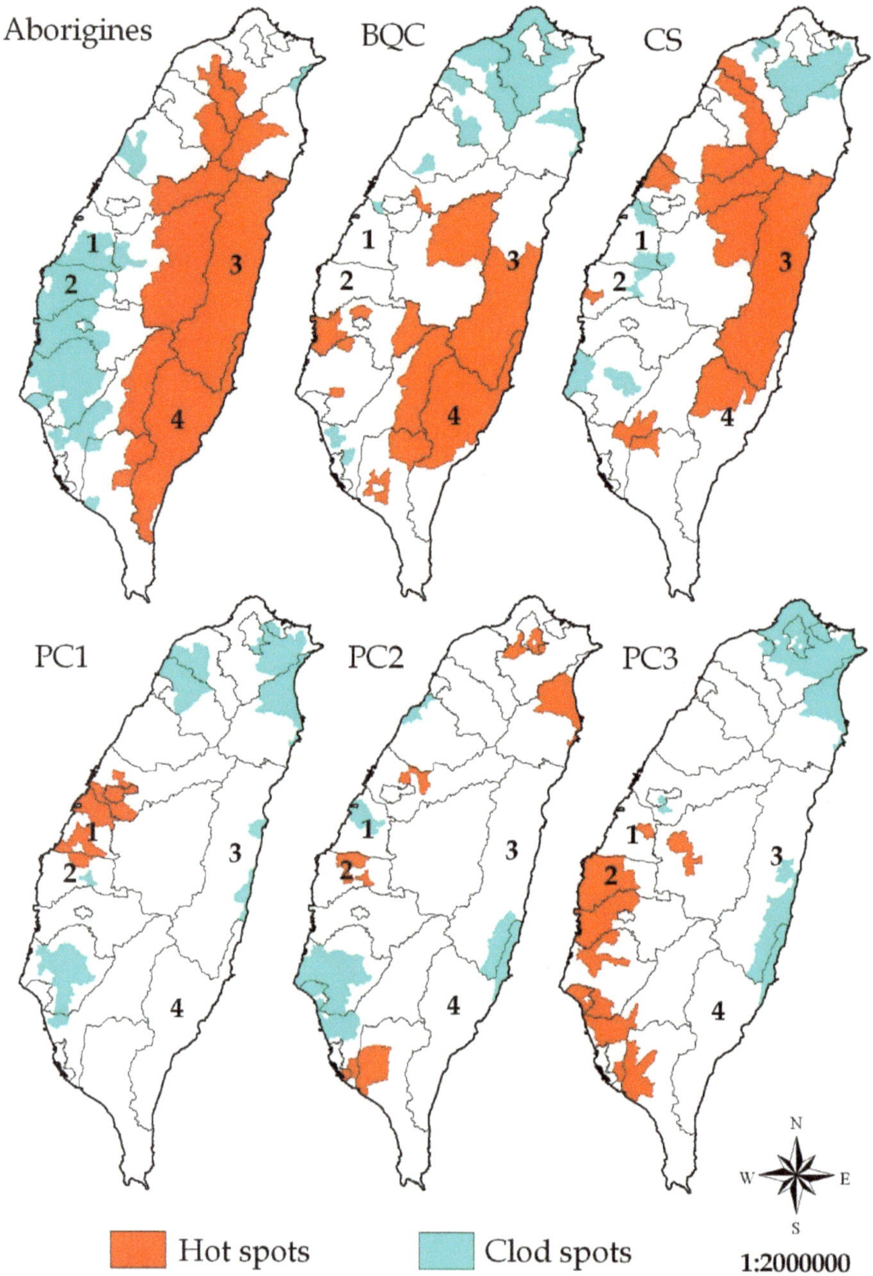

Fig. 3. Cluster locations of related potential factors identified by local indicator of spatial association (LISA). 1) Changhua County, 2) Yunlin County, 3) Hualien County, 4) Taitung County.

a hot spot for oral cancer can be approximately attributed to where the large numbers of aboriginal people reside and has high prevalence of BQC. But another hot spot for oral cancer is identified in central Taiwan, which is not the main distribution area of aboriginal people and BQC is not seem to be quite prevalent. Since the 1970s, the Taiwan government's policy was to promote "home into small factories," which has caused Changhua County to become a gathering place for electroplating and hardware manufacturing factories. Changhua County, located in central Taiwan, is a well-known Taiwanese "rice warehouse," and more than 60% of the county's total area has become arable land since 2001 (Council of Agriculture [COA], 2001). During the past few decades, farm soil has been seriously polluted by heavy-metal-contaminated wastewater discharged from factories through irrigation systems in Changhua County (Lin et al., 2002). Therefore, heavy metal pollution was to be considered as a potential risk factor for oral cancer, and three PCs obtained from the PCA were used to represent the overall soil pollution by heavy metals in Taiwan. The locations of hot spots for high PC1 and PC3 scores partially overlapped with a hot spot for oral cancer located in central counties of Taiwan. These findings legitimately suggested that soil pollution by heavy metal is an additional risk factor for oral cancer development.

3.5 Spatial regression analysis (SLM) for oral cancer mortality rates

This study further determined whether there is any correlation between the abnormally high-mortality rates of male oral cancer and related potential factors. Based on the results of above Sections 3.2 and 3.3, BQC prevalence rate, PC1 and PC3 had spatial autocorrelation and they correlated with oral cancer mortality. Thus, these three variables were included as predictors in a multiple regression model. The spatial autocorrelation in residuals for ordinary least squares (OLS) regression was found by the Moran's I statistic. Moreover, Lagrange multipliers (LM) and Robust LM for spatial lag were both statistically significant in favor of conducting SLM regression. Table 7 shows the estimation results of non-spatial and SLM regressions for male oral cancer mortality rates in four time periods. For non-spatial regression, PC1, PC3 and BQC prevalence rate significantly and positively spatially associated with oral cancer mortality rates for male in each period of time. In terms of SLM regression, a significantly spatial correlation between PC1 and male oral cancer mortality in the study period except the time period of 2001-2009. Only in the time period of 1992-2001, BQC prevalence rate associated with male oral cancer mortality. The estimation of all four SLM models had significantly positive values for spatial effect. In addition, the percentages of variance explained (R^2) by the SLM models were greater than that in the non-spatial regressions, indicating that spatial regression model was successful in accounting for spatial correlation in male oral cancer mortality rates.

BQC prevalence rates did not fully spatially correlated with oral cancer mortality rates in spatial regressions, but there was always a significant correlation between them in non-spatial regressions. It does not contradict that BQC is still the key culprit for causing oral cancer. The spatial regression results indicated that higher PC1 or PC3 scores in areas had higher male oral cancer mortality rates. The association between heavy metal pollution and oral cancer in Taiwan was further determined through regression analyses. Based on these highlights, environmental factors are strongly suspected to promote or cause oral cancer in Taiwan.

Variables	Non-spatial regression Regression coefficients				Spatial lag model regression Regression coefficients			
	Mortality (1972-1981)	Mortality (1982-1991)	Mortality (1992-2001)	Mortality (2001-2009)	Mortality (1972-1981)	Mortality (1982-1991)	Mortality (1992-2001)	Mortality (2001-2009)
constant	**2.661	**3.461	**7.511	**11.921	**1.216	**1.320	**2.171	**2.903
PC1	**0.651	**0.902	**1.406	**1.613	*0.289	**0.412	*0.436	0.435
PC3	**0.576	*0.412	**1.252	**2.177	0.195	0.135	*0.426	*0.605
BQC	*0.033	**0.044	**0.090	**0.207	0.010	0.017	0.022	**0.063
Rho (ρ)	–	–	–	–	**0.596	**0.632	**0.730	**0.745
R^2	0.115	0.149	0.210	0.278	0.356	0.438	0.609	0.646

Rho (ρ) denotes the spatial autoregressive coefficients. R^2 (the percentage of variation explained) is not directly provided for spatial model and model fit is thus assessed with a pseudo-R^2 value calculated as the squared Pearson correlation between predicted and observed values (Kissling & Carl, 2008).
* denotes significance at 0.05; ** denotes significance at 0.01.

Table 7. Regression analysis of oral cancer mortality rates in males and related potential factors.

4. Conclusion

In conclusion, by displaying the various data on maps, we found that the hot spots for male mortality rate of oral cancer partially overlapped with that for heavy metal pollution. Additionally, the male mortality rate of oral cancer is geographically associated with heavy metal pollution by conducting spatial regression analyses. In addition to the most well-known causative etiology of oral cancer, BQC, heavy metal pollution in the environment may be a promoting factor causing the development of oral cancer in Taiwan. Certain heavy metals are currently considered as known human carcinogens. Previous researches have uncovered a critical association between the abnormally high incidence or mortality rates for common types of cancer and the high content of soil heavy metals in the specified regions. Moreover, some epidemiological studies also have suggested that exposure to high levels of specific heavy metals in environmental media may be responsible for the high levels of that in human blood, urine and hair (Chang, Wang, Wang et al., 2006; Chang, Wang, Huang et al., 2006; Chiang et al., 2010; Rosas et al., 1989). More recently a case-control study on oral cancer and non-oral cancer patients living in central Taiwan has found that oral cancer patients' blood levels of heavy metal Cr, Ni, Cu and Zn were statistically significantly higher than those of non-oral cancer patients (Yuan et al., 2011); furthermore, these heavy metals are the same with the major components of PC1 influencing heavy metal pollution in Taiwan soil, which further indicates a tight link between heavy metal pollution in the environment and oral cancer. Obviously, spatial analysis is a relatively new and potentially valuable tool and it is believed that such techniques will gradually become an integral component of epidemiological research and risk assessment for oral cancer. Finally and most importantly, this study looks forward to providing a new direction in novel researches and issues in related fields such as clinical medicine and epidemiology in the future.

5. Acknowledgment

The authors are very grateful to the Department of Health (DOH), Executive Yuan, R.O.C (Taiwan) for providing the cancer registry database for the analyses and two anonymous reviewers for their valuable comments on an earlier draft of this paper.

6. References

Anselin, L. (1988). *Spatial Econometrics: Methods and Models (Studies in Operational Regional Science)*, Springer, ISBN 978-902-4737-35-2, Dordrecht, Boston

Anselin, L. (1995). Local Indicators of Spatial Association-LISA. *Geographical Analysis,* Vol. 27, No. 2, pp. 93-115, ISSN 1538-4632

Anselin, L. (1996). The Moran Scatterplot as an ESDA Tool to Assess Local Instability in Spatial Association, In: *Spatial Analytical Perspectives on GIS: GISDATA 4*. M. Fisher; H.J. Scholten & D. Unwin, (Eds), 111-125, Taylor & Francis, ISBN 978-0-7484-0339-4, London, UK

Anselin, L. & Rey, S. (1994). Properties of Tests for Spatial Dependence in Linear Regression Models. *Geographical Analysis,* Vol. 23, No. 2, pp. 112–131, ISSN 1538-4632

Ashley, D. (1969). Environmental Factors in the Aetiology of Gastric Cancer. *British Journal of Preventive & Social Medicine,* Vol. 23, No. 3, pp. 187-189, ISSN 0007-1242

NCI & NIEHS. (2003). Cancer and the Environment-What You Need to Know. What You Can Do, In: *National Cancer Institute (NCI) and National Institute of Environmental Health Sciences (NIEHS)*, 25.05.2011, Available from http://www.k4health.org/system/files/Cancer%20_Enviornment.pdf

Blot, W.; McLaughlin, J.; Winn, D.; Austin, D.; Greenberg, R.; Preston-Martin, S.; Bernstein, L.; Schoenberg, J.; Stemhagen, A. & Fraumeni, J. (1988). Smoking and Drinking in Relation to Oral and Pharyngeal Cancer. *Cancer Research,* Vol. 48, No. 11, pp. 3282-3287, ISSN 0008-5472

Cancela, M.; Ramadas, K.; Fayette, J.; Thomas, G.; Muwonge, R.; Chapuis, F.; Thara, S.; Sankaranarayanan, R. & Sauvaget, C. (2009). Alcohol Intake and Oral Cavity Cancer Risk among Men in a Prospective Study in Kerala, India. *Community Dentistry and Oral Epidemiology,* Vol. 37, No. 4, pp. 342-349, ISSN 1600-0528

Chang, F.; Wang, H.; Wang, S.; Wang, Y.; Hsieh, D.; Chang, L. & Ko, Y. (2006). Survey of Urinary Nickel in Residents of Areas with a High Density of Electroplating Factories. *Chemosphere,* Vol. 65, No. 10, pp. 1723-1730, ISSN 0045-6535

Chang, F.; Wang, S.; Huang, Y.; Tsai, M.; Yu, S. & Chang, L. (2006). Biomonitoring of Chromium for Residents of Areas with a High Density of Electroplating Factories. *Journal of Exposure Analysis and Environmental Epidemiology,* Vol. 16, No. 2, pp. 138-146, ISSN 1559-0631

Chang, T.; Hwang, K. & Shyu, G. (1997). Using Factor analysis to Evaluate Characteristic of Metals in Soil Pollution. *Journal of Chinese Agricultural Engineering,* Vol. 43, pp. 11-18, ISSN 0257-5744 (in Chinese)

Chang, T.; Shyu, G.; Lin, Y. & Chang, N. (1999). Geostatistical, Analysis of Soil Arsenic Content in Taiwan. *Journal of Environmental Science and Health Part a-Toxic/Hazardous Substances & Environmental Engineering,* Vol. 34, No. 7, pp. 1485-1501, ISSN 1093-4529

Chiang, C.; Hwang, Y.; Su, C.; Tsai, K.; Lian, I.; Yuan, T. & Chang, T. (2010). Elucidating the Underlying Causes of Oral Cancer through Spatial Clustering in High-risk Areas of Taiwan with a Distinct Gender Ratio of Incidence. *Geospatial Health,* Vol. 4, No. 2, pp. 230-242, ISSN 1970-7096

Choi, S. & Kahyo, H. (1991). Effect of Cigarette Smoking and Alcohol Consumption in the Aetiology of Cancer of the Oral Cavity, Pharynx and Larynx. *International Journal of Epidemiology,* Vol. 20, No. 4, pp. 878-885, ISSN 0300-5771

COA. (2001). Agricultural Statistics Yearbook 2001, In: *Council of Agriculture (COA), Executive Yuan, R.O.C. (Taiwan)*, 10.05.2011, Available from http://www.coa.gov.tw/view.php?catid=209

BHP. (2011a). Cancer Registry Annual Report of the Republic of China (Taiwan), 1995-2008, In: *Bureau of Health Promotion (BHP), Department of Health, R.O.C. (Taiwan)*, 10.05.2011, Available from http://www.bhp.doh.gov.tw/BHPnet/Portal/Statistics.aspx

BHP. (2011b). Interactive Query System for Cancer Registry, In: *Bureau of Health Promotion (BHP), Department of Health, R.O.C. (Taiwan)*, 15.05.2011, Available from https://cris.bhp.doh.gov.tw/

BHP. (2011c). Interactive Query System for Health Indicators, In: *Bureau of Health Promotion (BHP), Department of Health, R.O.C. (Taiwan)*, 16.05.2011, Available from http://olap.bhp.doh.gov.tw/

Dyomin, S.; Buldacov, L.; Ternovsky, I.; Tokarskaya, Z.; Fomina, T.; Tretyakov, F.; Ivanova, G.; Shevchenko, V.; Kolmogortsev, V. & Uralshin, A. (1994). Factors Effecting the Morbidity in Populations Living in the Vicinity of Atomic Industry Plants. *Science of the Total Environment*, Vol. 142, No. 1-2, pp. 105-109, ISSN 0048-9697

Green, C.; Hoppa, R.; Young, T. & Blanchard, J. (2003). Geographic Analysis of Diabetes Prevalence in an Urban Area. *Social Science & Medicine*, Vol. 57, No. 3, pp. 551-560, ISSN 0277-9536

Hotelling, H. (1933). Analysis of Complex Statistical Variables into Principal Components. *Journal of Educational Psychology*, Vol. 24, No. 6, pp. 417-441, ISSN 0022-0663

IARC. (1987). Overall Evaluations of Carcinogenicity: An Updating of IARC Monographs, In: *IARC Monographs on the Evaluation of Carcinogenic Risks to Humans, Volumes 1 to 42 (Supplement 7)*, World Health Organization International Agency for Research on Cancer, ISBN 978-928-3214-11-3, Lyon, France

IARC. (1988). Alcohol Drinking, In: *IARC Monographs on the Evaluation of Carcinogenic Risks to Humans, Volume 44*, World Health Organization International Agency for Research on Cancer, ISBN 978-928-3212-44-7, Lyon, France

IARC. (1990). Chromium, Nickel and Welding, In: *IARC Monographs on the Evaluation of Carcinogenic Risks to Humans, Volume 49*, World Health Organization International Agency for Research on Cancer, ISBN 978-928-3212-49-2, Lyon, France

IARC. (2003). Betel-quid and Areca-nut Chewing and Some Areca-nut-derived Nitrosamines, In: *IARC Monographs on the Evaluation of Carcinogenic Risks to Humans, Volume 85*, World Health Organization International Agency for Research on Cancer, ISBN 92-832-1285-1, Lyon, France

Kissling, W. & Carl, G. (2008). Spatial Autocorrelation and the Selection of Simultaneous Autoregressive Models. *Global Ecology and Biogeography*, Vol. 17, No. 1, pp. 59-71, ISSN 1466-822X

Kitron, U. & Kazmierczak, J. (1997). Spatial Analysis of the Distribution of Lyme Disease in Wisconsin. *American Journal of Epidemiology*, Vol. 145, No. 6, pp. 558-566, ISSN 0002-9262

Ko, Y.; Huang, Y.; Lee, C.; Chen, M.; Lin, L. & Tsai, C. (1995). Betel Quid Chewing, Cigarette Smoking and Alcohol Consumption Related to Oral Cancer in Taiwan. *Journal of Oral Pathology & Medicine*, Vol. 24, No. 10, pp. 450-453, ISSN 0904-2512

Lai, P.; So, F. & Chan, K. (2009). Areal Methods of Disease Analysis. In *Spatial Epidemiological Approaches in Disease Mapping and Analysis,* pp. 71-79, Taylor & Francis, ISBN 978-1-4200-4546-8, Boca Raton, FL

Lin, C.; Shiau, T.; Ko, Y.; Chen, P. & Wang, J. (2008). Prevalence and Determinants of Biochemical Dysfunction of the Liver in Atayal Aboriginal Community of Taiwan: Is Betel Nut Chewing a Risk Factor? *BMC Gastroenterology,* Vol. 8, pp. 1-8, ISSN 1471-230X

Lin, Y.; Teng, T. & Chang, T. (2002). Multivariate Analysis of Soil Heavy Metal Pollution and landscape Pattern in Changhua County in Taiwan. *Landscape and Urban Planning,* Vol. 62, No. 1, pp. 19-35, ISSN 0169-2046

Liu, C.; Lin, K. & Kuo, Y. (2003). Application of Factor Analysis in the Assessment of Groundwater Quality in a Blackfoot Disease Area in Taiwan. *The Science of the Total Environment,* Vol. 313, No. 1-3, pp. 77-89, ISSN 0048-9697

Merletti, F.; Boffetta, P.; Ciccone, G.; Mashberg, A. & Terracini, B. (1989). Role of Tobacco and Alcoholic Beverages in the Etiology of Cancer of the Oral Cavity/Oropharynx in Torino, Italy. *Cancer Research,* Vol. 49, No. 17, pp. 4919-4924, ISSN 0008-5472

Moran, P. (1950). Notes on Continuous Stochastic Phenomena. *Biometrika,* Vol. 37, No. 1-2, pp. 17-23, ISSN 0006-3444

Ogden, G. (2005). Alcohol and Oral Cancer. *Alcohol,* Vol. 35, No. 3, pp. 169-173, ISSN 0741-8329

Pearson, K. (1901). On Lines and Planes of Closest Fit to Systems of Points in Space. *Philosophical Magazine,* Vol. 2, pp. 559-572, ISSN 1941-5982

Petti, S. & Scully, C. (2005). Oral Cancer: The Association between Nation-based Alcohol-drinking Profiles and Oral Cancer Mortality. *Oral Oncology,* Vol. 41, No. 8, pp. 828-834, ISSN 1368-8375

Pfeiffer, D.; Minh, P.; Martin, V.; Epprecht, M. & Otte, M. (2007). An Analysis of the Spatial and Temporal Patterns of Highly Pathogenic Avian Influenza Occurrence in Vietnam Using National Surveillance Data. *The Veterinary Journal,* Vol. 174, No. 2, pp. 302-309, ISSN 1090-0233

Reichart, P. & Way, T. (2006). Oral Cancer and Pre-cancer in Myanmar: A Short Review. *Journal of Oral Pathology & Medicine,* Vol. 35, No. 4, pp. 193-196, ISSN 0904-2512

Rheeder, J.; Marasas, W.; Farina, M.; Thompson, G. & Nelson, P. (1994). Soil Fertility Factors in Relation to Oesophageal Cancer Risk Areas in Transkei, Southern Africa. *European Journal of Cancer Prevention,* Vol. 3, No. 1, pp. 49-56, ISSN 0959-8278

ROCEPA. (1985). Survey of Heavy Metals in the Soil Samples, In: *Yearbook of Environmental Protection Statistics Taiwan Area, the Republic of China,* Environmental Protection Administration, Executive Yuan, R.O.C. (Taiwan), Taipei

Rosas, I.; Belmont, R.; Baez, A. & Villalobos-Pietrini, R. (1989). Some Aspects of the Environmental Exposure to Chromium Residues in Mexico. *Water, Air, & Soil Pollution,* Vol. 48, No. 3-4, pp. 463-475, ISSN 0049-6979

Stocks, P. & Davies, R. (1964). Zinc and Copper Content of Soils Associated with the Incidence of Cancer of the Stomach and Other Organs. *British Journal of Cancer,* Vol. 18, pp. 14-24, ISSN 0007-0920

Su, C.; Yang, H.; Huang, S. & Lian, I. (2007). Distinctive Features of Oral Cancer in Changhua County: High incidence, Buccal Mucosa Preponderance, and a Close

Relation to Betel Quid Chewing Habit. *Journal of the Formosan Medical Association,* Vol. 106, No. 3, pp. 225-233, ISSN 0929-6646

Türkdoğan, M.; Kilicel, F.; Kara, K.; Tuncer, I. & Uygan, I. (2003). Heavy Metals in Soil, Vegetables and Fruits in the Endemic Upper Gastrointestinal Cancer Region of Turkey. *Environmental Toxicology and Pharmacology,* Vol. 13, No. 3, pp. 175-179, ISSN 1382-6689

Ward, M. & Carpenter, T. (2000). Techniques for Analysis of Disease Clustering in Space and in Time in Veterinary Epidemiology. *Preventive Veterinary Medicine,* Vol. 45, No. 3-4, pp. 257-284, ISSN 0167-5877

Wen, C.; Tsai, S.; Cheng, T.; Chen, C.; Levy, D.; Yang, H. & Eriksen, M. (2005). Uncovering the Relation between Betel Quid Chewing and Cigarette Smoking in Taiwan. *Tobacco Control,* Vol. 14, pp. I16-I22, ISSN 0964-4563

Yang, Y.; Chen, H.; Tseng, C. & Shieh, T. (2002). Prevalence Rates of Areca/Betel Quid Chewing in Counties of Taiwan. *Taiwan journal of Oral Medicine Health & Health Science,* Vol. 18, pp. 1-16, ISSN 1560-1587 (in Chinese)

Yuan, T.; Lian I.; Tsai, K.; Chang, T.; Chiang, C.; Su, C. & Hwang, Y. (2011). Possible Association between Nickel and Chromium and Oal cancer: A Case-control Study in Central Taiwan. *Science of the Total Environment,* Vol. 409, No. 6, pp. 1046-1052, ISSN 1879-1026

Zeng, D.; Yan, O. & Li, S. (2008). Spatial Regression-based Environmental Analysis in Infectious Disease Informatics, In: *Biosurveillance and Biosecurity,* D. Zeng; H.C. Chen; H. Rolka; B. Lober & M. Waterman, (Eds.), 175-181, Springer-Verlag, ISBN 978-354-0897-45-3, Berlin, Heidelberg

The Changing Aetiology of Oral Cancer and the Role of Novel Biomarkers to Aid in Early Diagnosis

Michael J. McCullough[1],
Gareema Prasad[1], Sarah Zhao[2,3] and Camile S. Farah[2,3]
[1]*The University of Melbourne, Melbourne Dental School, Melbourne*
[2]*The University of Queensland, School of Dentistry, Brisbane*
[3]*The University of Queensland, UQ Centre for Clinical Research, Herston*
Australia

1. Introduction

Head and Neck Squamous Cell Carcinoma (HNSCC) is the sixth most prevalent neoplasm in the world, with approximately 900,000 cases diagnosed worldwide (Chin, Boyle et al. 2006). The chronic use of tobacco and alcohol consumption has long been recognized as prominent risk factors in the development of oral cancer (Hashibe, Brennan et al. 2009). Oral Cancer is the 8th and 13th most common malignancy in the world for males and females respectively. Up to 80 % of these cancers occur in Asia (Cheong, Chandramouli et al. 2009). Precancerous and cancerous oral lesions may mimic any number of benign oral lesions, and as such may be left without investigation and treatment until well advanced.

The five year survival following the diagnosis of oral malignancy can be as low as 15-50% as most cancer are advanced and associated with lymphatic spread at the time of discovery (McCullough and Farah 2008). Most patients with oral cancer or a potentially malignant oral mucosal lesion are often asymptomatic at the time of diagnosis (Baranovsky and Myers 1986). Some patients do not seek care until pain, persistent ulceration, unexplained bleeding or an oral or neck mass is discovered at which time the disease is very advanced.

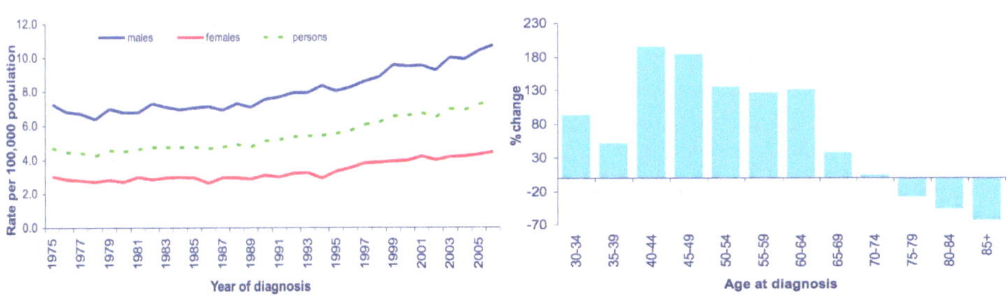

Most cancer deaths occur in patients 55 years or older (Silverman and Gorsky 1990). Thus, oral cancer is predominantly a disease of the elderly and for those with known epidemiologic risk factors, sufficient time exists to examine patients, detect precursor lesions and treat prior to the development of malignancy.

2. Aetiology

There are several known risk factors in the development of oral cancer with the most studied and well-established being the use of tobacco (Marder 1998; Hashibe, Brennan et al. 2009). In the developing world, tobacco and areca nut use, either alone or in combination, account for the majority of leukoplakias, whereas the majority of oral leukoplakias in the developed world are associated with just the use of tobacco (Napier and Speight 2008). Heavy smokers have been shown to be seven times more likely than non-smokers to have leukoplakias. Further, the importance of tobacco is reinforced by the regression and / or disappearance of many lesions following cessation with a recent study showing that 56% regressed at 3 months and 78% regressed a year after smoking cessation (Napier and Speight 2008).

2.1 Alcohol

There is increasing evidence of the role of alcohol consumption in the development of oral cancer (Hindle, Downer et al. 2000; Hashibe, Brennan et al. 2009). In a recent large pooled study undertaken by the International Head and Neck Cancer Epidemiology (INHANCE) consortium, analyzed 11,221 patients with head and neck cancer and 16,168 controls and showed a greater than multiplicative joint effect of both tobacco and alcohol (Hashibe, Brennan et al. 2009). Further, this study estimated the population attributable risks for smoking and drinking combined to be 64% (95% CI: 45-75%) showing that the joint effect of tobacco and alcohol is responsible for a large proportion of head and neck cancers (Hashibe, Brennan et al. 2009). Interestingly though, this study also concluded that a proportion of head and neck cancers cannot be attributed to either tobacco or alcohol, particularly for oral cavity cancer, among women and below age 45 (Hashibe, Brennan et al. 2009).

The ability of alcohol to cause protein denaturation and lipid dissolution, as well as its anti-microbial activity against most bacteria, fungi and viruses has resulted in alcohol being used in mouthwashes as a solvent, preservative and antiseptic agent. Studies have shown that high concentrations of alcohol in mouthwashes may have detrimental oral effects such as epithelial detachment, keratosis, mucosal ulceration, gingivitis, petechiae, and oral pain (Hsu TC, Furlong C et al. 1991; Warnakulasuriya S, Parkkila S et al. 2008) Furthermore, there is increasing evidence that there may be a direct relationship between the alcohol content of mouthwashes and the development of oral cancer, specifically, an increased risk of acquiring cancer (oral cavity, pharynx, larynx) by over 9 times for current smokers, over 5 times for those who also drink alcohol, and almost 5 times for those who neither smoke nor drink alcohol (Guha, Boffetta et al. 2007). A recent review of the literature suggested that it would be inadvisable for oral health care professionals to recommend the long-term use of alcohol-containing mouthwashes (McCullough and Farah 2008).

While alcohol was initially described as only a risk enhancer in smokers, there is now sufficient epidemiological evidence to suggest that chronic alcohol consumption is an independent risk factor (Rothman and Keller 1972; Herity, Moriarty et al. 1981; Maserejian, Joshipura et al. 2006). The exact mechanism of alcohol on the development of oral cancer remains unclear, as alcohol in itself is not clastogenic, mutagenic or carcinogenic. There is growing evidence that the local oxidation of alcohol to its toxic metabolite, acetaldehyde (AA), may be the ultimate mechanism for mediating the carcinogenic effect of alcohol in the mouth (Seitz, Matsuzaki et al. 2001).

AA is the first metabolite of alcohol and is a well-known mutagenic and carcinogenic agent (Feron, Kruysse et al. 1982). The 1999 International Agency for Research on Cancer Monographs evaluated the carcinogenic risk of AA and concluded that there was inadequate evidence in humans, but sufficient evidence in experimental animals of the carcinogenic nature of AA. Although the bulk of alcohol metabolism is carried out in the liver, extra-hepatic metabolism of alcohol to AA has been shown to occur elsewhere in the body including the oral cavity. An early study demonstrated considerable AA production in saliva (up to 143μM) after moderate consumption of alcohol (0.5g/kg body weight) (Homann, Karkkainen et al. 1997). The level of AA formed was well above endogenous AA level of 1μM (Lachenmeier, Kanteres et al. 2009) and was within the range that is capable of inducing mutagenic changes 50-150μM (Salaspuro 2007). Furthermore, studies have also found that ingested alcohol may in fact be metabolized to AA by commensal organisms in the oral cavity via microbial alcohol dehydrogenase. Microorganisms that have been documented to be significantly associated with higher AA production include *Streptococcus* spp., particularly *S. Salivarius*, *Neisseria* spp and *Candida albicans* (Homann, Tillonen et al. 2000; Muto, Hitomi et al. 2000; Kurkivuori, Salaspuro et al. 2007). The known toxic effect of AA as well as its local production in the mouth has led to increasing interest in the level of salivary AA formed after alcohol-containing mouthwash use and its association with oral cancer development.

Epidemiological studies have not led to a definitive consensus on the association of alcohol-containing mouthwashes and oral cancer. Lachenmeier et al (2009) tested the salivary AA content of four healthy individuals after rinsing with alcohol-containing mouthwash (Lachenmeier, Gumbel-Mako et al. 2009). Using headspace gas chromatography, this study found salivary AA concentrations significantly above endogenous levels.

To further our understanding of the level of salivary acetaldehyde after rinsing with alcohol containing liquids, we have recently completed an study with 30 healthy dentate dental students from the University of Melbourne participated in this study. They were selected based on the following criteria: 1) >18years of age; 2) good over-all health; 3) non-smoker; 4) non-intraoral prosthesis; 5) healthy dentition with no oral problems. The four test liquid samples selected were red wine (14% vol. alcohol), scotch whiskey (43% vol. alcohol), low alcohol mouthwash with chlorhexidene (11.5% vol. alcohol) and high alcohol mouthwash (26.9% vol. alcohol).

Saliva samples for each test liquid were collected on different days. Participants were randomly allocated a test liquid depending on the day of sampling. Participants were excluded if they had consumed food or drink, or performed oral hygiene in the previous 2 hours or consumed alcohol in the previous 24 hours.

Baseline salivary samples were collected before participants rinsed with any test liquid. Participants were then instructed to rinse 20ml of the selected test liquid vigorously for 30 seconds and expectorate immediately. Salivary samples were collected after 1 and 5 minutes after the expectoration of test liquid. Patients were required to chew on cotton rolls for 1 minute before sampling. The cotton rolls were centrifuged for 2 minutes at 3000 g in Salivette saliva collection tubes (Sarstedt, Australia Pty Ltd). A 450 μL sample of the clear saliva supernatant was then transferred to a 10 mL headspace vial containing 50 μL of perchloric acid (20% w/w) (Eriksson et al, 1982). The effect of sample storage conditions were tested by comparing AA concentrations in a set of spiked samples frozen for 2 days against a batch of freshly spiked samples.

Salivary AA concentrations were measured using headspace gas chromatography similar to previously reported methods (Lachenmeier, Gumbel-Mako et al. 2009). A gas chromatograph (GC-2010, Shimadzu) equipped with a flame ionization detector (FID) and headspace autosampler (AOC-5000, CTC analytics) was used for analysis. Data acquisition and analysis were performed using GC Solutions software. Sample vials were first incubated for 5 min at 50°C in the autosampler's oven to achieve a favourable vapour-liquid equilibrium of the AA in the headspace vials. Thereafter, 1 mL of sample headspace was automatically drawn into the injection syringe by means of the electropneumatic dosing system and injected into the GC using a split ratio of 10:1. The GC conditions used to separate the volatile components in the saliva were as follows: column: 30 m x 0.25 mm I.D. x 0.25 μm film thickness (DB-23, J&W Scientific Inc.); temperature program: 40°C hold for 2 min, 80°C/min up to 200°C and hold for 3 min; injection port temperature: 200°C; FID temperature: 250°C; carrier gas (He) flow rate: 30 cm/sec.

The suitability of the internal standards method, the calibration curve method and the standard addition method for calculating the unknown AA concentration in the saliva samples was studied. The results shown in Table 1 indicate that the analyte concentration detected from the saliva standards is in good correspondence to that with standards made up in deionized water. The calibration curve prepared from aqueous AA standards (1, 2, 5, 10 mg/L) was linear over the whole range and the limit of detection was 0.5 mg/L (11.4μM). Preliminary experiments indicated that the method developed had good reproducibility (%RSD = 1.05%, n = 6).

All mouthwashes caused a statistically significant ($p < 0.05$) increase in production of AA at both the 2 minutes and 5-minute samples when compared to the pre-mouthwash sample. Statistically significantly more AA was present at the 2-minute interval than at the 5-minute sample (Table 1). However, even 5 minutes after rinsing there was statistically significantly more AA present for all four mouthwashes when compared to the pre-mouthwash sample. There was no significant difference ($p = 0.218$) between the levels of AA produced 5 minutes after rinsing with any of the 4 solutions.

There are of course limitations to this preliminary study in particular the small sample size with only nine subjects for each test liquid. Nevertheless, these results indicate that rinsing with alcohol produced an increase in oral AA above endogenous levels and in the range capable of inducing mutagenic change (50-150μM) and that alcohol containing mouthwash has a similar effect on acetaldyde levels within the oral cavity as recreational alcohol containing liquids. These results indicate that further investigation is required into the levels of AA produced by a wide range of alcohol containing liquids, particularly those in common use.

	Alcohol (%)	Average AA concentration (μM)		
		Baseline	1 minute	5 minutes
Scotch	43	8.1 ± 8.1	97.0 ± 33.2	41.9 ± 21.2
Wine	14	11.2 ± 6.4	59.4 ± 31.0	33.8 ± 20.2
Listerine	26.9	9.1 ± 5.9	53.5 ± 19.3	25.1 ± 11.6
Savacol	11.5	18.5 ± 11.2	43.8 ± 13.8	31.4 ± 7.5

Table 1. Average AA concentration after rinsing with test liquids.

We have further assessed whether alcohol-containing mouthwashes (ACM) can induce cellular toxicity and/or genotoxicity in human cells in vitro with the single-cell gel (comet) assay and morphological assessment of apoptosis and mitosis, in order to clarify suggestive but inconclusive epidemiological data concerning a potential oral cancer risk associated with regular use of alcoholic mouthwash. Normal (OKF6/TERT-2 cells) (Dickson MA 2000) and dysplastic (DOK cells) (Chang Se 1992) human oral epithelial cells were treated for 30 seconds with a 1:5 alcohol-containing mouthwash (26% ethanol) dilution and equivalent concentration of ethanol (5.4%) for comparison. The negative control group was treated with phosphate buffered saline solution and the positive control group was treated with 650μM H2O2. Recovery time points of 5, 10 and 20 minutes were allowed before trypsinisation and layering onto slides with low-melting point agarose for electrophoresis. DNA damage was scored using the visual method established by Speit and Hartmann (Speit G 2006). Parameters from the comet assays and cytotoxicity testing were analysed by one-way ANOVA and Tukey's test.

ACM and ethanol treatment groups consistently demonstrated significantly greater DNA damage ($P < 0.001$) in the comet assay when compared to negative controls. No significant difference was noted between recovery time points. No significant differences in apoptosis and mitosis were noted between treatments and controls in the cytotoxicity assay, however OKF-6 cells (normal) were shown to have increased apoptosis and decreased mitosis when compared to DOK cells (dysplastic). These results indicate that ACMs do have a genotoxic effect in oral epithelial cells, however they do not induce cellular toxicity in these short-term laboratory conditions.

Although separate assays exist to detect damage through each specific mechanism discussed above, the comet assay is a general test for detection of DNA breakage- the end result of all damage pathways. It is sensitive to DNA single- and double-strand breaks, interstrand cross-links, and apurinic/apyrimidinic (AP) sites which relax the supercoiled structure of genomic DNA under alkaline conditions (Speit G 2006). Multiple studies have established that visual scoring is both efficient and accurate, bearing a linear correlation to computer scoring (Garcia O 2004) (Panayiotidis MI 2004). Results indicate that ACMs cause significant fragmentation of DNA, which over many cycles can lead to mutation. Furthermore, it was found that no DNA repair occurred within the 20 minutes allowed for recovery following treatments, allowing carcinogenic effects to compound more rapidly.

Selecting two cell lines (DOK and OKF-6) for experiments permitted testing of ACM effects on normal oral epithelial cells, as well as allowing comparisons to be made with dysplastic cells. Results from the comet assay indicate that DNA damage is significantly greater in

DOK cells compared to OKF-6 cells, supporting the idea that ACM use may be a greater risk in smokers or patients with pre-existing dysplasia. Previous research shows that risk associated with alcohol consumption is not necessarily constant over the multistage pathway to oral cancer (Franceschi S 2000) (Franceschi et al., 2000). Traditionally, alcohol has been thought to play a role in the later stages of oral cancer progression (Day & Brown, 1980), a view supported by our results. However newer studies are finding that drinking may exert earlier effects, as cessation does not lower oral cancer risk for up to 9 years (Franceschi S 2000) Temporal mechanisms of alcohol carcinogenicity may be more complex and multifactorial than previously thought. Although experiments used were not sensitive to a concurrent synergism between ACM and tobacco carcinogens, it was possible to ascertain the possibility of a sequential synergistic effect with tobacco because DOK cells were developed from the tongue mucosa of a smoker.

Thus, it would appear that the effect of alcohol consumption on oral epithelial cells is likely to be local, topical and temporally important in oral carcinogenesis.

2.2 Human Papilloma Virus

For many years, HPV has been accepted as an important cofactor in the development of cervical cancer, originating from a mucous membrane with similarities to the oral mucosa. It has long been postulated that oncogenic HPV subtypes (specifically, HPV 16 and 18) can have a tumorigenic effect on oral epithelia. Evidence to support a role for HPV was found in analysis of the presence of HPV in biopsy specimens, the majority concluding that it was likely that HPV may be a cofactor in the development of oral cancer (Nielsen, Norrild et al. 1996; D'Costa, Saranath et al. 1998; Al-Bakkal, Ficarra et al. 1999). The INHANCE consortium mentioned above reported on the analysis of a large cohort assessing links between cancer and specific sexual behaviours, including practice of oral sex, number of lifetime sexual partners and oral sex partners, age at sexual debut, a history of same-sex contact and a history of oral-anal contact. This study concluded that these sexual behaviours are associated with increased risk of cancer, particularly of the tongue, tonsil and oro-pharynx and reinforce the association with infection by HPV sub-types (Heck, Berthiller et al. 2009). Furthermore, it has been shown that there is an overall increase in the incidence of base of tongue cancer over the past 30 years and further that there is an increase in the prevalence of HPV in these tongue cancers (Attner, Du et al. 2009). Thus, it would appear that there is an increased understanding of the causative role for HPV in oral and oro-pharyngeal cancer with an urgent need for further research in the role of that this virus may play in the propagation of potentially malignant mucosal lesions.

A recent extensive collaborative study recently reported the prevalence of HPV types in the oropharynx in men who have sex with men (MSM) and compared sampling methods as well as identifying risk factors. This cross-sectional study enrolled 250 HIV negative and 250 HIV positive MSM who were sampled by either a self-collected flocked throat/mouth swab agitated in RNAlater or collected gargled saline. Further, a questionnaire about sexual behaviour, oral hygiene and smoking was collected.

HPV PCR was undertaken after DNA extraction using MagNA Pure LC (Roche Molecular Systems) the HPV DNA amplification was undertaken using L1 consensus primers & beta-globin control via PCR. An ELISA using biotin-labeled probe was used to identify PCR products and subsequently a line-blot hybridization (Linear array - Roche) used to genotype the PCR product.

The results of this study showed a prevalence of oral HPV with 74 positive in one or both samples. The self-collected flocked throat and mouth swab was positive in 33 of the 74 (44.6% sensitive) while the oral rinse was positive in 65 of the 74 positive samples (87.8% sensitive). High-risk genotypes (16 and 59) were found in 21 (4.2%) samples. The HPV prevalence in this MSM population depended on the HIV status with those HIV negative showed 8% (0.8% HPV 16) positive samples while those MSM who were HIV positive had 22% (4.8% HPV 16) positive samples. Oral rinse method of sample collection was nearly twice as sensitive as self-collected swab. Significant risk factors included smoking, age greater than 40 and lifetime oral sex partners greater that 100.

Thus, it would appear that high-risk HPV sub-types are present in the oral cavity, and this presence is associated with risk behaviours, in particular smoking and the number of lifetime oral sex partners. It could be postulated that there is synergism of these risk factors, particularly if alcohol consumption was also included. There is therefore a need for the development and clinical validation of a simple salivary method for the assessment of risk of developing oral cancer that is not associated with smoking as this is likely to enhance the effectiveness of oral cancer screening services and improving oral cancer outcomes.

3. Novel biomarkers

Currently the gold standard in diagnosis of malignant and potentially malignant oral mucosal lesions is incisional biopsy and histo-pathological assessment. However, histopathological examination has concerns related to sampling errors and errors in interpretation, and lacks sensitivity to determine lesion progression.(Holmstrup, Vedtofte et al. 2006) That is, the level of dysplasia of an oral lesion may not necessarily correlate with the lesion's potential for malignant transformation. Hence, there is a need for a more accurate system to predict the progression to cancer and currently there is significant work being undertaken in identifying markers in patients with oral cancer and pre-cancer that may serve as a valuable resource in finding markers for the early diagnosis of these conditions.

3.1 DNA ploidy

Several studies have already shown that DNA ploidy is of prognostic importance in some human malignancies such as carcinomas of the ovary (Brescia and et al. 1990), prostate (Badalament and et al. 1991), urinary bladder (Norming and et al. 1992) and malignant melanomas (Sorensen and et al. 1991). Importantly, DNA ploidy has been shown to be an early marker of malignant transformation in oral dysplasia (Sudbo and et al. 2001). DNA ploidy can be classified into three clinically relevant categories, diploid, tetraploid and aneuploid. The positive correlation that has been reported to exist between DNA ploidy and prognosis of oral dysplasia (Sudbo and et al. 2001), suggests that DNA ploidy may well be a key factor in the diagnosis, prognosis and treatment of oral malignancies in the future and thus requires full investigation.

The use of DNA ploidy for oral mucosal conditions has attracted considerable controversy (Curfman GD 2006; Reed KD 2007). There was considerable promise in the early part of this decade that the use of DNA ploidy could better predict outcome for potentially malignant oral mucosal disease. Irrespective of the controversies associated with a large portion of this work multiple independent and meticulous studies have been undertaken to attempt to put the investigations of the utility of oral mucosal DNA ploidy on a sound scientific basis. Interestingly, the results of these studies have been varied with some reporting guarded success at predicting outcome of malignant transformation (Torres-Rendon and et al. 2009 June), while others have shown little benefit from this technique in assessing the malignant potential of mucosal lesions (Neppelberg and Johannessen A.C. 2007).

The majority of previous studies assessing DNA ploidy in oral mucosal lesions have used nuclei isolated from formalin fixed, paraffin embedded, archival material 19-22. These nuclei were extracted, processed to form a monolayer on glass slides and, after Feulgen staining, individual nuclei selected for integrated optical density analysis. The number of nuclei analyzed was usually in the range of 200-300 per sample 22. In each of these retrospective studies, internal control nuclei within each monolayer, such as inflammatory cells or "unsuspicious" epithelial cells, were used to assess for significant variations from DNA diploidy (aneuploidy) of nuclei from each specimen. However, as a prospective clinical tool, such methodology is limited.

Over recent years there has been increased use of liquid-based cytology (LBC) for cervical smears and this method has been analyzed for utility with oral cytology (Kujan and et al. 2006). The initial study evaluating LBC for oral cytology assessed 150 specimens from 50 healthy volunteers and found that this technique distributed cells evenly, optimized fixation, improved and unbiased sampling, enhanced nuclear detail and eliminated air-drying artifacts. These researchers also reported that the specimens showed cells from two populations, superficial and intermediate cells with only six (4%) of specimens containing parabasal or basal cells (Kujan and et al. 2006). This latter finding has significant impact as these superficial cells represent keratinocytes that are terminally differentiating and thus nuclei have become non-functional with condensed and fragmented chromatin.

In a recent study (McCullough MJ 2009) assessing the variability of ploidy present in oral cytological material using nuclear analyses of integrated density via Feulgen staining, liquid based processing of oral cytological samples and the establishment of a large database of normality. This study found that there was more variabilitiy observed in patients with normal mucosa than in oral mucosal dysplasia and neoplasia. It may well be that these nuclear alterations present in the superficial cell layers resulted in increased optical integrated density after Feulgen staining observed and the observed lack of differentiation between normal and abnormal samples was likely to be due to sampling, with inadequate numbers of basal cells whose DNA could not be assessed separately from the large number of superficial nuclei (McCullough MJ 2009).

An attempt to circumvent this tissue-sampling problem has been reported by obtained representative tissue specimens by scraping with a dermatological curette (Navone R 2008), thus producing "micro-biopsies" rather than cytological samples from brushing mucosa. Such a technique, which included liquid cytology for tissue handling, has been reported to be a non-invasive, rapid method that has little patient discomfort and is able to sample a broader area than a single biopsy (Navone R 2008). Ideally, the analyses of the cells collected would include multiple markers, not only assessing the presence of basal cells in the sample, but also the extent of a number of genetic changes known to be linked to the development of oral neoplasia. This is unlikely to be feasible using ploidy assessment via the Feulgen reaction as this reaction requires acid hydrolysis of DNA significantly altering both cytological and nuclear attributes. Such markers may well include the recently reported centrosomal abnormalities reportedly to occur universally in oral dysplasia.

Thus, there still remains the need for a robust method to assess molecular changes known to be associated with the early changes in neogenesis to aid in the early detection of oral mucosal lesions with increased malignant potential.

3.2 mRNAs

The identification of tissue markers that aid assessment of malignant potential have been investigated, and reviewed by Scully (Scully 1993). Such markers include cell surface and cytoplasmic components.

Loss of Heterozygosity (LOH) is considered loss of genetic material at microsatellite loci, and has been shown to be an important event in tumorigenesis (Ng IO, Xiao L et al. 2000). Investigations of LOH in genes and chromosomal regions, has shown that defined regions are affected in oral carcinogenesis/HNSCC and that these may be used as a possible prognostic marker.

A model for HNSCC progression has been proposed suggesting deletions at 3q, 9q and 17q are associated with a morphological transition of cells from normal to dysplastic cells, and that carcinoma development was promoted by further deletions at 4q, 6p, 11q, 13q and 14q (Califano J, van der Riet P et al. 1996).

Single nucleotide polymorphisms (SNPs) are single base alteration or point mutations in DNA and are considered the most common form of genetic variation, occurring approximately every 1200 base pairs in human chromosomes (Sherry 2001). Hence, many studies have investigated the incidence of SNPs in particular genes to determine their role in HNSCC carcinogenesis.

TP53 is an extensively characterised TSG, which encodes the protein p53. TP53 is located on the short arm of chromosome 17 and has 11 exons, one of which is non functional (Liao PH, Chang YC et al. 2000). p53 is a sequence specific transcription factor that is important for DNA maintenance.

A study of 94 oral squamous cell carcinomas (OSSC) found that 43% had TP53 mutations (Ostwald, 2000), similarly another study observed 48.66% of OSSC had p53 mutations (Hsieh, Wang et al. 2001). An analysis of 18 oral tumours found 72% had TP53 mutation, however this high incidence may have been due to the small sample size (Partridge, 2000). Generally, TP53 mutations are considered a common genetic change, being evident in 40-50% of HNSCC (Nylander, 2000).

Other studies have documented associations between TP53 polymorphisms and HNSCC. One investigation observed the highest number of mutations occurred in exon 7 and that the type of SNP was characteristic of lesion location. Lip lesions exhibited G:C to A:T transitions while intra-oral lesions exhibited an equal frequency of transitions and transversions (G:C to T:A) (Ostwald C, Gogacz P et al. 2000). It has been proposed that these transversions are preferentially induced by breakdown products of benz[a]pyrenes, suggesting a strong correlation with tobacco usage (Ostwald C, Gogacz P et al. 2000). A study of sequential epithelial dysplasias and squamous cell carcinomas suggested TP53 mutations correlated with an invasive tumour phenotype (Shahnavaz SA, Regezi JA et al. 2000). A further study reported greater than 90% of HNSCC samples had TP53 mutations, with the type of mutation varying among tumours (van Oijen MG, Vd et al. 2000 Feb). They also demonstrated primary tumours and metastases showed the same TP53 mutation, suggesting that TP53 mutations are relatively stable within a given tumour.

SNPs in other genes have been investigated including the CYP1A1 polymorphism in the gene encoding cytochrome p450. This polymorphism results in an amino acid substitution from Isoleucine to Valine. It has been proposed that the Valine form of the enzyme has a greater catalytic and mutagenic activity towards benz[a]pyrenes and therefore may be associated with high risk of OSSC development (Sato M, Sato T et al. 2000; Sreelekha TT, Ramadas K et al. 2001). However, other studies have not observed an association between this polymorphism and HNSCC (McWilliams JE, Evans AJ et al. 2000).

3.3 MicroRNAs

An area of interest for markers of potentially malignant mucosal lesions is MicroRNAs (miRNAs). MiRNAs are small non coding RNAs that mediate gene expression at the post-transcriptional level by degrading or repressing target messenger RNAs (mRNAs). They act by binding to partially complementary sites in the 3` region of the mRNA target. MiRNAs are approximately 18 - 22 nucleotides in length and are predicted to regulate at least 30% of the mRNA transcripts (Gomes and Gomez 2008).

MiRNAs are transcribed by RNA polymerase II or III as an independent gene unit or as part of an intron on a larger mRNA molecule. This mRNA can be up to 1000 nucleotides in length and has a stem-loop structure. This initial transcript is cleaved into a shorter stem-loop structure of less than 100 nucleotides by a type III RNAse (Drosha). This pre - miRNA is exported out into the cytoplasm by exportin-5 where another RNAse III (Dicer) cleaves it, resulting in a 18 - 24 nucleotide long mature miRNA. The mature miRNA is bound to a protein complex called an RNA induced silencing complex (RISC - RNA) formed by four argonaute family proteins (Ago 1-4). This active miRNA - protein complex binds to specific sites present in a number of mRNA's resulting in their inactivation. To date, 1048 different human miRNAs have been identified in the miRBase database It has been shown that each mirNA regulates a number of mRNAs(Gomes and Gomez 2008).

MicroRNAs bind to the 3′ untranslated region (30 UTR) of target mRNA. Depending on the degree of sequence complementary, the mRNA is either inhibited or degraded. Studies conducted up to date suggest that miRNAs function either as oncogenes or tumor suppressors in various cancer types, as well as OSCC.

MiRNAs have been associated with almost all types of human malignancies including haematological and solid cancers. When the classification accuracy of types of cancer were compared, variation from the normal profile of miRNAs were shown to more pronounced in poorly differentiated tumors (Hui, Shi et al. 2009).

A reduction in miRNAs that suppress tumours is thought to result in an increase of oncogenic proteins and hence accelerates oncogenic transformation. On the other hand, an increase in miRNAs during oncogenises may be associated with inactivation of tumour suppressor genes thus accelerating oncogenic transformation as outlined in Fig.1. (Gomes and Gomez 2008).

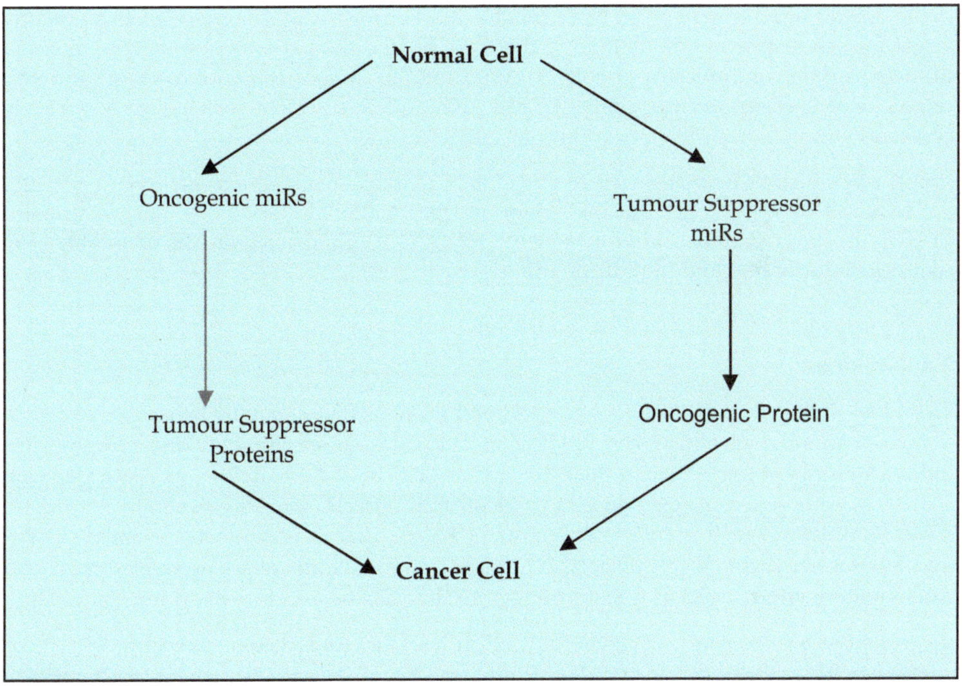

Fig. 1.

Abnormal regulation of these miRNAs in OSCC induces cell proliferation and anti-apoptosis, promotes cancer metastasis and potentiates resistance to chemotherapy. miRNA-regulated pathways in OSCC (Bo-hai Wua, Xue-peng Xiong et al. 2011).

In the past, a great deal of focus has been placed on messenger RNAs (mRNAs) and their ability to act as biological markers in cancer. Recent studies have shown that miRNAs more accurately cluster different types of solid tumors than mRNA, suggesting that miRNAs may be an alternative early marker of malignancy (J, G et al. 2005) Furthermore, the extent of change in mRNA between cancer cells and normal cells is relatively small, whereas, many miRNAs exhibit large changes between normal and cancer cells (in the order of ten to hundred fold changes) hence potentially enhancing detection of differences.(Jinmai Jiang, Eun Joo Lee et al. 2005)

It has been reported that miRNAs may be less prone to degradation and modification than mRNAs due to their small size, hence allowing the use of formalin fixed paraffin embedded (FFPE) samples (Martina, Magotra Amber A. et al. 2008). There is thus a potential rich source of retrospective information available for comparative genomics and investigation of potential biomarkers that is likely to provide biological insights far more expeditiously than the prospective collection of frozen samples.

Abnormal miRNA expression has been found in both premalignant and malignant cells (Clague j, Scott M. Lippman et al. 2010). Hence, there is a need for the investigation of miRNA expression in potentially malignant oral mucosal lesions as well as OSCC as deregulated miRNAs may be an early reliable marker for malignancy as well as a potential target for cancer prevention. Although there are no specific patterns of miRNA expression till date, certain core miRNAs should be considered in tumorigenesis of the head and neck region. This core set includes, mir -21, mir -205 and mir - 155 which have shown to be constantly upregulated (Tran, O'Brien et al. 2010).

It is evident further investigations to elucidate a marker or markers of malignant potential are required to aid detection of malignant and pre-malignant lesions, as well as to better predict the prognosis of individuals with HNSCC. With the advent of accessible gene sequence information and high throughput genetic methods, genetic alterations may act as such a marker.

3.4 Cytokines

Cytokines are a group of small, mainly secreted proteins that affect the behaviour of cells in a diverse number of ways. The binding of cytokines to specific cytokine receptors can induce a number of activities in the cell, such as growth, differentiation, or death (Janeway CA 1996). Although most cytokines have pleotrophic effects, some are generally considered pro-inflammatory, such as interferon-gamma (IFN-γ), tumour necrosis factor-alpha (TNF-α) and interleukin-1beta (IL-1β) (Dinarello CA 1997), whereas others are associated with anti-inflammatory effects, such as transforming growth factor-beta-1 (TGF-β1) (Ling EM 2002).

Over the last 5 years or so, a considerable effort has been undertaken analysing the salivary proteome. There has been a very large number of non-redundant proteins recognised in saliva with one study (Scarano E 2010) reporting over 1400, while a further (Xiao H 2011) almost 2,000, reflecting the potency of salivary biomarker profiles in the identification and management of a range of diseases (Bandhakavi S 2009). Salivary biomarkers have the potential to serve as non-invasive, widely available screening tools that do not rely on the localization of a lesion for diagnosis. This advantage over other detection methods gives salivary biomarker screening the potential to identify patients with premalignant lesions.

Of particular interest has been the use of salivary cytokine levels as markers of cell proliferation and oral cancer (Schapher M 2011) with the most studied cytokines including epidermal growth factor (EGF), interleukin 6 and 8, vascular endothelial growth factor (VEGF), interleukin 4 and 10, tumour necrosis factor (TNF) and endothelin.

A large body of work has assess interleukin 6 (IL-6), a multifunctional cytokine that participates in the inflammatory and immune responses shown to directly promote the growth of certain types of cancer as well as being associated with an increased rate of metastasis (St John MA 2004) (Brailo V, 2006 #143). Interestingly, IL-6 would appear to have different effects on different cell populations, stimulatory for some cell types, while inhibitory for others (Wang YF 2002) as well as demonstrable direct effect on cancer cells due to inactivation of the p53 tumour suppressor gene (Hodge DR 2005). Irrespective of the role of IL-6, there is an increasing body of evidence to support that there is higher level of IL-6 in saliva of patient with oral cancer as well as oral potentially malignant lesions, than in normal controls. In a recently trial of 29 consecutive patients being treated for oral cancer it was shown that these patients had much higher salivary concentration of IL-6 than in controls and that this concentration increased during the treatment period returning to baseline levels at discharge (Sato J 2010).

Other studies however have assessed a panel of pro-inflammatory cytokines as makers of malignancy. In a recent study of levels of IL-1a, IL-6, IL-8, VEGF-a and TNF-a in saliva were measured using quantitative ELISA in a grop of 18 patinets with tongue SCC. These biomarkers were increased in patients with oral cancer, significantly increased in a sub-group of patients with endophytic tongue cancer and IL-8 levels particularly shown to correlate with poor prognosis as well as controls who smoke and consumed alcohol daily (Korostoff A 2011).

These findings indicate that salivary cytokine levels is very likely to provide useful information of epithelial behaviour and carcinogenesis and the potential of a panel of these cytokines being able to be used as a screening tool for oral cancer is currently underway, the results of which are eagerly awaited as this is likely to have a profound impact on the early detection of oral cancer and thus morbidity and mortality.

3.5 Chemokines

Chemokines are a superfamily of structurally related cytokines, which share an ability to chemotactically attract their target cells along a concentration gradient. It is through this ability that these molecules play an integral role in the migration of immune cells to areas of pathogen challenge. Chemokines also mediate the movements of cells to allow interactions between immune cells that are essential for mounting immune responses (Zlotnik A 2000).

All chemokines are small proteins, ranging in weight from 6-14KDa. There are now over 40 identified chemokines which can be classified into 4 main structural families, dependent upon the position of cysteine residues near the N-terminus. These families are the CC, CXC, C and CX3C, with the X denoting the number of amino acids between the cysteine residues (Olsen TS 2002). Nearly all chemokines are secreted from the site of production and they often bind with glycosaminoglycans (Hoogewerf AJ, Kuschert GS et al. 1997 Nov 4). It is thought that this is the method in which the chemokines form the concentration gradient that target cells migrate towards, as a higher concentration is formed on the connective tissue nearest the area of chemokine production.

The function of chemokines can be subdivided into two main families; those that are induced after inflammatory stimuli, the inflammatory chemokines, and those produced constitutively in tissues, the homing chemokines (Kunkel EJ 2002). There appears to be some overlap between these chemokines as some of the inflammatory chemokines appear to be produced constitutively in some areas of the body (Izadpanah A 2001) and some of the chemokines designated as homing chemokines can be upregulated by inflammatory stimuli (Morales J 1999) .

Although the detection of chemokine levels by enzyme-linked immunosorbent assay (ELISA) has become a sensitive and specific method to determine the chemokine profile in patient fluids, this does not fully represent the actual inflammatory conditions in vivo. Indeed, many chemokines are post-translationally modified by proteolytic cleavage, which can render an agonist more active, inactive or even convert the active chemokine into a receptor antagonist of the intact molecule (Struyf S 2003).

A recent study analysed, using ELISA, the saliva of patients with oral cancer for the presence of both inflammatory chemokines (CXCL8, CXCL10 and CCL2) as well as homeostatic chemokines (CXCL4, CCL14 and CCL18) (Michiels K 2009). Patients with and without periodontitis were used as controls and it was found that H&N carcinomas give rise to a change in the chemokine composition of the oral fluid with a significant increase in CXCL8, CXCL10, and CCL14 before, but not after, therapy. However, the levels detectable by ELISA were very low and it is likely that more refined methods should indicate not only intact chemokines, but also those modified post-translationally. These authors conclude that it can be expected that specific truncated chemokines and the proteases involved are linked to a particular disease state and postulate that further proteomic analysis of biological fluids will help us to learn more about the pathogenesis of specific diseases and can provide solutions for new diagnostic and treatment options.

4. Conclusion

Oral cancer is a significant problem with low rates of mortality and an enormous impact on quality of life and morbidity. In the past this has been predominantly a disease of the elderly with known epidemiologic risk factors, however this appears to be changing. The principle recognized risk factor is smoking; however, there is growing evidence that the local effect of alcohol, most likely via its toxic metabolite acetaldehyde, may be increasing in importance. There is now evidence that alcohol containing mouthwash show similar oral acetaldehyde levels as recreational alcohol containing liquids. Further, these mouthwashes have been shown to have genotoxic effect in oral epithelial cells. Therefore be inadvisable for oral health care professionals to recommend the long-term use of alcohol-containing mouthwashes.

Particular high-risk HPV sub-types are now known to be implicated in a large proportion of oro-pharyngeal cancers and these same sub-types are present in the oral cavity. It has been postulated that there is synergism of risk factors, such as smoking and alcohol consumption. As these previously under-recognized risk factors may be becoming of increasing important aetiological agents, there is therefore a need for the development and clinical validation of a simple salivary method for the assessment of risk of developing oral cancer that is not associated with smoking as this is likely to enhance the effectiveness of oral cancer screening services and improving oral cancer outcomes. Identifying a combination of salivary biomarkers that predict at- risk and cancerous states with sufficient sensitivity and specificity for widespread use will have a profound impact on improving the morbidity and mortality of the disease.

A number of cellular and molecular markers are currently under ongoing investigation to aid in the detection of early changes to aid in the detection of oral mucosal lesions with increased malignant potential. With the advent of accessible gene sequence information and high throughput genetic methods, genetic alterations may act as such a marker. Furthermore, there is evidence that salivary cytokine levels can provide useful information of oral epithelial behaviour and carcinogenesis and the potential of a panel of these cytokines being able to be used as a screening tool for oral cancer is currently underway, the results of which are eagerly awaited as this is likely to have a profound impact on the early detection of oral cancer and thus morbidity and mortality. Finally, further genomic and proteomic analysis of oral tissue, whether oral biological fluids or cells, will help us to learn more about the pathogenesis of oral cancer and it is anticipated that this will provide solutions for new diagnostic and treatment options.

5. References

Al-Bakkal, G., G. Ficarra, et al. (1999). "Human papilloma virus type 16 E6 gene expression in oral exophytic epithelial lesions as detected by in situ rtPCR." *Oral Surg Oral Med Oral Pathol Oral Radiol Endod* 87(2): 197-208.

Attner, P., J. Du, et al. (2009). "The role of human papillomavirus in the increased incidence of base of tongue cancer." *Int J Cancer.*

Badalament, R. A. and et al. (1991). "DNA ploidy and prostate-specific antigen as prognostic factors in clinically resectable prostate cancer." *Cancer* 27(12): 3014-23.

Bandhakavi S, S. M., Onsongo G, Van Riper SK, Griffin TJ. (2009). "A dynamic range compression and three-dimensional peptide fractionation analysis platform expands proteome coverage and the diagnostic potential of whole saliva." *J Proteome Res.* 8(12): 5590-600.

Baranovsky, A. and M. H. Myers (1986). "Cancer incidence and survival in patients 65 years of age and older." *CA Cancer J Clin* 36(1): 26-41.

Bo-hai Wua, Xue-peng Xiong, et al. (2011). "MicroRNAs: New actors in the oral cancer scene, ." *Oral Oncology*

Brescia, R. J. and et al. (1990). "The prognostic significance of nuclear DNA content in malignant epithelial tumors of the ovary." *CANCER* 65(1): 141-7.

Califano J, van der Riet P, et al. (1996). "Genetic progression model for head and neck cancer: implications for field cancerization. ." *Cancer Res.* 56(11): 2488-92.

Chang Se, F. S., Betts D, Marnock WE (1992). "DOK, a cell line established from human dysplastic oral mucosa, shows a partially transformed non-malignant phenotype." *International Journal of Cancer* 52: 896-902.

Cheong, S. C., G. V. Chandramouli, et al. (2009). "Gene expression in human oral squamous cell carcinoma is influenced by risk factor exposure." *Oral Oncol* 45(8): 712-9.

Chin, D., G. M. Boyle, et al. (2006). "Head and neck cancer: past, present and future." *Expert Rev Anticancer Ther* 6(7): 1111-8.

Clague j, Scott M. Lippman, et al. (2010). "Genetic Variation in MicroRNA Genes and Risk of Oral Premalignant Lesions." *molecular carcinogenesis* 49: 183 - 189

Curfman GD, M. S., Drazen JM (2006). "Expression of concern: Sudbo J et al. DNA content as a prognostic marker in patients with oral leukoplakia. N Engl J Med 2001;344:1270-

8 and Sudbo J et al. the influence of resection and aneuploidy on mortality in oral leukoplakia. N Engl J Med 2004;350:1405-13." *N Engl J Med* 354(6): 638.

D'Costa, J., D. Saranath, et al. (1998). "Detection of HPV-16 genome in human oral cancers and potentially malignant lesions from India." *Oral Oncol* 34(5): 413-20.

Dickson MA, H. W., Ino Y, Ronfard v, Wu JY, Weinberg RA, Louis DN, Li FP, Rheinwald JG. (2000). "Human keratinocytes that express hTERT and also bypass a p16(INK4a)-enforced mechanism that limits life span become immortal yet retain normal growth and differentiation characteristics." *Mol Cell Biol* 20: 1436-47.

Dinarello CA (1997). "Role of pro- and anti-inflammatory cytokines during inflammation: experimental and clinical findings." *Journal of Biol Regul Homeost Agents* 11(3): 91-103.

Feron, V. J., A. Kruysse, et al. (1982). "Respiratory tract tumours in hamsters exposed to acetaldehyde vapour alone or simultaneously to benzo(a)pyrene or diethylnitrosamine." *Eur J Cancer Clin Oncol* 18(1): 13-31.

Franceschi S, L. F., Maso LD, Talamini R, Negru E, Vecchia CL (2000). "Cessation of alcohol drinking and risk of cancer of the oral cavity and pharynx. ." *International Journal of Cancer* 85: 787-790.

Garcia O, M. T., Lamadrid AI, Diaz A, Remiglo A, Gonzalez Y, Piloto J, Gonzalez JE, Alvarez A. (2004). "Sensitivity and variability of visual scoring in the comet assay: results of an inter-laboratory exercise with the use of silver staining." *Mutation Research* 556: 25-34.

Gomes, C. and R. Gomez (2008). "MicroRNA and oral cancer: Future Perspectives." *Oral Oncology* 44: 910 -914.

Guha, N., P. Boffetta, et al. (2007). "Oral health and risk of squamous cell carcinoma of the head and neck and esophagus: results of two multicentric case-control studies." *Am J Epidemiol* 166(10): 1159-73.

Hashibe, M., P. Brennan, et al. (2009). "Interaction between tobacco and alcohol use and the risk of head and neck cancer: pooled analysis in the International Head and Neck Cancer Epidemiology Consortium." *Cancer Epidemiol Biomarkers Prev* 18(2): 541-50.

Heck, J. E., J. Berthiller, et al. (2009). "Sexual behaviours and the risk of head and neck cancers: a pooled analysis in the International Head and Neck Cancer Epidemiology (INHANCE) consortium." *Int J Epidemiol.*

Herity, B., M. Moriarty, et al. (1981). "A case-control study of head and neck cancer in the Republic of Ireland." *Br J Cancer* 43(2): 177-82.

Hindle, I., M. C. Downer, et al. (2000). "The association between intra-oral cancer and surrogate markers of smoking and alcohol consumption." *Community Dent Health* 17(2): 107-13.

Hodge DR, P. B., Cherry JC, Hurt EM, Fox SD, Kelley JA, (2005). "Interleukin 6 supports the maintenance of p53 tumor suppressor gene promoter hypermethylation. ." *Cancer Res* 65: 4673-82.

Holmstrup, P., P. Vedtofte, et al. (2006). "Long-term treatment outcome of oral premalignant lesions." *Oral Oncol* 42(5): 461-74.

Homann, N., P. Karkkainen, et al. (1997). "Effects of acetaldehyde on cell regeneration and differentiation of the upper gastrointestinal tract mucosa." *J Natl Cancer Inst* 89(22): 1692-7.

Homann, N., J. Tillonen, et al. (2000). "Increased salivary acetaldehyde levels in heavy drinkers and smokers: a microbiological approach to oral cavity cancer." *Carcinogenesis* 21(4): 663-8.

Hoogewerf AJ, Kuschert GS, et al. (1997 Nov 4). "Glycosaminoglycans mediate cell surface oligomerization of chemokines." *Biochemistry.* 36(44): 13570-8.

Hsu TC, Furlong C, et al. (1991). "Ethyl alcohol as a cocarcinogen with special reference to the aerodigestive tract: a cytogenetic study." *Anticancer Res* 11: 1097-1101.

Hui, A. B., W. Shi, et al. (2009). "Robust Global micro - RNA profiling with formalin-fixed-paraffin-embedded breast cancer tissues." *Laboratory Investigation* 89: 597-606.

Izadpanah A, D. M., Eckmann L, Varki NM, Kagnoff MF, (2001). "Regulated MIP-3alpha/CCL20 production by human intestinal epithelium: mechanism for modulating mucosal immunity." *Am J Physiol Gastrointest Liver Physiol.* 280(4): 710-19.

J, L., G. G, et al. (2005). "MicroRNA expression profiles classify human cancers." *Nature* 435: 834–8.

Janeway CA, T. P. (1996). *Immunobiology: The Immune System in Health and Disease.* , Churchill Livingstone.

Jinmai Jiang, Eun Joo Lee, et al. (2005). "Real-time expression profiling of microRNA precursors in human cancer cell lines." *Nucleic Acids Research* 33: 5394 - 5403.

Korostoff A, R. L., Masood R, Sinha UK. (2011). "The role of salivary cytokine biomarkers in tongue cancer invasion and mortality." *Oral Oncol.* 47(4): 282-7.

Kujan, O. and et al. (2006). "Screening programmes for the early detection and prevention of oral cancer." *Cochrane Database Syst Rev* 3: CD004150.

Kunkel EJ, B. E. (2002). "Mini-review: Chemokines and the tissue-specific migration of lymphocytes. ." *Immunity* 16: 1-4.

Kurkivuori, J., V. Salaspuro, et al. (2007). "Acetaldehyde production from ethanol by oral streptococci." *Oral Oncol* 43(2): 181-6.

Lachenmeier, D. W., S. Gumbel-Mako, et al. (2009). "Salivary acetaldehyde increase due to alcohol-containing mouthwash use: a risk factor for oral cancer." *Int J Cancer* 125(3): 730-5.

Lachenmeier, D. W., F. Kanteres, et al. (2009). "Carcinogenicity of acetaldehyde in alcoholic beverages: risk assessment outside ethanol metabolism." *Addiction* 104(4): 533-50.

Liao PH, Chang YC, et al. (2000). "Mutation of p53 gene codon 63 in saliva as a molecular marker for oral squamous cell carcinomas. ." *Oral Oncol.* 36(3): 272-276.

Ling EM, R. D. (2002). "Transforming growth factor-beta1: its anti-inflammatory and pro-fibrotic effect. ." *Clinical and Experimental Allergy* 32: 175-178.

Marder, M. Z. (1998). "The standard of care for oral diagnosis as it relates to oral cancer." *Compend Contin Educ Dent* 19(6): 569-72, 574, 576 passim; quiz 584.

Martina, D., Magotra Amber A. , et al. (2008). "Evaluation and Validation of Total RNA Extraction Methods for MicroRNA Expression Analyses in Formalin-Fixed, Paraffin-Embedded Tissues." *Journal of Molecular Diagnostics* 10: 203-211.

Maserejian, N. N., K. J. Joshipura, et al. (2006). "Prospective study of alcohol consumption and risk of oral premalignant lesions in men." *Cancer Epidemiol Biomarkers Prev* 15(4): 774-81.

McCullough, M. J. and C. S. Farah (2008). "The role of alcohol in oral carcinogenesis with particular reference to alcohol-containing mouthwashes." *Aust Dent J* 53(4): 302-5.

McCullough MJ, F. C. (2009). "The assessment of the DNA content of oral cytology via virtual microscopy for the early detection of epithelial dysplasia and neoplasia in oral mucosal lesions." *Oral Oncol* 45(9): 114-5.

McWilliams JE, Evans AJ, et al. (2000). "Genetic polymorphisms in head and neck cancer risk." *Head Neck.* 22(6): 609-17.

Michiels K, S. E., Conings R, Lenaerts J-P, Put W, Nuyts S, Delaere P, Jacobs R, Struyf S, Proost P, Van Damme J, (2009). "Carcinoma cell-derived chemokines and their presence in oral fluid." *Eur J Oral Sci* 117(4):362-8.(4): 362-8.

Morales J, H. B., Vicari AP, Hudak S, Oldham E, Hedrick J, Orozco R, Copeland NG, Jenkins NA, McEvoy LM, Zlotnik A, (1999). "CTACK, a skin-associated chemokine that preferentially attracts skin-homing memory T cells." *Proc Natl Acad Sci U S A.* 96(25): 14470-5.

Muto, M., Y. Hitomi, et al. (2000). "Acetaldehyde production by non-pathogenic Neisseria in human oral microflora: implications for carcinogenesis in upper aerodigestive tract." *Int J Cancer* 88(3): 342-50.

Napier, S. S. and P. M. Speight (2008). "Natural history of potentially malignant oral lesions and conditions: an overview of the literature." *J Oral Pathol Med* 37(1): 1-10.

Navone R, P. M., Rostan I, Burlo P, Marsico A, Broccoletti R, Scully C, Gandolfo S (2008). "Oral potentially malignant lesions: first-level micro-histological diagnosis from tissue fragments sampled in liquid-based diagnostic cytology." *J Oral Pathol Med* 37(6): 358-63.

Neppelberg, E. and Johannessen A.C. (2007). "DNA content, Cyclooxygenase-2 expression and loss of E-cadherin expression do not predict risk of malignant transformation in oral lichen planus. ." *Eur Arch Otorhinolaryngol* 264(10): 1223-30.

Ng IO, Xiao L, et al. (2000). " Microsatellite alterations in squamous cell carcinoma of the head and neck - clustering of loss of heterozygosity in a distinct subset. ." *Oral Oncol.* 36(5): 484-490.

Nielsen, H., B. Norrild, et al. (1996). "Human papillomavirus in oral premalignant lesions." *Eur J Cancer B Oral Oncol* 32B(4): 264-70.

Norming, U. and et al. (1992). "Prognostic significance of mucosal aneuploidy in stage Ta/T1 grade 3 carcinoma of the bladder." *J Urol,* 148(5): 1420-7.

Olsen TS, L. K. (2002). "Chemokines and chemokine receptors in leukocyte trafficking. ." *American Journal of Physiol Regulatory Integrative Comp Physiol* 283: R7-R28.

Ostwald C, Gogacz P, et al. (2000). "p53 mutational spectra are different between squamous-cell carcinomas of the lip and the oral cavity." *Int J Cancer.* 88(1): 82-86.

Panayiotidis MI, R. R., Allen CB, Riddle SR, Scheider BK, Ahmad S, White CW. (2004). "Hyperoxia-induced DNA damage causes decreased DNA methylation in human lung epithelial-like A549 cells." *Antioxidants and Redox Signalling* 6: 129-136.

Reed KD, S.-S. S. (2007). "Retraction - Sudbo J. Novel management of oral cancer: a paradigm of predictive oncology." *Clin Med Res* 5(3): 203.

Rothman, K. and A. Keller (1972). "The effect of joint exposure to alcohol and tobacco on risk of cancer of the mouth and pharynx." *J Chronic Dis* 25(12): 711-6.

Salaspuro, M. (2007). "Interrelationship between alcohol, smoking, acetaldehyde and cancer." *Novartis Found Symp* 285: 80-9; discussion 89-96, 198-9.

Sato J, G. J., Murata T, Kitamori S, Yamazaki Y, Satoh A, Kitagawa Y (2010). "Changes in saliva interleukin-6 levels in patients with oral squamous cell carcinoma." *Oral Surg Oral Med Oral Pathol Oral Radiol Endod* 110: 330-336.

Sato M, Sato T, et al. (2000). "Genetically high susceptibility to oral squamous cell carcinoma in terms of combined genotyping of CYP1A1 and GSTM1 genes." *Oral Oncol.* 36(3): 267-71.

Scarano E, F. A., Picciotti PM, Passali GC, Calò L, Cabras T, Inzitari R, Fanali C, Messana I, Castagnola M, Paludetti G (2010). "Proteomics of Saliva, Personal Experience." *Acta Otorhinolaryngol Ital.* 30(3): 125-30.

Schapher M, W. O., Gröschl M, (2011). "Salivary cytokines in cell proliferation and cancer." *Clin Chim Acta.* 412(19-20): 1740-8.

Scully (1993). "Oncogenes, tumor suppressors and viruses in oral squamous carcinoma. ." *J Oral Pathol Med.* 22(8): 337-47.

Seitz, H. K., S. Matsuzaki, et al. (2001). "Alcohol and cancer." *Alcohol Clin Exp Res* 25(5 Suppl ISBRA): 137S-143S.

Shahnavaz SA, Regezi JA, et al. (2000). "p53 gene mutations in sequential oral epithelial dysplasias and squamous cell carcinomas. ." *J Pathol.* 190(4): 417-22.

Silverman, S., Jr. and M. Gorsky (1990). "Epidemiologic and demographic update in oral cancer: California and national data--1973 to 1985." *J Am Dent Assoc* 120(5): 495-9.

Sorensen, F. B. and et al. (1991). "DNA level, tumor thickness, and stereological estimates of nuclear volume in stage I cutaneous malignant melanomas. A comparative study with analysis of prognostic impact." *Am J Dermatopathol* 13(1): 11-19.

Speit G, H. A. (2006). "The comet assay: a sensitive genotoxicity test for the detection of DNA damage and repair." *Methods in Molecular Biology* 314: 275-286.

Sreelekha TT, Ramadas K, et al. (2001). "Genetic polymorphism of CYP1A1, GSTM1 and GSTT1 genes in Indian oral cancer." *Oral Oncol.* 37(7): 593-98.

St John MA, L. Y., Zhou X, Denny P, Ho CM, Montemagno C, Shi W, Qi F, Wu B, Sinha U, Jordan R, Wolinsky L, Park NH, Liu H, Abemayor E, Wong DT. (2004). "Interleukin 6 and interleukin 8 as potential biomarkers for oral cavity and oropharyngeal squamous cell carcinoma." *Clin Cancer Res.* 10(24): 8442-50.

Struyf S, P. P., Van Damme J. (2003). "Regulation of the immune response by the interaction of chemokines and proteases. ." *Adv Immunol* 81: 1-44.

Sudbo, J. and et al. (2001). "Comparison of histological grading and large-scale genomic status (DNA ploidy) as prognostic tools in oral dysplasia. ." *J Pathol,* 194(3): 303-10.

Torres-Rendon, A. and et al. (2009 June). "DNA ploidy analysis by image cytometry helps to identify oral epithelial dysplasias with a high risk of malignant progression. ." *Oral Oncol* 45(6): 468-73.

Tran, N., C. O'Brien, et al. (2010). "Potential Role of Micro - RNAs in head and Neck Tumorigenesis." *Wiley InterScience (www.interscience.wiley.com). DOI: 10.1002/hed.21356.*

van Oijen MG, L. Vd, et al. (2000 Feb). "The origins of multiple squamous cell carcinomas in the aerodigestive tract. ." *Cancer.* 88 (4): 884-93.

Wang YF, C. S., Tai SK, Li WY, Wang LS, (2002). "Clinical significance of interleukin-6 and interleukin-6 receptor expressions in oral Squamous cell carcinoma. ." *Head Neck* 24: 850-858.

Warnakulasuriya S, Parkkila S, et al. (2008). "Demonstration of ethanol-induced protein adducts in oral leukoplakia (pre-cancer) and cancer." *J Oral Pathol Med* 37: 157-65.

Xiao H, W. D. (2011). "Proteomics and its applications for biomarker discovery in human saliva." *Bioinformation.* 5(7): 294-6.

Zlotnik A, Y. O. (2000). "Chemokines: a new classification system and their role in immunity." *Immunity* 12: 121-127.

8

p53 Mutation and Multiple Primary Oral Squamous Cell Carcinomas

Nur Mohammad Monsur Hassan[1,2] et al.*
[1]*Department of Oral and Maxillofacial Surgery, Division of Oncological Science, Okayama University Graduate School of Medicine, Dentistry and Pharmaceutical Sciences, Okayama,*
[2]*Division of Cancer-Related Genes, Institute for Genetic Medicine, Hokkaido University, Sapporo, Japan*

1. Introduction

Oral squamous cell carcinoma (OSCC) is a worldwide malignancy and is ranked the sixth most common cancer. At current rates, approximately 45,000 cases in the United States and more than 650,000 cases worldwide will be diagnosed each year (Jemel et al., 2008). One promising strategy for the treatment of OSCC and other cancers, which has developed as a result of breakthroughs in the fields of molecular biology, cancer genetics, and cancer biology, is molecular targeted therapy. Patients with a head-and-neck squamous cell carcinoma (HNSCC) often develop multiple malignant lesions. The oral sites that give rise to the majority of HNSCCs undergo cornification and shed squames during terminal differentiation, a process that is impaired in malignancies. The lymph nodes of the head and neck region form the principle site of primary metastasis, and perineural invasion marks tumours with a poor prognosis. Genetic changes correlate with lymph node metastasis in SCC. It is frequently observed that genetic damage persists beyond the histological border of precancerous lesions and tumours often develop far from the precancerous site (Braakhuis et al., 2003).

The p53 gene is the most frequent target of genetic alterations being, mutated in half of human cancers (Nylander et al., 2000, Iwakuma et al., 2005). Loss of p53 function leads to enhanced accumulation of mutations in other genes and reduced apoptotic responses, processes important to cancer progression and response to treatments. Using laser capture

---

* Mitsuhiro Tada[2], Jun-ichi Hamada[2], Masanobu Shindoh[4], Haruhiko Kashiwazaki[3], Yutaka Yamazaki[5], Yuichi Ashikaga[6], Tetsuya Moriuchi[2], Nobuo Inoue[3] and Akira Sasaki[1]
1 Department of Oral and Maxillofacial Surgery, Division of Oncological Science,
Okayama University Graduate School of Medicine, Dentistry and Pharmaceutical Sciences, Okayama, Japan,
2 Division of Cancer-Related Genes, Institute for Genetic Medicine, Japan,
3 Department of Geriatric Stomatology, Japan,
4 Department of Oral Pathology, Japan,
5 Department of Oral Diagnosis and Oral Medicine, Division of Oral Health Science, Japan,
6 Department of Oral and Maxillofacial Surgery, Division of Oral Health Science,
Hokkaido University Graduate School of Dental Medicine, Sapporo, Japan.

microdissection of tumour cells, p53 mutations were found in 100% of SCC (Agar et al., 2004). The p53 gene is mutated in more than 70% of oral SCC (Kashiwazaki et al., 1997, Hassan et al., 2008). In this article, we demonstrate that p53 statuses were diverse in the oral SCCs and leukoplakias, which indicated independent origins of the tumors in the multiple cancers. It is necessary to individual follow-up to each precancerous lesions based on the molecular alteration by the molecular analysis. However, the development of targeted approaches to OSCC requires understanding of the molecular pathogenesis of the disease, as well as further characterization of the specific molecular events involved in multiple cancers. The first part of this chapter will discuss on the molecular mechanisms of multiple carcinoma and the current status of targeted therapies directed toward critical molecular alterations in OSCC and the second part will evaluate a critical analysis of the various technological aspects of p53 analysis and the third part will present a case report with multiple carcinoma and molecular analysis of p53.

2. Molecular pathogenesis of OSCC

OSCC arises as a result of multiple molecular events that develop from the combined influences of an individual's genetic predisposition and exposure to environmental carcinogens (Califano et al., 1996). Chronic exposure to carcinogens such as tobacco, alcohol, oncogenic viruses, and inflammation can damage individual genes as well as larger portions of the genetic material, including chromosomes. Accumulation of such genetic alterations can lead to the development of premalignant lesions and subsequent invasive carcinoma. These genetic alterations include mutations, amplification or translocation of oncogenes that promote cell survival and proliferation, as well as inactivation of tumor suppressor genes involved in the inhibition of cell proliferation. From these alterations of oncogenes and tumor suppressor genes, tumor cells acquire autonomous self-sufficient growth and evade growth-inhibitory signals, resulting in uncontrolled tumor growth. Tumor cells thereby escape programmed cell death and replicate infinitely through the immortalization process by telomere lengthening. As OSCCs grow, invade, and metastasize, new blood vessel formation is critical. OSCCs, like most tumors, are able to create a blood supply by stimulating endothelial cell proliferation and new blood vessel formation. During oral carcinogenesis, there is selective disruption of this process, such that pro-angiogenic factors predominate (Hanahan & Weinberg, 2000). This angiogenesis is an essential part of solid tumor formation. The subsequent progression of OSCC includes tissue invasion and metastasis. Invasion of adjacent normal tissue requires that cellular adhesion molecules, such as integrin and cadherins, are lost, to allow cancer cells to leave their primary site. OSCCs develop through a complex process, as mentioned above. Here, we discuss those processes involving genetic alteration during multistep carcinogenesis, growth regulation, apoptosis, immortalization, angiogenesis, invasion, and metastasis.

2.1 Genetic alterations during development of OSCC

Califano, Sidransky, and colleagues have developed a genetic progression model based on their studies of gene alterations in squamous cell carcinomas of the head and neck (SCCHN) (Sidransky, 1995; Califano et al., 1996). They found that the most common genetic alteration in SCCHN is loss of chromosomal region 9p21, which occurs in 70–80% of dysplastic lesions of the oral mucosa, suggesting that this loss is an early event in oral carcinogenesis (van der Riet et al., 1994; Califano et al., 1996; Mao et al., 1996a). This region of chromosome 9p21, known as the CDKN2A locus, encodes the tumor suppressors p16 and $p14^{ARF}$, which frequently are inactivated by promoter hypermethylation (Reed et al., 1996). Loss of the chromosome 3p region is another common early genetic alteration in oral carcinogenesis (Garnis et al., 2003; Masayesva et al., 2004). The chromosome 3p region includes FHIT (fragile histidine triad gene) and RSSFIA, tumor suppressor genes inactivated by exonic deletion and hypermethylation (Mao et al., 1996a; Kisielewski et al., 1998; Dong et al., 2003). Loss of heterozygosity (LOH) of chromosome region 17p and mutation of the p53 gene are genetic alterations that occur in the later stage of progression from dysplasia to invasive squamous carcinoma. Alterations of p53, including mutation or deletion, are associated with increased genomic instability in oral dysplasia and may accelerate the rate of genetic alterations in oral carcinogenesis. Amplification of 11q13 and overexpression of cyclin D1 have been described in 40% of cases of oral squamous dysplasia (Rousseau et al., 2001). In general, loss of chromosomal material at 9p, 3p, and 17p is observed in relatively high proportions of dysplastic lesions, indicating that those events are early markers of oral carcinogenesis, whereas losses at 13q and 8p are observed more frequently in carcinomas than in dysplasia and are associated with later stages of carcinogenesis (Califano et al., 1996).

2.2 Multiple carcinomas

Individuals with one carcinoma of the head and neck region have an increased risk of developing a second malignancy (Schwartz et al., 1994); the frequency of that event varies from 16% to 36%. When a second malignancy occurs at the same time as the initial lesion, it is called a synchronous carcinoma. Metachronous neoplasm, on the other hand, is additional primary surface epithelial malignancies that develop in a later time period than the original tumor. About 40% of second malignancies of the upper aero digestive tract arise simultaneously and represent a synchronous tumor. The remaining multiple cancers in this population represent metachronous disease and usually develop within 3 years of the initial tumor (Schwartz et al., 1994). Second primary tumors are the chief cause of death in patients with an early -stage diagnosis (Hong et al., 1990). The tendency to develop multiple carcinomas in the upper aero digestive region is known as "field cancerization" (Slaughter et al., 1953). Prolonged and diffuse exposure to local carcinogens, particularly tobacco combined with alcohol, appears to increase the malignant transformation potential of exposed epithelial cells in the upper aero digestive tract and lungs (Franco et al., 1991). The overall risk for developing a second head and neck malignancy is 10 to 30 times higher in populations that use tobacco and alcohol than in the general population (Fijuth et al., 1992).

2.3 Field cancerization

Since the epithelial layer of the upper aero digestive tract is exposed to carcinogenic insult, such as tobacco products and alcohol, the entire area is at increased risk for the development of malignant lesions from the accumulation of genetic alterations of oncogenes and tumor suppressor genes. This led Slaughter and colleagues to develop a theory of "field cancerization", based on their extensive histological examination of dysplastic epithelium adjacent to invasive oral cancers; this dysplasia accounts for the relatively high incidence of second primary tumors in patients treated for OSCC (Slaughter et al., 1953). Many of these second primary tumors are associated with a lower rate of survival than the original tumor (Day et al., 1994; Cianfriglia et al., 1999). In this field cancerization model, multiple oral cancers develop from separate, independent cell clones, and this hypothesis has been supported by data from chromosome X inactivation studies, microsatellite analysis, and p53 mutational analysis (Bedi et al., 1996; Lydiatt et al., 1998; Tabor et al., 2002). More recent genetic analyses have shown, however, that second or multiple cancers distant from the abnormal fields can be clonally related and derived from expansion of an original clone (Braakhuis et al., 2003).

To reconcile this finding, Braakhuis *et al.* proposed a progression model, in which a stem cell located in the basal cell layer of the epithelium acquires a genetic alteration and subsequently give rise to a clonal unit, consisting of the stem cell with its daughter cells, all of which share the DNA alteration. Next, this patch of cells progresses into an expanding field as a result of additional genetic alterations (Braakhuis et al., 2004). This mucosal field pushes the normal epithelium aside and can expand to a size of several centimeters. These fields are often macroscopically undetectable, but they can also appear as oral lesions such as leukoplakia or erythroplakia. Ultimately, clonal selection leads to the development of carcinoma within this field of preneoplastic cells. The mechanism of this clonal expansion may be intra-epithelial migration of transformed cells or inoculation through saliva.

From these data, it has become clearer that the multifocality of oral carcinogenesis is an important cause of treatment failure in oral cancer. Although primary excision can completely remove an oral carcinoma, the altered field may remain, and the patient can develop a second primary tumor nearby, in the same field, that may be clinically indistinguishable from a local recurrence. Understanding of this field cancerization concept led Hong, Lippman, and other investigators to develop a strategy called 'chemoprevention', in which systemic therapy is administered with the intent of preventing epithelium from the entire upper aero digestive tract from progressing along the multistep pathway of carcinogenesis (Lippman et al., 2005).

2.4 Tumor suppressor genes

Tumor suppressor genes encode proteins that typically transduce negative growth-regulatory signals (Weinberg, 1991). These genes are often involved in cell-cycle regulation, including cell-cycle arrest and apoptosis. Unlike oncogenes, which can be activated by mutation of only one of the two gene copies, tumor suppressor genes are inactivated by any of several mechanisms, including point mutations and/or deletion, in both alleles of the gene, in a "two hit" fashion (Knudson, 1977; Vogelstein & Kinzler, 1993; Yokota & Sugimura, 1993). Once these genes are inactivated, the cell escapes tight cell-cycle control, predisposing it to uncontrolled growth and division, which contributes to the malignant phenotype (Levine, 1997).

2.4.1 p53

p53 is a tumor suppressor gene, located on chromosome 17p13.1, which plays a role in cell-cycle progression, cellular differentiation, DNA repair, and apoptosis. A major function of p53 is to serve as a guardian of the genome. Endogenous or exogenous stresses, such as DNA damage, hypoxia, and oncogene activation, increase p53 levels, leading to cell-cycle arrest that enables DNA repair to occur (Hartwell & Kastan, 1994). The induction of p53 expression can also occur through oncogenic stimulation that leads to $p14^{ARF}$ activation (Vogelstein et al., 2001) or DNA double-strand breaks that activate the ATM/Chk2-dependent pathway (Levine, 1997). p53 is the most commonly mutated gene and is altered in over 50% of all cancers, including 25–70% of oral cancers (Levine et al., 1991; Kashiwazaki et al., 1997, Baral et al., 1998). Most TP53 alterations are missense mutations, localized in the DNA-binding domain, and abolish the transcriptional activity via p53-responsive elements. The residues such as R175, G245, R248, R249, R273 and R282 in the p53 protein are frequently mutated, and are therefore called "hot spots (Brachmann et al., 1996).

Immunohistochemical positivity or various mutation analyses of the DNA-binding domain of p53 are known to be useful markers for predicting prognosis of patients with oral SCC (Hassan et al., 2008, Yamazaki et al., 2003, De Vicente et al., Marx et al., 2007). Mutation most often occurs at a 'hot spot' region from codon 238 to codon 248 (Somers et al., 1992; Hainaut et al., 1998; Kropveld et al., 1999) and causes defects in the binding of specific DNA sequences and the transactivation of genes whose expression is up-regulated by the wild-type protein (Vogelstein et al., 2001). Some human tumor-associated p53 mutants possess unique properties not found in the wild-type protein (Sigal & Rotter, 2000). Based on functional interactions with the remaining wild-type (WT) p53 allele, the p53 mutations are classified into two types, recessive and dominant-negative (DN) mutations. The most frequent p53 mutations are dominant negative (DN). Such "gain of function" activities include the ability to transform cells, increase tumorigenicity, and modulate the sensitivity of cancer cells to drugs (Sigal & Rotter, 2000; Song & Xu, 2007). We have found that oral SCC patients with DNp53 mutations have a significantly worse outcome than patients with recessive mutations, in terms of recurrence free survival [Hassan et al., 2008]. This has also been noted in other cancers (Marutani et al., 1999; Sakuragi et al., 2005). The over-representation of DN mutants, accounting for about 27% of all p53 mutations (6414 of all 23,544 in the IARC database R11), suggests an advantage for tumour development of the cancer cell harbouring a DN mutation. But why does this occur? The mechanism responsible for the poor clinical outcome in DNp53 mutants is unknown at present. One explanation is that the DNp53 allele suppresses the remaining wild-type p53 allele, promoting tumour progression. Another explanation is that DNp53 mutant proteins often possess a gain-of-function (GOF) related to malignancy, other than transdominance over WT p53 function. Indeed, some DN p53 mutants are known to bind to other transcription factors and to transactivate or repress specific target genes, such as MYC (Frazier et al., 1998), MDR-1 [Sampath et al., 2001], CD95 (Fas/APO-1) (Zalcenstein et al., 2003) and EGR1 (Weisz et al., 2004). It is important to understand malignant properties acquired by GOF activity in each mutation to enable better use of genetic information for diagnosis and therapy. Interestingly, we recently showed that different p53 mutants have a different quality in gain-of-function (GOF) activities even for different mutations occurring at the same codon (Yoshikawa et al., 2010).

Even in the absence of p53 mutations, p53 function can be inactivated by other mechanisms, such as infection with an "oncogenic" human papillomavirus type, such as HPV16 or HPV18. In HPV-positive SCCHN, p53 interacts with the E6 protein, which leads to increased ubiquitin-dependent proteolysis of p53 (Min et al., 1994; Nagpal et al., 2002). Another mechanism of p53 inactivation is elevation of expression of the MDM2 protein, which binds to p53 and promotes ubiquitination of the C-terminus of p53 and subsequent degradation (Oliner et al., 1993). p14^{ARF} interacts with MDM2, preventing association of p53 and MDM2 and thereby stabilizing p53 (Pomerantz et al., 1998). Therefore, degradation of p53 may be inappropriately stimulated by over expression of MDM2 or by deletion or epigenetic silencing of p14^{ARF}.

p53 mutations commonly arise as a result of alcohol and/or tobacco exposure, and their presence is associated with the early recurrence and development of second primary tumors (Shin et al., 1996). Wild-type p53 gene therapy has been attempted in preclinical studies and in clinical trials in heavily treated patients. These studies demonstrated the feasibility of delivering the wild-type p53 gene to human tumors and yielded some clinical response and induction of apoptosis in the tumors (Clayman et al., 1998, 1999). However, difficulty in obtaining uniform delivery of the gene throughout the tumor has limited the utility of this therapeutic strategy. Other reports have demonstrated associations between p53 mutation and unfavorable responses to chemotherapy or radiation therapy (Temam et al., 2000; Warnakulasuriya et al., 2000).

Inactivation of the p53 gene is essentially due to small mutations (missense and nonsense mutations or insertions/deletions of several nucleotides), which lead to either expression of a mutant protein (90% of cases) or absence of protein (10% of cases). No inactivation of p53 gene expression by hypermethylation of transcription promoters has been demonstrated at the present time, which supports the hypothesis of a function for p53 mutants. We can analyse p53 gene alteration in cancer in different way.

3. Analyse p53 gene alterations in cancers

3.1 Molecular analysis

Direct sequencing of the p53 gene after PCR amplification remains the "Gold Standard" of molecular analysis. For the p53 gene, this approach is facilitated by the fact that the 10 coding exons are smaller than 350 bp and can therefore be easily amplified individually. Mutations involving partial or total gene deletions are relatively rare. Unfortunately, although considerable progress has been made in the field of DNA sequencing in terms of throughput, its sensitivity still remains limited. The major problem of molecular analysis of tumour specimens is the presence of normal cells (lymphocytes, stromal cells) that contaminate the tumour samples. According to the type of tumour or the type of sample, the rate of contamination can range from several percent (surgical tumour sample) to 50% (biopsies) or even more than 95% (urine, stools or bronchial lavage). It is generally accepted that direct sequencing requires at least 20% of mutant alleles, but this can vary considerably according to the quality of the sample. This qualitative aspect is generally underestimated. The quantity and quality of DNA obtained varies considerably according to the origin of the sample (frozen tumour, formalin- or paraffin-embedded tissues). This variability can lead to the generation of PCR artifacts, which can be falsely interpreted as mutations. In the case of heavily contaminated samples, microdissection can be performed in order to enrich the tumour cell content, but this complicates the manipulations and cannot be performed routinely at the present time. The application of molecular technologies to routine analysis in hospital is a very important aspect. Many extremely sensitive molecular analysis methodologies have been developed, but their clinical application is generally limited because of the complex installation, their low throughput, the use of radioactivity or the need for highly qualified personnel.

Up until now, molecular analyses have been performed on exons 5-8 of the p53 gene, as the majority of mutations are located in these regions. It is generally established that 90% of mutational events are missense mutations leading to the synthesis of an abnormal protein that is not degraded and which accumulates in the nucleus of tumour cells. The remaining 10% of mutational events are nonsense mutations or small deletions that do not lead to accumulation of p53. This type of mutation excludes the possibility of using molecular methodologies such as PTT (Protein truncature test) based on expression of truncated proteins. More recently, molecular studies have been extended to the other exons, as exons 4, 9 and 10 have been found to contain a considerable number of mutations (about 15%) (Soussi & Béroud, 2001). Analysis of molecular events also shows a high proportion of nonsense mutations in these exons. Analysis of the latest version of the p53 gene mutation database shows that about 20% to 25% of mutations do not lead to the synthesis of a p53 protein. These mutations also present a marked variability as a function of the type of cancer: they are more frequent in lung cancers and breast cancers than in colon cancers (Soussi & Béroud, 2001).

About 280 of the 393 codons of the p53 gene can be affected by a mutation. Furthermore, as each codon comprises 3 bases, which can each be altered generating a different amino acid, there are a very large number of theoretical combinations. 1,300 different variants have been identified in the p53 mutation database, which comprises more than 15,000 mutations derived from as many tumours (Béroud et al., 2000).

Many prescreening methodologies have been used to increase the sensitivity of detection of mutations and to concentrate the sequencing exclusively on the mutant exon. Unfortunately, many of these methods, possibly with the exception of DHPLC (denaturing high-performance liquid chromatography), remain confined to specialized laboratories and the sensitivity of detection of some of them is incompatible with the needs of clinical diagnosis. However, they present the advantage of being able to detect mutations in samples heavily contaminated by normal DNA.

3.2 Immunohistochemical analysis

Immunohistochemical studies concerning p53, as for other markers, suffer from a lack of standardization, leading to very heterogeneous results. The sources of heterogeneity are multiple: i) the various antibodies used; ii) methodological aspects (amplification, epitope unmasking); iii) the initial material (paraffin block, frozen tumour) and storage conditions; iv) the positive cut-off value, which can vary from 1% to 20% according to the authors; and v) individual variability of interpretation of the results (McShane et al., 2000; Schmitz-Drager et al., 2000).

Nonsense or frame shift mutations do not lead to accumulation of p53 protein. This is certainly due to instability of truncated proteins, which are generally not detectable despite the use of monoclonal antibodies which recognize an epitope situated in the amino-terminal domain of p53. It is beyond the scope of this chapter to present an exhaustive review of the literature concerning immunohistochemical analysis of p53 and its clinical applications (Hall & Lane, 1994; Save et al., 1998).

3.3 Serological analysis of p53 gene alterations

Since 1992, a new series of studies has shown that p53-Abs can be found in the serum of patients with various types of cancer, whereas the prevalence of these antibodies in the normal population remains very low. To date, the majority of published studies suggest that most patients with p53 antibodies have a p53 mutation leading to p53 accumulation. It is also clear that not all patients with a p53 alteration develop p53 antibodies. Comparison of the frequency of p53 alterations in the literature indicates that 30% to 40% of patients with an alteration of the p53 gene develop p53 antibodies (Lubin et al., 1995a).

The majority of the literature clearly demonstrates the specificity of this serological analysis, as such antibodies are very rare in the normal population. The specificity of this assay can be estimated to be 95%. This high specificity is supported by the fact that p53 specifically accumulates in the nucleus of tumour cells after gene mutation. One of the disadvantages of this assay is its lack of sensitivity, as only 20% to 40% of patients with p53 mutations develop p53-Abs. This lack of sensitivity totally precludes the use of the assay to evaluate p53 alterations in human tumour. Nevertheless, if we estimate that there are 8 million patients with various types of cancer throughout the world, and 50% of them have a mutation in their p53 gene, then we can deduce that about 1 million of these patients would have p53- Abs.

3.4 FASAY functional assay

FASAY (Functional Assay in Yeast) is used for the detection of mutations in tumour samples (Flaman et al., 1995; Ishioka et al., 1993). Here cDNA obtained from tumour RNA. PCR amplification of this cDNA, using primers corresponding to codons 52to 364 (68% of exons 4 to 10), followed by introduction of the PCR product into an indicator yeast, where it recombines with an expression vector, can be used to define the transactivating activity of the protein expressed. Red yeast colonies express mutant p53, while white colonies express wild-type p53 (Fronza et al., 2000). The amplified region corresponds to 95 % of the mutations identified to date, which makes FASAY a very good approach for exhaustive analysis of p53 gene mutations. All alterations leading to absence of RNA expression will obviously not be detected, but this is a relatively rare situation for p53. The only criticism that can be formulated in relation to this methodology is that it provides no information about the type of mutation, so that sequencing must always be performed subsequently. As sequencing is performed on DNA extracted from red colonies (mutant p53), problems of sensitivity are eliminated. This methodology can also be used to demonstrate splicing alterations. Waridel et al. have modified the FASAY technique to increase its sensitivity and robustness (Waridel et al., 1997).

In addition, the DN potential of the detected *p53* mutant was tested using a yeast-based transdominance assay as described previously (Marutani et al., 1999). Briefly, yIG397 was transformed with both a plasmid with wild-type *p53* and a plasmid with the mutant *p53* that had been sequence-verified. For each transformation, 50 µl of yeast suspension were mixed with 100 ng of pTSHP53 (Trp 1 marker), 100 ng of mutant *p53*-containing pSS16 (Leu 2 marker), 50 µg of sonicated single-stranded salmon sperm DNA and 300 µl of LiOAc containing 40% polyethylene glycol 4000. The mixture was incubated at 30 °C for 30 min and heat-shocked at 42 °C for 15 min. Yeast was then plated on SD medium minus leucine and tryptophan, but with a limited amount of adenine (5µg/ml). The plates were then incubated for 48 hr in a 30 °C-humidified atmosphere. Double-transformant clones (Leu^+, Trp^+) giving rise to white (Ade^+) or pink/red (Ade^-) colonies were interpreted as expressing recessive and DN mutant, respectively.

Recently, we used this approach to detect p53 gene mutations in biopsies containing only 5% of tumour cells (Fouquet et al., 2004). These mutations could not be detected by direct sequencing. In addition to this high level of sensitivity, the FASAY technique also presents the advantage of being simple and robust. FASAY avoids selecting active variants (see below for problems related to this biological activity). It also has the advantage of being the only method able to rigorously demonstrate codon 72 polymorphism linked to the mutant allele (see beginning of the chapter for the significance of this polymorphism) (Tada et al., 2001). The cloning and sequencing of cDNA in the indicator yeast provide a non-fragmented molecule corresponding to the initial RNA expressed by the p53 gene. New indicator yeasts allowing more accurate evaluation of p53 activity have been developed. It remains to be seen whether the use of these yeasts can help to increase the sensitivity of this test.

4. Case report

This study reported on a patient with multiple primary carcinomas, consisting of five separate carcinomas and three leukoplakias of the head and neck region. To determine whether the individual head and neck carcinomas were of multiple origins but genetically related, or whether they were metastases, analysis of p53 mutation by yeast functional assay and subsequent sequencing analysis were performed. The yeast p53 functional assay tests the ability of p53 to activate transcription in vivo in yeast (Flaman et al., 1995). It was demonstrated that the p53 status is diverse in oral SCCs and leukoplakias, suggesting that the tumours in a multiple carcinoma may have independent origins.

A 67-year-old man was referred to the Outpatient Clinic of Hokkaido University Dental Hospital in September 2003. He had an ulcerative lesion at the right (lesion 1) and left (lesion 2) lower gingiva and left side of the tongue (lesion 3) with a continuous dull pain in the most part of the mandibular area. He also had white patches (leukoplakia) in the upper left (lesion 4) and right (lesion 5) gingiva and left side (lesion 6) of the buccal mucosa (Figure 1).

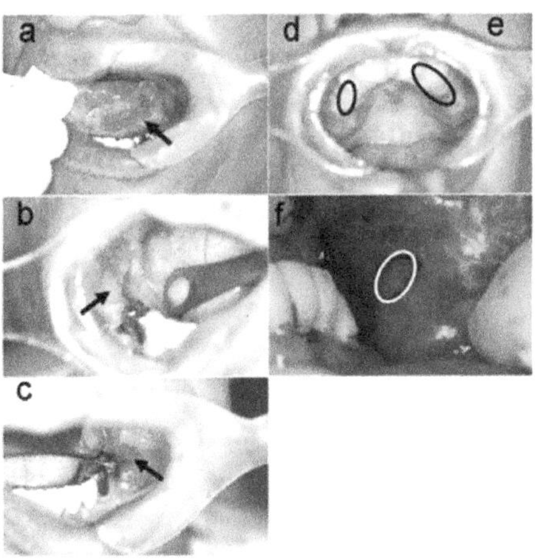

Fig. 1. Preoperative state of the tumors. Arrows indicate cancerous ulcerations; on left side of the tongue (a), right side of the lower gingiva (b) and left side of the lower gingiva (c). Circles indicate leukoplakic lesions in the right (d) and left upper gingiva (e) and left side of buccal mucosa (f).

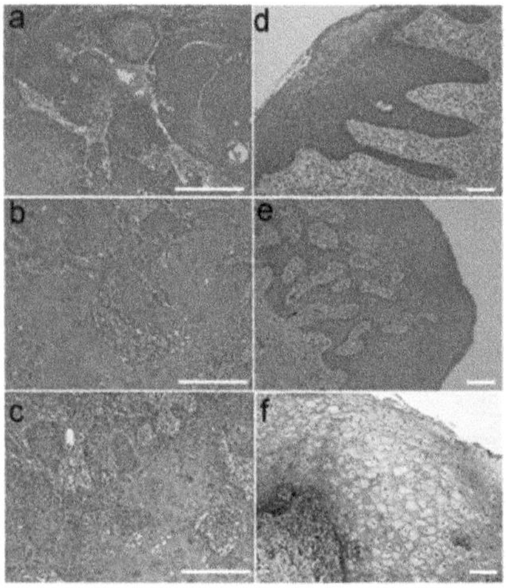

Fig. 2. Histopathology of the biopsy specimens corresponding to the lesions in Figure 1. Well differentiated squamous cell cancers (a, b, c), and leukoplakias (d, e, f) showing hyperkeratosis with low grade dysplasia but no evidence of malignancy (H&E stain, bar indicates 100 micrometer)

He had a long history of cigarette smoking (20 cigarettes a day) and alcohol intaking (beer 500 ml + sake 300 ml a day) for about 48 years. Family history was unremarkable except that his mother had died of gall bladder carcinoma. Physical examination disclosed hard swelling of sub-mandibular lymph nodes at both sides of the neck: one at the right sub-mandibular, two in the right jugulo-digastric area, two in the left submandibular and one in the left jugulo-digastric area. Magnetic resonance imaging (MRI) revealed ill-defined, hypointense masses in the lower right and left gingival regions and in the left side of the tongue. Both lesions in the gingival regions showed invasion of the medial surface of the mandible and extension into the bone marrow (Figure 3).

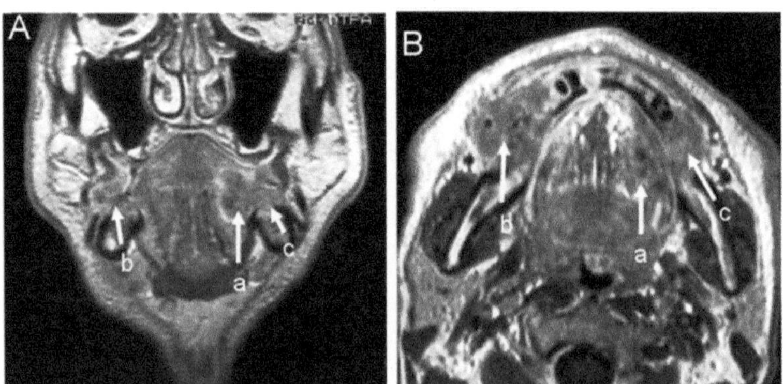

Fig. 3. T1- weighted coronal (**A**) and axial (**B**) magnetic resonance images showing ill-defined, hypo-intense masses surrounded by a Gd-enhanced outer margin in left side of the tongue (a), right molar region (b), and the left molar region (c).

After being admitted to the Department of Oral Maxillofacial Surgery, the patient received 40 Gy preoperative irradiation in 20 sessions over 4 weeks along with chemotherapy consisting of CDDP (6 mg/m2, four times a week) and TXT (15 mg/m2, once a week).

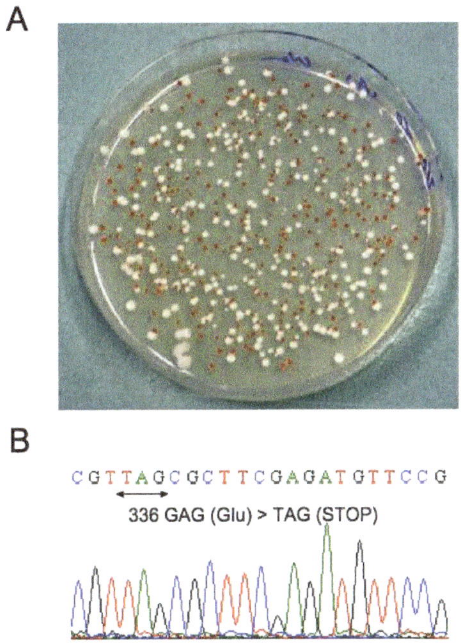

Fig. 4. **A**, A representative result of the yeast p53 functional assay. Colonies containing mutant- type p53 are red due to accumulation of ADE2 substrate, while colonies containing wild type p53 are white. Tumor specimen (left side of the tongue) gave 62.5% red colonies, indicating 62.5% p53 mRNA in the tumor specimens were mutant.
B, Sequence chromogram of the p53 cDNA recovered from a red colony. Wild-type sequence was CGT GAG CGC TTC GAG ATG TTC, in which the underlined glutamic acid changed into a stop codon at the codon 336 (GAG > TAG).

In December 2003, removal of the tumours and radical neck dissection were carried out under tracheostomy and general anaesthesia. Resection of the left half of the tongue and segmental resection of the most part of mandible body were performed. The mandible was reconstructed with titanium plates and the defects of the oral mucosa were repaired with rectus abdominis myocutaneous free flap. After the surgery, the patient was observed without adjuvant therapy. Lesions 1, 2 and 3 were pathologically diagnosed as squamous cell carcinomas. The final TNM staging was pT4N2cM0. The patient was discharged in May 2004. Four months after discharge, he was admitted to a local hospital for terminal care, where he died of sudden severe bleeding due to a locally recurrent invasive tumour. The histopathological study of the surgical specimens confirmed that lesions 1 and 3 were well - differentiated SCC, while lesion 2 was a moderately differentiated SCC. Leukoplakias (lesions 4, 5 and 6) showed hyperkeratosis with a low-grade dysplasia but no evidence of malignancy (Figure 3, Table I).

Lesion ID	Location Size	HPV infection	Histological type	Red colony %	p53 status	Mutated Codon#
a	Tongue 3.9 x 1.7cm	Negative	SCC?	62.5	Mutant	336 GAG (E) > TAG (STOP)
b	Rt* lower gingival 3.0 x 3.2 cm	Negative	SCC	64.6	Mutant	285 GAG (E) > AAG (K)
c	Lt+ lower gingival 2.0 x 2.2 cm	Negative	SCC	4.3	Wild type	
d	Rt upper gingival 2.0 x 2.0 cm		Low grade dysplasia	53.4	Mutant	273 CGT (R) > CAT (H)
e	Lt upper gingival 1.0 x 1.0 cm		Low grade dysplasia	9.5	Wild type	
f	Rt buccal mucosa 2.0 x 2.5 cm		Low grade dysplasia	16.4	Wild type	

*Rt, right side; + Lt, left side; ? SCC, squamous cell carcinoma; # Mutated Codon, codon number, wild type codon (amino acid) > mutant codon (substituted amino acid)

Table 1. p53 mutational status and HPV status.

Specimens of the tumors and leukoplakic lesions were subjected to yeast functional assay. The yeast assay which screens human p53 function in yeast is now described (6). The reporter yeast strain (yIG397) contains an integrated plasmid with the ADE2 open reading frame under the control of a human p53-responsive promoter. When the strain is transformed with a plasmid encoding mutant p53, the yeast strain becomes defective in adenine synthesis due to a mutation in the endogenous ADE2 gene. Therefore, colonies expressing mutant p53 are red, whereas colonies expressing wild-type (WT) p53 become white. In this system, when more than 20% of colonies are red the sample is considered positive for a p53 gene mutation (Kashiwazaki et al., 1997) and plasmids recovered from at least five red colonies are sequenced for verifying the presence of clonal mutation(s). p53 mutation was observed in two of the three SCCs and one of the three leukoplakias. In the SCCs, one missense mutation (lesion 1) at codon 285 (GAG>AAG, Glu>Lys) and one nonsense mutation (lesion 3) at codon 336 were observed. In the leukoplakias, one missense mutation (lesion 5) at codon 273 (CGT>CAT, Arg>His) was observed (Table I). All mutations were identified as clonal because the sequences from the five red colonies were identical. These results showed that two of the three mutations were G to A transition, being consistent with the record in the IARC TP53 database (http; //www.p53.iarc.fr), showing that the G: C to A: T transition is the most prevalent in oral SCCs in smokers (detailed in Discussion).

In addition, to detect human papillomavirus (HPV) infection of SCC samples, genomic DNA extracted from the tumour specimens was tested by multiplex PCR (8). No HPV infection was detected in any form of HPV subtypes (genotypes 6, 11, 16, 18, 30, 31, 33, 35, 39, 45, 51, 52, 56, 58, 59, and 66) (Table I).

SCC is thought to progress through a series of well defined histopathological stages that run parallel to specific genetic changes. Patients with primary malignancy (especially in the head and neck (HN) area) are at high risk for developing additional primary malignancies.

The oral cavity presents a field, which, if exposed to carcinogens may allow multiple precancerous and tumorous lesions to develop synchronously and metachronously. Generally multiple primary tumors are encountered in 3-5% of malignant tumors. They are most often met with secondary malignant tumors; triple tumors occur in 0.5%, quadruple tumors in 0.3% of malignant tumors (Moertel et al., 1958).

The criteria for diagnosing multiple primary tumors are (a) each of the tumors must present a definite picture of malignancy, (b) each must be distinct, (c) the probability that one may be a metastatic lesion from the other one must be excluded and (d) tumors are multicentric when they are formed at the same site and have the same histological type (Moertel et al., 1977). The histological verified cancers (SCC) in the present case were proven distinct by the MRI findings (Figure 3) and macroscopic findings during surgery. It was impossible to exclude the possibility that the tumors might be metastatic or dissemination from one tumor by image diagnosis or pathological findings. The different p53 mutations were found in the tumors (Table 1), which, strongly suggested that the tumors were of different clonal origins. Therefore, the tumors in the present case were defined multiple and multicentric, fulfilling the above criteria (a) to (d).

It is widely accepted that alterations in multiple oncogenes and tumor suppressor genes are the genetic basis for human carcinogenesis (Weinberg et al., 1989). The p53 gene is the most frequent target of genetic alterations, being mutated in half of human cancers. The p53 mutation usually shows clonality in a cancer and therefore suggests that the mutation has occurred in the very beginning stage of carcinogenesis, which is likewise in oral SCC (kashiwazaki et al., 1997). It means that distinct clonal p53 mutation works as a molecular tag that denies the metastatic dissemination of a single-tumor-origin cells (Tjebbes et al., 1999). This was seen in the present case, as the yeast functional assay and sequence analysis showed a distinct but the same (clonal) mutational status in each SCC: 285K in Lesion 1, wild-type p53 in Lesion 2, 336X in Lesion 3. In addition, other genetic alterations such as PTEN or PIK3CA can activate p53-dependent growth suppression in human cells (kim et al., 2007). So, it has been considered that the other gene alterations are also involved in wild type p53 (lesion 2).

The sequences of appearance of multiple tumors is defined as simultaneous (all malignant tumors are observed at the same time), as synchronous (the second tumor appears within 6 months after the first), or metachronous (the multiple tumor is diagnosed more than 6 months after the recognition of the previous one (Németh et al., 1999). In our case, according to the patient statement, three SCCs and leukoplakias of the oral cavity developed within six months. Different p53 mutation and histology proved their distinctness. So that our patient fulfilled the criterion of synchronous multiple primary malignant neoplasm.

Most of the multiple oral carcinomas are associated with leukoplakia, (Moertel et al., 1977) however, in pre-malignant lesion p53 alteration has not been described frequently (kashiwazaki et al., 1997). Perhaps tobacco uses as in the present case have a high incidence of p53 mutations.[12] We can explain by that way the p53 gene alteration has occurred before the carcinogenetic change. In the present case, we also found in each leukoplakias: wild-type p53 in lesion 4, 273H in lesion 5, and wild type p53 in lesion 6 (Table 1).

The concept of field cancerization is to explain that have strong tendency those who are exposed repeatedly to carcinogenic factors such as tobacco and alcohol, to develop multiple primary tumors, being consistent with the present case. Mutations of p53 gene occur during early stages in the development of HN SCCs because they are already present in premalignant lesions (Lazarus et al., 1995). In our study, we found hot spot p53 mutation in codon 273 in one leukoplakia. It has been shown that the malignant potential of leukoplakia is as high as 23-38% (Silverman et al., 1984); hence mutations of p53 gene may be indicative of the potential of these lesions to develop into SCC. G to A transition is the predominant mutations observed in oral SCCs caused from tobacco (tobacco specific N-nitrosomines) (IARC database new version12, $p < 0.002$) (Shin et al., 1994; Petitjean et al., 2007). The most prevalent type of p53 mutation is G: C to A: T transitions found in our study were double times within three mutations. The rest one mutation G: C to T: A transition was also found in our study, which is also frequently mutated in tobacco smokers, although it is not significant in IARC data ($p < 0.11$). The overrepresentation of DN mutants, accounting for about 27% of all p53 mutations (6414 of all 23,544 in the IARC database R11) and suggests an advantage of the cancer cell harbouring a DN mutation in tumour development. In this study we found R273H mutant, which is the most common hotspot DN mutations to the IARC TP53 database (release 11, containing a total of 1093 oral SCC). Studies using mouse models of Li-Fraumeni syndromes have reported gain of functions in R175H and R273H mutants (Lang et al., 2004), which were identified as DN mutants in our study (Hassan et al., 2008). R248W and R273 H mutants interfere with recruiting MRE11-RAD50- NBS1 (MRN) complex to the site of DNA damage, leading to inactivation of ATM (Song et al., 2007). It further enhances genomic instability, which is caused by the loss of p53 function. The gain of-function property of p53 mutants is considered to lend further malignant phenotypes to the tumour cells, such as enhancement of tumourigenicity, metastatic potential and therapy resistance and also new function in conferring the increased cell growth and inhibition of apoptosis (Dittmer et al., 1993; kim et al., 2004; Wong et al., 2007).

Some tumors including oral cancer, inherit gene mutation (Patrikidou et al., 2002) but there are no published reports of germ line p53 mutation. To single out the specific cause of multiple primary malignant tumors is difficult. It is possible that exposure to carcinogens capable of causing multiple genetic abnormalities could develop cancers independently each other throughout the entire anatomic region.

5. Future directions

A longer follow-up in a larger number of patients would further confirm and strengthen the usefulness of DN p53 mutation as a predictor of early recurrence in oral cancer. It should warrant further investigations regarding specific types of DN p53 mutations in relation to the prognosis and responses to therapy in patients with oral SCC. In addition, identification of the dominant-negative property of p53 mutation may be useful for tailoring the treatment of oral cancer. Readers can refer to the database for all the known DN p53 mutation at-http://www.igm.hokudai.ac.jp/crg/DNbase/DNp53.html.

6. Conclusions

Multiple cancers can occur after successfully treating tumors. Genetic analysis of one patient who had simultaneously three SCCs and three dysplasia lesions provided important information on molecular mechanisms of oral cancer development and for its therapeutic strategy. In this particular case, p53 mutation was observed in two of three SCCs and one of the three dysplasias. and these three mutations were at different sites in the p53 gene. These findings indicate that p53 mutations occurs even at a precancerous lesion and that precancerous and cancerous lesions have different genetic backgrounds for their development. Depending on the molecular findings, we should make a multidisciplinary plan for multiple cancer patients, which will give a valuable insight in future cancer prognosis. We should take extra care with awareness of a patient with risk factors of carcinogenesis. It is further necessary to monitor the effects of single p53 mutation-transduction on a global gene expression by using a cDNA microarray or a tilling array combined with chromatin-immunoprecipitation in order to discover the molecules responsible. Such case provides useful information for predicting the risk for multiple cancers. A more detailed understanding of the p53-related mechanisms that lead to cancer will contribute to the development of more effective, tailored intervention strategies. In particular, detailed information of the p53 status, including transdominancy and GOF activity is expected to be useful for diagnosis and therapeutic strategy fitting each individual patient with multiple carcinomas. Elucidating its role and targets in DNp53 function in cancer cells will open up a new avenue for treatment design in the coming years.

7. References

Agar, N.S., Halliday, G.M., Barnetson, R.S., Ananthaswamy, H.N., Wheeler, M. & Jones, A.M. (2004). The basal layer in human squamous tumor harbors more UVA than UVB fingerprint mutations : A role for UVA in human skin carcinogenesis. *Proc Nat Acad Sci, USA*, 101, (14), pp.4954-4959, ISSN 1091-6490

Baral, R., Patnaik, S. & Das, B.R. (1998). Co-overexpression of p53 and c-myc proteins is linked with advance stages of betel and tobacco related oral squamous cell carcinoma from Eastern India. *Eur J Oral Sci*, 106, (5), pp. 907–913, ISSN 1600-0722

Bedi, G.C., Westra, W.H., Gabrielson, E., Koch, W. & Sidransky, D. (1996). Multiple head and neck tumors: evidence for a common clonal origin. *Cancer Res*, 56, (11), pp. 2484–2487, ISSN 1538-7445

Béroud, C., Collod-Béroud, G., Boileau, C., Soussi, T., & Junien, C. (2000). UMD (Universal Mutation Database): A generic software to build and analyze locus-specific databases. *Hum Mutat*, 15, (1), pp. 86-94, ISSN 1098-1004

Braakhuis, B.J., Tabor, M.P., Kummer, J.A., Leemans, R. & Brakenhoff, R.H. (2003). A genetic explanation of Slaughter's concept of field cancerization: evidence and clinical implications. *Cancer Res*, 63, (8), pp. 1727–1730, ISSN1538-7445

Braakhuis, B.J., Brakenhoff, R.H. & Leemans, C.R. (2004). A genetic progression model of oral cancer: current evidence and clinical implications. *J Oral Pathol Med*, 33, (6), pp. 317–322, ISSN 1600-0714

Braakhuis, B.J.M., Tabor, M.P., Kummer, J.A., Leemans, C.R. & Brakenhoff, R.H. (2003). A genetic explanation of Slaughter's concept of field cancerization: evidence and clinical implications. *Cancer Res*, 63, (8), pp. 1727-1730, ISSN 1538-7445

Brachmann, R.K., Vidal, M. & Boeke, J, D. (1996). Dominant-negative p53 mutations selected in yeast hit cancer hot spots. *Proc Natl Acad Sci U S A*, 93,(9), pp. 4091-4095, ISSN 1091-6490

Califano, J., van der Riet, P., Westra, W., Nawroz, H., Clayman, G., Piantadosi, S., Corio, R., Lee, D., Greenberg, B., Koch, W. & Sidransky, D. (1996). Genetic progression model for head and neck cancer: implications for field cancerization. *Cancer Res*, 56, (11), pp.2488–2492, ISSN 1538-7445

Cianfriglia, F., DiGregorio, D.A. & Manieri, A. (1999). Multiple primary tumours in patients with oral squamous cell carcinoma. *Oral Oncol*, 35, (2), pp.157-163, ISSN1368-8375

Clayman, G.L, el-Naggar, A.K., Lippman, S.M., Henderson, Y.C., Frederick, M., Merritt, J.A., Zumstein, .LA., Timmons, T.M., Liu, T.J., Ginsberg, L., Roth, J.A., Hong, W.K., Bruso, P. & Goepfert, H. (1998). Adenovirus-mediated p53 gene transfers in patients with advanced recurrent head and neck squamous cell carcinoma. *J Clin Oncol*, 16, (6), PP. 2221-2232, ISSN 1527-7755

Clayman, G.L., Frank, D.K., Bruso, P.A. & Goepfert, H. (1999). Adenovirus-mediated wild-type p53 gene transfer as a surgical adjuvant in advanced head and neck cancers. *Clin Cancer Res*, 5, (7), pp. 1715-1722, ISSN 1078-0432

Day, G.L., Blot, W.J., Shore, R.E., McLaughlin, J.K., Austin, D.F., Greenberg RS, Liff, J.M, Preston-Martin, S, Sarkar, S. & Schoenberg, J.B. (1994). Second cancers following oral and pharyngeal cancers: role of tobacco and alcohol. *J Natl Cancer Inst*, 86, (2), pp.131-137, ISSN 1460-2105

De Vicente, J.C., Gutiérrez, L.M.J., Zapatero, A.H., Forcelledo, M.F.F., Hernández-Vallejo, G. & Arranz J.S.L. (2004). Prognostic significance of p53 expression in oral squamous cell carcinoma without neck node metastases. *Head Neck*, 26, (1), PP. 22-30, ISSN 1097-0347

Dong, S.M., Sun, D.I., Benoit, N.E., Kuzmin, I., Lerman, M.I. & Sidransky, D. (2003). Epigenetic inactivation of RASSFIA in head and neck cancer. *Clin Cancer Res*, 9, (10), pp. 3635-3640, ISSN 1078-0432

Fijuth, J., Mazeron, J.J., Le Pechoux, C., Piedbois, P., Martin, M., Haddad, E., Calitchi, E., Pierquin, B. & Le Bourgeois, J.P. (1992). Second head and neck cancers following radiation therapy of T1 and T2 cancers of the oral cavity and oropharynx. *Int J Radiat Oncol Biol Phys*, 24, (1), pp. 59-64, ISSN 1879-355X

Flaman, J.M., Frebourg, T., Moreau, V., Charbonnier. F, Martin, C., Chappuis, P., Sappino, A.P., Limacher, J.M., Bron, L., Benhattar, J., Tada, M., Van Meir, E.G., Estreicher, A. & Iggo, R.D. (1995). A simple p53 functional assay for screening cell lines, blood, and tumors. *Proc Natl Acad Sci USA*, 92, (9), pp. 3963-3967, ISSN 1091-6490

Fouquet, C., Antoine, M., Tisserand, P., Favis, R., Wislez, M., Como, F., Rabbe, N., Carette, M. F., Milleron, B., Barany, F., Cadranel, J, Zalcman, G. & Soussi, T. (2004). Rapid and sensitive p53 alteration analysis in biopsies from lung cancer patients using a functional assay and a universal oligonucleotide array: a prospective study. *Clin Cancer Res*, 10, (10), pp. 3479-89, ISSN 1078-0432

Franco, E.L., Kowalski, L.P. & Kanda, J.L. (1991). Risk factors for second cancers of the upper respiratory and digestive system: a case-control study. *J Clin Epidemiol*, 44, (7), pp. 615-25, ISSN1878-5921

Frazier, M.W., He, X., Wang, J., Gu, Z., Cleveland, J.L. and Zambetti, G.P. (1998). Activation of c-myc gene expression by tumor-derived p53 mutants requires a discrete C-terminal domain. *Mol Cell Biol*, 18, (7), pp. 3735-3743, ISSN 1098-5549

Fronza, G., Inga, A., Monti, P., Scott, G., Campomenosi, P., Menichini, P., Ottaggio, L., Viaggi, S., Burns, P. A., Gold, B. & Abbondandolo, A. (2000). The yeast p53 functional assay: a new tool for molecular epidemiology. Hopes and facts. *Mutat Res*, 462, (2-3), pp. 293-301,ISSN 1873-135X

Garnis, C., Baldwin, C., Zhang, L., Rosin, M.P. & Lam, W.L. (2003). Use of complete coverage array comparative genomic hybridization to define copy number alterations on chromosome 3p in oral squamous cell carcinomas. *Cancer Res*, 63, (24), pp. 8582–8585, ISSN 1538-7445Hanahan, D. & Weinberg, R.A. (2000). The hallmarks of cancer. *Cell*, 100, (1), pp. 57–70, ISSN 1097-4172

Hainaut, P., Hernandez, T., Robinson, A., Rodriquez-Tome, P., Flores, T., Hollstain, M., Harris, C.C. & Montesano, R. (1998). IARC database of P53 gene mutation in human tumors and cell lines: updated compilation, revised formats and new visualization tools. *Nucleic Acids Res*, 26, (1), pp. 205–213, ISSN 1362-4962

Hall, P. A., & Lane, D. P. (1994). P53 in tumour pathology - can we trust immunohistochemistry - revisited. *J Pathol*, 172,(1), pp. 1-4, ISSN 1096-9896

Hassan NM., Tada, M., Hamada, J., Kashiwazaki, H., Kameyama, T., Akhter, R., Yamazaki, Y., Yano, M., Inoue, N. & Moriuchi, T. (2008). Presence of dominant negative mutation of TP53 is a risk of early recurrence in oral cancer. *Cancer Lett*, 270, (1), pp. 108-119, ISSN1872-7980.

Hartwell, L.H. & Kastan, M.B. (1994). Cell cycle control and cancer. *Science*, 266, (5192), pp. 1821–1828, ISSN 1095-9203

Hong, W.K., Lippman, S.M., Itri, L.M., Karp, D.D, Lee, J.S, Byers, R.M, Schantz, S.P, Kramer, A.M., Lotan, R. & Peters, L.J. (1990). Prevention of secondary primary tumors with isotretinoin in squamous cell carcinoma of the head and neck. *N Engl J Med*, 323, (12), pp. 795-801, ISSN 1533-4406

Hsieh, L.L., Wang, P.F., Chen, I.H., Liao, C.T., Wang, H.M., Chen, M.C., Chang, J.T. & Cheng, A.J. (2001). Characteristics of mutations in the p53gene in oral squamous cell carcinoma associated with betel quid chewing and cigarette smoking in Taiwanese. *Carcinogenesis*, 22, (9), pp. 1497-1503, ISSN 1460-2180

Ishioka, C., Frebourg, T., Yan, Y., Vidal, M., Friend, S. H., Schmidt, S, & Iggo, R. (1993).Screening patients for heterozygotous p53 mutations using a functional assay in yeast. *Nature Genetics*, 5, (2), pp. 124-129, ISSN 1546-1718

Jemal A, Siegel R, Ward E, Hao Y, Xu J, Murray T & Thun MJ. (2008). Cancer statistics. *CA Cancer J Clin*, 58, pp. 71–96, ISBN 1542-486

Iwakuma, T., Lozano, G. & Flores, E.R. (2005). Li-Fraumeni syndrome: a p53 family affair. *Cell Cycle*, 4, (7), pp. 865-867, ISSN 1551- 4005

Kashiwazaki, H., Tonoki, H., Tada, M., Chiba, I., Shindoh, M., Tosuka, Y., Iggo, R. & Moriuchi, T. (1997). High frequency of p53 mutations in human oral epithelial dysplasia and primary squamous cell carcinoma detected by yeast functional assay. *Oncogene* ,15, (22), pp. 2667-2674, ISSN1476-5594

Kisielewski, A.E., Xiao, G.H., Liu, S.C., Klein-Szanto, A.J., Novara, M., Sina, J., Bleicher, K, Yeung, R.S. Goodrow, T.L. (1998). Analysis of the FHIT gene and its product in squamous cell carcinomas of the head and neck. *Oncogene*, 17, (1), pp. 83–91, ISSN 1476-5594

Kim, E & Deppert W. (2004) Transcriptional Activities of mutant p53: when mutations are more than a loss. *J Cell Biochem*, 93, (5), pp. 878-886, ISSN 1097-4644.

Kim, J.S., Lee, C., Bonifant, C.L., Ressom, H. & Waldman, T. (2007). Activation of p53-dependent growth suppression in human cells by mutations in PTEN orPIK3CA. *Mol Cell Biol*, 27, (2), pp. 662-677, ISSN 1471-0080

Knudson, A.G. Jr. (1977). Genetics and the etiology of human cancer. *Adv Hum Genet*, 8, pp. 1–66, ISSN 0065-275X

Kropveld, A., Rozemuller, E.H., Leppers, F.S., Scheidel, K.C., de Weger, R.A., Koole R, Hordijk, G.J, Slootweg, P.J. & Tilanus, M.G. (1999). Sequencing analysis of RNA and DNA of exons 1 through 11 shows p53 gene alterations to be present in almost 100% of head and neck squamous cell cancers. *Lab Invest*, 79, (3), pp. 347-353, ISSN 037-6617

Lang GA, Iwakuma T, Suh YA, Liu G, Rao VA, Parant JM, Valentin-Vega YA, TerZian T, Caldwell LC, Strong LC, El-Neggar AK & Lozano G. (2004). Gain of function of a p53 hot spot mutation in a mouse model of Li-fraumeni syndrome, Cell, 119, (6) pp. 861-872, ISSN 1097-0215

Lazarus, P., Garewal, H.S., Sciubba, J., Zwiebel, N., Calcagnotto, A., Fair, A., Schaefer, S. & Richie, J.P. Jr (1995). A low incidence of p53 mutations in pre-malignant lesions of the oral cavity from non-tobacco users. *Int J Cancer*, 60, (4), pp. 458-463, ISSN 1097-0215

Levine, A.J (1997). p53, the cellular gatekeeper for growth and division. *Cell*, 88, (3), PP. 323-331, ISSN 1097-4172

Levine, A.J., Momand, J. & Finlay, C.A. (1991). The p53 tumor suppressor gene. *Nature*, 351, (6326), pp. 453-456, ISSN 1476-4687

Lippman, S.M., Sudbo, J. & Hong, W.K. (2005). Oral cancer prevention and the evolution of molecular-targeted drug development. *J Clin Oncol*, 23, (2), pp. 346-356, ISSN 1527-7755

Lubin, R., Schlichtholz, B., Bengoufa, D., Zalcman, G., Tredaniel, J., Hirsch, A., Caron de Fromentel, C., Preudhomme, C., Fenaux, P., Fournier, G., Mangin, P., Laurent-Puig, P., Pelletier, G., Schlumberger, M., Desgrandchamps, F., Le Duc ,A., Peyrat, J.P., Janin, N., Bressac, B., Soussi, T. (1993). Analysis of p53 antibodies in patients with various cancers define B-Cell epitopes of human p53 -distribution on primary structure and exposure on protein surface. *Cancer Res*, 53, (24), pp. 5872-5876, ISSN 1538-7445

Lydiatt, W.M., Anderson, P.E., Bazzano, T., Casale, M., Hughes, C.J., Huvas, A.J., Lydiatt, D.D. & Schantz, S.P. (1998). Molecular support for field cancerization in the head and neck. *Cancer*, 82, (7), pp. 376-1380, ISSN1097-0142

Mao, L., El-Naggar, A.K., Fan, Y.H., Lee, J.S., Lippan, S.M., Kayser, S., Lotan, R. & Hong, W.K. (1996b). Telomerase activity in head and neck squamous cell carcinoma and adjacent tissues. *Cancer Res*, 56, (24), pp. 5600-5604, ISSN 1538-7445

Marutani, M., Tonoki, H., Tada, M., Takahashi, M., Kashiwazaki, H., Hida, Y., Hamada, J-I, Asaka, M. & Moriuchi. T. (1999). Dominant-negative mutations of the tumor suppressor p53 relating to early onset of glioblastoma multiforme. *Cancer Res*, 59, (19), pp. 4765-69, ISSN 1538-7445

Marx, J. (2007). Recruiting the cell's own guardian for cancer therapy. *Science*, 315, (5816), PP. 1211-3, ISSN1095-9203

Masayesva, B.G., Ha, P., Garrett-Mayer, E., Pilkington, T., Mao, R., Pevsner J, Speed, T., Benoit, N., Moon, C.S., Sidransky, D., Westra, W.H. & Califano, J. (2004). Gene expression alterations over large chromosomal regions in cancers include multiple genes unrelated to malignant progression. *Proc Natl Acad Sci USA*, 101, (23), pp. 8715-8720, ISSN 1091-6490

McShane, L. M., Aamodt, R., Cordon-Cardo, C., Cote, R., Faraggi, D., Fradet, Y., Grossman, H. B., Peng, A., Taube, S. E., & Waldman, F. M. (2000). Reproducibility of p53 immunohistochemistry in bladder tumors. National Cancer Institute, Bladder Tumor Marker Network [In Process Citation]. *Clin Cancer Res,* 6, (5), pp. 1854-1864, ISSN 1078-0432

Min, B.M., Baek, J.H., Shin, K.H., Gujulava, C.N., Cherrick, H.M. & Park, N.H. (1994). Inactivation of the p53 gene by either mutation or HPV infection is extremely frequent in human oral squamous carcinoma cell lines. *Eur J Cancer B Oral Oncol,* 30, (B), pp. 338–345, ISSN 1368-8375

Moertel, C.G. (1977). Multiple primary malignant neoplasms: Historical perspectives. *Cancer,* 40, (4), pp. 1786-1792, ISSN 1097-0142

Moertel, C.G. & Foss, E.L. (1958). Multicentric carcinomas of the oral cavity. *Surg Gynecol Obstet* , 106, (6), pp.652-4, ISSN 0039-6087

Nagpal, J.K., Patnaik, S., Das, B.R. (2002). Prevalence of high-risk human papilloma virus types and its association with p53 codon -72 polymorphism in tobacco addicted oral squamous cell carcinoma (OSCC) patients of Eastern India. *Int J Cancer,* 97, (5), pp. 649–653, ISSN 1097-0215

Németh, Z.S., Czigner, J., Iván, L., Ujpál, M., Barabás, J. & Szabó, G. (2002). Quadruple cancer, including triple cancers in the head and neck region. *Neoplasma,* 4, (6), pp. 412-414, ISSN 0028-2685

Nishiwaki, M., Yamamoto, T., Tone, S., Murai, T., Ohkawara, T., Matsunami, T., Motoiki, K., Takagi, Y., Yamaguchi, J., Kondo, N., Nishihira, J., Horikawa, T. & Yoshiki, T. (2008). Genotyping of human Papillomaviruses by a Novel One-Step Typing Method with Multiplex PCR and Clinical Applications. *J Clin Microbiol,* 46, (4), pp. 161-1168, ISSN 1098-660X

Nylander, K., Dabelsteen, E. & Hall, P.A. (2000). The p53 molecule and its prognostic role in squamous cell carcinomas of the head and neck. *J Oral Pathol Med,* 29, (9), pp. 413-425, ISSN 1600-0714

Oliner, J.D., Pietenpol, T.A., Thiagalingam, S., Gyuris, J., Kinzler, K.W. & Vogelstein, B. (1993). Oncoprotein MDM2 conceals the activation domain of tumour suppressor p53. *Nature,* 362, (6423), pp. 857–860, ISSN 1476-4687

Patrikidou, A., Bennett, J., Abou-Sleiman, P., Delhanty, J.D.A & Harris, M, (2002). A novel, de novo germline TP53 mutation in a rare presentation of the Li-Fraumeni syndrome in the maxilla. *Oral Oncol,* 38, (4), pp. 383-390, ISSN1368-8375

Parkin, D.M., Läärä, E., & Muir, C.S. (1988). Estimates of the worldwide frequency of sixteen major cancers in 1980. *Int J Cancer,* 41, (2), pp. 184-197, ISSN 1097-0215.

Petitjean, A., Mathe, E., Kato, S., Ishioka, C., Tavtigian, S.V., Hainaut, P. & Olivier, M. (2007). Impact of mutant p53 functional properties on TP53 mutation patterns and tumor phenotype: lessons from recent developments in the IARC TP53 database. *Hum Mutat,* 28, (6), pp. 622-629, ISSN 1098-1004

Pomerantz, J., Schreiber-Agus, N., Liegeois, N.J., Silverman, A., Alland, L., Chin, L., Potes, J., Chen, K., Orlow, I., Lee, H.W., Cordon-Cardo, C. & DePinho, R.A. (1998). The Ink4a tumor suppressor gene product, p19Arf, interacts with MDM2 and neutralizes MDM2's inhibition of p53. *Cell,* 92, (6), pp. 713–723, ISSN 1097-4172

Reed, A.L., Califano, J., Cairns, P., Westra, W.H., Jones, R.M., Koch, W., Ahrendt, S., Eby, Y., Sewell, D., Nawroz, H., Bartek, J. & Sidransky, D. (1996). High frequency of p16(CDKN2/MTS-1/INK4A) inactivation in head and neck squamous cell carcinoma. *Cancer Res,* 56, (16), pp. 3630–3633, ISSN- 1538-7445.

Rousseau, A., Lim, M.S., Lin, Z. & Jordan, R.C. (2001). Frequent cyclin D1 gene amplification and protein overexpression in oral epithelial dysplasias. *Oral Oncol*, 37, (3), pp. 268–275, ISSN 1368-8375

Sakuragi, N., Watari, H., Ebina, Y., Yamamoto, R., Steiner, E., Koelbl, H., Yano, M., Tada, M. & Moriuchi, T. (2005). Functional analysis of p53 gene and the prognostic impact of dominant-negative p53 mutation in endometrial cancer. *Int J Cancer*, 116, (4), pp. 514–519, ISSN 1097-0215

Sampath, J., Sun, D., Kidd, V.J., Grenet, J., Gandhi, A., Shapiro, L.H., Wang, Q., Zambetti, G.P. & Schuetz, J.D. (2001). Mutant p53 cooperates with ETS and selectively up-regulates human MDR1 not MRP1. *J Biol Chem*, 276, (42), pp.39359-39367, ISSN 1083-351X

Save, V., Nylander, K., & Hall, P. A. (1998). Why is p53 protein stabilized in neoplasia? Some answers but many more question! *J Pathol*, 184, (4), pp. 348-350, ISSN1096-9896

Schmitz-Drager, B. J., Goebell, P. J., Ebert, T., & Fradet, Y. (2000). p53 immunohistochemistry as a prognostic marker in bladder cancer. playground for urology scientists? [In Process Citation]. *Eur Urol*, 38, (6). pp. 691-700, ISSN 1873-7560

Schwartz, L.H., Ozsahin, M., Zhang, G.N., Touboul, E., De Vataire, F., Andolenko, P., Lacau-Saint-Guily, J., Laugier, A. & Schlienger, M. (1994). Synchronous and metachronous head and neck carcinomas. *Cancer*, 74, (7), PP. 1933-8, ISSN 1097-0142

Shin, D.M., Ro, J.Y., Hong, W.K. & Hittelman, W.N. (1994). Dysregulation of epidermal growth factor receptor expression in premalignant lesions during head and neck tumorigenesis. *Cancer Res*, 54, (12), pp. 3153–3159, ISSN 1538-7445

Shin, D.M., Kim, J., Ro, J.Y., Hittelman, J., Roth, J.A., Hong, W.K. & Hittelman, W.N. (1994). Activation of p53 gene expression in premalignant lesions during head and neck tumorigenesis. *Cancer Res*, 54, (2), pp. 321-326, ISSN1538-7445

Sigal, A. & Rotter, V. (2000). Oncogenic mutations of the p53 tumor suppressor: the demons of the guardian of the genome. *Cancer Res*, 60, (24), Pp. 6788–6793, ISSN 1538-7445

Sidransky, D. (1995). Molecular genetics of head and neck cancer. *Curr Opin Oncol* 7, (3), pp. 229–233, ISSN 1531-703X

Silverman, S. Jr., Gorsky, M. & Lozada, F. (1984). Oral leukoplakia and malignant transformation. A follow-up study of 257 patients. *Cancer*, 53, (3), pp. 563-568, ISSN 1097-0142

Slaughter, D.P., Southwick, H.W., & Smejkal, W. (1953). Field cancerization in oral stratified squamous epithelium: clinical implication of multicentric origin. *Cancer*, 6, (5), pp. 963–968, ISSN 1097-0142

Somers, K.D., Merrick, M.A., Lopez, M.E., Incognito, L.S., Schechter, G.L. & Casey, G. (1992). Frequent p53 mutations in head and neck cancer. *Cancer Res*, 52, (21), pp. 5997–6000, ISSN 1538-7445

Song, H. Hollstein M, and Xu, Y. (2007). p53 gain -of function cancer mutants induce genetic instability by inactivating ATM. Nat Cell Biol, 9, (5), pp. 573–580, ISSN 1476-4679

Song, H. & Xu, Y. (2007). Gain of function of p53 cancer mutants in disrupting critical DNA damage response pathways. *Cell Cycle*, 6, (13), pp. 1570–1573, ISSN 1551-4005

Soussi, T., & Béroud, C. (2001). Assessing TP53 status in human tumours to evaluate clinical outcome. *Nat Rev Cancer*, 1, (3), pp. 233-240, ISSN 1474-1768

Tabor, M.P., Brakenhoff, R.H.,, Ruijter-Schippers H.J., van der Wal, J.E., Snow, G.B., Leemans, C.R. & Braakhuis, B.J. (2002). Multiple head and neck tumors frequently originate from a single preneoplastic lesion. *Am J Pathol*, 161, (3), pp. 1051-1060, ISSN 1525-2191

Tada, M., Furuuchi, K., Kaneda, M., Matsumoto, J., Takahashi, M., Hirai, A., Mitsumoto, Y., Iggo, R. D., & Moriuchi, T. (2001). Inactivate the remaining p53 allele or the alternate p73? Preferential selection of the Arg72 polymorphism in cancers with recessive p53 mutants but not transdominant mutants. *Carcinogenesis*, 22, (3), pp. 515-517, ISSN 1460-2180

Temam, S., Flahault, A., Périé, S., Monceaux, G., Coulet, F., Callard, P., Bernaudin, J.F, St Guily, J.L. & Fouret , P. (2000). p53 gene status as a predictor of tumor response to induction chemotherapy of patients with locoregionally advanced squamous cell carcinomas of the head and neck. *J Clin Oncol*, 18, (2), pp. 385-394, ISSN 1527-7755

Tjebbes, G.W.A., Leppers, V.D straat, F.G.J., Tilanus, M.G.J., Hordijk, G.J. & Slootweg, P.J. (1999). p53 tumor suppressor gene as a clonal marker in head and neck squamous cell carcinoma: p53 mutations in primary tumor and matched lymph node metastases. *Oral Oncology*, 35, (4), pp. 384-389, ISSN 1368-8375

van der Riet, P., Nawroz, H., Hruban, R.H., Corio, R., Tokino, K., Koch, W. & Sidransky, D. (1994). Frequent loss of chromosome 9p21-22 early in head and neck cancer progression. *Cancer Res*, 54, (5), pp.1156-1158, ISSN 1538-7445

Vogelstein, B. & Kinzler, K.W. (1993). The multistep nature of cancer. *Trends Genet*, 9, (4), pp. 138-141, ISSN 0168-9525

Vogelstein, B., Lane, D. & Levine, A.J. (2001). Surfing the p53 network. *Nature*, 408, (6810), pp. 307-310, ISSN 1476-4687

Warnakulasuriya, S., Jia, C., Johnson, N. & Houghton, J. (2000). p53 and P-glycoprotein expression are significant prognostic markers in advanced head and neck cancer treated with chemo/radiotherapy. *J Pathol*, 191, (1), pp. 33-38, ISSN 1096-9896

Waridel, F., Estreicher, A., Bron, L., Flaman, J. M., Fontolliet, C., Monnier, P., Frebourg, T. & Iggo, R. (1997). Field cancerisation and polyclonal p53 mutation in the upper aero digestive tract. *Oncogene* 14, (2), pp. 163-169, ISSN 1476-5594

Weinberg, R.A. (1991). Tumor suppressor genes. *Science*, 254, (5035), pp. 1138-1146, ISSN 1095-9203

Weinberg, R.A. (1989). Oncogenes, antioncogenes, and the molecular basis of multistep carcinogenesis. *Cancer Res*, 49, (14), pp. 3713-3717, ISSN 1538-7445

Weisz, L., Zalcenstein, A., Stambolsky, P., Cohen, Y., Goldfinger, N., Oren, M. & Rotter, V. (2004). Transactivation of the EGR1 gene contributes to mutant p53 gain of function. *Cancer Res*, 64, (22), pp. 8318-8327, ISSN 1476-5594

Yamazaki, Y., Chiba, I., Hirai, A., Satoh, C., Sakakibara, N., Notani, K-I, Kashiwazaki, H., Tei, K., Totsuka, Y. & Fukuda, H. (2003). Specific p53 mutations predict poor prognosis in oral squamous cell carcinoma, *Oral Oncol*, 39, (2), PP. 163-169, ISSN 1368-8375

Yokota, J. & Sugimura, T. (1993). Multiple steps in carcinogenesis involving alteration of multiple tumour suppressor genes. *FASEB J*, 7, (10), pp. 920-925, ISSN 1530-6860

Yoshikawa, K., Hamada, J., Tada, M, Kameyama, T., Nakagawa, K., Suzuki, Y., Ikawa, M., Hassan, N.M.M., Kitagawa, Y. & Moriuchi, T. (2010). Mutant p53 R248Q but not R248W enhances in vitro invasiveness of human lung cancer NCI-H1299 cells. *Biomedical Research*, 31, (6), pp. 401-411, ISSN. 1880-313X

Zalcenstein, A., Stambolsky, P., Weisz, L., Muller, M., Wallach, D., Goncharov, T.M., Krammer, P.H., Rotter, V. & Oren, M. (2003). Mutant p53 gain of function: repression of CD95(Fas/APO-1) gene expression by tumor-associated p53 mutants. *Oncogene*, 22, (36), pp. 5667-5676, ISSN1476-5594.

Part 2

Diagnosis and Management

9

Diagnostic Aids in Oral Cancer Screening

Pegah Mosannen Mozafari, Zahra Delavarian and Nooshin Mohtasham
Oral and Maxillofacial Diseases Research Center, Mashhad Dental Faculty, Mashhad University of Medical Sciences, Mashhad, Iran

1. Introduction

At the world level, head and neck cancer is the sixth most common cancer (Fedele 2009). Oral squamous cell carcinoma (OSCC) accounts for about 40% of head and neck and 90-95% of oral malignancies (Neville et al. 1995; Pektas et al. 2006). OSCC is proceeded by visible changes in the oral mucosa, such as: white plaque, redness, ulcer or exophytic lesion, with no other signs/symptoms. (Delavarian et al. 2010). If OSCC is diagnosed and treated in this stage, it will be curable and inexpensive to treat with excellent treatment outcomes and survival (Rosenberg and Cretin 1989).

Five-year survival is about 76% to 80% if diagnosis is performed in stage 1 and 2. Late diagnosis in stage 3 and 4 can decrease this value to 41% and 9% respectively (Mashberg and Feldman 1988; Neville et al. 1995; Maraki, Becker, and Boecking 2004; Pektas et al. 2006). At this time, metastasis to regional lymph nodes has occurred and cancer cannot be treated without undesirable complications and morbidity (such as mucosities, xerostomia, surgical defect, etc....). Unfortunately majority of cases are diagnosed at stage 3 and 4 with more than 50% of them exhibiting metastatic lymphadenopathy (Eisenbud and Sciubba 1978). Despite advances in diagnostic procedures in medical practice, mortality of OSCC has remained unchanged in the past 40 years and and a significant diagnostic delay (up to 8 months)has persisted over time. (Abdo et al. 2007; Peacock, Pogrel, and Schmidt 2008) For example, the mortality rate for oral cancer is similar to that of colon cancer even though it is much easier to screen and detect oral cancers than it is for colon cancer. The most important factor in patient survival and prognosis is early diagnosis. Studies have shown that most OSCC could have been detected 3 to 7 month earlier by a trained dentist (Bruun 1976), but as mentioned, 50% of patients have regional or distant metastasis at the time of diagnosis (Acha 2005; Fedele 2009). There are some reasons for this delay (Wood and Goaz 1997;Abdo et al. 2007; Peacock, Pogrel, and Schmidt 2008;):

1. Lack of public awareness about signs, symptoms and risk factors of oral cancer.
2. Absence of routine oral examination in at least 50% of public.
3. Absence of symptoms in early stages of oral cancer.
4. Development of cancer in parts of oral cavity which normally scape inspection by the patients and/or physician (e.g. floor of the mouth).
5. Similarity of lesions to benign ones (e.g.; candidiasis, recurrent aphthous stomatitis, etc.).
6. Absences of prevention and early detection by heath care providers (e.g. lack of knowledge and ability to recognize oral cancer in early stages and absence of generally accepted screening tests which can be easily performed by general dentists).

OSCC very often arises from an oral premalignant lesion (OPL). OPL is defined as a benign, morphologically altered tissue that has a greater than normal risk of malignant transformation((Neville et al. 1995). Erythroplakia, leukoplakia, oral lichen planus and oral submucous fibrosis are examples of OPL. Erythroplakia either isolated or concomitant with leukoplakia may show severe dysplasia or carcinoma *In Situ*. Indeed 90% of erthroplakia lesions are histologically diagnosed as carcinoma *In Situ* or cancer (Mashberg and Feldman 1988; Mills and Carter 2004; Maraki, Becker, and Boecking 2004; Kujan et al. 2005).

Leukoplakia is the most common OPL in the oral cavity with a 4-40% chance for malignant changes (Waldron and Shafer 1975; Sciubba 1999; Maraki, Becker, and Boecking 2004). A new cohort showed that 17.9% of leukoplakia lesions developed into oral cancer with a mean duration of 5.2 years. (Liu et al. 2010). Oral lichen planus may become cancerous in 0.4 to 2.5% of cases (Sciubba 1999;Maraki, Becker, and Boecking 2004). A new retrospective study in Spain revealed 0.9% chance of malignancy in oral lichen planus with the tongue as the most common location (Bermejo-Fenoll et al. 2009).

Sometimes oral cancer develops *de novo*- from a normal mucosa- and is not preceded by an OPL, but usually a small part of an OPL may undergo dysplasia or malignant changes. Early removal of this part can prevent emergence of malignant lesions. But the question is- how can we find early malignant changes in an apparently benign lesion? To answer this question we must be familiar with adjunctive diagnostic aids which if employed properly, can enhance diagnosis and improve treatment outcomes. In the next section we introduce the diagnostic aids in oral Cancer screening or diagnosis.

2. Diagnostic aids in screening of oral cancer

Diagnostic aids can help the physician to decide whether the suspicious lesion needs biopsy or removal for cancer detection. Sometimes malignant changes occur without any clinical evidence of malignancy. In this situation even an expert eye may overlook malignant changes. Diagnostic aids can reveal these occult changes. In other word, diagnostic aids can be used as screening or as adjunctive tools. The decision whether to screen for oral cancer or not depends on many factors. Table1 shows the criteria for implementation of a screening program. (Lingen et al. 2008) when screening is indicated for oral cancer in a certain population, a suitable test should be employed. Table2 illustrates the characteristics of a good screening test. (Lingen et al. 2008)

The disease must be an important health problem
An accepted treatment must be available for patients with recognized disease
Facilities for diagnosis and treatment must be available
There must be a recognizable latent or early symptomatic stage
A suitable test must be available
The test should be acceptable to the population
The natural history of the condition should be adequately understood
There should be an agreed policy on whom to treat as patients
The screening program should be cost-effective
The screening process should be a continuing process and not a 'once and for all' project

Table 1. Criteria for the implementation of a screening program (Lingen et al. 2008)

There are different screening tests for oral cancer with variable indications, limitations and implications. Yet the gold standard for cancer diagnosis is surgical biopsy and histopathologic examination. But not every suspicious lesion should be surgically biopsied. There is a spectrum ranging from clinical examination to surgical biopsy. Diagnostic tests are located in the middle of this spectrum and have their own indications. Here we discuss diagnostic procedures, which can be employed in early detection of oral cancer.

A screening test should:
Be simple, safe and acceptable to the public
Detect disease early in its natural history
Preferentially detect those lesions which are likely to progress
Detect lesions which are treatable or where an intervention will prevent progression
Have a high positive predictive value and low false negatives (high sensitivity)

Table 2. Characteristics of a good screening test (Lingen et al. 2008)

Screening test must be evaluated with respect to their diagnostic value. This value includes sensitivity (SN), specificity (SP), positive predictive value (PPV) and negative predictive value (NPV). If calculating of these values is considered the results must be compared to the gold standard. The gold standard of oral cancer diagnosis is yet scalpel biopsy (surgical biopsy). The gold standard is used to classify subjects as to their true state of disease. Table 3 shows the SN, SP, PPV and NPV and the way to calculate them.

$$SN = \frac{a}{a+c}$$

$$SP = \frac{d}{d+b}$$

$$PPV = \frac{a}{a+b}$$

$$NPV = \frac{d}{d+c}$$

		Gold Standard		Total
		Disease present	Disease absent	
Diagnostic test	+	a True positive	d False positive	a+d
	-	c False negative	b True negative	c+b
Total		a + c	b + d	a+b+c+d

Table 3. Standard 2X2 table for the calculation of sensitivity(SN), specificity(SP), positive predictive value(PPV) and negative predictive value(NPV)

2.1 Clinical examination

Diagnosis of oral cancer begins with a complete history taking followed by a thorough clinical examination. Oral cavity is the most accessible site of alimentary track for clinical examination. (Chiodo, Eigner, and Rosenstein 1986)Precise inspection of all parts of oral mucosa using an incandescent light can reveal abnormal changes. The physician must examine the whole oral cavity accurately. Posterior portions and floor of the mouth must be surveyed meticulously. Even self-examination of oral cavity can be performed by the individuals for early detection of oral cancer (Elango et al. 2011). Any symptom or sign must be assessed exactly. The teeth must be examined for any evidence of mobility or tilting. Sometimes radiographic examination is necessary to complete the clinical examination. The clinician must palpate any lesion to find induration or firmness. Apparently normal mucosa must be palpated to reveal any mass or abnormal change (e.g. roughness, altered texture…). Cervical lymph nodes must be palpated to find metastatic lymphadenopathy in occult oropharynx malignancy

At the time of evaluating an OPL, any evidence of roughness, ulceration, redness and induration must be further examined by histopathologic examination. Diagnostic value of clinical examination has been reported in literature. (Sankaranarayanan et al. 2005; Downer et al. 1995; Nagao et al. 2000; Jullien et al. 1995; Downer et al. 2004; Mignogna and Fedele 2005). A Meta analysis on different studies of oral cancer screening showed an overall sensitivity of 0.857. (95% CI 0.73, 0.92) and specificity of 0.97(95%. CI 0.93, 0.98), Indicating a satisfactory test performance for oral examination (Downer et al. 2004). This study also suggested that trained auxiliaries are able to screen with a degree of accuracy similar to dental practitioner.

Mortality of oral cancer can be decreased by clinical examination. One study reported a 32% reduction in mortality of OSCC in high risk individuals, suggesting that about 40000 deaths can be prevented by oral examination worldwide (Mignogna and Fedele 2005; Sankaranarayanan et al. 2005). Even self examination can improve early detection of oral cancer, although compliance to seek treatment is still low (32%).(Elango et al. 2011; Warnakulasuriya et al. 1984) . False positive referrals for definite diagnosis can result in anxiety which can be decreased by public education for the individuals who receive oral examination. (Patton 2003)

To increase cost effectiveness of oral cancer screening programs, it is better to perform targeted clinical examinations of high-risk subjects (opportunistic screen) than mass screening (Speight et al. 2006; Patton 2003). A Cochrane systematic review found that there is no evidence to recommend inclusion or exclusion of screening for oral cancer using a visual examination unless randomized controlled trials provide the most reliable information for decision in clinical practice (Kujan et al. 2005).

Despite benefits of clinical examination, it has been demonstrated that between 4.5 and 15.3% of OPL and early stage oral cancers can not be adequately identified by visual inspection alone and may be overlooked even by highly trained professionals, potentially increasing the false negative rate (Moles, Downer, and Speight 2003). Because of this innate pitfall of visual inspection, other diagnostic aids can be employed to improve early detection of oral cancer.

2.2 Cytopathologic studies

2.2.1 Oral exfoliative cytology

Cythopathology is the microscopic study of cell samples collected from mucosal surfaces obtained by exfoliative cytology (via smears, scraping or lavage) or by fine needle aspiration (Sarah Freygang et al. 2011). Cytology has been applied to diagnose human diseases, since Papanicolaou and Traut validated it for diagnosis of cervical cancer (Papanicolaou GN 1941). Since then cytology of the oral cavity began to be used as a cytopathologic diagnostic technique. In early studies on this technique no satisfactory results were obtained, mainly due to its limitations and improper application. In this technique a collecting devise (swab, spatula and brush) is placed and rotated against the mucosal surface and the cells are collected.

The next step is to prepare a smear by spreading the cells onto a glass slide. After fixation and papanicolaou staining the slide is examined by pathologist. Interpretation of the results must be performed by an expert pathologist familiar with cytopathology. Sometimes cells are collected by a cytobrush. Diagnostic values of exfoliative cytology have a wide range due to kind of sampling instrument. A positive result is defined as definitive cellular evidence of epithelial dysplasia or carcinoma and atypical result is defined as abnormal epithelial changes of uncertain diagnostic significance (Maraki, Becker, and Boecking 2004). Studies from 1950 to 1970s reported high false negative results for exfoliative cytology (Folsom et al. 1972; Shklar, Cataldo, and Meyer 1970; Rovin 1967). For example Folsom et all reported 37% false negative result in 148 oral lesions (Folsom et al. 1972).

Recent studies have reported better results (Navone et al. 2004) due to combining molecular analysis with exfoliative cytology which will be discussed in a separate section. Some researchers have analyzed the reliability of oral cytology and it's cytometric analysis in the early detection of oral cancer. The SN 98.2%, SP100%, PPV of 100% and NPV of 99% have been reported (Remmerbach et al. 2003). Mehrotra et al Reviewed 22 articles and found SN and SP of oral exfoliation cytology to be 76.8% - 100% and 88.9% - 100% respectively (Mehrotra et al. 2009).

2.2.2 Brush biopsy

Oral CD-x brush is a kind of specialized oral brush, which can penetrate the thickness of the mucosa and collect representative sample of the lesion. (Acha 2005)Basal and parabasal cells- which are the precursor of malignant changes- are collected by this specially designed brush. "Brush biopsy" employs oral CD-x brush, which is then analyzed by computer. Some studies have used oral CD-x brush, but have analyzed the result by visual histopathology examination and not by computer (Mehrotra et al. 2006;Delavarian et al 2010).

The diagnostic value of brush biopsy has been reported in several studies. SN from 71 to 100 percent, SP varied from 27 to 94 percent, PPVs ranged from 38 to 88 percent and NPVs from 60 to 100 percent have been reported. According to a systematic review by Patton et all, oral CD-x cytological test has advantages in detecting dysplastic changes in high risk mucosal lesions but in low risk populations or clinical innocuous lesions its application remains in doubt. This technique can not be performed in place of surgical biopsy.(Patton, Epstein, and

Kerr 2008) It seems that OralCDx technique overestimates dysplastic lesions and has a low PPV(Bhoopathi, Kabani, and Mascarenhas 2009)

2.2.3 Liquid based cytology (LBC)

Since 1990, liquid-based cytology (LBC) has been designed to improve slide quality and quantity of conventional cytology (Davey et al. 2006). LBC is an improvement in cytology technique that can compensate many disadvantages of conventional exfoliate cytology. Instead of a unique smear, a suspension of cells is obtained and several slides could be prepared. In LBC the sample collector with the sample is immersed in a tube containing preservative fluid, which fixes the cells immediately and can be a useful source of cells for upcoming researches. The fluid is placed on a centrifugal force and the cells make a thin high cellular confined zone on the glass slide, which can be assessed easily by the pathologist. Many artifacts of conventional cytology do not occur in LBC technique. By employing this technique unsatisfactory slides and false negative results have been reduced and the diagnostic value of cytology has improved. Up to now, only few studies in oral cavity -based on LBC technique- have been published in English literature. In Hayama study; 44 different oral lesions were examined by both conventional and liquid based (Autocyte Inc) cytological examination using a cytobrush -not specified for oral mucosa. It was concluded that the two techniques led to the same diagnosis and the same papanicolaou class was assigned in all adequate cases. Three conventional smears were hypocellular, hence making the cytological diagnosis impossible. The LBC preparations showed a satisfactory higher improvement in slide quality (thinness, even cell distribution, absence of overlapping and bleeding) (Hayama et al. 2005).

In Navone study 2006, results of conventional exfoliative cytology and LBC (by using dermatologic curette) were compared with scalpel biopsy. Both sensitivity and specificity were higher in LBC group than in conventional cytology. The false negative and positive results were 7/89 and 2/89 in conventional smear group and 4/384 and 3/384 in LBC group. Upon these results, it can be concluded that LBC gives better results and enhances SN and SP (Navone et al. 2007). Recently Navone reported a 95.1% SN and 99% SP for LBC technique. (Navone 2009)

2.2.4 A modified liquid-based cytology using OralCDx® Brush

Although the diagnostic values of brush biopsy or LBC technique have been published previously there are some pitfalls: First, in many brush biopsy studies not all of samples with different brush results underwent scalpel biopsy so the reported values for sensitivity, specificity, etc., could be questionable. Second, in the case of performing both brush and biopsy, there are few, if ever, studies which both techniques are done simultaneously and exactly from the same area. Third, all of LBC studies in oral cavity are performed using cervical or dermatological tools for sample collection and never a specialized oral tool (e.g.CDx brush) has been employed (Hayama et al. 2005; Navone et al. 2007). Because of non rigid nature of cervical brushes, inadequate results are expected. This leads to false negative results and significant diagnostic delay (Potter, Summerlin, and Campbell 2003).

So, we planned a study to use LBC technique employing a specialized oral brush (OralCDx® Brush), simultaneously and exactly from the same area to determine the diagnostic value (sensitivity, specificity, positive and negative predictive values and positive and negative likelihood ratios) of modified LBC technique in detection of dysplasia /malignancy in oral potentially malignant and cancerous lesions and to evaluate diagnostic agreement between this technique and scalpel biopsy. (Delavarian et al. 2010)

Since only a few laboratories evaluate the OralCDx® results by computer-assisted analysis, we examined microscopic slides visually. First, we designed a pilot study on 3 normal mucosa and 7 epithelial lesions to qualify slide properties, using standard protocol of OralCDx® kits. After manipulation of standard protocol neither the quality nor the quantity of slides were suitable for cytopathologic diagnosis, so we applied an LBC technique and modified the conventional protocol in this way:

First, instead of spreading the brush onto a glass slide, the brush was placed in the supplied glass tube, containing formalin (10%), and sent to the cytopathology laboratory. There the brush and the formalin, containing cells dispersed from brush were placed in a vortex for 5 minutes in 4000 RPM. This centrifugal force helped to sediment the cells and taken them off from the brush hairs. Then 100 λ (mm3) of this sediment was placed onto the cup of Cytospine (Shandon UK) centrifuge in 1000RPM(similar to power recommended in this vortex for vaginal samples). Two to 4 samples were obtained from each cellular sediment. The more the sediment was rich in cellular material or blood component, the more glass slides were prepared.

The study group consisted of 25 patients with 26 lesions which had been visited from Oct 2005 to Jan 2007, at Oral Medicine Department of Mashhad Faculty of Dentistry and Otorhinolaryngology Departments of QAEM, IMAM REZA and OMID hospitals, Mashhad, Iran. (Table 4)The study protocol was approved by the committee on ethics of Mashhad University of the Medical Sciences (MUMS) on the basis of the Helsinki consent 2005.Patients were informed with regard to the research objectives, methods, possible benefits and potential risks and a written consent was obtained from all participants.

Inclusion criterion was: lesions clinically diagnosed as oral potentially malignant (leukoplakia, OLP) or malignant lesions (OSCC and verrucous carcinoma) and requiring an incisional (scalpel) biopsy for definite diagnosis. Exclusion criteria were: A) History of any treatment for the lesion (drug, radiation and chemotherapy) and B) A systemic contraindication for scalpel biopsy.

The most appropriate site of biopsy was determined upon the most probable site of dysplasia/malignancy (e.g. presence of firmness and indurations and roughness or red surface or high risk areas for dysplasia/malignancy (e.g. Ventral tongue and floor of the mouth) or the most surgically accessible site.

Demographic data were recorded. After determination of the site of biopsy, under local anesthesia, needed for scalpel biopsy, the Oral CDx brush was placed in the selected area and turned 5 to 10 times until appearing pinpoint bleeding-upon to manufacturer's recommendation. The brush was sent to cytopathology laboratory immersing in supplied 10 %formalin glass tube. The scalpel biopsy was also done immediately in site of pinpoint bleeding.

In cytopathology laboratory, the slides were prepared by Modified Liquid Based Techniques. By using cytospine vortex the cells were compacted in a 20mm2 area ,then they were fixed in 96° alcohol for 20 minutes and papanicolaou staining was done. They were examined by a pathologist informed about clinical diagnosis, but blind to the histopathological results; using Leica BME (Leica Buffalo state, US) microscopes in 100X and 400X magnifications.

The cytopathological findings were categorized as three groups: 1) Positive: dysplastic epithelial changes. 2) Negative: absence of any evidence suggesting dysplasia.3) Inadequate sampling: means two entities:A) Inadequate depth of sampling -absence of basal and parabasal cell layers in slide.B) Inadequate quantity of cells-hypocellularity.

The histopathologic preparations were observed by the same pathologist blind to cytopathological study and informed about clinical diagnosis. The Pindborg criteria (Warnakulasuriya et al. 2008) for detecting dysplasia and malignancy were used and the histopathologic diagnosis was made .The presence of dysplasia/malignancy in histopathology(P.D.M.H) was classified as normal(no dysplasia/malignancy),mild, moderate and severe dysplasia (level 1 to 3),carcinoma *In Situ*(level 4) and carcinoma(level 5)(table 4).

Quantitative variables were analyzed by T test as $\overline{X}$ ±SD and for qualitative variables $\chi 2$ and Exact Fisher tests were done using SPSS11.5 software. SN, SP, PPV and NPV were calculated for modified technique and clinical examination. Positive likelihood ratio (LR+) and negative likelihood ratio (LR-) were calculated for modified technique. Kappa value was calculated to determine diagnostic agreement between the modified technique and scalpel biopsy, the gold standard.

Thirteen male and 12 female contributed to this study (Table 4).In one female patient (Table 4 -pt (patient) No 25) two sites with two different clinical diagnoses (one proved to be severely dysplastic and one OSCC in histopathologic assessment) were biopsied (Fig 1). The mean age of patients was 54.00±17.38 (12 females; 54.23±19.77and 13 males; 53.77±15.43 years).T test revealed senile contingency in two groups. Six lesions were clinically diagnosed as OLP, six as leukoplakia, 13 as OSCCs and one as verrucous carcinoma (Table 4).

The Modified LBC results showed 10 negative and 16 positive results ,without any inadequate results, hence all the specimens were included basal and parabasal layers and enough quantity. Histopathologic results were as follow : (Table 4) 7 lesions diagnosed as OLP, 5 as leukoplakia, 11 as OSCC and one as verrucous carcinoma, two lesions(pt Nos 9 and 23) , were diagnosed as Granular Cell Tumors (GCT) of tongue.

Clinical diagnosis was in agreement in 88.4% (23/26) with histopathological findings. One lichenoid reaction clinically diagnosed as leukoplakia and two granular cell tumors clinically diagnosed as OSCCs. In 92.3 %(24/26, p<0.001) results of modified LBC were in agreement with presence of malignancy/dysplasia in histopathology. The two false negative results were outcomes of histopathologically focal dysplasia (one mild and one moderate dysplasia).

Kappa value (an index of diagnostic agreement) was calculated 0.806 for modified LBC and scalpel biopsy. In our study, SN, SP, PPV and NPV of modified LBC technique were calculated as follows: 88.8%, 100%, 100% and 80%. All the samples contained cells of all epithelial layers (including basal and parabasal layers) because of specialized designed rigid hairs of CDx brush. This is an advantage, which can resolve the problem of false negative and inadequate results and help to improve sensitivity. It is the first attempt to apply Liquid Based Cytology (LBC) using a specialized oral cytology instrument (OralCDx® Brush), hence other LBC studies in oral cavity have used cervical or dermatologic tools for sample collection(Hayama et al. 2005; Navone et al. 2007).

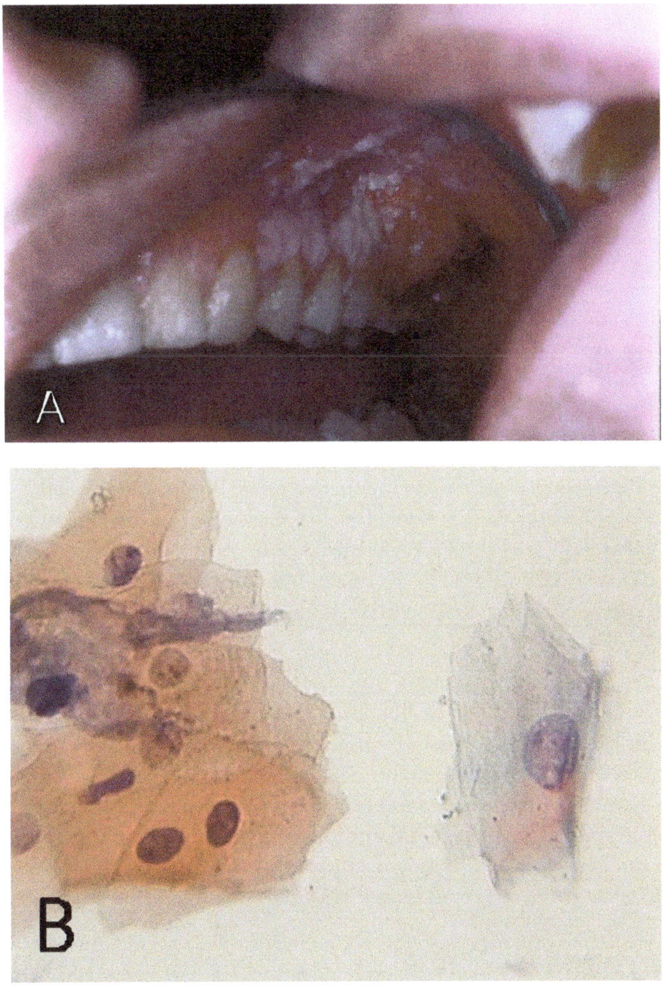

Fig. 1. Patient NO.25. **A)** malignant changes (posterior portions) in a severely dysplastic leukoplakia(anterior portions) on maxillary gingiva. **B)**LBC prepared cytologic slides revealed dysplasia in leukoplakic area ,note to different nucleus size and high protein synthesis activity (100X magnification - Papanicolaou staining)

False negative ratio (11%=2/18) was slightly higher than other studies (3.5%, 1.9%, 5%) (Christian 2002;Potter, Summerlin, and Campbell 2003; Scheifele et al 2004; Navone et al 2004). Because of small sample size, especially in premalignant lesions, it is not possible to compare researches. Svirsky reported 4 false negatives but three out of four false negative results seemed to originate from incompatible site and time of both biopsy techniques; indeed only 1 " false negative" was reported which could be the result of the technique *per se*. Other negative results seemed to originate from (Svirsky et al. 2002). In our study, performing brush biopsy simultaneously on the exact biopsy site could compensate this shortcoming.

Two clinically diagnosed malignancies (OSCCs)-proved to be granular cell tumors of tongue- had negative brush results. This suggests more specificity for brush compared to clinical diagnosis. SN 88.8% was almost similar to some results of oral exfoliative cytology researches (86.5%, 71.4% and 92.3%) (Scheifele et al. 2004; Navone et al. 2004; Poate et al. 2004; Sciubba 1999) and in contrast to results of other study with extremely high SN (100%) (Sciubba 1999).100% PPV was higher than previous studies (38.3% 7.4%and 7.9%) (Bhoopathi, Kabani, and Mascarenhas 2009; Svirsky et al. 2002), which can be due to higher prevalence of dysplasia and malignancy in our sample group.

LR+ and LR- are two tools that combine information about the SN and SP of a test and are not commonly reported in oral medicine's literature. LR+ >10 and LR- <0.1 makes a test suitable for clinical use. They were infinity and 0.11 respectively that empress positive results may be always true .It seems that this finding is because of great prevalence of disease in study group and larger sample size can near this result to more realistic value. LR- =0.11 shows "moderate decrease in the likelihood of the disease".

There was a high diagnostic agreement between brush biopsy and histopathologic examination. In two dysplastic lesions the brush could not reveal atypical changes, so contingency coefficient was 92.3%. Kappa value was calculated to show diagnostic agreement. Based on literature review Kappa value has not been calculated for brush biopsy yet. Kappa result (0.806) was greater than 0.7 and shows substantial agreement between brush biopsy and scalpel biopsy.

Based on our study, high SN,SP, LR+ and Kappa value, showed that modified LBC is a suitable test for clinical use. Our modification can eliminate some of the disadvantages of conventional, brush and liquid -based cytology, previously attempted in oral cavity. This study has some great advantages:1)All subjects under went scalpel biopsy so we could compare our results with gold standard so the reported SN,SP,PPV and NPV are reliable.2)Both samples were obtained from the same site.3)The special oral brush was used to collect cells for LBC. It seems that our study combines the benefits of brush biopsy and LBC in early detection of oral premalignant and malignant changes.

2.3 Vital tissue staining

2.3.1 Vital iodine stain

Vital iodine stain (3% lugol solution) has been used to determine the best site for biopsy in endoscopy of alimentary tract and cervix.(Navone 2009).This technique works on binding of iodine to glycogen granules in the cytoplasm, resulting in a black brown tissue color(Maeda et al. 2010; Maeda et al. 2009) . In a study of 54 patients with oral cancer or OPL, this dye was used to determine surgical margins. The results showed a significantly low(<2%) recurrence rate(Navone 2009).

Patient number	*Age(Yrs.)*	*Sex**	*Clin Dia. †*	*Brush Results*	*Histo Dia. ‡*	*(P.D.M.H) §*
1	65	M	SCC¶	Pos	SCC	level 5
2	48	M	LEUK**	Pos	LEUK	level 3
3	71	M	SCC	Pos	SCC	level 5
4	67	F	SCC	Pos	SCC	level 5
5	74	M	LEUK	Pos	LEUK	level 1
6	40	M	LEUK	Neg	LEUK	level 2
7	79	F	LEUK	Neg	OLP‡‡	level 1
8	70	F	SCC	Pos	SCC	level 5
9	49	F	SCC	Neg	GCT	Normal
10	74	F	SCC	Pos	SCC	level 5
11	73	F	Ver.car††	Pos	Ver.car	level 5
12	55	F	OLP‡‡	Pos	OLP	level 2
13	70	M	OLP	Neg	OLP	Normal
14	47	F	SCC	Pos	SCC	level 5
15	36	M	OLP	Neg	OLP	Normal
16	36	M	OLP	Neg	OLP	Normal
17	39	M	SCC	Pos	SCC	level 5
18	69	M	SCC	Pos	SCC	level 5
19	35	F	SCC	Pos	SCC	level 5
20	64	M	SCC	Pos	SCC	level 5
21	35	M	OLP	Neg	OLP	Normal
22	52	M	OLP	Neg	OLP	Normal
23	42	F	SCC	Neg	GCT	Normal
24	70	F	LEUK	Neg	LEUK	Normal
25(Lesion1)	22	F	LEUK	Pos	LEUK	level 3
25(Lesion2)	22	F	SCC	Pos	SCC	level 5

Abbreviations: *sex is defined as Male(M) and Female(F),†Clinical diagnosis,‡ histopathological diagnosis, § presence of dysplasia/malignancy in histopathology, ¶ squamous cell carcinoma, **leukoplakia, †† verrucous carcinoma,,‡‡ oral lichen planus or lichenoid reaction .Brush biopsy results are defined as Positive (Pos),Negative(Neg),and in adequate results(IAR)

Table 4. Demographic data in addition to clinical ,modified(Liquid-Based) brush biopsy and histopathological diagnosis.

2.3.2 Toluidine blue staining

Toluidine blue (TB) is a metachromatic dye that binds to nucleic acids(DNA or RNA) and can help to better visualization of high risk areas-with rapid cell proliferation of oral SCC or OPL.This will guid the clinician to :

- Detect carcinoma in situ and early invasive OSCC
- Delination of surgical fields for biopsy sites
- Detection of second primary cancers or satellite tumors
- Recognition of post-treatment recurrence(Rosenberg and Cretin 1989)

There have been some studies about diagnostic accuracy of TB staining (Epstein et al. 2008; Epstein and G¸neri 2009; Lingen et al. 2008; Patton, Epstein, and Kerr 2008; Rhodus 2009).These studies have addressed some limitations. Ligen et al reviewed these studies and concluded that absence of randomized clinical trials and histological diagnosis as gold standard and variability of methods of applications are the major factors in exact diagnostic value of TB. (Lingen et al. 2008)In other reported studies, SN is high but SP is low due to dye absorption by inflammatory lesions. It is a cheap, easy and none-invasive technique. (Epstein and G¸neri 2009; Epstein et al. 2007; Rhodus 2009). SN and SP are calculated at 38-100% and 9-100 %,respectively .(Awan, Morgan, and Warnakulasuriya 2011; Epstein and G¸neri 2009; Epstein et al. 1997; Martin, Kerawala, and Reed 1998; Warnakulasuriya and Johnson 1996)

It seems that SN in detecting dysplasia is still low. A high false positive result is a great limitation of clinical implication as a screening method. Sometimes subjective interpretation of the mucosal staining (dark royal blue compared to pale blue) cause differences in results(Lingen et al. 2008).A comprehensive review on clinical effectiveness of TB showed that TB is not a cost-effective method of picking up OSCC in primary care setting (Gray et al. 2000).

ViziLite plus is a system which uses TB in combination with ViziLite pens- a disposable chemiluminescent light device- to enhance the malignant changes of oral mucosa (see light-based detection systems)

2.3.3 Other staining methods

Methylene blue has been used for detection of oral cancer and OPL.SN, SP, PPV and NPV has been reported 90%, 69%, 74% and 87% respectively (Chen, Lin, Fong, et al. 2007; Chen, Lin, Wu, et al. 2007).

Rose bengal RB has been used to detect non-healthy epithelial mucosa such as ocular epithelium specially neoplasms(Kim 2000; Khan-Lim and Berry 2004; Wilson 2nd 1976; Singh et al. 2004) . One study was conducted in 132 cases of oral OPLs and oral SCC with a refined 4-grades shade guide. The results showed SN, SP, PPV and NPV to be 93.9%, 73.7%, 55.4% and 97.2% respectively. Six lesions with normal appearance in clinical examination were disclosed by RB staining. The authors concluded that RB staining can be used as a valuable diagnostic procedure in hospital-based population (with a high prevalence of malignancy dysplasia). Further research is necessary to reveal its benefits as a screening test (Du et al. 2007).

2.4 Light-based detection systems

2.4.1 Chemluminescence (reflective tissue fluorescence)

In this technique the mouth is rinsed with 1% acetic acis wash, which helps to remove debris and increase the visibility of epithelial cell nuclei as a result of mild cellular dehydration. The blue white illumination will be reflected by abnormal tissue, making occult lesion distinguishable from normal mucosa (Lingen et al. 2008). The normal mucosa appears blue whereas abnormal mucosal lesions reflect the light and appear more aceto-white with brighter, sharper and more distinct margins (Epstein et al. 2006; Farah and McCullough 2007; Kerr, Sirois, and Epstein 2006; Ram and Siar 2005).

In a clinical survey of 150 patients visiLite system was used to examine oral lesions. Since all lesions were not biopsied and compared with gold standard, diagnostic accuracy was not achieved (Huber, Bsoul, and Terezhalmy 2004).One case with normal clinical appearance was detected by ViziLite. All cases of leukoedema were aceto-white. These finding suggest that despite high SN of ViziLite, SP is still low. Several studies about viziLite examination for case-finding or screening of oral cancer (Farah and McCullough 2007; Huber, Bsoul, and Terezhalmy 2004; Oh and Laskin 2007) but the majority of them lack histopathologic correlation, which questions the diagnostic value. Most researchers found that this device has little benefit in discriminating Occult lesions. In addition distracting highlights produced by ViziLite system may make oral examination more difficult than with normal operating light (Oh and Laskin 2007). If well controlled clinical trials can show it's benefit in differentiating lesions, from normal appearing mucosa, this technology can be used as a true screening tool (Lingen et al. 2008).

Some studies(Bhalang et al. 2008; Oh and Laskin 2007) showed benefit with the use of acetic acid 1% or vinegar (5% acetic acid) prerinse for better visualization of oral mucosa, so acetic acid can be used without the accompanying light system.

2.4.2 Tissue fluorescence imaging

In this technique an intense blue excitation light (400-460 nm) is illuminated to oral mucosa and the abnormal tissue emits fluorescence due to altered structure and metabolism of epithelium and subepithelial stroma. Normal mucosa emits a pale green autofluorescence while abnormal tissue appears darker in comparison to surrounding healthy tissue. Microlux, orascoptic and veloscope are examples of this technique. Case series have found high sensitivity (98-100%) and specificity (3-100%) of veloscope in identifying areas of dysplasia and cancers that extended beyond the clinically evident tumors(Abdo et al. 2007; De Veld et al. 2005; Lingen et al. 2008; Onizawa et al. 1999; Patton, Epstein, and Kerr 2008).To date there are no puplished studies about using veloscope as a diagnostic adjunct in screening low risk population or in patients examined by primary health care providers (Lingen et al. 2008).

2.4.3 Tissue fluorescence spectroscopy

This technique consists of a small optical fiber that produces various excitation wave lengths and a spectrograph which receives and records on a computer and analyzes via a dedicated software, the spectra of reflected fluorescence from the tissue (De Veld et al. 2005; Inaguma and Hashimoto 1999; Lingen et al. 2008; Patton, Epstein, and Kerr 2008). This technique is very accurate in distinguishing normal mucosa from different lesions, but due to small size of optical fiber it is not practical to scan large areas of oral mucosa. Also it can not distinguish benign lesions from malignancy (De Veld et al. 2005; Inaguma and Hashimoto 1999; Lingen et al. 2008; Patton, Epstein, and Kerr 2008).

2.4.4 Other light-based techniques

Contact endoscopy and endoscopic high frequency ultra sound are promising new imaging systems which have been used in nasopharyngeal lesions. These techniques has been used in oral cavity and a SN=91.3% and SP=100% have been reported (Mallia et al. 2008). Narrow band imaging is a novel technique which uses narrow-band spectrum optical filters to enhance the visualization of mucosal and sub-mucosal microvascular patterns. (Piazza et al. 2010) SN, SP, PPV and NPV for this technique in combination with a high definition television have been reported as 96%, 100%, 100% and 93% respectively (Piazza et al. 2010).Further research is necessary to better understand the diagnostic value of these new technologies (Andrea et al. 1997; Andrea, Dias, and Santos 1995; Speight et al. 1995).

2.5 Cellular and molecular techniques

There are many diagnostic aids which can detect premalignant and malignant changes in cellular and molecular level at early stages. Examples are cytomorphometric and histomorphometric analysis, molecular analysis and genetic alteration assessment. These methods employ immunohistochemistry, histochemistry and immunologic techniques in detection of early changes. Yet these techniques are used for research purposes and are not clinically applicable. (Bourhis et al. 1996 ;Remmerbach et al. 2001; Maraki, Becker, and Boecking 2004; Maraki, Hengge, et al. 2006; Maraki, Yalcinkaya, et al. 2006; Yamazaki et al. 2008 ; Nagamani et al. 2010;Mohtasham et al. 2010; OHTA et al. 2010;Böcking et al. 2011).In addition these methods are expensive and are not widely accessible and only expert clinicians can use them for early diagnosis. More studies must be conducted to evaluate these techniques as screening methods of oral cancer.

3. Conclusion

There are many diagnostic aids for early detection of oral cancer. Yet the gold standard of oral cancer diagnosis is surgical biopsy, which can be performed by a trained dentist/physician. Diagnostic aids can be used in different situations specially when a surgical biopsy is not indicated and can help the clinician to:

1. Choose the best site for biopsy
2. Follow up a patient with a premalignant lesion
3. Screen for oral cancer in high risk patients or high risk sites of oral cavity (e.g. ventral tongue, floor of the mouth etc.)
4. Make a preliminary diagnosis when there is a systemic contraindication for surgical biopsy
5. Differentiation of pseudoepitheliomatous hyperplasia from a real malignancy.

4. Acknowledgement

The authors are most grateful to Prof. Dr Abbas Javadzadeh, who not only served as an excellent scientific consultant, but also encouraged and challenged us throughout our academic activity. The authors also would like to extend their appreciation to the Vice Chancellor For Research, MUMS (Mashhad University of Medical Sciences) and Oral And Maxillofacial Diseases Research Center (OMFDRC) for their support.

5. References

Abdo, E.N., A. de Almeida Garrocho, A.A. Barbosa, E.L. de Oliveira, L. França-Filho, S.L.C. Negri, and I.A. Pordeus. 2007. Time elapsed between the first symptoms, diagnosis and treatment of oral cancer patients in Belo Horizonte, Brazil. *Med oral patol oral cir bucal (Internet)* 12(7):E467-73.

Acha, A. 2005. Applications of the oral scraped (exfoliative) cytology in oral cancer and precancer. *Med oral patol oral cir bucal* 10(2):95-102.

Andrea, M., O. Dias, C. Macor, A. Santos, and J. Varandas. 1997. Contact endoscopy of the nasal mucosa. *Acta oto-laryngologica* 117 (2):307-311.

Andrea, M., O. Dias, and A. Santos. 1995. Contact endoscopy during microlaryngeal surgery: a new technique for endoscopic examination of the larynx. *Ann oto, rhinol laryngol* 104 (5):333.

Awan, KH, PR Morgan, and S. Warnakulasuriya. 2011. Utility of chemiluminescence (ViziLite™) in the detection of oral potentially malignant disorders and benign keratoses. *J Oral Pathol Med* 40(7): 541–544.

Bermejo-Fenoll, A., M. Sanchez-Siles, P. López-Jornet, F. Camacho-Alonso, and N. Salazar-Sanchez. 2009. Premalignant nature of oral lichen planus. A retrospective study of 550 oral lichen planus patients from south-eastern Spain. *Oral oncol* 45 (8):e54-e56.

Bhalang, K., A. Suesuwan, K. Dhanuthai, P. Sannikorn, L. Luangjarmekorn, and S. Swasdison. 2008. The application of acetic acid in the detection of oral squamous cell carcinoma. *Oral Surg Oral Med Oral Pathol Oral Radiol and Endod* 106 (3):371-376.

Bhoopathi, V., S. Kabani, and A.K. Mascarenhas. 2009. Low positive predictive value of the oral brush biopsy in detecting dysplastic oral lesions. *Cancer* 115 (5):1036-1040.

Böcking, A., C. Sproll, N. Stöcklein, C. Naujoks, R. Depprich, N.R. Kübler, and J. Handschel. 2011. Role of Brush Biopsy and DNA Cytometry for Prevention, Diagnosis, Therapy, and Followup Care of Oral Cancer. *J Oncol* Article ID 875959, 7 pages doi:10.1155/2011/875959.

Bourhis, J., R. Lubin, B. Roche, S. Koscielny, J. Bosq, I. Dubois, M. Talbot, P. Marandas, G. Schwaab, and P. Wibault. 1996. Analysis of p53 serum antibodies in patients with head and neck squamous cell carcinoma. *J National Can Ins* 88 (17):1228.

Bruun, J.P. 1976. Time lapse by diagnosis of oral cancer. *Oral Surg Oral Med Oral Pathol* 42 (2):139-149.

Chen, Y.W., J.S. Lin, J.H.J. Fong, and I. Wang. 2007. Use of methylene blue as a diagnostic aid in early detection of oral cancer and precancerous lesions. *Br J Oral Maxillofac Surg* 45 (7):590-591.

Chen, Y.W., J.S. Lin, C.H. Wu, M.T. Lui, S.Y. Kao, and Y. Fong. 2007. Application of in vivo stain of methylene blue as a diagnostic aid in the early detection and screening of oral squamous cell carcinoma and precancer lesions. *J Chinese Med Assoc* 70 (11): 497-503.

Chiodo, GT, T. Eigner, and DI Rosenstein. 1986. Oral cancer detection. The importance of routine screening for prolongation of survival. *Postgraduate med* 80 (2):231.

Christian, D.C. 2002. Computer-assisted analysis of oral brush biopsies at an oral cancer screening program. *J Am Dent Assoc* 133 (3):357.

Davey, E., A. Barratt, L. Irwig, S.F. Chan, P. Macaskill, P. Mannes, and A.M. Saville. 2006. Effect of study design and quality on unsatisfactory rates, cytology classifications, and accuracy in liquid-based versus conventional cervical cytology: a systematic review. *Lancet* 367 (9505):122-132.

De Veld, D. C., M. J. Witjes, H. J. Sterenborg, and J. L. Roodenburg. 2005. The status of in vivo autofluorescence spectroscopy and imaging for oral oncology. *Oral Oncol* 41 (2):117-31.

Delavarian, Z., N. Mohtasham, P. Mosannen-Mozaffari, A. Pakfetrat, M.T. Shakeri, and R. Ghafoorian-Maddah. 2010. Evaluation of the diagnostic value of a modified liquid-based cytology using OralCDx® brush in early detection of oral potentially malignant lesions and oral cancer. *Med Oral Patol Oral Cir Bucal* 15 (5):e671-6.

Downer, M.C., D.R. Moles, S. Palmer, and P.M. Speight. 2004. A systematic review of test performance in screening for oral cancer and precancer. *Oral oncol* 40 (3):264-273.

Downer, MC, AW Evans, CM Hallett, JA Jullien, PM Speight, and JM Zakrzewska. 1995. Evaluation of screening for oral cancer and precancer in a company headquarters. *Commun dent oral epidemiol* 23 (2):84-88.

Du, G., C. Li, H. Chen, X. Chen, Q. Xiao, Z. Cao, S. Shang, and X. Cai. 2007. Rose bengal staining in detection of oral precancerous and malignant lesions with colorimetric evaluation: A pilot study. *Int j cancer* 120 (9):1958-1963.

Eisenbud, L., and JJ Sciubba. 1978 .Oral cancer: a multidisciplinary challenge. *J hosp dent practice* 12 (3):96.

Elango, K.J., N. Anandkrishnan, A. Suresh, S.K. Iyer, S.K. RamaIyer, and M.A. Kuriakose. 2011. Mouth self-examination to improve oral cancer awareness and early detection in a high-risk population. *Oral Oncol* 47(7): 620-624.

Epstein, J. B., M. Gorsky, S. Lonky, S. Silverman, Jr., J. D. Epstein, and M. Bride. 2006. The efficacy of oral lumenoscopy (ViziLite) in visualizing oral mucosal lesions. *Spec Care Dentist* 26 (4):171-4.

Epstein, J.B., and P. G¸neri. 2009. The adjunctive role of toluidine blue in detection of oral premalignant and malignant lesions. *Cur opin otolaryng head neck surg* 17 (2):79.

Epstein, J.B., C. Oakley, A. Millner, S. Emerton, E. van der Meij, and N. Le. 1997. The utility of toluidine blue application as a diagnostic aid in patients previously treated for upper oropharyngeal carcinoma. *Oral Surg Oral Med Oral Pathol Oral Radiol and Endod* 83 (5):537-547.

Epstein, J.B., J. Sciubba, S. Silverman Jr, and H.Y. Sroussi. 2007. Utility of toluidine blue in oral premalignant lesions and squamous cell carcinoma: continuing research and implications for clinical practice. *Head neck* 29 (10):948-958.

Epstein, JB, S. Silverman Jr, JD Epstein, SA Lonky, and MA Bride. 2008. Analysis of oral lesion biopsies identified and evaluated by visual examination, chemiluminescence and toluidine blue. *Oral oncol* 44 (6):538-544.

Farah, C. S., and M. J. McCullough. 2007. A pilot case control study on the efficacy of acetic acid wash and chemiluminescent illumination (ViziLite) in the visualisation of oral mucosal white lesions. *Oral Oncol* 43 (8):820-4.

Fedele, S. 2009. Diagnostic aids in the screening of oral cancer. *Head Neck Oncology*. 1(5): doi:10.1186/1758-3284-1-5.

Folsom, T.C., C.P. White, L. Bromer, H.F. Canby, and G.E. Garrington. 1972. Oral exfoliative study:: Review of the literature and report of a three-year study. *Oral Surg Oral Med Oral Pathol* 33 (1):61-74.

Gray, M., L. Gold, A. Burls, K. Elley, K. House, W. Bromwich, and M. Bosworth. 2000. The clinical effectiveness of toluidine blue dye as an adjunct to oral cancer screening in general dental practice. *Birmingham: University of Birmingham, Department of Public Health and Epidemiology. A West Midlands Development and Evaluation Service Report.*

Hayama, F.H., A.C.F. Motta, A.P.G. Silva, and D.A. Migliari. 2005. Liquid-based preparations versus conventional cytology: specimen adequacy and diagnostic agreement in oral lesions. *Med oral patol oral cir bucal* 10(2):115-122.

Huber, M. A., S. A. Bsoul, and G. T. Terezhalmy. 2004. Acetic acid wash and chemiluminescent illumination as an adjunct to conventional oral soft tissue examination for the detection of dysplasia: a pilot study. *Quintessence Int* 35 (5):378-84.

Inaguma, M., and K. Hashimoto. 1999. Porphyrin-like fluorescence in oral cancer: In vivo fluorescence spectral characterization of lesions by use of a near-ultraviolet excited autofluorescence diagnosis system and separation of fluorescent extracts by capillary electrophoresis. *Cancer* 86 (11):2201-11.

Jullien, JA, MC Downer, JM Zakrzewska, and PM Speight. 1995. Evaluation of a screening test for the early detection of oral cancer and precancer. *Commun dent health* 12 (1):3.

Kerr, A. R., D. A. Sirois, and J. B. Epstein. 2006. Clinical evaluation of chemiluminescent lighting: an adjunct for oral mucosal examinations. *J Clin Dent* 17 (3):59-63.

Khan-Lim, D., and M. Berry. 2004. Still confused about rose bengal? *Current eye research* 29 (4-5):311-317.

Kim, J. 2000. The use of vital dyes in corneal disease. *Curr Opin Ophthalmol* 11 (4):241-7.

Kujan, O., A.M. Glenny, J. Duxbury, N. Thakker, and P. Sloan. 2005. Evaluation of screening strategies for improving oral cancer mortality: a Cochrane systematic review. *J Dent Edu* 69 (2):255.

Lingen, M.W., J.R. Kalmar, T. Karrison, and P.M. Speight. 2008. Critical evaluation of diagnostic aids for the detection of oral cancer. *Oral oncol* 44 (1):10-22.

Liu, W., Y.F. Wang, H.W. Zhou, P. Shi, Z.T. Zhou, and G.Y. Tang. 2010. Malignant transformation of oral leukoplakia: a retrospective cohort study of 218 Chinese patients. *BMC cancer* 10 (1):685.

Maeda, K., T. Suzuki, Y. Ooyama, K. Nakakuki, M. Yamashiro, N. Okada, and T. Amagasa. 2010. Colorimetric analysis of unstained lesions surrounding oral squamous cell carcinomas and oral potentially malignant disorders using iodine. *Int J Oral and Maxillofac Surg* 39 (5):486-492.

Maeda, K., M. Yamashiro, Y. Michi, T. Suzuki, Y. Ohyama, N. Okada, and T. Amagasa. 2009. Effective staining method with iodine for leukoplakia and lesions surrounding squamous cell carcinomas of the tongue assessed by colorimetric analysis. *J Med Dent Sci* 56 (4):123-3.

Mallia, R.J., S.S. Thomas, A. Mathews, and R. Kumar. 2008. Laser induced autofluorescence spectral ratio reference standard for early discrimination of oral cancer. *Cancer* 112 (7):1503-1512.

Maraki, D., J. Becker, and A. Boecking. 2004. Cytologic and DNA cytometric very early diagnosis of oral cancer. *J Oral Pathol Med* 33 (7):398-404.

Maraki, D., UR Hengge, J. Becker, and A. Boecking. 2006. Very early cytological and DNA cytometric diagnosis of in situ carcinoma in an immunosuppressed liver transplant recipient. *J Oral Pathol Med* 35 (1):58-60.

Maraki, D., S. Yalcinkaya, N. Pomjanski, M. Megahed, A. Boecking, and J. Becker. 2006. Cytologic and DNA cytometric examination of oral lesions in lichen planus. *J Oral Pathol Med* 35 (4):227-232.

Martin, IC, CJ Kerawala, and M. Reed. 1998. The application of toluidine blue as a diagnostic adjunct in the detection of epithelial dysplasia. . *Oral Surg Oral Med Oral Pathol Oral Radiol and Endod* 85 (4):444-446.

Mashberg, A., and L.J. Feldman. 1988. Clinical criteria for identifying early oral and oropharyngeal carcinoma: Erythroplasia revisited+. *Am J Surg* 156 (4):273-275.

Mehrotra, R., A. Gupta, M. Singh, and R. Ibrahim. 2006. Application of cytology and molecular biology in diagnosing premalignant or malignant oral lesions. *Mol Cancer* 5 (1):11.

Mehrotra, R., M. Hullmann, R. Smeets, T. E. Reichert, and O. Driemel. 2009. Oral cytology revisited. *J Oral Pathol Med* 38 (2):161-6.

Mignogna, M.D., and S. Fedele. 2005. Oral cancer screening: 5 minutes to save a life. *Lancet* 365 (9475):1905-1906.

Mills, S.E., and D. Carter. 2004. *Sternberg's diagnostic surgical pathology*. Vol. 1: Lippincott Williams & Wilkins Philadelphia, PA.

Mohtasham, N., N. Mahdavi-Shahri, J. Salehinejad, H. Ejtehadi, M. Torabi-Parizi, and N. Ghazi. 2010. Detection of nucleoproteins in squamous cell carcinoma, and dysplastic and normal mucosa in the oral cavity by methyl green-pyronin staining. *J Oral Sci* 52 (2):239-243.

Moles, D.R., M.C. Downer, and P.M. Speight. 2003. Oral cancer and precancer screening studies have high discriminatory ability. Evidence-Based Dentistry, 2000; 3: 79-80. *Evid Based Dent* 4 (2):45-45.

Nagamani, N., G. Julie, S. Tyler, T. Daniel, T. Gavin, and K. James. 2010. Desmosomal Component Expression in Normal, Dysplastic, and Oral Squamous Cell Carcinoma. *Dermatol Res Pract* Article ID 649731, 7 pages; doi:10.1155/2010/649731.

Nagao, T., N. Ikeda, H. Fukano, H. Miyazaki, M. Yano, and S. Warnakulasuriya. 2000. Outcome following a population screening programme for oral cancer and precancer in Japan. *Oral oncol* 36 (4):340-346.

Navone, R. 2009. Cytology of the oral cavity: a re-evaluation. *Pathologica* 101 (1):6-8.

Navone, R., P. Burlo, A. Pich, M. Pentenero, R. Broccoletti, A. Marsico, and S. Gandolfo. 2007. The impact of liquid based oral cytology on the diagnosis of oral squamous dysplasia and carcinoma. *Cytopathol* 18 (6):356-360.

Navone, R., A. Marsico, I. Reale, A. Pich, R. Broccoletti, M. Pentenero, and S. Gandolfo. 2004. Usefulness of oral exfoliative cytology for the diagnosis of oral squamous dysplasia and carcinoma]. *Minerva stomatologica* 53 (3):77.

Neville, B.W., D.D. Damm, C.M. Allen, and J.E. Bouquot. 1995. Oral & maxillofacial pathology. Vol. 620: Saunders Philadelphia.

Oh, E. S., and D. M. Laskin. 2007. Efficacy of the ViziLite system in the identification of oral lesions. *J Oral Maxillofac Surg* 65 (3):424-6.

Ohta, K., I. Ogava, S. Ono, M. Taki, K. Mizuta, M. Miyauchi, M. Takechi, H. Shigeishi, T. Takata, and N. Kamata. 2010. Histopathological evaluation including cytokeratin 13 and Ki-67 in the border between Lugol-stained and-unstained areas. *Oncol rep* 24 (1):9-14.

Onizawa, K., H. Saginoya, Y. Furuya, H. Yoshida, and H. Fukuda. 1999. Usefulness of fluorescence photography for diagnosis of oral cancer. *Int J Oral Maxillofac Surg* 28 (3):206-10.

Papanicolaou GN, Traut HF. 1941. The diagnostic value of vaginal smears in carcinoma of the uterus. *Am J Obstet Gynecol* 42:193-205

Patton, L. L., J. B. Epstein, and A. R. Kerr. 2008. Adjunctive techniques for oral cancer examination and lesion diagnosis: a systematic review of the literature. *J Am Dent Assoc* 139 (7):896-905; quiz 993-4.

Patton, L.L. 2003. The effectiveness of community-based visual screening and utility of adjunctive diagnostic aids in the early detection of oral cancer. *Oral oncol* 39 (7):708-723.

Peacock, Z.S., M.A. Pogrel, and B.L. Schmidt. 2008. Exploring the reasons for delay in treatment of oral cancer. *J Am Dent Assoc* 139 (10):1346.

Pektas , Z.Ö., A. Keskin, Ö. Günhan, and Y. Karsliog lu. 2006. Evaluation of nuclear morphometry and DNA ploidy status for detection of malignant and premalignant oral lesions: quantitative cytologic assessment and review of methods for cytomorphometric measurements. *J Oral Maxillofac surg* 64 (4):628-635.

Piazza, C., D. Cocco, F. Del Bon, S. Mangili, P. Nicolai, A. Majorana, A. Bolzoni Villaret, and G. Peretti. 2010. Narrow band imaging and high definition television in evaluation of oral and oropharyngeal squamous cell cancer: a prospective study. *Oral oncol* 46 (4):307-310.

Poate, TWJ, JAG Buchanan, TA Hodgson, PM Speight, AW Barrett, DR Moles, C. Scully, and SR Porter. 2004. An audit of the efficacy of the oral brush biopsy technique in a specialist Oral Medicine unit. *Oral oncol* 40 (8):829-834.

Potter, T.J., D.J. Summerlin, and J.H. Campbell. 2003. Oral malignancies associated with negative transepithelial brush biopsy. *J Oral Maxillofac Surg* 61 (6):674-677.

Ram, S., and C. H. Siar. 2005. Chemiluminescence as a diagnostic aid in the detection of oral cancer and potentially malignant epithelial lesions. *Int J Oral Maxillofac Surg* 34 (5):521-7.

Remmerbach, T.W., H. Weidenbach, C. Muller, A. Hemprich, N. Pomjanski, B. Buckstegge, and A. Bocking. 2003. Diagnostic value of nucleolar organizer regions (AgNORs) in brush biopsies of suspicious lesions of the oral cavity. *Analytical Cellular Pathology* 25 (3):139-146.

Remmerbach, T.W., H. Weidenbach, N. Pomjanski, K. Knops, S. Mathes, A. Hemprich, and A. Bocking. 2001. Cytologic and DNA-cytometric early diagnosis of oral cancer. *Analytical Cellular Pathology* 22 (4):211-222.

Rhodus, N. L. 2009. Oral cancer and precancer: improving outcomes. *Compend Contin Educ Dent* 30 (8):486-8, 490-4, 496-8 passim; quiz 504, 520.

Rosenberg, D., and S. Cretin. 1989. Use of meta-analysis to evaluate tolonium chloride in oral cancer screening. *Oral Surg Oral Med Oral Pathol* 67 (5):621-627.

Rovin, S. 1967. An assessment of the negative oral cytologic diagnosis. *J Am Dent Assoc* 74 (4):759.

Sankaranarayanan, R., K. Ramadas, G. Thomas, R. Muwonge, S. Thara, B. Mathew, and B. Rajan. 2005. Effect of screening on oral cancer mortality in Kerala, India: a cluster-randomised controlled trial. *The Lancet* 365 (9475):1927-1933.

Sarah Freygang, M., R. Grasieli de Oliveira, R. Elena Riet Correa, M. Filipe, and G. Liliane Janete. 2011. Techniques for Precancerous Lesion Diagnosis. *J Oncol* Article ID 326094, 5 pages doi:10.1155/2011/326094.

Scheifele, C., A.M. Schmidt-Westhausen, T. Dietrich, and P.A. Reichart. 2004. The sensitivity and specificity of the OralCDx technique: evaluation of 103 cases. *Oral oncol* 40 (8):824-828.

Sciubba, J.J. 1999. Improving detection of precancerous and cancerous oral lesions: computer-assisted analysis of the oral brush biopsy. *J Am Dent Assoc* 130 (10):1445.

Shklar, G., E. Cataldo, and I. Meyer. 1970. Reliability of cytologic smear in diagnosis of oral cancer: a controlled study. *Archives of Otolaryngology- Head and Neck Surgery* 91 (2):158.

Singh, J. K., F. E. Dhawahir, A. F. Hamid, and P. B. Chell. 2004. The use of dye in ophthalmology. *J Audiov Media Med* 27 (2):62-7.

Speight, PM, AE Elliott, JA Jullien, MC Downer, and JM Zakzrewska. 1995. The use of artificial intelligence to identify people at risk of oral cancer and precancer. *Br Dent J* 179 (10):382-387.

Speight, PM, S. Palmer, DR Moles, MC Downer, DH Smith, M. Henriksson, and F. Augustovski. 2006. The cost-effectiveness of screening for oral cancer in primary care. *Health Technol Assess* 10 (14):1-144.

Svirsky, JA, JC Burns, WM Carpenter, DM Cohen, I. Bhattacharyya, JE Fantasia, DA Lederman, DP Lynch, JJ Sciubba, and SL Zunt. 2002. Comparison of computer-assisted brush biopsy results with follow up scalpel biopsy and histology. *Gen dent* 50 (6):500.

Waldron, C.A., and W.G. Shafer. 1975. Leukoplakia revisited. A clinicopathologic study 3256 oral leukoplakias. *Cancer* 36 (4):1386-1392.

Warnakulasuriya, K., ANI Ekanayake, S. Sivayoham, J. Stjernswärd, JJ Pindborg, LH Sobin, and K. Perera. 1984. Utilization of primary health care workers for early detection of oral cancer and precancer cases in Sri Lanka. *Bulletin of the World Health Organization* 62 (2):243.

Warnakulasuriya, K., and N.W. Johnson. 1996. Sensitivity and specificity of OraScanÆ toluidine blue mouthrinse in the detection of oral cancer and precancer. *J Oral Pathol Med* 25 (3):97-103.

Warnakulasuriya, S., J. Reibel, J. Bouquot, and E. Dabelsteen. 2008. Oral epithelial dysplasia classification systems: predictive value, utility, weaknesses and scope for improvement. *J Oral Pathol Med* 37 (3):127-133.

Wilson 2nd, FM. 1976. Rose bengal staining of epibulbar squamous neoplasms. *Ophthalmic surgery* 7 (2):21.

Wood, N.K., and P.W. Goaz. 1997. Differential diagnosis of oral and maxillofacial lesions. Mosby: St. Louis, London.

Yamazaki, Y., I. Chiba, M. Ishikawa, C. Satoh, K. Notani, Y. Ohiro, Y. Totsuka, S. Mizuno, and Y. Kitagawa. 2008. Serum p53 antibodies as a prognostic indicator in oral squamous cell carcinoma. *Odontol* 96 (1):32-37.

10

Salivary Diagnostics in Oral Cancer

S. Gokul
YMT Dental College and Hospital
India

1. Introduction

Saliva is a complex fluid produced by the major and minor salivary glands and is a mixture of several constituents of non-salivary origin such as gingival crevicular fluid, expectorated bronchial and nasal secretions, serum and blood derivatives from oral wounds, microorganisms, desquamated epithelial cells, other cellular components and food debris (Kaufmann & Lamster, 2002).

Saliva is considered a mirror of body health and is composed of variety of analytes from systemic sources that reach the oral cavity through various pathways. Because water is a major constituent, saliva plays a key role in the lubrication and repair of oral mucosa, formation and swallowing of food bolus, digestion of starch, facilitation of food tasting and control of oropharyngeal microbial population (Lawrence, 2002).

Salivary constituents comprises both organic and inorganic components in generally small quantities that vary with changes in flow, yet continually providing an array of functions. The components, especially proteins are multifunctional, redundant, and amphifunctional as research into the complex roles of proteins and mucins support this theory. The multifarious components within the saliva not only protect the integrity of oral tissues, but also provide clues to various local and systemic conditions and diseases. These salivary components are constantly being explored as markers of various diseases and to monitor general health. Despite not being one of the popular bodily fluids as it is lacks the drama of blood, sincerity of sweat and emotional appeal of tears; a growing number of researchers from various fields including oncology are finding saliva as a useful diagnostic tool (Mandel, 1990).

The role of saliva as a diagnostic tool has advanced exponentially over the past decade. The ability to measure a wide range of molecular components in saliva and compare them with serum coupled with the easy and non-invasive method of collection has made it feasible to study microbes, chemical and immunological markers. As a consequence these advances in technology have helped to move saliva beyond measuring oral health characteristics to where it may now be used to measure essential features of overall health (Streckfus & Bigler, 2003)

The scientific literature on using human saliva as a diagnostic tool began to emerge in 1960's. Early attempts at the usage of saliva as a diagnostic tool was confusing as the studies were not precise and lacked uniformity. Over the years, identification of important constituents in the saliva, invention of more sensitive techniques for their detection aided with the description of various methods of saliva collection and the type of saliva to be collected, contributed in transforming saliva as a major diagnostic tool.

A large number of diagnostic analytes have been shown to be present in saliva including steroid hormones and HIV antibody. The past few years have seen the development of salivary diagnostic tools to monitor various oral diseases ranging from periodontal diseases, dental caries to infections and autoimmune diseases. The challenge of salivary diagnostics is to discover its potential and optimizing engineering technologies for the use of this biofluid. The challenge of making salivary diagnostics a clinical reality is in establishing the scientific foundation and clinical validations needed to position it as a highly accurate and feasible technology that can achieve definite point of care assessment of health and diseases states (Wong, 2006).

The various conditions where saliva has been used as a diagnostic tool includes autoimmune diseases like Sjogrens syndrome (Kalk et al., 2002; Tishler et al., 1997), head and neck cancer and cancer of other systemic sites, infectious diseases inclusive of viral, bacterial and fungal diseases, hereditary diseases like cystic fibrosis, drug and hormone monitoring and also for the diagnosis of systemic diseases like cardiovascular diseases, respiratory diseases, renal diseases and psychosomatic disorders. Of the lot, use of saliva as a diagnostic aid in oral cavity cancer is gaining immense popularity due to the close anatomic proximity of saliva to both pre-malignant and malignant neoplasms making it ideal for screening of these lesions.

Oral squamous cell carcinoma (OSCC) is one of the most common epithelial malignancies with significance morbidity and mortality. Inspite of diagnostic and therapeutic advances over the decades, the disease still remains a challenge for medical professionals with the five year survival rate being 30%-50% (Li et al., 2004). Recent observations indicate that the clinical and histological appearance of oral mucosa may not truly depict the damage occurring at the genetic level. This phenotypic and genotypic disparity may account in part for the failure to establish effective screening and surveillance protocols based on traditional clinical and microscopic examination (Li et al., 2004). Carcinogenesis is multistep process involving initiation, promotion and progression and evidence indicates that these are driven by accumulation of specific gene alterations (Sun, 1990). An understanding of the molecular mechanisms involved in OSCC is helpful in providing a more complete picture of the ways in which tumor arise and advance and a rationale for novel strategies of cancer detection. The oral cavity is particularly conducive to such strategies, given the ease with which saliva and exfoliated cells can be collected (Westra & Califano, 2004).

Tumor cells inhabit or produce biochemical substances referred to as tumor markers. These can be normal endogenous products that are produced at a greater rate in cancer cells or the products of newly switched on genes that remain quiescent in the normal cells (Malati, 2007). Tumor marker may be present as intracellular substances in tissues or as released substances in circulating body fluids such as serum, urine, CSF, and saliva. Until recently, analysis for tumor markers were carried out in fluids other than saliva such as CSF, blood and urine. With recent diagnostic technological advances however, the role of saliva as a tool for diagnosis has advanced exponentially.

The source of information is largely derived from the variety of DNA's, RNA's and proteins present in the saliva. Salivary DNA represents the genetic information of the hosting human body, the oral microbiota and the infecting DNA-viruses. Salivary RNA provides information on the transcription rates of the host genes and those of oral microbiota. Salivary proteins represent genetic information and help to understand the translational regulation of the host body and the oral microbiota (Fabian et al., 2008). In addition, saliva is also useful in detection of other markers such as cell cycle markers (p16, p53 etc), growth factors (Epidermal growth factor, transforming growth factor etc), cell surface markers, oxidant and antioxidants among others.

2. Properties of saliva

Saliva is a complex hypotonic fluid composed of secretions from the major and the minor salivary glands. The major glands are the parotid, submandibular and sublingual glands which are located outside the oral cavity and the secretions are transported to the mouth through the duct system. The minor salivary glands are numerous and are scattered throughout the oral cavity. Saliva is formed in two stages, the formation of the primary saliva by acinar cells and intercalated ducts which is isotonic plasma like containing most of the organic components and all of the water secreted by salivary glands. The second stage involves the modification of the primary saliva by the removal or addition of various ions in the salivary ducts to produce a hypotonic fluid that enters the mouth (Turner & Sugiya, 2002).

A normal healthy adult produces 1-1.5liters/day of saliva composing of mixture of serous and mucinous material at a rate 0.5ml/min. Resting saliva is mainly composed of submandibular secretion while stimulated saliva is made of mainly parotid saliva. Each individual type of salivary gland secretes a characteristic type of saliva such as the secretion of serous saliva from parotid gland.

Salivary output and composition depends on the activity of the autonomic nervous system through the sympathetic and parasympathetic systems. The parasympathetic supply is through the branch of facial nerve to sublingual and submandibular gland and a branch of IXn to the parotid gland. The sympathetic supply is through the fibers arising from first and the fourth thoracic segment and relaying in the superior sympathetic ganglion (Jenkins 1978). Parasympathetic stimulation results in a high flow of saliva containing low levels of organic and inorganic compounds. Sympathetic stimulation produces a low volume of protein rich and potassium rich saliva (Chiappin et al, 2007).

Saliva is composed of 99.5% water and 0.5% solid material which is inclusive of organic and inorganic constituents. The inorganic constituents are made of sodium, potassium, chlorine, bicarbonate, magnesium, calcium, phosphate, Thiocyanate, fluoride, lead, cadmium, copper, nitrite and nitrate. Sodium, potassium and chlorine contribute to the osmolarity of saliva and their concentration give diagnostic information related to the efficiency of ductal transport system. Bicarbonates are the most important buffer present in saliva resisting changes in salivary pH. Calcium, phosphate and fluoride have anti-caries activity. Thiocyanate acts as a anti-bacterial agent (Fergusson, 1994). Nitrate estimation in saliva provides a means of monitoring nitrate uptake and may also predict the future development of carcinoma.

The organic constituents are made up of proteins which include mucins and proline rich proteins which have lubricating properties, amylase and lipase with digestive properties, proteins such as sialoperoxidase, lysozyme (Thorn et al., 1989), lactoferrins, chitinase, cystatins, histatins, defensins, salivary leukocyte proteinase inhibitors, calprotectin, peroxidase, acid phosphatase, chromogranin A, sialin, agglutinin which have anti-microbial properties (Lamkin & Oppenheim, 1993). Other proteins include statherin, mucoproteins and glycoproteins. The rest of the organic constituents is made of blood group substances, enzymes such as aldolase, β-glucoronidase, succinic dehydrogenase, kallikrein, hormones, cacrbohydrates, lipids, nitrogen containing compounds, vitamins, oral microorganisms, various gases like oxygen, nitrogen and carbon dioxide, growth factors like epidermal growth factor and cells of desquamated epithelium (Jenkins, 1978).

The components present in the saliva could either be the inherent component of the saliva itself or the metabolites transferred from the plasma. The passage of plasma components into saliva involves several processes like, ultrafilteration through gap junctions between cells of secretory units, transudation of plasma compounds into oral cavity, from crevicular fluid or directly from oral mucosa and selective transport through cellular membranes by passive diffusion of lipophilic molecules or by active transport through protein channels (Chiappin et al., 2007).

2.1 Collection and storage of saliva

Saliva can be collected under both resting and stimulated conditions. The duration of the collecting period is important because flow rates vary with time. It is therefore important to standardize the collection procedure during the whole sampling period to keep the secretion rate as constant as possible. The methods of saliva collection comprise of collection of whole saliva and collection of glandular saliva. Among these, whole saliva collection is easiest and most feasible method. Specific glandular saliva can be collected with less easy methods.

The common methods of resting-saliva collection include draining method, spitting method, suction method and swab method. Methods of stimulated saliva collection include masticatory and gustatory method. For collection of specific saliva, following methods can be used; a) for parotid saliva, saliva can be collected in a two-chambered type of suction and collection cup according to Lashley (Hu et al., 2004) and b) for submandibular saliva, saliva is collected by placing the tip of collection device at the orifice of the Wharton's duct after occluding the parotid and sublingual ducts (Chiappin et al., 2007).

Various oral fluid collector devices are currently available which aid in collection of unstimulated saliva. These include Orasure HIV 1, Uplink, Salivette, Toothette plus, BBL culture swabs, transorb wicks, oral diffusion sink and ultrafilterate saliva collector (Hansen et al., 2004).

Saliva specimens after collection should preferably be kept on ice, aliquoted and frozen as soon as possible to maintain the sample integrity. The refrigeration prevents the degradation of some molecules in saliva and when necessary, bacterial growth may also be prevented (Chiappin et al., 2007). Storage procedure and time from the collection mainly affect the analysis of the biochemical variables characterized by temperature instability and bacterial growth. Some salivary compounds can have a very short half-life so that the sample to be analyzed needs a narrow range of time after collection, other substances can remain stable for a longer time and may be detected and quantified after sometime (Nurkka et al., 2003).

Certain approaches to store saliva in order to prevent degradation of salivary compounds include (Chiappan et al., 2007)

- Immediate storage without any processing; if analysis is to be done within 30-90min, saliva can be stored at room temperature; for analysis after 3 to 6hrs from collection, storage is to be done at +4^{0}C and if analysis is to done after days to months after collection, storage is to be done at -20^{0}C or still better at -80^{0}C.
- Snap freezing of saliva in liquid nitrogen
- Inhibition of enzyme activity in saliva by mixing with certain enzyme inhibitors
- Addition of sodium azide to retard bacterial growth
- Addition of trifluor acetate to denature salivary enzymes that could degrade salivary compounds such as proteins and steroid hormones.

For salivary DNA analysis, since the main source is from desquamated oral mucosal cells, pre-clearing of saliva before analysis is not recommended. In appropriate buffers of DNA extraction kits, saliva can be stored at room temperature for atleast one year. However before adding such buffer, saliva should be stored on ice to prevent microbial growth and to decrease salivary DNAase activity. Saliva can also be frozen and stored at -20^{0}C or -80^{0}C before extraction or after extraction before use (Fabian et al., 2008).

For RNA analysis, saliva sample is usually centrifuged because the majority of RNAs in the centrifuged whole saliva are genuine human RNA's (Park et al., 2007). For RNA studies focusing on oral microbiota, any kind of pre-clearing of saliva should be avoided. In order to avoid destruction of salivary RNA, the use of RNAase inhibitors are recommended. With the use of inhibitors, mRNA can be stabilized for longer run even in room temperature although cooling of saliva in ice is useful. RNA can be preserved in saliva by freezing at -80^{0}C also (Fabian et al., 2008).

For saliva protein analysis, centrifugation and/or microfiltration can be done. Pre-cleared saliva can be stored on ice without significant protein degradation for only few hours. Addition of protease inhibitors is advantageous especially for time consuming analysis procedures. Samples can be stored for few days at -20^{0}C. However prolonged storage at any temperature may lead to significant protein precipitation (Fabian et al., 2008).

3. Technologies for saliva based diagnosis

The complex nature of saliva consisting of mixture of various components makes it difficult to identify specific constituents. Recently, significant inroads have been made in discovery of a range of technologies which have high specificity and sensitivity in detection of salivary components. For assessment of the diagnostic technologies, a hierarchial model exist which consist of five basic levels of analysis at which the effectiveness of any diagnostic test should be evaluated. These include, analytic (precision and accuracy), diagnostic (sensitivity and specificity), patient outcome efficacy (medical decision making), operational (predictive value and efficiency) and cost / benefit (societal efficacy). This section discusses the various technologies available for saliva based diagnosis followed by the application aspect in oral cancer.

3.1 Proteomics

The proteome represents the complete set of proteins encoded by genome and proteomics is the study of the proteome that investigates the cellular levels of all the isoforms and post-translational modifications of proteins that are encoded by the genome of the cell under a given set of circumstances. Whilst a genome is more or less static, the protein levels in a cell can change dramatically as genes get turned on and off during the cells response to its environment. The proteomic analysis can ascertain function by either looking for changes in the expression of either all or subset of proteins, or by identifying binding partners for particular proteins and seeing how their interaction is affected by biological perturbation (Crocker & Murray, 2003).

The proteomics in bodily fluids are valuable tool for diagnosis due to their high clinical potential as sources of disease markers. In principle a global analysis of the human salivary proteomes can provide a comprehensive spectrum of oral and general health. Furthermore, analysis of salivary proteomes over the course of complications may unveil morbidity signatures in the early stage and monitor disease progression (Lee & Wong, 2009). The total amount of protein in whole saliva ranges between 0.5-3mg/ml. This proteome consist of roughly 1000 protein sequences from which around 300 sequences are of human origin (Fabian et al., 2008).

Proteomic analysis involves the following stages (Crocker & Murray, 2003):

i. Separation of proteins: Before analyzing protein expression and abundance levels, proteins have to be isolated into a purified state. This is generally done by using two-dimensional polyacrylamide gel electrophoresis (2D-PAGE). To resolve the complex composition of saliva, 2D- PAGE, allows separation not only of different molecules of similar molecular weights, but also of different modification patterns or isoforms of the same protein (Lee & Wong, 2009).
ii. Analysis of comparative expression: Once separated, it is necessary to carry out some form of analysis to assess the relative abundance of the protein present.
iii. Identification of protein species: Once a set of proteins showing differences in abundance between two or more states has been identified, mass spectrometric analysis is to be used to determine their identities. Proteins that are primarily identified by mass spectrometry (MS) can be further characterized by ionization methods such as electrospray ionization (ESI) and matrix assisted laser desorption ionization (MALDI) (Lee & Wong, 2003).
iv. Confirmatory experiments.

Two main methods are used to resolve the protein mixture and then to visualize the individual components in such a way that their relative abundance can be quantified. The two methods are i) 2D gel electrophoresis followed by a variety of in-gel staining methods and ii) liquid chromatographic separation with subsequent UV &/or mass spectrometric detection.

In 2D-PAGE, the proteins are initially separated by isoelectric focusing in the first dimension according to charge and then by SDS-PAGE in the second dimension according to size. This type of separation has the capacity to resolve complex protein mixtures, thus permitting analysis of hundreds of proteins at a time. For visualization, staining methods like

Coomassie staining, silver staining or Sypro post- electrophoretic fluorescent stains can be used.

The non-gel based methods are used to overcome the problems associated with 2D-PAGE such as the difficulty in detecting low abundance proteins particularly integral membrane proteins. Two dimensional high performance liquid chromatography (2D-HPLC) is recently employed which uses a capillary HPLC column with a strong cation exchange matrix at the front end of the column which is followed by a reverse phase packing at the back end. Their approach involves the tryptic digestion of soluble and insoluble protein fractions of the entire yeast proteome, followed by the application of total tryptic peptides from the two fractions onto the strong cationic exchange matrix at the top of the column. A salt step gradient is then used to displace a fraction of the peptides onto the reverse phase packing. Displaced peptides are then eluted into the mass spectrometer using a solvent gradient which generates fragmented data that are used for automated searches against protein databases and identification. This procedure is than repeated in steps, each time using an increasing amount of salt to release further peptides from cation exchange to the reverse phase packing.

Mass spectrometry is a powerful technique used for the identification of proteins from two dimensional cells. The ionization methods such as MALDI and ESI were developed by Karas & Hillenkomp (1988) and Fenn et al (1989) respectively. The combination of either of the above mass spectrometric techniques with the separation of proteins by 2D-PAGE is an established method of proteome analysis. In both the cases identification takes place at the peptide level and is therefore necessary to convert proteins in the excised gel pieces into peptides which can be extracted for analysis. Peptides can also be analyzed by MALDI to produce peptide mass fingerprints which are then matched against protein databases in order to identify corresponding proteins. It is also useful to identify which peptides in a tryptic digest have undergone post-translational modification like phosphorylation and glycosylation that are mediated by kinases and glycosyl transferases. An alternative mass spectrometric based method for protein identification is nanoelectrospray. This utilizes very fine glass capillaries with gold coated tips in order to produce a very fine spray which subsequently enables extremely low levels of protein digest mixtures to be analyzed at flow rated of approximately 20-50nl/min.

3.2 Transcriptomics

Salivary transcriptome diagnostics constitutes a novel clinical approach where a large panel of human RNAs can be readily detected in saliva. The large panel of human mRNA is determined by the use of microarray technology and after profiling, validation of transcriptome biomarkers will be done by quantitative real time PCR. Sometimes multiplex reverse transcriptase PCR are used to overcome problems with quantitative real time PCR (Lee & Wong, 2009).

Microarray technologies have the advantage of simultaneously detecting and quantifying the expression of large number of genes health and disease. The technology involves the use of robotic automated miniaturized microscopic spots of aliquots of cDNAs or oligonucleotides from specific genes in a standardized high density gridded arrangement on glass (Muelker & Young, 2004).

The steps involved in microarray analysis consist of RNA extraction, sample labeling, hybridization and processing, image capture analysis and data analysis. RNA is first extracted from tissues or cells of interest. The quality of RNA extracted is paramount to the overall success of the microarray experiment as impurities in the sample can affect both the probe labeling efficiency and also stability of the fluorescent label. Further extraction of mRNA from the total RNA can be done resulting in a purer starting material (Crocker & Murray, 2003).

The mRNA is transcribed in vitro with the concomitant inclusion of labeled nucleotides. The labels may be fluorescent or radioactive. After labeling, the cDNA is purified (to remove unincorporated nucleotides), mixed with a hybridization buffer and then applied to a cDNA microarray slide. The sample and the slide are heated prior to hybridization in order to separate double stranded DNA. A coverslip is applied or preferably a hybridization chamber is used to avoid evaporation and enable even hybridization. The hybridization and subsequent wash steps are carried out at a buffer stringency and temperature that enables hybridization of complementary strands of DNA but reduces non-specific binding. After hybridization, the microarray slides are scanned using either a laser or a phosphorimager. The images are analyzed using software that measures the intensity of the signal from the hybridized spotted genes which provide a measurement of the amount of cDNA bound. Thus, the initial concentration of mRNA is inferred. After the profiling of RNA by microarray, quantitative polymerase chain reaction is used to validate a subset of differently expressed transcripts that are identified by microarray analysis (Crocker & Murray, 2003).

3.3 Polymerase chain reaction (PCR)

PCR is a simple in-vitro method for amplification of specific short segments of DNA or cDNA reverse transcribed from RNA. The technique greatly simplifies genetic analysis and permits the study of all types of clinical samples. Oligonucleotide primers binding to the flanking regions of target sequence are used to initiate specific copying of DNA strands by DNA polymerase. The requirement for the reactions are template DNA to be studied, short single strand DNA primers, complementary to opposite strands of the flanking regions of the fragment of interest, the four nucleotide triphosphatases, a thermostable DNA polymerase and an appropriate buffer solution (Crocker & Murray, 2003).

PCR involves three major steps which are denaturation at 94-96^{0}C for 30 seconds, annealing at 50-60^{0}C for 30 seconds and extension at 70-72^{0}C for one minute. The procedure begins with isolation of DNA from the sample. Heating separates complementary double stranded DNA into single strand forms intended to act as a template dictating nucleotide sequence in vitro. Two short oligonucleotides primers are designed to anneal to the template and flank the region of interest. A thermostable DNA polymerase known as Taq polymerase catalyzes the sequential addition of the four nucleotides to the primers. Cooling the solution permits the primers to bind to template DNA and then Taq polymerase catalyzes the addition of dNTPs to the template between the primers. Salt and buffers permit the Taq polymerase to catalyze the reaction. The reaction is repeated for around 35 to 40 cycles (Jordan et al., 2001).

Reverse transcriptase-PCR (RT-PCR) is a modification of PCR which is important in transcriptomics as it permits analysis of mRNA and thus the study of gene transcription and easier analysis of multiple exons. RNA is extracted and mRNA reverse transcribed using reverse transcriptase. The standard PCR is then carried out after generation of cDNA to amplify the desired region. Quantitative PCR (qPCR) is used for accurate quantification. The generated PCR products can be monitored during the reaction process using fluorescent labeled probes (Crocker & Murray, 2003).

The visualization of amplification is done by agarose gel electrophoresis, southern blot, dot blot and reverse blot assays. The simplest method is agarose gel or polyacrylamide gel electrophoresis followed by ethidium bromide staining and viewing under UV illumination. The choice depends in the product size and the amount of resolution required (Crocker & Murray, 2003).

3.4 Genomics

Genomic analysis is one of the recent advances in the diagnosis of oral cancer and considerable research is being performed in this field. With the availability of high thoroughput technologies to harness genetic information from various sources like blood, saliva, etc., their usage has advanced exponentially. Stable cell free circulating DNA in plasma was first observed almost 60yrs ago. Plasma DNA were shown to exhibit tumor specific characteristics such as somatic mutations in tumor suppressor genes or oncogenes, microsatellite alterations, abnormal protein methylation, mitochondrial DNA mutations and presence of tumor related viral RNA (Zimmermann et al., 2007). These DNA related changes were also found in saliva, the identification of which helps a great deal in diagnosis of oral cancer. The techniques that are available for detection of genetic changes are discussed below.

3.4.1 Hybridization methods

Hybridization refers to the pairing of complementary DNA or RNA strands to produce double stranded nucleic acids. This method uses a radio-labeled or fluorescence labeled DNA or RNA probe that binds to the target molecule of interest, permitting visualization. The target nucleic acids can either be immobilized in a membrane (blotting) or examined in tissue sections (in situ) (Jordan et al., 2001).

Blotting technique involves the isolation of cell free mixture containing the biomolecules of interest, resolving the mixture into its component parts, transfer of the component parts onto a suitable membrane and detection of the biomolecules of interest. The blots are named according to the type of molecule that is blotted on the membrane i.e. DNA, RNA or protein as Southern, Northern and Western blotting respectively (Crocker & Murray, 2003).

The southern blot technique is used to detect specific sequences within the mixture of DNA; this was first described by Southern in 1975. The DNA is size fractioned by gel electrophoresis and then transferred by capillary action to a membrane. The technique involves the transfer or blotting of DNA fragments onto a membrane. DNA is first enzymatically cleaved into smaller pieces by restricted endonucleases, then size separated by gel electrophoresis. After fragment separation, the DNA is transferred from the gel to nylon or nitrocellulose membrane through capillary action of a buffer as it is absorbed by blotting paper. Then the DNA is bound to the membrane by baking the membrane in a vacuum oven or by ultra-violet light cross linking. Finally specific DNA fragments can be identified by hybridizing the membrane with labeled complementary DNA probes followed by detection of label by autoradiography or chemiluminescence (Jordan et al., 2001).

The northern blot analysis is used for RNA detection wherein RNA as a target molecule are size separated by agar gel electrophoresis, transferred to nylon or nitrocellulose membrane and hybridized with specific probes (Jordan et al., 2001). However, precautions should be taken to prevent RNA degradation that can be caused by the presence of ribonucleases (Crocker & Murray, 2003).

Western blotting detects antigenic determinants on protein molecules using polyclonal or monoclonal antibodies and often is described as immunoblotting. The first step involves solubilization of protein samples using sodium dodecyl sulphate and reducing agents like dithiothreitol or 2-mercaptoethanol. Individual proteins are then resolved by SDS polyacrylamide gel electrophoresis prior to electrophoretic transfer. Following blotting, conjugation with antibodies is performed and markers are visualized by autoradiography or chemiluminescence. The molecular weight of proteins is determined by comparison with a set of molecular weight markers which are co-electrophoresed (Crocker & Murray, 2003).

3.4.2 Flow cytometry

Flow cytometry is an important method used to analyze cell kinetics and protein expression in normal and tumor cells (Jordan et al., 2001). It is routinely used to measure DNA content of cells using dyes whose fluorescence is enhanced by binding to nucleic acids and accurately reflecting DNA content (Crocker & Murray, 2003). The dye most commonly used is propidium iodide. It can be excited by the blue line (488nm) of an argon ion laser, fitted into flow cytometers. When bound to double stranded nucleic acids, the dye fluoresces red. Other dyes that can be used are ethidium bromide, 7-aminoactinomycin, DRAQ5, Acridine orange etc. The labeled cells are then directed in a single file along a charged column through a laser beam which excites the fluorescent dye bound to the cell. The fluorescent emission from the excited cells are then collected by a fluorescence detector and analyzed. Cell size can also be detected by using data from the forward scatter of the excitation laser passing through the stream of single cells (Jordan et al., 2001).

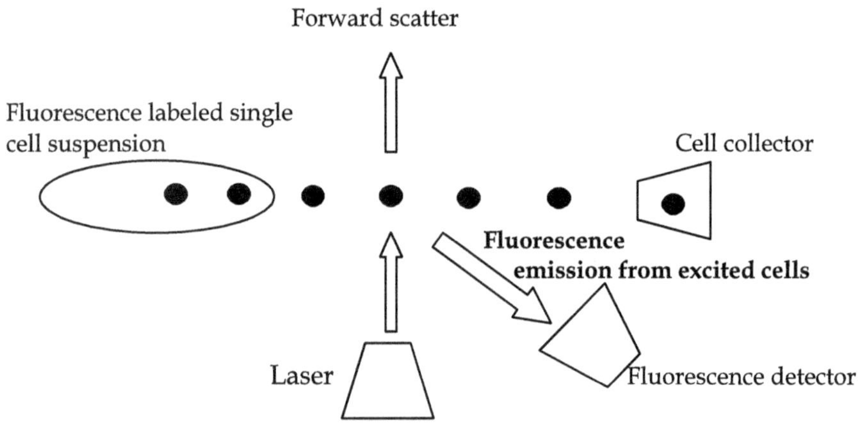

Diagrammatic representation of flow cytometric analysis

3.5 Point of care diagnostics

In recent years, the concept and practice of Point of Care Testing (POCT) is gathering growing interests and remains an important discovery of the present century. POCT is advantageous over standard laboratory procedures by providing timely information to medical teams, facilitating rational, time critical decisions and has been demonstrated to improve patient outcomes in critical care settings. POCT facilitates personalized medicine allowing the caregiver to customize the therapy according to the patient needs. It reduces turnaround time for results which avoids the patients not following up with their caregiver after a test. POCT avoids some of the cost associated with sample handling, packaging, tracking and shipping to centralized labs and reduces the likelihood of samples being contaminated, mixed up, lost &/or degraded. POCT assays must be highly automated to minimize error, sample contamination and sample degradation. Early POCT were based on lateral flow (LF) assays. Recently microfluidics has been known to offer greater functionality and sophisticated flow control than lateral flow assays. The field is often referred to as micro-total analysis or lab on a chip (LOC). POCT microfludic devices are classified as instrumented or un-instrumented devices. Instrumented devices consist of a disposable cassette accompanied by a portable, durable analyzer. Un-instrumented devices are a reincarnation of the LF strips with added capabilities and sophistication. POCT can be used for detection of proteins and nucleic acids. For immunoassay test for small molecules and proteins, enzyme linked immunosorbent assay (ELISA) is the gold standard which shows high specificity and sensitivity. They utilize the high specificity of antibody binding to their target antigen ligand. The most ubiquitous point of care immunoassay is the LF strip also known as immunochromatographic strip. Another assay that is employed at point of care is based on microbeads. Microbeads with various functionalization are ubiquitous solid supports for capturing target molecules in both bench top and microfluidic system (Hart et al., 2011).

In 1999, The NIDCR initiated a research workshop aimed at applications of microfluidics and micro/nanoelectromechanical system (MEMS/NEMS) to saliva based diagnostics. MEMS/NEMS is an integrated system that consists of a central unit for processing data and several other components that connect with the outside interface like microsensors. In continuation of development of saliva diagnostic technologies, in 2002, the NIDCR funded seven projects that explored different point of care systems to detect salivary analytes and provide an overall profile that correlated with a particular disease states. Electrochemical sensing, on chip PCR/RTPCR, microsphere based nano-biochip, microsphere based optical fiber assay, high thoroughput DNA microarray, surface plasmon resonance optical system and microchip electrophoretic immunoassay (Lee & Wong, 2009).

Point of care microfluidic systems are being developed for diagnosis of oral and breast cancers. They permit concurrent detection of multiple salivary analytes including protein and nucleic acid. Oral fluid nanosensor test (OFNASET) is a handheld, automated, easy to use integrated system that will enable simultaneous and rapid detection of multiple salivary proteins and nucleic acids (Wong, 2006).

4. Salivary tumor markers in oral cancer

4.1 Protein markers

Protein biomarkers in saliva are being analyzed both individually and as a panel of markers to aid in early detection of oral cancer and in implementing appropriate therapeutic regime.

Hu S et al (2008) tried to discover and validate differentially expressed proteins in saliva of oral squamous cell carcinoma (OSCC) patients which could serve as potential markers in its detection. The study was performed using subtractive proteomics approach to profile salivary proteins from oral cancer and matched healthy subjects followed by validation by immunoassay to identify a co-panel of candidate protein biomarkers for OSCC detection. 461 and 438 non-redundant proteins were identified in OSCC and control groups respectively. Of these, 409 proteins were found in both the groups while the rest were specific for individual groups. Among the large number of proteins, many of them were differentially expressed as reflected by the differential number of mass spectrometric analysis. Proteins like MRP14 which is a calcium binding protein were significantly overexpressed in OSCC group. Polymeric immunoglobulin receptor (PIGR) was significantly downregulated in saliva of OSCC patients.

The study showed up-regulation of 12 markers in OSCC group. Among these, 5 showed significant difference which included M2BP, MRP14, CD59, catalase and prolifin. Some proteins which were downregulated include clusterin (protein involved in apoptosis) that was absent in OSCC and present in control group. MRP14 expression which is also a calcium binding protein was found to be increased in OSCC group. MRP14 was show to have increased expression in another study performed in tongue cancer by He QY et al (2004). CD 59 (protectin) which was overexpressed in OSCC group enables the tumor cells to escape from complement dependent and antibody mediated killing (Ravindranath & Shuler, 2007). Profilin 1, another upregulated protein is a regulator of microfilament system and is involved in various signaling pathways via interaction with cytoplasmic and nuclear ligands. It may be secreted into tumor microenvironments during the early progressive stage of tumor formation. Catalase protects the cell against oxidative stress and altered levels of catalase are involved in carcinogenesis and tumor progression (Hu et al., 2008).

Protein	Functions
M2BP	Tumor antigen
MRP14	Calcium binding protein
CD 59	Enables the tumor cells to escape from complement dependent and antibody mediated killing
Prifilin 1	Regulator of microfilament system and is involved in various signaling pathways
Catalase	Protects against oxidative stress

Table 1. Overexpression of proteins in OSCC and their functional role.

Analysis of salivary epithelial markers was performed in a study which included CA125, CA19-9, tissue polypeptide antigen (TPA), carcino-embryonic antigen (CEA), SCC and Cyfra 21-1. The study found that the salivary concentration of all these markers was increased in cancer patients than in normal controls. However concentration of SCC, CA19-9 and CEA showed statistically significant differences while the others did not (Nagler et al., 2006).

Contucci et al., (2005) analyzed statherin levels in oral pre-cancer and cancer and found decreased statherin levels compared to healthy controls. Statherin possess high affinity for calcium and phosphorus minerals and provides protective effect which can delay and decrease the level of proliferation induced by carcinogen and reduction of this protective effect is associated with an increased penetration of environmental carcinogens through the mucosal surface.

Cyfra 21-1 is a soluble fragment of cytokeratin 19, which is a component of cytoskeletal protein with a molecular weight of 40kDa. Cleavage of CK19 through caspases 3 activity releases cyfra21-1 into the extracellular space. A study evaluated salivary cyfra21-1 levels in OSCC using ELISA kits and compared with normal and found significantly increased levels in OSCC group. The study also found that the pre-operative saliva Cyfra 21-1 levels were significantly higher in patients suffering from tumor recurrence than in patients without recurrence. The study highlights the usefulness of Cyfra 21-1 for tumor detection and predicting recurrence. It has been postulated that increased Cyfra 21-1 could be due to increased CK19 expression in tissues (Ping et al., 2007).

Salivary soluble CD44 levels were evaluated in head and neck squamous cell carcinoma compared with controls (Franzmann et al., 2005). CD44 are adhesion molecules expressed on normal T-lymphocytes and is used by these cells to migrate to selective sites in the lymphoid tissue. Such migration is accompanied by binding of CD44 to hyaluronate on high endothelial venules and overexpression of this molecule may favor metastatic spread (Kumar et al., 2005). These isoforms arise from alterative splicing of a variable exon present in CD44 mRNA. Franzmann et al., (2005) performed the study using ELISA and western blotting and demonstrated increased value in head and neck squamous cell carcinoma than in controls, suggesting their usage in early detection of cancer.

P53 gene is lovated on chromosome 17p and functions as a critical gatekeeper against development of cancer. They also function as critical modulator of the cellular response to exogenous and endogenous stress. The main functional activity of p53 protein is cell cycle arrest and initiation of apoptosis in response to DNA damage. In a study by Liao et al., (2000), mutation of p53 was observed in DNA extracted from saliva of OSCC patients suggesting a potential use as biomarker for oral cancer detection. The study concentrated on p53 exon 4 codon 63 mutations which was significantly higher.

Hyaluronic acid (HA) is a non-sulfated glycosaminoglycan made of repeating disaccharide units, D-glucoronic acid and N-acetyl- D- glucosamine responsible for regulation of cell adhesion, migration and proliferation. They support metastasis by promoting tumor cell migration offering protection against immune surveillance and causing a partial loss of contact mediated inhibition of cell growth and migration. Hyaluronidase is an endoglycosidase that degrades HA into small angiogenic HA fragments. HAase is shown to alter the expression of CD44 isoforms which may be involved in tumor progression (Franznmann et al., 2003). Franznmann et al., (2003) in their study showed statistically significant rise in HA and HAase in OSCC patients than normal controls suggesting their role as potential marker for diagnosis and prognosis of head and neck SCC.

Balicki et al., (2005) estimated EGF levels in saliva of oral cancer and compared with controls and found significantly decreased EGF levels in OSCC patients. It was suggested that the impaired ability to heal oral mucosal damage in neoplastic diseases may be related to low EGF concentration in saliva. The weaker mitogenic effect due to decreased EGF concentration reduces the reconstructive potential of oral mucus membrane epithelium in patients suffering from oral cavity cancer.

Analysis of interleukin 6 & 8 in OSCC patients revealed significantly higher values than in normal controls. Increased interleukin 6 has been shown to promote immune unresponsiveness and induction of wasting, cachexia and hypercalcemia. Interleukin 8 plays a role in stimulation of angiogenesis, proliferation and chemotaxis of granulocytes and mecrophages which are prominent constituents in the stroma of OSCC (St. John et al., 2004).

Estimation of salivary sialic acid as a tumor marker was considered as aberrant glycosylation are universal features of cancer. A study performed to evaluate salivary sialic acid, total protein and total sugar in OSCC patients found significantly increased levels in OSCC patients than in healthy controls (Sanjay et al., 2008, Debensteen et al., 1991). Another protein evaluated was statherin and results have shown increased levels in OSCC group than in normal controls (Contucci et al., 2005).

Free radical generation result in production of reactive oxygen species which at high levels are known to cause DNA based alteration, strand breaks, damaged tumor suppressor genes and enhanced expression of proto-oncogenes. Numerous anti-oxidants exist in the body that protects from the damaging effects of reactive oxygen species and reactive nitrogen species. Any imbalance in oxidant-antioxidant balance contributes to cancer development and hence determination of salivary oxidant and antioxidant levels may be helpful in early detection, treatment planning and prevention of tumor recurrence.

Salivary nitrites are produced by tobacco and fungal organisms which are of special importance in carcinogenesis as they form nitrosamines. Studies have shown that salivary DNA and proteins to be profoundly oxidized with increased salivary reactive nitrogen species while all salivary antioxidants were significantly reduced (Bahar et al., 2007). Studies by Rai et al., (2008) showed significantly elevated levels of malondialdehyde in pre-cancer and cancer.

In addition to the use of saliva in oral cancer detection, evidence support the usage of saliva in diagnosis of cancer from other sites such owing to the fact that many markers which are identified in other cancers can be isolated from saliva. Markers such as C-erbB2 and CA15-3 for breast cancer, CA125 for ovarian cancer, kallikrein and epidermal growth factor for breast cancer have been evaluated and found to be very useful in the detection of distant tumors (Streckfus & Bigler, 2005)

4.2 Genomic markers

Tumor specific genomic markers consisting of DNA and RNA markers can be identified in saliva for detection of oral cancer considering that the initiation and progression of malignant tumors is driven by the accumulation of specific genetic alterations. DNA shows tumor specific characteristics such as somatic mutations in tumor suppressor genes and p53, microsatellite alteration, abnormal promoter methylation, mitochondrial DNA mutations and presence of tumor related viral DNA. In addition transcript levels of mRNA, microRNA levels are also considered as diagnostic markers for oral cancer.

Microsatellite DNA consist of tandem repeats of one to six nucleotides scattered throughout the genome. DNA microsatellites are highly polymorphic and vary between every individual. These microsatellite sequences are fixed for an individual and same in every tissue. Any error in mismatch repair, creates microsatellite instability which has been successfully used as molecular markers for analysis of tumorigenesis in head and neck cancer (Kumar et al, 2004). Loss of heterozygosity (LOH) is a term used to describe a condition where the cell becomes homozygous to a mutant allele resulting in cancer development. LOH can occur through mechanisms such as loss of a chromosome through mitotic non-disjunction, deletion on the chromosome carrying the corresponding allele and cross over between two homologous genes leading to homozygosity for the mutant allele (Muelker & Young, 2004).

Studies using microsatellite markers from different chromosomal arms in head and neck SCC have shown alterations at certain regions on chromosome 3p, 9p, 17p & 18q to be associated with development of tumors (El- Naggar et al, 2001). El- Naggar et al., (2001) evaluated salivary samples to analyze DNA and showed highest incidence of microsatellite LOH of chromosome 9p, 3p &17p.

Methylation is the main epigenetic modification in humans and changes in methylation pattern plays a main role in tumorigenesis. Epigenesis is the alteration of gene activity without change in their structure (Kumar et al., 2004). Certain tumor suppressor genes are inactivated by hypermethylation of promoter sequences without a change in DNA base sequence resulting in loss of expression.

p16INK4A also known as CDKN2A is a cyclin dependent kinase inhibitor which is critical in cyclin D-Rb pathway for maintaining Rb protein in its active, non-phosphorylated state. It blocks CDK4 binding to cyclin thus helping in cell cycle regulation. Any mutation of p16INK4A occurring in tumors result in inability to block cyclin D-CDK4 activity and preventing Rb phosphorylation during cell cycle. O-methylguanine-DNA-methyltransferase (MGMT) is DNA repair gene for guanosine methyl adduct; death associated protein kinase (DAP-K) is a novel serine/ threonine kinase whose expression is required for interferon induced apoptosis which functions as a potential metastasis inhibitor (Rosas et al., 2001).The study by Rosas et al., (2001) determined the promoter hypermethylation of the above three markers in saliva of patients with head and neck SCC and normal controls and found that 56% of the cases exhibited promoter hypermethylation in atleast one of the genes. Among the cases, 47% exhibited hypermethylation at p16, 33% at DAP-K and 23% at MGMT. The authors suggested that these alterations can be used for early detection of cancer and also for detection of natural progression from neoplasia to cancer in at risk population.

Righini et al., (2007) tried to define a gene methylation profile in head and neck SCC tumors and saliva for diagnosis and follow up by analyzing eleven genes. They found that six methylated genes were most frequently found which included tissue inhibitors of metalloproteinase (TIMP 40%), ECAD (36%), MGMT (29%), p16(29%), DAPK (27%) & RASSF1A (20%). It was suggested that aberrant methylation of these 6 genes in exfoliated malignant cells of the saliva reflects tumor status. TIMP3 encodes for metalloproteinase inhibitor that suppresses tumor growth, angiogenesis, invasion and metastasis.

Detection of telomerase activity in saliva of OSCC was performed by Zhong et al., (2005) and they detected telomerase positivity in 75% of cases suggesting that telomerase detection could be used as assistant marker in OSCC. Telomerase is a ribonucleoprotein aid to elongate repeat sequence at the end of the chromosomes. Reactivation of telomerase is considered to be a pre-requisite for development of malignant tumor cells from somatic cells.

Adenosine deaminase (ADA) and 5′- nucleotidase (5′-NT) are important enzymes participating in purine and DNA metabolisms. Defect in ADA results in intracellular accumulation of adenosine and deoxyadenosine which are toxic to living cells. Deoxyadenosine causes dATP accumulation which is strong inhibitor of ribonucleotide reductase and cause some aberrations in DNA synthesis. They also interfere with critical methylation dependent process such as synthesis, maturation or function of DNA. Saracoglu et al., (2005) found decreased ADA in oral cancer patients and suggested that it may be a compensatory mechanism against rapid purine and DNA metabolism in cancer cells. Decreased ADA activities cause higher dATP and AMP concentration in the cell, thereby lowering dATP and dAMP ratio and leading to decreased energy production. This may be a limiting factor against rapid proliferation of cancer cells.

In a study conducted by Yang et al., (2004), microarray analysis of salivary transcriptome showed that there are 1679 genes exhibiting different expression levels between cancer patients and controls. Of these, seventeen cancer related biomarkers showed significant elevation (3.5 fold) and quantitative PCR was performed to validate these findings. Nine markers were then selected based on their reported cancer association (DUSP 1, GADD45B, H3F3A, IL1B, IL8, OAZ1, RGS2, S100P & SAT). The results confirmed that seven of these nine markers showed significant elevation in saliva of OSCC patients. The validated seven genes could be classified in three ranks by the magnitude of increase into highly upregulated mRNA (IL-8), moderately upregulated mRNA (H3F3A, IL1B, S100P) and low upregulated mRNA (DUSP1, OAZ1 &SAT).

Gene symbol	Gene name	Functions
DUSP-1	Dual specificity phosphatase 1	Protein modification, signal transduction, oxidative stress
H3F3A	H3 histone, family 3A	DNA binding activity
IL1 β	Interleukin-1β	Signal transduction, proliferation, inflammation, apoptosis
IL 8	Interleukin-8	Angiogenesis, replication, Ca++ mediated signaling pathway, cell adhesion, chemotaxis, cell cycle arrest, immune response
OAZ-1	Ornithine decarboxylase antizyme-1	Polyamine synthesis
S-100P	S-100 Ca^{++} binding protein P	Protein binding, Ca++ ion binding
SAT	Spermidine / Spermine N1-acetyl transferase	Enzyme, transferase activity.

Table 2. Salivary mRNA showing significant changes in oral cancer with their functions.

MicroRNAs (miRNA) are a group of small RNAs, 19-25 nucleotides in length, involved in the regulation of development and cell differentiation, proliferation and survival. They exert their effects by two mechanisms; mRNA degradation and inhibition of translation. A single miRNA is capable of regulating the translation of a multitude of genes by targeting specific regions in their mRNA transcript. As a single miRNA can regulate hundreds of genes and may act as a master regulator of processes; select subsets of miRNAs can be used as biomarkers of physiological and pathological states (Micheal et al., 2010).

Analysis of miRNA from saliva of OSCC patients was performed by Park et al., (2009). Of the total number of miRNA analyzed, four potential miRNA were identified as being present in statistically significant levels between the two groups. These included miR-200a, miR-125a, miR-142-3p & miR-93. Further analysis of these miRNA in a separate set of OSCC and normal patients suggested that miR-200a and miR-125a were present in significantly lower levels in OSCC than in healthy controls. These findings suggested that the detection of miRNA in saliva can be used as a non-invasive and rapid diagnostic tool for oral cancer detection. These were considered as the third diagnostic alphabet in saliva (Park et al., 2009).

4.3 Salivary microbiota

A multitude of microorganisms thrive in the oral cavity interacting with each other and at times causing clinical diseases. Oral cavity plays host to a wide array of microorganisms inclusive of variety of bacteria, viruses and fungi. This natural microflora is essential for the normal development of host physiology and contributes to host defenses by excluding exogenous microorganisms. Certain alterations in diet, medications, habits and host immune status may lead to overgrowth of minor components of oral microflora which can predispose the site to disease. Organisms such as candida act as opportunistic pathogens contributing to various oral diseases. The role of bacteria in oral cancer is currently being investigated to determine if the role is a causal or it is a co-incidental finding.

Kang et al., (2009) evaluated the salivary levels of group of organisms (cariogenic, periodontopathic and fungal) and demonstrated significant increase in the levels of *P. Gingivalis, T. Forsythia* & *C. albicans* in cancer group than in normal controls. The study also found that the prevalence of *S. sobrinus* in healthy group was significantly lower than in healthy head and neck tumors.

Mager et al., (2005) determined salivary counts of forty common oral bacteria in OSCC and normal controls using DNA hybridization techniques. They found significantly elevated levels of *P. gingivalis, P. melaninogenica* & *S.mitis* in saliva of OSCC patients thereby suggesting the role of salivary microbiota as a diagnostic indicator in OSCC.

Candida species are normal commensals of the oral cavity and evidence suggest their involvement in oral cancer development primarily through nitrosation of nitrosobenzene compounds (Krogh, 1990). Studies have found increased candidal carriage in salivary samples of OSCC group than in normal controls (Kang et al., 2009). This indicates that the salivary analysis of candida species might be useful as diagnostic and prognostic indicator of oral pre-cancer and cancer.

5. Conclusion

Saliva has been considered as the mirror image of blood for a long time and its various components acts as a mirror of body's health. Since the ancient times, saliva has been used for detection of various diseases ranging from autoimmune diseases to infections and cancer among others. The identification of many new components along with the introduction of newer technologies has led researchers to believe that saliva could be used as an attractive tool. Salivary analysis is advantageous due to the easy and non-invasive method of collection, safety and the possibility of repeated collection without discomfort to the patient. However, saliva analysis was not considered to be effective owing to the inability to isolate minor components as a result of technological barriers. Emerging technologies with high sensitivity and specificity developed in the recent past have overcome these problems giving a new dimension to the use of saliva as a diagnostic tool.

Saliva is normally composed of many organic and inorganic constituents and identification of these proteins in disease states were considered useful from a diagnostic perspective. Salivary proteins, nucleic acids and microbiota have been studied in oral cancer with an aim to identify specific components that could serve as a useful marker for cancer detection as well as treatment planning. Advances like proteomics which is used to detect a panel of proteins, transcriptomics for DNA and RNA and genomics for determination of genetic damage are helpful for characterization of disease states. With point of care diagnostics being the requirement of the day salivary analysis could become a routine procedure for cancer detection.

6. References

Bahar, G.; Feinmesser, R.; Shpitzer, T.; Popovtzer, A.; Nagler, RM. (2007). Salivary analysis in oral cancer patients: DNA and protein oxidation, reactive nitrogen species and antioxidant profile. *Cancer*, Vol. 109, pp. 54-59, ISSN 1097-0142

Balicki, R.; Grabowksa, SZ. & Citko A. (2005). Salivary epidermal growth factor in oral cavity cancer. *Oral Oncol*, Vol. 45, pp. 48-55, ISSN 1368-8375

Chiappin, S.; Antonelli, G.; Gatti,R. & De Palo, EF. (2007). Saliva specimen: A new laboratory tool for diagnostic and basic investigation. *Clin Chim Acta*, vol. 383, pp. 30-40, ISSN 0009-8981

Contucci, AM.; Inzitari, R.; Agostino, S.; Fiorita, A.; Cabras, T. et al. (2005). Statehrin levels in saliva of patients with pre-cancerous and cancerous lesions of oral cavity: a preliminary report. *Oral Oncol*, Vol.11, pp. 95-99, ISSN 1368-8375

Contucci, AM.; Inzitari, R.; Agostino, S.; Vitali, A.; Fiorita, A. et al. (2005). Statherin levels in saliva of patients with precancerous and cancerous lesions of the oral cavity: a preliminary report. *Oral Dis*, Vol.11, pp. 95-99, ISSN 1601-0825

Dabensteen, E.; Clausen, H. & Mandel, U. (1991). Aberrant glycosylation in oral pre-malignant and malignant lesions. *J Oral Pathol Med*, Vol. 20, pp. 361-368, ISSN 1600-0714

El- Naggar, AK.; Mao, L.; Staerkel, G.; Coombes, MM.; Tucker, SL. & Luna, MA. (2001). Genetic heterogenecity in saliva form patients with oral squamous cell carcinoma. *J Mol Diag*, Vol. 3, pp. 164-170, ISSN 1432-1440

Fabian, TK.; Fejerdy, P. & Csermely P. (2008). Salivary genomics, transcriptomics and proteomics: the emerging concept of oral ecosystem and their use in the early diagnosis of cancer and other diseases. *Current Genomics*, Vol. 9, pp. 11-21, ISSN 1389-2029

Fergusson, BD. (1994), 1st edition. *Oral Bioscience*, Churchill livingstone, ISBN-9780755202294, Place- United Kingdom

Franzmann, JE.; Reategue, EP.; Carraway, KL.; Hamilton, KL.; Weed, DT. et al. (2005). Salivary soluble CD44: a potential marker for head and neck cancer. *Cancer Epidemiol Biomarkers Prev*, Vol. 14, No. 3, pp. 735-739, ISSN 1055-9965

Franzmann, JE.; Schroeder, GL.; Goodwin, WJ.; Weed, DT.; Fisher, P & Lokeshwat, VB. Expression of tumor markers hyaluronic acid and hyaluronidase in head and neck tumors. *Int J Cancer*, Vol. 106, No. 3, pp. 438-445, ISSN 1097-0215

Hansen, CH.; Tong, G.; Davis, C.; Abrams, RW. & Malamud, D. (2004). Comparison of oral fluid collectors for use in point of care diagnostic device. *Clin Diagn Lab Immunol*, Vol. 11, No. 5, pp. 909-912, ISSN 1556-6811

Hart, RW.; Mauk, MG.; Liu. C.; Qiu, X.; Thompson, JA.; et al. (2011). Point -of- care oral-based diagnostics. *Oral Dis*, doi:10.1111/j.1601-0825.2011.01808.x

He, QY.; Chen, J.; Tsang, NM.; et al. (2004). Identification of tumor associated proteins in oral tongue squamous cell carcinoma by proteomics. *Proteomics*, Vol. 4, pp. 271-278, ISSN 1615-9861

Hu, S.; Arellano, M.; Boontheung, P.; Wang, J.; Zhou, H et al. (2008). Salivary proteomics for oral cancer biomarker discovery. *Clin Cancer Res*, Vol. 14, No. 19, pp, 6246-6252, ISSN 1078-0432.

Hu, S.; Denny,P.; et al. (2004). Differentially expressed protein markers in human submandibular and sublingual secretions. *Int J Oncol*, Vol. 25, pp. 1423-1430, ISSN 1791-2423

Jenkins, NG. (1978). 4th edition. *The physiology and biochemistry of the mouth*, Blackwell scientific publications, ISBN- 0632001380, Place- Oxford, Philadelphia

Jordan, RCK.; Daniells, TE.; Greenspan, JS. & Regezi, JA (2001). Advanced diagnostic aids in oral and maxillofacial pathology. Part I: Molecular methods. *Oral Med Oral Surg Oral Path Oral Rad Endod*, Vol. 92, No. 6, pp. 650-659, ISSN 1079-2104

Kalk, WWI.; Vissink, A.; Spijkervet, FKL.; Bootsma, H.; Kallenberg, CGM. & Amerongen, AVN. (2001). Sialometry and siaolochemistry: Diagnostic tools for Sjogren's syndrome. *Ann Rheum Dis*, Vol. 60, pp. 1110-1116, ISSN 1468-2060

Kalk, WWI.; Vissink, A.; Stegenga, B.; Bootsma, H.; Amerongen, AVN. & Kallenberg, CGM. (2002). Sialometry and sialochemistry: A non invasive approach for diagnosing Sjogren's syndrome. *Ann Rheum Dis*, Vol.61, pp. 137-144, ISSN 1468-2060

Kang, M.; Oh, J.; Kim, H.; Lee, I.; Choi, H. et al. (2009). Prevalence of oral microbes in the saliva of oncological patients. *J Bacteriol Virol*, Vol. 39, No. 4, pp. 277-85, ISSN 1598-2467

Kaufmann, E. & Lamster, B. (2002). The diagnostic applications of saliva- A review. *Crit Rev Oral Biol Med*, Vol. 13, No.2, pp. 197-212, ISSN 1045-4411

Krogh P. (1990). The role of yeasts in oral cancer by means of endigenous nitrosation. *Acta Odontol Scand*, Vol. 48, pp. 85-88, ISSN 0001- 6357

Kumar, V.; Abbas, AK. & Fausto, N. (2007). 4th edition. *Pathological basis of disease*, Saunders, ISBN- 0-8089-2302-1, Pennsylvania.

Lamkin, MS & Oppenheim, GF. (1993). Structural features of salivary function. *Crit Rev Oral Biol Med*, Vol. 4, No. 3/ 4, pp. 251-259, ISSN 1045-4411

Lavelle, CLB. (1988). *Applied oral physiology*, Buttersworth and Co Ltd, ISBN 0-7236-0818-0.

Lawrence, PH. (2002). Salivary markers of systemic disease: Noninvasive diagnosis of disease and monitoring of general health. *J Can Dent Assoc*, Vol. 68, No. 3, pp. 170-174, ISSN 0008-3372

Lee, Y & Wong DT. (2009). Saliva: An emerging biofluid for early detection of diseases. *Am J Dent*, Vol. 22. No. 4. pp. 241-248, ISSN 0894-8275

Li, Y.; St. John, MAR.; Zhou, X.; Kim, Y & Sinha, U. et al. (2004). Salivary transcriptome diagnostics for oral cancer detection. *Clin Cancer Res*, Vol. 10, (December), pp. 8442-8450, ISSN- 1078-0432

Liao, PS.; Chang, YC.; Huang, MF.; Tai, KW. & Chou, MY. (2000). Mutation of p53 gene codon 63 in saliva as a molecular marker for oral squamous cell carcinomas. *Oral Oncol*, Vol. 36, pp. 272-276, ISSN 1368-8375

Mager, DL.; Haffajee, AD.; Devlin, PM.; Norris, CM.; Posner, MR. & Goodson, JM. (2005). The salivary microbiota as a diagnostic indicator of oral cancer: A descriptive, non-randomized study of cancer-free and oral squamous cell carcinoma subjects. *J Translational Medicine*, Vol.3, pp.27-34, ISSN 1939-067x

Malati, T. (2007). Tumor markers: An overview. *Ind J Clin Biochem*, Vol. 22, No. 2, pp. 17-31, ISSN 0970-1915

Mandel, ID. (1990). The diagnostics uses of saliva. *J Oral Pathol Med*, Vol. 19, pp. 119-125, ISSN 1600-0714

Michael, A.; Bajracharya, SD.; Yuen, PST.; Zhou, H.; Star, RA.; et al. (2010). Exosomes from human saliva as a source of microRNA biomarkers. *Oral Dis*, Vol.16, pp-34-38, ISSN-1601-0825

Muelker, RF. & Young, DI. (2004). 12th edtn. *Emery's elements of medical genetics*. Churchill Livingstone. ISBN 978-0-7020-2917-2, Exeter, UK.

Nagler, R.; Bahar, G.; Shpitzer, T. & Feinmesser R. (2006). Concomitant analysis of salivary tumor markers-A new diagnostic tool for oral cancer. *Clin Cancer Res*, Vol. 12, No. 13, pp. 3979- 3984, ISSN 1078-0432

Nurkka,A.; Obiero, J.; Kaythy, H. & Sscott, AG. (2003). Effects of sample collection and storage methods on antipneumococcal immunoglobulin A in saliva. *Clin Diagn Lab Immunol*, Vol. 10, No. 3, pp. 357-362, ISSN 1556-6811

Park, NJ.; Zhou, A.; Elashoff, D.; Henson BS.; Kastratovic DA.; et al. (2009). Salivary microRNA: Discovery, characterization and clinical utility for oral cancer detection. *Clin Cancer Res*, Vol. 15, No. 17, pp. 5473-5477, ISSN- 1078-0432

Rai, B.; Kharb, S.; Jain, R.; Anand, SC. (2008). Salivary lipid peroxidation product malonaldehyde in pre-cancer and cancer. *Advances in medical and dental sciences*, Vol. 2, No. 1, pp. 7-8, ISSN- 1995-0764

Ravindranath, NM. & Shuler C. (2007). Cell surface density of complement restriction factors (CD46, CD55 and CD59): oral squamous cell carcinoma versus other solid tumors. *Oral Surg Oral Med Oral Pthol Oral Radiol Endod*, Vol. 103, pp. 231-239, ISSN 1079-2104

Righini, CA.; De Fraipont, F.; Timsit, J.; Faure, C.; Brambilla E. et al. (2007). Tumor specific methylation in saliva: A promising biomarker for early detection of head and neck cancer recurrence. *Clin Cancer Res*, Vol. 13, pp. 1179-1185, ISSN- 1078-0432

Rosas, SLB.; Koch, W.; Carvalho, MGC.; Wu, L.; Califano. et al. (2001). Promoter hypermethylation patterns of p16, O-methylguanine-DNA-methyltransferase and death associated protein kinase in tumors and saliva of head and neck cancer patients. *Cancer Res*, Vol. 61, pp. 939-942, ISSN 1573-7217

Sanjay, PR.; Hallikeri K, Shivasankara, AR.; (2008). Evaluation of salivary sialic acid, total protein and total sugar in oral cancer: A preliminary report. *Ind J Dent Res*, Vol. 19, No. 4, pp. 288-291, ISSN 1998-3603

Saracoglu, U.; Guven, O.; Durak, I.; Adenosine deaminase and 5'- nucleotidase activities in saliva from patients with oral and larungeal cancer. *Oral Dis*, Vol. 11, pp.323-325, ISSN 1601-0825

St. John, MAR.; Li, Y.; Zhou, X.; Denny, P.; Ho, C. et al. (2004). Interleukin 6 and interleukin 8 as potential biomarkers of oral and oropharyngeal squamous cell carcinoma. *Arch Otlaryngol Head Neck Surg*, Vol. 130, Aug, pp. 929-935, ISSN 1538-361x

Streckfus, C.; Bigler, L. (2005). The use of soluble salivary c-erbB-2 for the detection and post-operative follow up of breast cancer in women: the result of five year translational research study. *Adv Dent Res*, Vol.18, pp. 17-24, ISSN 1544-0737

Streckfus, CF. & Bigler, LR. (2002). Saliva as a diagnostic fluid. *Oral Dis*, Vol. 8, pp. 69-76, ISSN 1601-0825

Sun Y. (1990). Free radicals, antioxidant enzymes and carcinogenesis. *Free Radic Biol Med*, Vol. 8, pp. 583-99, ISSN 0891-5849

Tenovuo, JO. (1989). *Human saliva: Clinical chemistry and microbiology*, CRC Press, ISBN 0849363926

Thorn, JJ.; Prause, JU. & Oxholm P. (1989). Sialochemistry in Sjogrens syndrome: A review. *J Oral Pathol Med*, Vol. 18, pp.457-466, ISSN 1600-0714

Tishler, M.; Yaron, I.; Shiraz, I. & Yaron, M. (1997). Saliva an additional diagnostic tool in Sjogren's syndrome. *Semin Arthritis Rheum*, Vol. 27, pp. 173-179, ISSN 1462-0332

Turner, JR. & Sugiya H. (2002). Understanding salivary fluid and protein secretion. *Oral Dis*, Vol.8, No. 1, pp. 3-11, ISSN 1601-0825

Westra, WH. &Califano J. (2004). Toward early oral cancer detection using gene expression profiling of saliva: A thoroughfare or dead end. *Clin Cancer Res*, Vol. 10, (December), pp. 8130-8131, ISSN- 1078-0432

Wong, DT. (2006). Salivary diagnostics powered by nanotechnologies, proteomics and genomics. *J Am Dent Assoc*, Vol. 137, (March), pp.313-320, ISSN 0002-8177

Yang, L.; Maie, SR.; St. John.; Zhou, X.; Kim, Y. et al. (2004). Salivary transcriptome diagnostics for oral cancer detection. *Clin Cancer Res*, Vol. 10, pp. 8442-8450, ISSN-1078-0432

Zhong, L.; Zhang, C.; Zheng, J.; Li, J.; Chen W. et al. (2007). Increased Cyfra 21-1 concentration in saliva from primary oral squamous cell carcinoma patients. *Arch Oral Biol*, Vol. 52. pp. 1079-1087, ISSN 0003-9969

Zhong, LP.; Chen, GF.; Xu, ZF.; Zhang, X.; Ping, FY. & Zhao, SF. (2005). Detection of telomerase activity in saliva from oral squamous cell carcinoma patients. *Int J Oral Maxillofac Surg*, Vol. 34, pp. 566-570, ISSN- 0901-5027

Zimmermann, BG.; Park, NH. & Wong, DT. (2007). Genomic targets in saliva. *Ann N Y Acad Sci*, Vol. 1098, pp. 184-91, ISSN 1384.002

11

Timing of Oral Cancer Diagnosis: Implications for Prognosis and Survival

Pablo Varela Centelles, Juan Manuel Seoane-Romero, Iria Gómez, Pedro Diz-Dios, Nilce Santos de Melo and Juan Seoane
[1]*University of Santiago de Compostela*
[2]*University of Brasilia*
[1]*Spain*
[2]*Brazil*

1. Introduction

Oral cancer has become a global health problem (Parkin, 2005; Gillison, 2007) and its increasing incidence and mortality rates are particularly relevant in certain parts of Europe (France, Hungary, Spain and Croatia), Brazil, and South-Eastern Asia (Sri Lanka, Pakistan, Bangladesh and India) (Warnakulasuriya, 2009). These geographical variations seem to reflect disparities in tobacco, areca nut and alcohol consumption (Warnakulasuriya, 2009). Worldwide, oral cancer has one of the lowest survival rates that remains unaltered despite recent therapeutic advances. Young adults seem to be growingly affected by tongue cancer in Brazil, several European countries and USA (Llewellyn, 2004). However, current reports describe a trend -more marked for tongue carcinomas- towards improved survival at each stage and at all ages but ≥75 years (Pulte, 2010).

Search for prognostic markers for oral cancer has been extensive and thorough with diverse results: age, gender, immunological or nutritional status, size and location of the tumour, disease stage, nodal status, oncogene expression, proliferation markers, or DNA content have been allocated independent prognostic value (Johnson, 1996); but tumour stage at diagnosis remains the most important prognostic maker for oral squamous cell carcionoma (Garzino-Demo, 2006). Unfortunately, almost half of the oral neoplasms are diagnosed at stages III or IV, with 5-year survival rates ranging from 20% to 50% depending upon tumour sites (Holmes, 2003; Brandizzi, 2005).

Early detection is widely recognised as the cornerstone to reduce diagnostic delay and, thus, to improve survival (De Faria , 2003; McDowell, 2006). However, this term (early detection) is not free from confusion as can be understood either as "a relative small tumour in size at the time of detection" or as "short time interval since cancer onset to diagnosis" (diagnostic delay) (van der Waal, 2011).

2. Early detection. Diagnosis of small-size oral carcinoma

Tumour size influences therapy and prognosis of oral cancer. Diagnosis of larger oral carcinomas has been linked to an increased risk of neck-node metastases and poor survival

(Woolgar, 1999). Lately, this variable (plain clinical or pathological tumour size) has been replaced by tumour thickness or depth of invasion as more significant prognostic factors (Gonzalez-Moles, 2002; O-charoenrat, 2003). Moreover, tumour thickness has proved independent predictive value for subclinical node metastases, local recurrence and survival (Po Wing Yuen, 2002). Accordingly, a critical thickness of 4 mm has been proposed, above which the risk for metastases is 4 times the risk of tumours with minor invasion depth (Ambrosch, 1995). Generally speaking, a small-size tumour should present a diameter inferior than 2 cm, less than 4 mm of invasion depth and usually asymptomatic (Woolgar, 2006). Thus, clinicians are recommended to be watchful on the signs of potentially malignant lesions or early stage cancers in all patients, but particularly on heavy smokers and alcohol consumers. These signs include indurations, bleeding, exophytic growths larger than 1 mm, chronic ulcerations with irregular, dirty or spotty appearance in lesions that do not disappear after the hypothetical causal agents have been removed, together with texture changes or granulation on the surface of the lesion. Moreover, keeping in mind that persistent erythroplastic lesions are the most frequent clinical presentation of early carcinomas (Mashberg, 1977; Mashberg, 1988; Bouquot, 1995) (Figure 1) along with erythro-leukoplastic (23%) and leukoplastic lesions (21%) may ease an early diagnosis of oral cancer (Mashberg, 1995).

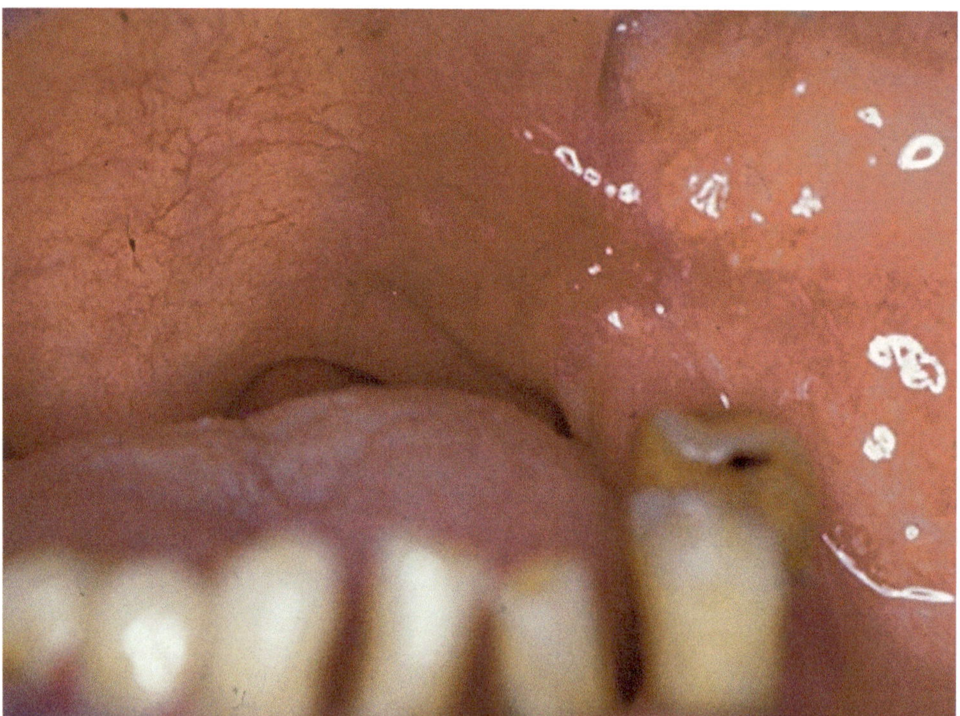

Fig. 1. Erythroplastic oral squamous cell carcinoma.

3. Diagnostic delay in oral cancer. Concept

The concept of diagnostic delay would comprise the time since first sign or symptom to definitive diagnosis. This fairly clear concept has been studied from different points of view with heterogeneous criteria (Allison, 1998a; Allison, 1998b; Allison, 1998c), resulting in categorisations that include: "patient delay": the period between the patient first noticing a symptom and the first consultation with a health professional about the symptom; and "professional delay": the period from patient's first consultation with a clinician to the definitive pathological diagnosis". This categorisation can be broken down further to include the "delay by patients": time until consultation due to inaccessibility to the healthcare provider (Allison, 1998a; Allison, 1998b; Allison, 1998c; Onizawa, 2003) -which is not always due to the patients-. To overcome this ambiguity, the term "scheduling delay" (period between the patient making an appointment and actually seeing a healthcare professional) was introduced (Diz-Dios, 2005) (Figure 2).

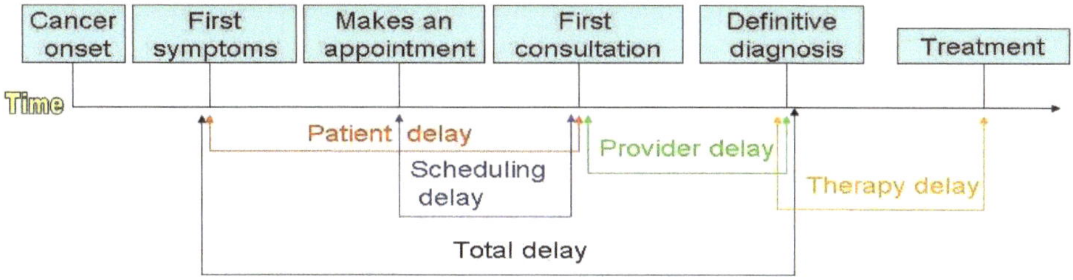

Fig. 2. Types of diagnostic delay in oral cancer.

Despite these efforts, to date there is no consensus on a time-point beyond which a cancer diagnosis can be considered delayed. Several research groups have used the mean or the median of the time distribution to categorise diagnostic delay (Andersen, 1995; Pitiphat, 2002; Carvalho, 2002; Gorsky, 1995), the latter being more frequent as it is not affected by the extreme values of distributions that usually show very wide ranges. Other authors choose an arbitrary time-point (more than thirty days) to discriminate between delayed and non-delayed cases (Allison, 1998a; Allison, 1998b; Allison, 1998c; Brouha, 2005), in order to allow time for the patient to identify the symptoms, seek consultation, for a follow up of 7-10 days and a second consultation and biopsy, and, finally for the pathologist to report the results back to the clinician (Gorsky, 1995).

Other criteria include a first stage: since the first symptom until the first contact with the clinician; a second stage: since the first visit until a referral letter is written; a third stage: since the patient gets the referral letter until the first consultation at a specialised service; and a 4th stage, since the first consultation to a specialist until a definitive diagnosis is reached (Onizawa, 2003). As can be inferred, this approach introduces some degree of complexity and limits the external validity of the studies performed under this scheme.

Regardless of the importance of this topic, it is somehow surprising the limited number of reports dealing with the influence of diagnostic delay in head and neck carcinomas retrievable from scientific databases, particularly when compared to melanoma or colorectal, breast, and bladder carcinomas.

4. Causes of oral cancer diagnostic delay

The proportion of patients receiving a delayed definitive diagnosis of oral cancer remains high worldwide, with wide variations in the values reported: in Greece more than a half of oral cancer patients are diagnosed with delays longer than 3 weeks (Pitiphat, 2002), whereas Dutch and Spanish patients are diagnosed with an average delay of 1.5 months (Kowalsky, 1994; Seoane, 2006); series published from Canada, Italy, Denmark or Israel report medians of diagnostic delays ranging from 3 to four months (Allison, 1998a; Allison, 1998b; Allison, 1998c; Wildt, 1995; Gorsky, 1995).

Undoubtedly, there are potential factors responsible for late diagnosis of oral cancer: on the one hand, psychosocial factors related to the patient may well condition the perception of the cancer symptoms by the individual and lead him/her to erroneous behavioural responses that may adversely affect his/her demands and access to care. This may explain why the use of traditional herbal medication before visiting a healthcare professional is recognised as a significant independent predictor for patient delay in Thailand (Kerdpon, 2001a; Kerdpon, 2001b).

On the other hand, the accessibility (ability to obtain services based on oral health needs) can be limited by financial, structural and personal barriers (beliefs, language) and thus decisively conditioning the timing of oral cancer diagnosis (Seoane, 2010). Disparities in access to oral health services across Europe and USA are well known, particularly for low-income populations (uninsured, migrant, homeless, etc). Ethno-regional differences have also been identified in terms of incidence and mortality rates of oral cancer, which may result from the variation in the access to oral care but also from the different exposition to risk factors or from the limited resources in detection and prevention methods available to these individuals.

The causes of diagnostic delay related to the clinician are particularly interesting, and can be basically due to not to practice a full clinical examination (Bruun, 1976), the presence of unspecific or banal clinical signs (Bruun, 1976), low index of suspicion and lack of familiarity and experience with the disease (Guggenheimer, 1989). Co-morbidity has also been suggested (Allison, 1998a; Allison, 1998b; Allison, 1998c), as clinicians in these situations tend to focus their attention on the existing disorders.

Lack of oral cancer knowledge has also been described to influence delays in referral and treatment (Colella, 2008; Seoane 2010), and this situation has been detected internationally as a worrying lack of knowledge on diagnostic procedures, main locations of oral cancer (Alonge, 2003) and on leuko- or erythroplakia-like carcinomas as primary oral cancer lesions, as well as on the effects of vegetable intake on the incidence of oral cancer. Conversely, facts like squamous cell carcinoma being the most common histopathologial type or oral cancer, criteria for referral of patients with suspicious lesions, that early detection improves the 5-year survival rate and that tobacco and alcohol are risk factors for oral cancer (Seoane 2010) are well known by the healthcare professionals.

In short, diagnostic delay is a complex concept conditioned by tumour biology, patient behaviour, clinician awareness and attitudes, as well as by the healthcare system performace.

5. Other factors related to late stage diagnosis of oral squamous cell carcinoma

Although recognition of predictors for advanced-stage diagnosis could permit the implementation of strategies for increasing the number of oral carcinomas diagnosed at an early stage, there is no much information on this issue.

The most frequently studied variables (age, gender, and tobacco and alcohol intake) are not linked to late-stage diagnosis, as were not previously associated to professional or patient-related delays (Boing, 2010; Guggenheimer 1989). Neither precancerous lesions connected to the tumour seem to modify the spread of the disease at diagnosis, even when proliferative verrucous leukoplakia or the presence of mild to moderate epithelial dysplasia at the margins of a surgically removed oral squamous cell carcinoma carries a significant risk of local recurrence and modifies the prognosis of the disorder (Thomsom, 2007).

Ulcerated-type oral squamous cell carcinomas are usually diagnosed at stages III or IV (Jaulerry, 1985) (Figure 3). Although the predictive value of the clinical appearance of the primary lesion remains controversial, it is accepted that ulcerated lesions imply poorer survival rates (Jaulerry, 1985).

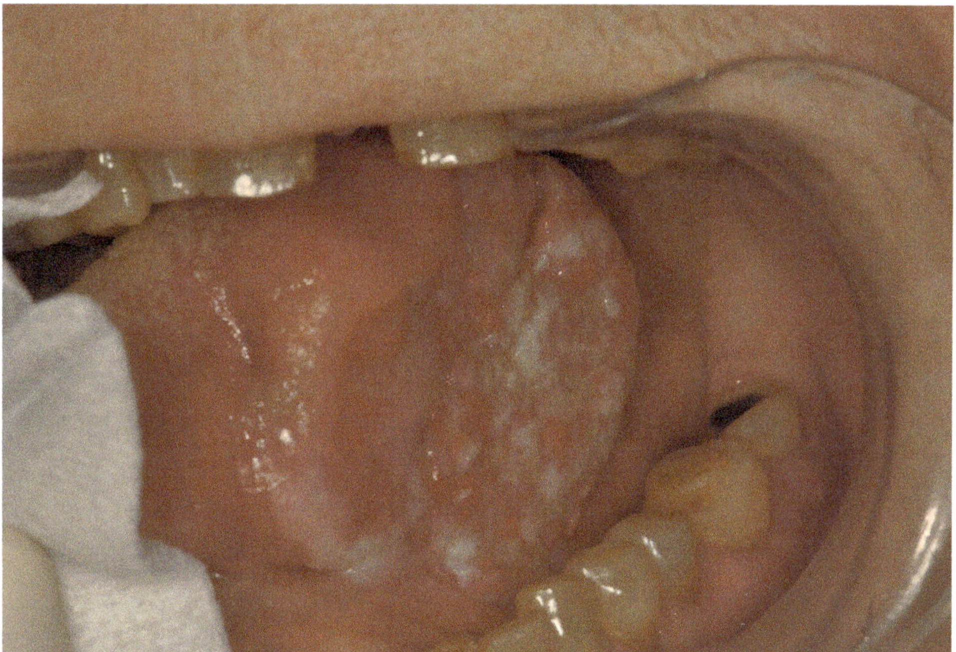

Fig. 3. Ulcerated-type tongue squamous cell carcinoma.

The site of the primary lesion has been also linked either to delayed diagnosis or diagnosis at advanced stages (Brouha, 2005): tongue, buccal mucosa and lip carcinomas seem to be diagnosed at earlier stages (Gorsky, 1995) than floor of the mouth and retromolar trigone neoplasms; whereas palate or gingival tumours showed contradictory results (Gorsky, 1995). Accordingly, the floor of the mouth, gingivae and retromolar trigone have recently been identified as independent prognostic factors for late-stage diagnosis, which may well be explained by the fact that patients' self-perception and self-exploration abilities are conditioned by the site of the tumour (Andersen, 1995); the presence of the gingivae within this group would be due to the association of gingival locations to advanced stage at diagnosis (late diagnosis) caused by the early invasion of the nearby bone (T4 primary tumour) (Seoane, 2006).

Late diagnosis of neoplasms, particularly in oral cancer, has been conventionally ascribed to delays in reaching a diagnosis, as patients at advanced tumour stages are more likely to have experienced longer patient and professional delays than those diagnosed at earlier stages (Sargeran, 2009). Surprisingly, there is an evident lack of sound scientific evidence supporting this traditional association between diagnostic delay and disease extension (III-IV TNM stages) (Gomez, 2009; Gomez, 2010).

The biological behaviour of the tumour has also been investigated as an hypothetical predictor for a late-stage diagnosis, with positive results, as poorly differentiation of a tumour (biologically more aggressive) proved to be an independent risk factor for diagnosis at stages III and IV, which may suggest that the TNM stage of a tumour when diagnosed could be affected more by the biology of the cancer (degree of differentiation) than by a delay in the diagnosis.

6. Relationships between diagnostic delay in primary oral cancer and disease extension

Tumour size and nodal status seem to correlate well with tumour growth chronology in oral cancer (Spiro, 1986; Brown, 1989; Parker, 1996). This paradigm leaded to investigations on the feasibility that diagnostic delay contributes to the spread of the disease. Despite this theory could be proved for certain tumours (Erwenne, 1989; Porta , 1991; Faccione, 1993), no definitive conclusions could be drawn for oral cancer, where disagreements between the groups who discard an association (Allison et al, 1998; Kantola et al, 2001; Kerdpon et al, 2001b) and those who endorse it (O'Sullivan, 2001; Brouha et al, 2005b, Gomez et al., 2009) are evident.

The paper by Guggenheimer et al (1989) was one of the first in considering this hypothetical relationship in a mixed sample of 149 oral and pharyngeal cancers and failed to identify an association even after considering patient and professional delays separately. From then on, this has been a common conclusion in the literature (Jovanovic et al, 1992; Amir et al, 1999; Hollows et al, 2000; Kerdpon et al, 2001a; Kerdpon et al 2001b) until 1994, when Kowalski et al. significantly related professional delay and tumour stage, but not between overall delay and spread of the disease, which may suggest the relevance of memory bias in this particular type of research.

The control of biases is a challenging issue for researchers in this field. The consideration of patient survival as the research outcome and the use of multivariate analysis to adjust for confounding factors (Wildt et al, 1995) meant an improvement in the design of these studies but the sought association could not still be identified for oral cancer (Wildt et al , 1995) or for mixed samples of head and neck carcinomas (Gorsky & Dyan, 1995). Research designs were further improved by the combination of data collection methods to include prospective and retrospective data for reducing memory bias: McGurk et al (2005) gathered a sample of 613 cases over 40 years and failed to unveil a relationship between delay in diagnosis and tumour stage but they used an arbitrary time point of three months to distinguish between delayed and non-delayed cases in their mixed sample of head and neck cancers that, combined with a vague definition of diagnostic delay, compromise their conclusions.

The composition of the study sample may be relevant, since Scott et al (2005) found no relationship between diagnostic delay and tumour stage, but discovered a trend in this direction for certain oral sites. Carvalho et al (2002) somehow confirmed this trend in their series of 676 head and neck squamous cell carcinomas when observed that laryngeal and hypopharyngeal cancers were more prone to be diagnosed at advanced stages than lip, oral and oropharyngeal neoplasms. Additional light in this course was provided by Allison et al (1998c) who demonstrated that patients with upper aerodigestive tract carcinomas with professional delays longer than 1 month had an increased risk to be diagnosed at late stage.

When dealing with diagnostic delay, the beginning of any study is, unavoidably, the recognition of the signs and symptoms by the patient, and this recognition is undoubtedly affected by his/her psychosocial characteristics. The first group in considering these variables was that of Kumar et al (2001) who identified a significant relationship between overall diagnostic delay and tumour stage in their sample of 79 patients. Similar findings were reported by Pitiphat et al (2002) from a case-control study, demonstrating that the length of diagnostic delay was significantly greater in patients with advanced tumour stages (TNM stage IV).

There is no sound scientific evidence supporting an association between diagnostic delay in oral cancer, extension of the disease diagnosed at advancer stages (TNM III-IV) and lower survival rates. However, this fact is probably due to methodological flaws in the published reports to date (Allison, 1998a; Allison, 1998b; Allison, 1998c). These reports use different conceptions of diagnostic delay and are thus liable to misclassifications; use retrospective designs without strategies to diminishing patients' memory bias and often break down diagnostic delay classifications to groups with insufficient sample size. Moreover, the study of samples with heterogeneous cancer sites introduce confounding factors in the analysis, as the patient's self-perception and self- exploration abilities depend on the site of the tumour (Allison et al, 1998a; Tromp et al, 2005; Wildt et al, 1995; O'Sullivan, 2001). For example, gingival locations are associated with advanced stages at diagnosis due to the early invasion of the adjacent bone tissue (T4 primary tumour) (Seoane et al., 2006) yet could present without time delay. Additional difficulties come from the type of data collected (e.g.: continuous variables (Wildt et al, 1995; Hollows et al 2000; Kumar et al, 2001; Kantola et al, 2002) versus categorical (Allison et al 1998b; Kerdpon et al 2001a), from the different sources of patient data (questionnaires, interviews, clinical records) and also from the already mentioned patient memory bias.

Different velocities of tumour growth may well also explain why some tumours remain small in size in spite of delay. Even though some studies related diagnostic delay and tumour stage (Brouha et al 2005), it is possible that the relationship between delay and advanced tumour stage is veiled by the fact that certain cancers remain silent during the initial stages and induce symptoms only when they reach and advanced phase (Scott, 2005).

This being, tumour growth rate would act as a confounding factor in the relationship between diagnostic delay and tumour stage, since patients with aggressive tumours and poor prognosis do not usually present diagnostic delay, while tumours with low proliferation rates demonstrate good prognosis despite long diagnostic delays (Kaufman, 1980; Evans, 1982; Allison, 1998a).

A recent meta-analytical study has shown that diagnostic delay is broadly associated to more advanced stages in oropharyngeal cancers. This association resulted to be specially strong when the analysis was restricted to oral cancer (pooled RR, 1.47; 95% CI: 1.09-1.99) and when the delay was longer than one month (pooled RR, 1-69; 95%CI: 1.26-2.77) (Gomez et al 2009). The probability for delayed patients to present an advanced stage of oral cancer at diagnosis in this report was 25% higher than that of non-delayed patient. Nevertheless these data should be interpreted with caution since all 9 studies considered in the analysis were cross-sectional in nature, with retrospective designs and a potential for recall bias.

Study	Tumour site	Age-range (years)	Gender M/F	Delay Non-advanced/Advanced	OR (95%CI)
Guggenheimer, 1989	Oral & OPH	NS	NS	54/19	0.5 (0.2-1.2)
Gorsky,1995	Oral & OPH	10-99	363/180	259/1323	1.0 (0.5-2.1)
Allison, 1998	Oral & Pharynx	34-91	134/54	67/84	3.0 (1.8-4.8)
Kerdpon, 2000	Oral	32-93	117/44	42/78	1.7 (1.0-2.9)
Kantola, 2001	Tongue	26-85	34/41	6/20	3.4 (1.0-11.7)
Pitiphat, 2002	Oral & Pharynx	26-91	65/40	38/15	0.8 (0.3-2.3)
Carvalho, 2002	Oral & OPH	15-82	363/54	78/224	0.8 (0.5-1.4)
Onizawa, 2003	Oral	33-96	100/52	41/32	0.7 (0.3-1.4)
Scott, 2004	Oral	22-89	157/88	48/59	1.3 (0.8-2.2)

NS: not stated; OPH: Oropharynx; M: male; F: female; OR: odds ratio; CI: confidence interval

Table 1. Association between diagnostic delay and advanced disease stage for oro pharyngeal carcinomas.

7. Diagnostic delay and survival to oral cancer

The number of studies focusing on the relationship between diagnostic delay and survival to oral cancer are scarce (Table 2), and their results show substantial discrepancies: on the one hand the strength of the association did not reach signification (Ho, 2004), but on the other hand there seems to exist a strong relationship when referral delay is considered (Kantola, 2001; Sandoval, 2009), more specifically: when longer than month, these delays worsen survival to oral and oropharyngeal cancer (Sandoval. 2009), however when tumour aggressiveness is considered, the role of diagnostic delay could not be demonstrated (Seoane, 2010).

Reports on tongue cancer are particularly paradoxical, as referral delays worsen survival, but professional delay behaves as a protective prognostic factor with shorter delays showing a trend towards impaired survival (Kantola, 2001; Teppo 2008). The impact of delays on survival was apparently unreasonable, as shorter delays impaired survival. This paradoxical circumstance, where diagnostic delay, tumour stage and tumour prognosis are inversely related, has been previously described in breast, cervix, lung, colon, renal and urethral cancer and seems to suggest that stage at diagnosis and survival are affected more by the biology of the cancer (rapid tumour growth) than by a delayed diagnosis.

These conclusions demand more studies assessing the impact of diagnostic delay on the course of oral squamous cell carcinomas with sound epidemiologic design (prospective), standardised criteria for diagnostic delay and protocols to minimise recall bias. These future investigations would also benefit from considering in their statistical analyses the biological features of the tumour and treatment delays.

Author	Country	Data collection	Tumor Site	SS	TNM n (%)	P D RR (95%CI)	Prof D RR (95%CI)	Ref D RR (95%CI)	T D RR (95%CI)
Kantola	Finland	1974-1994	Tongue	75	I 9 (12%) II 22 (29.3%) III 33 (44%) IV 11 (14.7%)	-	-	6.3 (1.7-22.9)	-
Teppo	Finland	1986-1996	Tongue	62	I 8 (13%) II 22 (35%) III 25 (40%) IV 7 (11%)	0.58 (0.36-0.93)	1.07 (0.68-1.70)	-	-
Seoane	Spain	1997-2002	Oral	63	I 9 (14.3%) II 20 (31.7%) III 10 (15.9%) IV 24 (38.1%)	-	-	-	1.0 (0.9-1.1)
Sandoval	Spain	1996-1999	Oral & OPH	146	I 15 (10.3%) II 30 (20.5%) III 35 (24%) IV 66 (45.2%)	-	-	2.1 (1.0-4.3)	-

SS: sample size; PD: patient delay; Prof D: professional delay; Ref D: referral delay; TD: Total Delay; RR: relative risk; OPH: oropharyngeal

Table 2. Reports on the association between diagnostic delay in oral cancer an survival.

This is important, as the clarification of this hypothetical relationship between diagnostic delay and survival to oral cancer may condition early oral cancer detection strategies either by strengthening programmes for diminishing diagnostic delay or favouring oral cancer and precancer screening strategies.

8. Strategies to minimise diagnostic delay in oral cancer

A delay when dealing with oral cancer diagnosis is unacceptable. Despite the quickness in obtaining a diagnosis does not ensure an early-stage tumour, it is essential for reducing cancer mortality (Horowitz, 1995). Specific educational interventions on the population, focused on risk groups (self-exploration) and on the clinicians (index of suspicion) are needed to achieve this goal. These interventions should provide sound knowledge of the disease presentation and competences for visual/tactile diagnosis. Additional improvements to ease accessibility to health care and the implementation of clear referral schemes for patients with suspicious lesions would also contribute to this purpose. An example of these schemes would be the "Two weeks wait", rolled out in December 2000 in the United Kingdom for referral of head and neck cancer patients from primary care to specialised centres (Department of Health, 2000). The audit of this programme showed a high proportion of non-malignant lesions being referred through the fast-track system, highlighting a low sensitivity among the general practitioners and stressing need for better visual detector guidelines. This assessment stressed the need for the primary care clinician to know which kind of cases should be sent to the specialist (all suspicious lesions and all suspicious borderline lesions). As it is difficult to detect oral cancer lesions at early stage, several ancillary diagnostic tests have been developed to improve diagnostic performance, such as toluidine blue staining, chemiluminiscence and autofluorescence (Trullenque -Eriksson, 2009).

8.1 Toluidine blue

Tolonium chloride (toluidine blue) has been assessed as diagnostic aid for diagnosis of oral malignant and premalignant lesions by a number of studies (Epstein, 2007; Epstein, 2008; Epstein, 2009). These results were studied from a meta-analytical perspective in 1989, revealing sensitivities ranging from 93.5% to 97.8% and specificities from 73.3% to 92.9% (Rosenberg, 1989), this good performance of the product was somehow spoiled by the serious methodological limitations observed in some of the original reports. A more recent report by Lingen (2008) described sensitivities for the detection of oral cancer ranging from 0.78 to 1.00, and specificities of 0.31 to 1.00. A comprehensive analysis of the current evidence suggest that toluidine blue ins good at detecting carcinomas, but its sensitivity in detecting dysplasia is significantly lower (Epstein, 2008; Lingen, 2009).

8.2 Light-based detection systems

These systems are based upon the structural and metabolic changes the oral mucosa undergoes during the carcinogenesis process. These phenomena induce different absorbance and refractance profiles when exposed to different sources of light or energy (Epstein, 2009).

8.2.1 Vizilite® (Zila Pharmaceuticals, Phoenix, AZ)

A number of cross-sectional studies assessed this chemiluminiscence device with high scores in sensitivity (100%), as every patient had previously visualized mucosal lesions, but low specificity values (0-14.2%) with high percentages of false positives. This device has proved a high capacity to emphasize certain visual features of the lesion, such as brightness and lesions limits (Epstein, 2009), but it does not aid in the identification of a premalignant or malignant oral lesion (Farah, 2007). A combination of Vizilite and toludine blue (ViziLite Plus) has been introduced to reduce the number of false positives but, although both specificity and predictive positive values improved, the scientific evidence on this combination published to date is scarce (Epstein, 2008).

A different system based on the same principles of ViziLite (Microlux/DL, Danbury,USA) has been designed, which illuminates the lesion with a diffused light from a light-emitting diode. When assessed prospectively, it showed a sensitivity of 77.8% and a specificity of 70.7% (McIntosh, 2009). Some reports point that chemoluminiscence could be useful to identify lesions hidden to incandescent light sources, but no evidence supports this theory.

8.2.2 Tissue fluorescence imaging

The VELscope® system (Visually Enhanced Lesion Scope; LED Dental Inc., White Rock, USA) uses autoflorescence technology to detect the loss of fluorescence in visible and non-visible oral lesions. Its sensitivity ranged from 97 to 100%, and proved useful to establish safer surgical margins in tumour excision (Huber, 2009), but no methodologically sound studies back the usefulness of this system as ancillary diagnostic tool when dealing with malignant or premalignant lesions in lower-risk, primary care patients (Lingen, 2008; Epstein, 2009).

8.2.3 Tissue fluorescence spectroscopy

This system produces various excitation wavelengths that are received by a spectrograph and recorded on a computer (Fedele, 2009). Its main advantage is the elimination of the subjective interpretation of the changes in the fluorescence of the tissues, but its main indication is limited to the exploration of previously visually-diagnosed small lesions. This device has shown a high sensitivity and specificity to differentiate healthy mucosa from malignant oral lesions (De Veld, 2005).

Regardless of these promising technologies, the path until these systems enhance visual detection beyond what is achieved through conventional visual and tactile examinations is still to be covered.

9. Oral cancer diagnosis at asymptomatic phases of the disease

The studies on diagnostic delay consider only the symptomatic stage of the disease, which represents a minor part of the disease natural history. The equivocal relationship between diagnostic delay and certain outcomes of interest, like tumour stage and survival to the disease, suggest the need to prioritise the early diagnosis of oral cancer through screening programmes aimed at detecting the disease during its asymptomatic phases, as there is evidence demonstrating that oral visual inspection is satisfactorily sensitive to detect oral precancers and that can improve oral cancer stage at diagnosis. Moreover, community-based screening on these bases may thus decrease oral cancer specific mortality amongst people who use tobacco, alcohol or both (Kujan, 2006).

However, it has to be born in mind that these kind of approaches can also be affected by biases, like the so-called "length-time bias", where the possibility to detect aggressive oral carcinomas by screening is low due to the fact that the period until symptoms arise is short. On the other hand, less aggressive tumours with longer periods until symptoms are easier to detect by screening; this phenomena may make think that an early diagnosis improves prognosis, when what actually happens in that this approach detects mostly tumours biologically less aggressive (van der Waal, 2011).

Another potential bias affecting this kind of programmes would be the "lead-time bias", where survival to oral cancer may seem better when cases are diagnosed early but what actually happens is that cases are detected earlier though patients do not live longer than would live if the neoplasm were diagnosed during the symptomatic period of the disease (van der Waal, 2011).

A different approach would be the case-search: the patient is explored searching for subclinical disease. This procedure is not so demanding but in any situation, the screening test should be easy, safe, reproducible and valid, as well as accepted by the population and by the healthcare workers involved, and should also assess risks, nuisances and costs. In areas with low prevalence of oral cancer, screening programmes result in a reduced detection rate. However, opportunistic high-risk screening (involves offering patients a screen when they attend a clinic for some other, unrelated reason), particularly in general dental practice, may be cost-effective (Conway, 2006). This screening may be more effectively targeted to younger age groups, chiefly 40-60 years old (Conway, 2006). Moreover, new educational strategies are needed to identify populations at particular risk; younger people (Farshadpour, 2007) and non-smoking and non-drinking oral cancer patients (females, old at disease presentation). Thus, the range of ages for systematic oral examination should be broaden.

Opportunistic screening by general dentists includes a systematic review of the oral mucosa during regular dental care. About 83%-86% of European and American GDPs declared to perform a systematic exploration of oral soft tissues to rule out oral cancer. Despite this fact, their ability to make a correct positive detection of oral cancer (sensitivity) remains low, as reported scores varied from 0.4 to 1.0. The specificity ranged from 0.31 to 0.92; these low values would mean that patients with oral carcinomas would not be adequately referred for the decisive diagnosis and treatment (Downer, 2006). Despite that, selective opportunistic screening may be a realistic and effective solution, as detections of oral and oropharyngeal squamous cell carcinomas during a non-symptom-driven examination has demonstrated to be related to lower stages at diagnosis although there is insufficient evidence to determine whether screening by visual and tactile examination in asymptomatic patients alters disease-specific mortality (Downer, 2006). Of course, it has to be kept in mind that "insufficient evidence" only means that there are no methodologically sound studies available to support a given technique or approach.

10. References

Alonge OK, & Naredran S. Opinions about oral cancer prevention and early detection among dentists practising along the Texas-Mexico border. *Oral Dis.* 2003;9:41-45.

Allison P, Franco E, & Feine J. Predictors of professional diagnostic delays for upper aerodigestive tract carcinoma. *Oral Oncology* 1998(a);34:127-132.

Allison P, Franco E, Black M, & Feine J. The role of professional diagnostic delays in the prognosis of upper aerodigestive tract carcinoma. *Oral Oncology* 1998(b);34:147- 153.

Allison P, locker D, & Feine J. The role of diagnostic delay in the prognosis of oral cancer: a review of the literature. *Oral Oncology* 1998(c); 34: 161-170.

Ambrosch P, Kron M, & Fischer G. Micrometastases in carcinoma of the upper aerodigestive tract: detection, risk of metastasizing, and prognostic value of depth of invasión. *Head Neck* 1995; 17: 473–479.

Amir Z, Kwan SYL, Landes D, Feber T, & Williams SA. Diagnostic delays in head and neck cancers. *European Journal of Cancer Care* 1999;8:198-203.

Andersen BL, & Cacioppo JT. Delay in seeking a cancer diagnosis: delay stages and psychophysiological comparison processes. *British Journal of Social Psychology* 1995;34:33-52.

Boing AF, Ferreira Antunes JL, et al.. How much do smoking and alcohol consumption explain socioeconomic inequalities in head and neck cancer risk?. *J Epidemiol Community Health.* 2010 Aug 18.

Bouquot JE, & Ephros H. Erythroplakia: the dangerous red mucosa, *Pract Periodontics Aesthet Dent* 1995; 7:59–67.

Brandizzi D, Chuchurru J, Lanfranchi H, & Cabrini R. Analysis of the epidemiological features of oral cancer in the city of Buenos Aires. *Acta Odontol Latinoam* 2005; 18: 31-5.

Brouha XDR, Tromp DM, Hordijk GJ, Winnubst JAM, & Leeuw RJ. Oral and pharyngeal cancer: analysis of patient delay at different tumor stages. *Head and Neck* 2005;27:939-945.

Brown B, Barnes L, Mazariegos J, Taylor F, Johnson J, & Wagner RL. Prognostic factors in mobile tongue and floor of the mouth carcinoma. Cancer 1989;64:1195-1202.

Bruun JP. Time lapse by diagnosis of oral cancer. *Oral surg Oral Med Oral Pathol* 1976; 42: 139-49.

Carvalho AL, Pintos J, Schlecht NF, et al. Predictive factors for diagnosis of advanced-stage squamous cell carcinoma of the head and neck. *Arch Otolaryngol Head Neck Surg* 2002;128:313-318.

Conway DI. To screen or not to screen? Is it worth it for oral cancer? *Evid Based Dent.* 2006;7:81-2.

De Faria PR, Cardoso SV, De A Nishioka S, et al. Clinical presentation of patients with oral squamous cell carcinoma when first seen by dentist or physician in a teaching hospital in Brazil. *Clin Oral Invest.* 2003;7:46-51.

De Veld DC, Witjes MJ, Sterenborg HJ, & Roodenburg JL. The status of in vivo autofluorescence spectroscopy and imaging for oral oncology. *Oral Oncology* 2005;41:117–31.

Diz -Dios P, Padrón N, Seoane J, Tomas I, LimeresJ, & Varela-Centelles P. "Scheduling delay" in oral cancer diagnosis: a new protagonist. *Oral Oncology* 2005; 41:142-6.

Downer M, Moles D, Palmer S, & Speight P. A systematic review of measures of effectiveness in screening for oral cancer and precancer.*Oral Oncology.* 2006;42(6):551-60.

Epstein JB, & Güneri P. The adjunctive role of toluidine blue in detection of oral premalignant and malignant lesions. *Curr Opin Otolaryngol Head Neck Surg* 2009;17:79–87.

Epstein JB, Sciubba J, Silverman S, & Sroussi HY. Utility of toluidine blue in oral premalignant lesion and squamous cell carcinoma: continuing research and implications for clinical practice. *Head Neck* 2007;29:948–58.

Epstein J, Silverman S, Epstein J, Lonky S, & Bride M. Analysis of oral lesion biopsies identified and evaluated by visual examination, chemiluminescence and toluidine blue. *Oral Oncology* 2008;44:538–44.

Erwenne CM, & Franco ELF. Age and lateness of referral as determinants of extra-ocular retinoblastoma. *Opthal Pediatr Genetics* 1989;10:179-184.

Evans SJW, Langdon JD, Rapidis AD, & Johnson NW. Prognostic significance of STNMP and velocity of tumour growth in oral cancer. *Cancer* 1982;49:7773-776.

Faccione N. Delay versus help seeking for breast cancer symptoms: a critical review of the literature on patient and provider delay. *Social Science and Medicine* 1993;36:1521- 1534.

Farah CS, & McCullough MJ. A pilot case control study on the efficacy of acetic acid wash and chemiluminescence illumination (ViziLite) in the visualisation of oral mucosa white lesions. *Oral Oncology* 2007;43:820–4.

Fedele S. Diagnostic aids in the screening of oral cancer. *Head Neck Oncol* 2009;I:5.

Garzino-Demo P, Dell´Acqua A, Dalmasso P et al. Clinicopathological parameters and outcome of 245 patients operated for oral squamous cell carcinoma. *J Craniomaxillofac Surg* 2006; 34: 344-50.

Gillison ML. Current topics in the epidemiology of oral cavity and oropharingeal cancers. *Head & Neck* 2007. Jan 17.

Gómez I, Seoane J, Varela-Centelles P, Diz P, & Takkouche B. Is diagnostic delay related to advanced-stage oral cancer? A meta-analysis.Eur J Oral Sci. 2009 (b);117(5):541-6.

Gómez I, Warnakulasuriya S, Varela-Centelles PI, López-Jornet P, Suárez M, Diz-Dios P, & Seoane J. Is early diagnosis of oral cancer a feasible objective? Who is to blame for diagnostic delay? *Oral Dis.* 2010 (a);16(4):333-42.

Gonzalez-Moles. MA, Esteban F, Rodriguez-Archilla A, Ruiz-Avila I, & Gonzales-Moles S. Importance of tumour thickness measurement in prognosis of tongue cancer, *Oral Oncol* 2002; 38:394–397.

Gorsky M, & Dayan D. Referral delay in diagnosis of oro/oropharyngeal cancer in Israel. *Oral Oncol, Eur J Cancer* 1995;31B:166-168.

Guggenheimer J, Verbin RS, Johnson JT, Horkowitz CA, & Myers EN. Factors delaying the diagnosis of oral and oropharingeal carcinomas. *Cancer* 1989;64:932-935.

Hollows P, McAndrew PG, & Perini MG. Delays in the referral and treatment of oral squamous cell carcinoma. *Br Dent J* 2000;188:262-265.

Holmes JD, Dierks EJ, Homer LD, & Potter BE. Is detection of oral and oropharyngeal squamous cancer by a dental health care provider associated with a lower stage at diagnosis? *J Oral Maxillofac Surg* 2003;61:285-291.

Horowitz AM, Drury TF, & Canto MT. Practices of Maryland dentists: oral cancer prevention and early detection-baseline from 1995. Oral Dis. 2000;6:282-288.

Huber MA. Assessment of the VELscope as an adjunctive examination tool. *Tex Dent* 2009;126:528–35.

Jaulerry C, Bataini JP, Brunin F, Rodríguez J, & Brugère J. Prognostic factors and results of external irradiation of cancers of the base of the tongue. *Ann Otolaryngol Chir Cervicofac.* 1985;102:519-24.

Johnson NW, Warnakulasuriya S, & Tavassoli M. Hereditary and environmental risk factors: clinical and laboratory risk markers for head and neck specials oral, cancer and precancer. *Eur J Can Prev* 1996; 5: 5-17.

Jovanovic A, Kostense PJ, Schulten EAJM, Snow GB, & van der Waal I. *Oral Oncol, Eur J Cancer* 1992;28B, 37-38.

Kantola S, Jokinen K, Hyrykangas K, Mäntyselkä P, & Alho OP. Detection of tongue cancer in primary care. *British Journal of General Practice* 2001; 51: 106-111.

Kaufman S, Grabau JC, & Lore JH. Symptomatology in head and neck cancer; a quantitative review of 385 cases. *American Journal of Public Health* 1980;70:520-522.

Kerdpon D, & Sriplung H. Factors related to delay in diagnosis of oral squamous cell carcinoma in southern Thailand. *Oral Oncology* 2001(a);17:127-131.

Kerdpon D, & Sriplung H. Factors related to advanced stage oral squamous cell carcinoma in Southern Thailand. *Oral Oncology* 2001(b);37:216-221.

Kowalski LP, Franco EL, Torloni H, et al. Lateness of diagnosis of oral and oropharyngeal carcinoma: factors related to the tumour, the patient and health professionals. *Oral Oncol Eur J Cancer* 1994;30B:167-173.

Kujan O, Glenny AM, Oliver RJ, Thakker N, & Sloan P. Screening programmes for the early detection and prevention of oral cancer. *Cochrane Database Syst Rev.* 2006 Jul 19;3:CD004150

Kumar S, Heller RF, Pandey U, Tewari V, Bala N, & Oanh KTH. Delay in presentation of oral cancer: a multifactor analytical study. *Natl Med J India* 2001;14:13-17.

Lingen MW, Kalmar JR, Karrison T, & Speight PM. Critical evaluation of diagnostic aids for the detection of oral cancer. *Oral Oncology* 2008;44:10–22.36.

Llewellyn CD, Johnson NW, & Warnakulasuriya KA. Risk factors for oral in newly diagnosed patients aged 45 years and younger: a case-control study in Southern England. *J Oral Pathol Med* 2004: 33: 525-332.

Mashberg A. Eritroplasia vs. Leukoplakia in the diagnosis of early asymptomatic oral squamous cell carcinomas. *N Engl J Med* 1977;297:109-110.

Mashberg A, & Feldman LJ. Clinical criteria for identifying early oral and oropharyngeal carcinoma: Eritroplasia revisited. *Am J Surg* 1988; 156:273-275.

Mashberg A, & Samit A. Early diagnosis of asymtomatic oral and oropharyngeal squamous cancer. *CA-A Cancer Journal for Clinicans* 1995; 45: 328-351

McDowell JD. An overview of epidemiology and common risk factors for oral squamous cell carcinoma. *Otolaryngol Clin North Am* 2006;39:277-94.

McGurk M, Chan C, Jones J, O'Regan E, & Sherriff M. Delay in diagnosis and its effect on outcome in head and neck cancer. *British Journal of Oral and Maxillofacial Surgery* 2005;43:281-284.

McIntosh L, McCullough MJ, & Farah CS. The assessment of diffused Light illumination and acetic acid rinse (Microlux/DL) in the visualisation of oral mucosal lesions. *Oral Oncology* 2009;45:E227–31.

O-charoenrat P, Pillai G, Patel S, et al. Tumour thickness predicts cervical nodal metastases and survival in early tongue cancer. *Oral Oncology* 2003; 39:386–390.

O'Sullivan EM. Some insights into the potential for the earlier detection of oral cancer: a population-based study. In: 7th International Congress on Oral Cancer, April 2001, The Hague, Netherlands. Oral Oncol 2001;37:553.

Onizawa K, Nishihara K, Yamagata K, et al. Factors associated with diagnostic delay of oral squamous cell carcinoma. *Oral Oncology* 2003;39:781-788.

Parker SL, Tong T, Bolden S, & Wingo PA. Cancer statistics 1996. *CA-A Cancer Journal for Clinicians* 1996;46:5-28.

Parkin DM, Bray F, Ferlay J, & Pisani P. Global cancer statistics, 2002. *CA-A Cancer Journal for Clinicans* 2005; 55: 74-108.

Pitiphat W, Diehl SR, Laskaris G, Cartsos V, Douglass CW, & Zavras AI. Factors associated with delay in the diagnosis of oral cancer. *J Dent Res* 2002;81:192-197.

Po Wing Yuen A, Lam KY, et al. Prognostic factors of clinically stage I and II oral tongue carcinoma—a comparative study of stage, thickness, shape, growth pattern, invasive front malignancy grading, Martinez-Gimenco score, and pathologic features, Head Neck 2002; 24:513–520

Porta M, Gallen M, Malats N, & Planas J. Influence of diagnostic delay upon cancer survival: an analysis of 5 tumour sites. *Journal of Epidemiology and Community Health* 1991;45:225-230.

Pulte D, & Brenner H. Changes in survival in head and neck cancers in the late 20th and early 21st Century, a period analysis. *The oncologist* 2010; 15: 994-1001.

Rosenberg D, & Cretin S. Use of meta-analysis to evaluate tolonium chloride in 287oral cancer screening. *Oral Surg Oral Med Oral Pathol* 1989;67:621–7.

Sargeran K, Murtomaa H, Safavi SM, & Teronen O. Delayed diagnosis of oral cancer in Iran: challenge for prevention. *Oral Health Prev Dent.* 2009;7:69-76.

Scott SE, Grunfeld EA, & McGurk M. The idiosyncratic relationship between diagnostic delay and stage of oral squamous cell carcinoma. *Oral Oncology* 2005;41:396-403.

Seoane J, Pita S, Gómez I, Vazquez I, et al. P.Proliferative activity and diagnostic delay in oral cancer. *Head Neck.* 2010 (b); 32(10):1377-84.

Seoane J, Varela-Centelles PI, Walsh TF, et al. Gingival squamous cell carcinoma: diagnostic delay or rapid invasion? *J Periodontol.* 2006 Jul;77:1229- 33.

Seoane J, Velo J, Warnakulasuriya S, Varela-Centelles P, et al. Knowledge of oral cancer and preventive attitudes of Spanish dentists. Primary effects of a pilot educational intervention. *Med Oral Patol Oral Cir Bucal.* 2010 (a) May

Spiro R, Huvos A, Wong G, et al. Predictive value of tumour thickness in squamous carcinoma confined to the tongue and floor of the mouth. *Am J Surg* 1986;152:345- 350.

Teppo H, & Alho OP. Relative importance of diagnostic delays in different head and neck cancers.*Clin Otolaryngol.* 2008 Aug;33(4):325-30.

Thomsom PJ, & Hamadah O. Cancerisation within the oral cavity: the use of field mapping biopsies in clinical management. *Oral Oncology* 2007;43:20-6.

Tromp DM, Brouha DR, Hordijk GJ, Winnubst JAM, & Leeuw RJ. Patient and tumour factors associated with advanced carcinomas of the head and neck. *Oral Oncology* 2005;41:313-319.

Trullenque -Eriksson A, Muñoz-Corcuera M, Campo-Trapero J, et al. Analysis of new diagnostic methods in suspicious lesions of the oral mucosa. *Med Oral Patol Oral Cir Bucal* 2009;14:E210–6.360

van der Waal I, de Bree R, Brakenhoff R, & Coebergh JW. Early diagnosis in primary oral cancer: is it possible? *Med Oral Patol Oral Cir Bucal.* 2011 May 1;16(3):e300-5.

Warnakulasuriya S. Global epidemiology of oral and oropharyngeal cancer. *Oral Oncology* 2009 Apr-May;45(4-5):309-16. Epub 2008 Sep 18

Wildt J, Bundgaard T, & Bentzen SM. Delay in the diagnosis of oral squamous cell carcinoma. *Clin Otolaryngol* 1995;20:21-25.

Woolgar J. Histopathological prognosticators in oral and oropharyngeal squamous cell carcinoma. *Oral Oncology* 2006; 42: 229-239

Woolgar JA, Rogers S, West C, et al. Survival and patterns of recurrence in 200 oral cancer patients treated by radical surgery and neck dissection, *Oral Oncology* 1999; 35:257– 265

12

Microsurgical Reconstruction of the Oral Cavity and Oropharynx After Cancer Ablation

Mônica Lúcia Rodrigues, Hugo Fontan Köhler and Luiz Paulo Kowalski
Department of Head and Neck Surgery and Otolaryngology, A. C. Camargo Hospital
Brazil

1. Introduction

1.1 A brief history of head and neck reconstruction

Head and neck cancer treatment may cause significant functional and esthetic morbidity with quality-of-life limiting sequelae. Factors like lesion's topography and extension as well as the function of the compromised structures will determine the characteristics of the defect; the reconstruction modality chosen, the multidisciplinary rehabilitation work and the patient's adaptation capacity will determine the impact of oral cancer treatment on overall life quality. Therefore, it's necessary to perform a critical appraisal of the available methods for reconstruction and its interaction with rehabilitation on each patient in order to ensure optimal results (Gal & Futran, 2002).

Pedicled fasciocutaneous flaps from the trunk were the major form of head and neck reconstruction until 1963 (Pagedar & Gilbert, 2009). These flaps have significant limitations due to unreliable perfusion, limited skin island flap, absence of muscle or bone and the need for at least two operations.They were followed by local flaps, with a defined vascular pedicle and a greater extension of available tissue for transfer. They allowed for better functional and cosmetic outcomes and the realization of a wider range of surgeries. Among these flaps we may cite McGregor (McGregor, 1963) and Bakamjian (Bakamjian, 1965) flaps which were the major form of reconstruction after head and neck ablative surgery in the period from 1963 to the end of the seventies.

A major development in head and neck reconstruction was the introduction of the pectoralis major flap by Ariyan (Ariyan, 1979a, 1979b). The pectoralis major flap presented major advantages over the local and random flaps such as: blood supply from a well-defined and calibrous vascular pedicle; the possibility to include skin, muscle and bone in a single flap; long pedicle, allowing for coverage of distant sites like the maxillary sinus and parietal area; primary closure of the donor area; and adequate coverage of the neck vessels after neck dissection.

The development of microvascular surgery parallels that of pedicled flaps with the description by Seidenberg of autologous jejunal transplantation for esophageal reconstruction (Seidenberg, 1959). But the initial large series of microsurgical flaps were not published until the 1970's (O'Brien et al, 1974). Since then, free flaps have become the workhorse of head and neck reconstruction with and expanding role and a significant impact on treatment outcome.

1.2 Advantages of free flaps over pedicled flaps

We believe that free flaps possess major advantages over pedicled flaps, allowing for better reconstructions and, therefore, a better rehabilitation. The successful reconstruction allows for improved dental and prosthetic rehabilitation with a significant impact on the patient's quality of life.

A major difference between free and pedicled flaps is the available donor areas. While pedicled flaps are restricted to the transplantation of nearby tissues of the ablation site, such limitation is not significant for free flaps, with more than twenty different donor areas already described. It allows for considerations on the cosmetic of the donor area to be evaluated and considered as part of the decision process. A critical example of this advantage is the possibility of sparing thoracic scars and breast deformity in young female patients.

Free flaps also allow for tailor-made reconstructions with the use of flaps that are ideally suited to that specific region and defect. Factors like tissue malleability, thickness and hair coverage may be planned ahead and designed to best suit the defect. A major example is the use of the radial forearm free flap for oral reconstruction when compared to the pectoralis major flap (Jacobsen et al, 1995).

An interesting feature of free flaps is the possibility of reinnervation, with recovery of sensation at the defect area. Previous research demonstrated that nervous ingrowth may occur in noninnervated flaps (Sebesan et al, 2008), but this finding is controversial (Vries et al, 1996). In a case-control study comparing oral tongue resection patients after antebrachial cutaneous nerve-lingual nerve anastomosis and healthy controls, recovery of some sensory ability was demonstrated in all patients but significant differences were noted when compared to controls in mastication, speech intelligibility and sensory capabilities of the neotongue (Loewen et al, 2010).

The risk of recurrence is inherent to any malignant neoplasm and a significant proportion of oral cancer patients will present some form of it during their follow-up. Local recurrences may occur in 25 to 48 % of patients with oral cavity or oropharynx squamous cell carcinomas, depending on their TNM stage and other pathological factors (Agra et al, 2006). When free flaps are used on the initial ablative procedure, the pectoralis major flap and other regional and local flaps are preserved for the eventuality of salvage surgery. This is a major advantage considering the impact of local tumor recurrence on patient performance and its capability to support a major procedure like microvascular flap surgery. The risk of a second primary head and neck cancer is also significant and may be another useful situation to have a local/regional flap available.

1.3 Considerations on patient selection

We consider all patients at their first ablative surgery as potential candidates for free flap reconstruction but, in a set of patients, we still perform local or regional flaps. The most significant decision criterion is the performance status of the patient (Rodrigues et al, 2009).

Patients with a Karnofsky performance-status (KPS) below 60 % aren't considered for free flap reconstruction. We also consider absence of suitable arterial recipient vessels in the neck as a major contraindication. The lack of venous recipient vessels is more easily managed by rotation of the cephalic vein or the use of interposition grafts. Finally, prior carotid surgery, as endarterectomy, is considered a contraindication for free flap transfer.

Importantly, age is not a contraindication to free flap surgery. The population's longevity is increasing worldwide and more and more patients get at the seventh decade of life and beyond in good overall health conditions. Also, the development of anesthetic techniques and intensive care support added to the security of performing major surgeries on these patients.

Nao et al analyzed the results of free flap reconstruction for elderly patients (>70 yrs) and showed that advanced patient age had a significant impact on overall, disease-free, and specific survival on univariate analysis but on multivariate analysis, only overall survival was affected. Most importantly, the functional outcomes were similar between old and young patients (Nao et al., 2011). In an article investigating the impact of age on patients submitted to major head and neck procedures, age wasn't considered as a major prognostic factor for surgical outcome (Boruk et al, 2005). In our own experience, age is no longer considered as significant when considering the reconstruction modality to be employed, being replaced by performance-status evaluation. This option is supported by several reports on the literature in which adequate control of preoperative comorbidity is performed (Bridger et al, 1994; Beausung et al, 2003).

In the salvage setting, free flaps are the first option for reconstruction. In this situation, patients usually have a lower KPS than at primary treatment and the possibility of vessel-depleted necks is higher. Therefore, we believe that reliability of the flap is a major concern with the radial forearm free flap and the anterolateral thigh flap being considered the first options due to their long and calibrous vascular pedicles. The need for vein grafting is more frequent in this setting. Finally, the major indication for free flap reconstruction in patients submitted to salvage is the functional improvement it may represent over conventional, pedicled flaps.

The surgeon must account for factors that may hinder tissue healing when planning the reconstruction. These factors are related both to patient and wound characteristics and may alter the healing progression and jeopardize patient recovery (table 1) (Pagedar & Gilbert, 2009).

Patient-related factors	Wound-related factors
Denutrition	Radiotherapy
Immunodeficiency	Contamination
Diabetes mellitus	Infection
Tobacco abuse	
Advanced age	

Table 1. Factors that may impact on healing in patients with oral cancer.

An interesting point is made by Hanasono et al when comparing the impact of microsurgery on the outcomes of surgical oral cancer. They state that even after the availability of free flaps, a significant percentage of patients where still been reconstructed by regional or local pedicled flaps (Hanasono et al, 2009). We also believe that free flaps don't replace other modalities of reconstruction but should be considered as an addition to the options at disposal.

2. Reconstruction of specific sites

2.1 Reconstruction of the oral cavity and oropharynx

The upper aerodigestive tract is formed by multiple structures that possess complex and interdependent functions. They are essential for breathing and feeding as well as for the speech capabilities and their compromise may significantly impact on basic, survival capabilities as well as in personal communication. The resection of oral cancer implies in the interruption, at least temporarily, of these functions, adding morbidity to these patients. The reconstruction and rehabilitation phases of treatment aim at restoring function and self-image as similar as possible to those before treatment (Vos & Burkey, 2004). The evolution of reconstructive surgery transformed the treatment of oral cancer from a highly disfigurative procedure, usually in multiple stages to a single stage procedure with adequate results. Nowadays, we cannot consider the treatment of the tumor as the final and unique objective to be pursued or be satisfied with quicker and easier reconstruction techniques if this will cause functional or cosmetic sequelae (Brennan & Cummings, 1999).

A significant advantage of free flaps and the first step in the reconstruction is the choice of the donor area and the design and planning of the flap. It allows for tailor-made flaps designed to allow the preservation of the non-resected tissues' anatomy with improved function preservation and coverage of vessels and bone. A major example is the oral tongue in patients submitted to partial pelveglossectomies. Primary closure using a tongue flap will cause such decrease in mobility that the patient behaves like one submitted to total glossectomy. A fasciocutaneous microsurgical flap allows the preservation of tongue mobility along aside intraoral volume. This results in better functional results even for patients with small post-resection defects.

We standardized the following four flaps for reconstruction of the oral cavity and oropharynx: the radial forearm free flap (RFFF), the lateral arm flap (LAF), the rectus abdominis flap and the anterolateral thigh flap (ALTF). The choice among them depends on the extent of the defect, its location, the availability of recipient vessels and the patient body profile.

The main staples of oral tongue and oropharyngeal reconstruction are the LAF and the RFFF. They are chosen if the defect encompasses no more than 70 % of the tongue. In these cases, a pliable, flexible and thin flap will allow adequate movements of the remaining tongue with good overall function.

The LAF has become our workhorse in patients that need a thin, pliable fasciocutaneous flap. Its main indications are (Faria el al, 2007):

- Provide enough skin island for defect closure without tension;
- Primary closure of the donor area is possible;
- Good recipient vessels without the need for vein grafting;
- Compatible thickness of the flap with defect area;

The advantages of the LAF for oral reconstruction were also demonstrated in another article with assessment of donor site morbidity and esthetic outcome. The authors report an excellent esthetic outcome with a patient's satisfaction of 6.58 for the primary site and 7.13 for the donor area in a 0 to ten scale. They also remark that all patients had intelligible speech (Thankappan et al, 2011).

Otherwise, our second choice is the RFFF (Rodrigues et al, 2007). It possesses several disadvantages when compared to the lateral arm flap like the need to graft the donor area causing a cosmetic defect in an exposed area and the sacrifice of the radial artery. Its main indications in our routine are:

- Need of long, calibrous pedicle;
- Vein graft interposition in vessel depleted necks;
- Thickness more constant and predictable than LAF, which may be unsuitable in obese patients due to adipose tissue.

The anterolateral thigh flap may also be used for reconstruction of small defects in the oral cavity as demonstrated by Bussu et al. In a quality of life analysis, they found similar functional outcomes between the ALTF and other flaps after oral reconstruction, including the mobile tongue (Bussu et al, 2011). In a specific comparison of the ALTF and the RFFF for hemiglossectomy defects, both groups had similar functional outcomes regarding speech and swallowing. The donor area of the ALTF group were primarily closed without complications while the RFFF patients were all submitted to skin grafts with a 40 % loss rate (de Vicente et al, 2008). Also, the ALTF donor area may provide more soft tissue, with a significant difference in flap area when compared to the RFFF ($p=0.005$) at a lower complications rate ($p=0.035$), the only significant disadvantage being the longer flap-harvesting time ($p=0.020$) (Kesting et al, 2011). In an analysis of functional results after RFFF (17 patients) or ALTF (31 patients) for oral and oropharyngeal reconstruction, no significant differences could be demonstrated (Camaioni et al, 2008).

Patients that more than 70 % of tongue removal are, in our opinion, better candidates for a bulky, thick flap that provides more intraoral volume and is less pliable. Resections involving the base of tongue has a significant impact on quality of life, especially in the oral feeding domain, and its restoration through free flap reconstruction seems to improve the effect of tissue loss (Hartl et al, 2009). Our choices in these cases are the anterolateral thigh flap and the rectus abdominis flap. The ALTF is usually preferred due to the large and long vascular pedicle and its flexible composition allowing transfer as a fasciocutaneous or a myocutaneous flap. In our experience, this flap had a significantly higher complication rate at the donor site than the RAFF but these most related to fluid accumulation and wound dehiscence with minimal impact on morbidity while the RAFF presented usually with more significant complications like bleeding and abdominal wall weakness. Also fasciocutaneous flaps pose less strain on the recipient vessels due to their lower blood flow. (Rodrigues et al,

2006). A third option, no longer in routine use at our service, is the latissimus dorsi flap. Its indications were similar to those of the two previous flaps but the need to mobilize the patient during the procedure increased operative time and flap ischemia time. These bulky flaps allow for adequate oral intake and emission of a greater number of phonemes (in native Portuguese speakers) even after total removal of the tongue.

The planning of a bulky flap must consider its volume loss over time. In a recent article with serial volume evaluation by CT scan or magnetic resonance imaging, the estimated volume decrease was 20.9% and 24.8 % for the ALTF at 12 and 24 months after the procedure (Cho et al, 2011). The use of adjuvant radiotherapy must also be remembered since it will have a major impact on fat tissue atrophy and therefore volume change (Fujioka et al, 2011). Another option for these patients is the gracilis myocutaneous flap. It allows for reinnervation with microsurgical anastomosis of the obturator nerve to the gracilis with the hypoglossus. This may preserve muscular tonus and decrease volume loss over time. The intention is to replace the motor function of the genioglossus muscle, that is significant for deglutition, and the mylohyoid muscle, that elevates the larynx and prevents aspiration (Yoleri & Mavioglu, 2000).

A significant contribution for the rehabilitation of the oral cancer patient and its return to everyday life is made by the speech therapist. The first postoperative evaluation is performed immediately after patient dismissal from the intensive care unit and therapy is started as soon as possible. A major concern is to start oral feeding and remove the tracheostomy tube before the beginning of adjuvant therapy (radiotherapy or chemoradiation). We strongly believe that early rehabilitation will have a significant impact on late quality of life.

2.2 Reconstruction of the mandible

The resection of the mandible is an integral part of oral cancer treatment and may be caused by direct tumor invasion or to allow oncologic margins to be achieved. The mandible is essential for mastication, deglutition, speech and oral continence. Mandible reconstruction is therefore essential in obtaining adequate functional recovery and aims at preserving facial contour and better rehabilitation of both speech and oral feeding. Resections affecting the anterior arch are most prone to produce significant sequelae. Another significant factor when considering mandible reconstruction is future dental rehabilitation.

Free flaps were a major revolution for mandible reconstruction allowing long segments of vascularized bone to be used. They are more resistant to radiotherapy than bone grafts and present little resorption. Also, they allow for immediate dental rehabilitation using osteointegrated implants. Four flaps are commonly used for mandible reconstruction: the fibular flap, the iliac crest flap, the scapular flap and the radium flap. We will briefly discuss the first two since they are our usual choices.

The fibular osteocutaneous flap represents our first option for mandible reconstruction. It allows for a long segment (up to 25 centimeters) of vascularized bone to be transferred to the head and neck region with minor morbidity to the donor site. We consider as major advantages of this flap its long and reliable vascular pedicle and its location far away from the oncologic surgery site allowing for a two-team approach. A major drawback is the limited amount of soft tissue available in the traditional flap design although a technique with simultaneous transfer of the soleus muscle is described, allowing its use to reconstruct soft tissue defects or improving neck contour by replacing the sternocleidomastoid muscle after its removal en bloc with the neck dissection specimen (Ersoy et al, 2011). In our experience, we prefer a second flap when the fibular flap can't satisfy the need for soft tissue. In these patients we use either the pectoralis major myocutaneous flap or the microvascular ALTF. This finding is also demonstrated in he literature. In a review of patients with multiple free flap reconstructions at M.D. Cancer Center from 2001 to 2007, thirty-four patients (87 %) had defects involving the mandible associated with extensive soft tissue resections. The reconstruction had a satisfactory functional result in most patients (Hanasono et al, 2008). The use of double simultaneous free flaps should be performed in selected patients due to the high complication rate of the procedure and usually limited functional outcome (Andrades et al, 2009). We prefer to reserve this reconstruction option in patients with low comorbidity index and good oncologic prognosis.

In a series of 117 patients submitted to free fibular flaps, the quantity of available bone, the height of the bone at reconstruction site, and the possibility of dental rehabilitation are the major advantages of the fibular flap. They point to a 8.5 % failure rate and calf paresthesias as a major donor site morbidity, affecting 21 % of patients (López-Arcas et al, 2010).

The iliac crest flap main indication is actually a contraindication to the fibular flap. Patients with previous history of lower limb fracture or signs of arterial vascular insufficiency are considered unsuitable for the fibular flap. Also, we perform this flap in patients with limited bone defect when the split iliac crest will suffice.

Although not in our routine use, the scapular flap is a good option when we consider the amount of soft tissue that may be taken along the bone flap. Its most significant feature is the possibility of two separate skin paddles, allowing for greater flexibility in flap suturing at the defect area. The osteocutaneous radial forearm free flap is presented as an alternative to the fibular flap. In a comparison, this flap presented a lower but not statistically significant ($p=0.13$) complication rate at the donor site and comparable rates of oral diet intake ($p=0.49$), bony malunion ($p=0.26$) and dental implants, although they were at a very low rate (2.3 % of all patients). Also, only patients with segmental mandible defects were included (Virgin et al, 2010).

3. Oncologic results

The reconstruction is usually implied in the functional results of the treatment although recently authors have investigated its role in the oncologic outcomes of oral cancer treatment. Series of patients submitted to free flap reconstruction focused on showing their survival results without effectively comparing different treatment modalities. The main focus was stating the acceptable survival rates obtained by free flap reconstruction and encouraging their use (Podrecca et al, 2006). These articles presented contradictory results due to different settings, patient selection and statistical analysis.

In our opinion, a major impact of free flaps on the ablative procedure is the amount of tissue available for transfer. The oncologic surgeon has more freedom to extend the surgery beyond the limits of what could be safely reconstructed using the pectoralis major flap or local flaps. Also, the level of specialization necessary for microsurgery requires, usually, a two-team approach. This allows each team to focus on a single part of the procedure with greater freedom of action.

In a retrospective cohort of 98 patients submitted to either free flap or regional flap reconstruction, a significant difference in survival was noted between the two groups (67.3% or free flaps and 47 % for pedicled flaps, p=0.03). In univariate analysis, compromised surgical margins and recurrence were significant for survival in the free flap group. At final analysis, the modality of reconstruction was not significant but showed a trend toward better survival (de Vicente et al, 2011). The impact of free flap was more evident in a retrospective study of 773 patients with oral squamous cell carcinoma. A direct comparison between the groups and a matched-pair were performed. In the first analysis, a significant impact of microsurgical reconstruction was observed (HR: 0.66, 95% CI: 0.52 - 0.83, p<0.001) that was magnified by the matched-pair analysis (HR: 0.58, 95% CI: 0.44 - 0.73, p<0.001). The benefit of microsurgical reconstruction in these patients was observed mostly for patients with primary tumors staged as T3/T4a (HR: 0.46, 95% CI: 0.31 - 0.69, p<0.001) and the benefit for patients with T1/T2 tumors was less clear although a trend towards better results was shown (HR: 0.74, 95% CI: 0.53 - 1.04, p=0.08). A significant characteristic from this article is that patients with close or compromised surgical margins were excluded from analysis. The authors consider free flap reconstruction recommended, especially when postoperative functional deficits are expected (Mücke et al, 2010). A small study also designed to evaluate the impact of microsurgical reconstruction on survival didn't show any significant improvement only a trend towards better prognosis (Marchetti et al, 2008). This study didn't directly compare the results of free flaps and pectoralis major pedicled flaps.

In a series from M.D. Anderson, the authors show the possible impact of free flap reconstruction on patient survival. They don't direct compare the impact of free flap reconstruction with pedicled flaps but rather of those patients operated before and after the establishment of microsurgical reconstruction. They report a higher rate of advanced tumors both at the primary site and in the neck after the availability of free flaps. In this series, free flaps didn't have a significant impact on local recurrence (p=0.48), overall survival (p=0.63) and disease-specific survival (pp=0.124), but caused a significant decrease in compromised surgical margins rate. A major observation is that even after free flap introduction, approximately one-third of all patients receive pedicled flap reconstruction (Hanasono et al, 2009).

In a retrospective analysis of our experience including 605 patients (Rodrigues et al, 2011) we could confirm the two above-mentioned facts. After their introduction, free flaps became the main modality for reconstruction after oral cancer ablation (figure 1). A significant impact of free flaps occurred on the rate of compromised surgical margins (p<0.0001). This increase in free margins rate in surgery had a significant impact on local recurrence rate (figure 2) and disease-specific survival (figure 3). Microvascular flaps also had a significant impact on the interval for adjuvant treatment, allowing its timelier introduction (p=0.03).

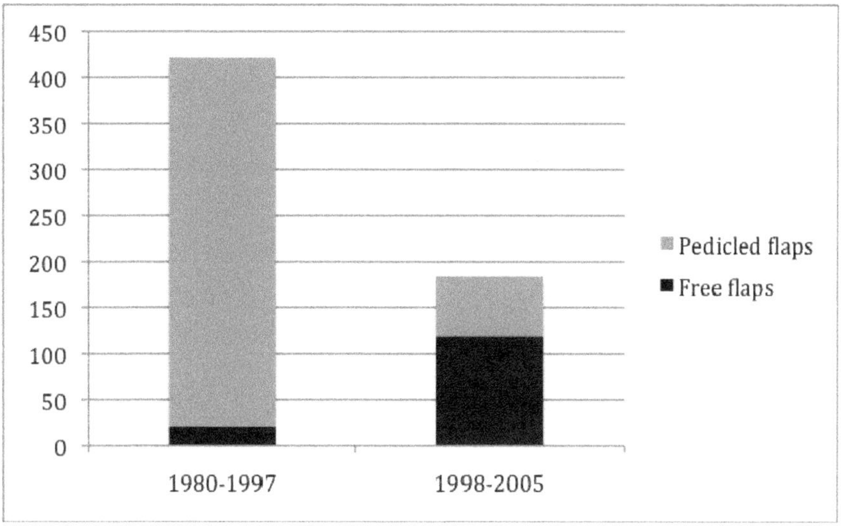

Fig. 1. Time period distribution of free and pedicled flaps in A C Camargo Hospital, São Paulo, Brazil.

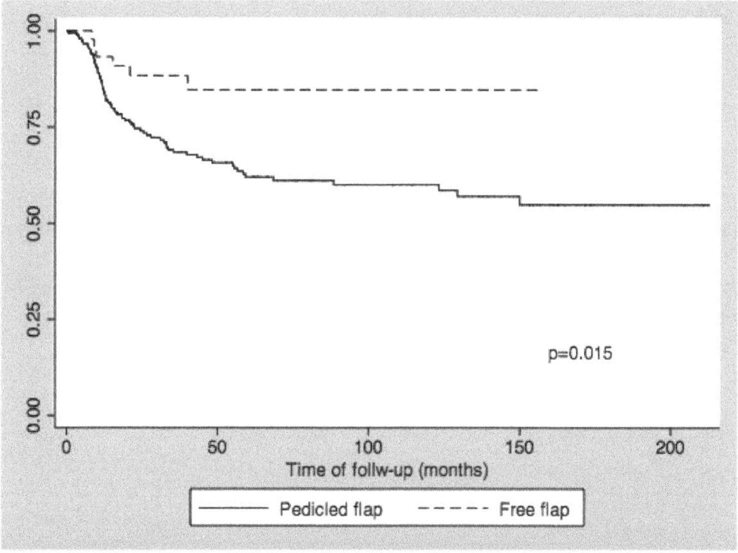

Fig. 2. Local recurrence in patients with advanced-stage (T3/T4) primary tumors submitted to pedicled or free flaps.

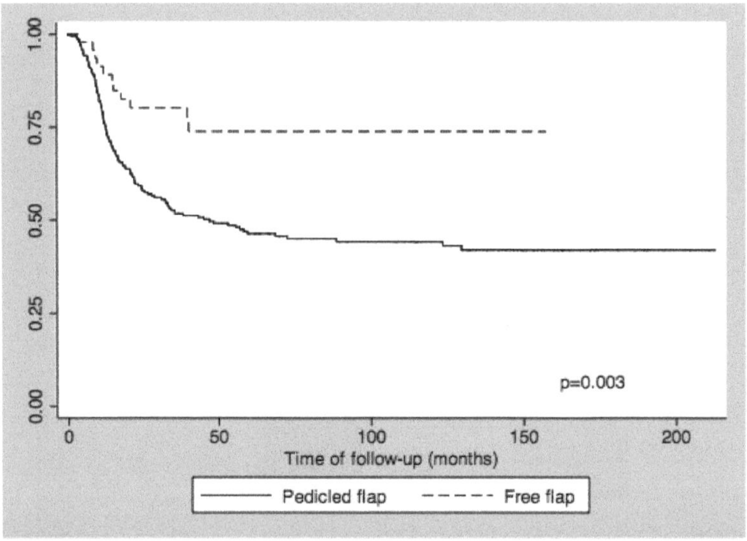

Fig. 3. Disease-specific survival in oral cancer patients according to reconstruction modality. Only patients with T3/T4 primary tumors were included.

Based on data from these different studies, we believe that oral cancer reconstructive surgery should be based on a two-team approach and make extensive use of free flaps. Its indication for patients with high-risk tumors has been challenged by cost-effectiveness analysis of these patients and their risk of recurrence. Some even argue that free flaps should be reserved for selected patients, excluding patients with features like advanced tumor stage, clinically compromised neck lymph nodes and other poor prognosis markers. These patients would derive the least benefit from the reconstructive procedure (Schusterman et al, 1991). Our opinion is exactly the opposite. All patients with oral cancer should be considered candidates for free flap reconstruction and adverse prognostic characteristics shouldn't be considered a counter indication. Usually, these patients are those that have extensive soft tissue or mandible defects and whose rehabilitation will be significantly improved by free flaps. As demonstrated by our experience (Rodrigues et al, 2011) and the article by Mücke et al (Mücke et al, 2010), the choice of reconstruction modality may even have a significant impact on their oncologic outcome. Although the three studies that compare he impact of microsurgical flaps on survival have different inclusion criteria, the sum of their results in a meta-analysis, favors the use of free flaps over pedicled flaps in oral cancer patients (table 2).

Study	RR	95 % CI	Weight
de Vicente, 2011	1.139	0.898 - 1.445	7.54
Rodrigues, 2011	1.233	1.137 - 1.336	37.31
Mücke, 2010	1.087	1.004 - 1.177	55.15
Pooled RR	1.145	1.083 - 1.211	100.00

Table 2. Meta-analysis of the oncologic outcome of free flaps reconstruction on oral cancer patients.

4. Functional outcomes

Good functional outcomes are a major objective of head and neck reconstructive surgery. They mean not only quality of life but also survival. In a previously published study, good general physical health, ability to oral feed communication and absence of pain were strongly correlated with survival (Karvonen-Gutierrez et al, 2008). The return to preoperative status is the ultimate goal, allowing resumption of a normal, productive life with adequate social interaction and quality of life.

In a prospective study of quality of life using the University of Washington - Quality of life and the Head and Neck Performance Status Scale a significant impact of the reconstruction modality is observed. A significant decrease of the scores is observed after 3 months, with progressive improvement until 1 year after treatment, achieving normal or near normal function in 77 % of patients. In multivariate analysis, segmental mandibulectomy and free flap reconstruction were significant, with significant improvement when compared to other reconstruction modalities (Villaret et al, 2008). This finding is confirmed by another study that evaluates quality of life before and after surgery and free flap reconstruction of advanced stage head and neck cancer. A significant decrease is observed immediately after treatment with significant improvement and return to preoperative levels after six months (Rizvi et al, 2009).

The removal of the mobile tongue is perhaps the main cause of disability and functional limitation after oral cancer ablation. The use of the RFFF may significantly improve the outcome of such patients. Longitudinal analysis of swallowing function and tongue mobility in a group of 15 patients and comparison against patients without tongue involvement shows a significant decrease in liquid swallowing and posterior tongue motility after one month of treatment. But all measures returned to baseline level after 12 months, indicating a good capacity of functional recovery over time. The role of post-treatment rehabilitation through a multi-specialty team is specially indicated as it provides the best results (Brown et al, 2010). In an analysis of patients submitted to oral cancer ablation and RFFF reconstruction, high comorbidity index, large flap surface, radiotherapy and involvement of the mobile tongue were significant for poorer functional outcomes. Despite this, 87 % were on exclusive oral diet and 80 % had intelligible speech (Bozec et al, 2009). The RFFF may be transferred as an innervated flap. In this case, limited recovery of sensorial function is possible, although not full recovery.

Videofluoroscopy (VF) has been used for assessment of deglutition after free flap reconstruction for oral cancer in 20 patients. It demonstrated an 89.4 % of good neotongue mobility with adequate control of he food bolus in 73.6 % of patients. In 85 % of patients, oral diet could be resumed and 75 % had intelligible speech and were able to effectively communicate. It is concluded that free flaps significantly improve life quality with adequate rehabilitation of swallowing and speech capabilities (Archontaki et al, 2010). VF evaluation in patients submitted to base of tongue resection and RFFF reconstruction also show a good functional recovery. In a prospective series of 20 consecutive patients, nineteen were able to resume oral feeding with good swallowing function without signs of aspiration. The flap allows for good apposition of the base of tongue and posterior pharyngeal wall preserving deglutition mechanics (O'Connell et al, 2008). Using a barium swallow in a series of 100 consecutive patients, tongue base resection and preoperative radiotherapy were the only significant factors for post-treatment aspiration in patients submitted to microsurgical flap reconstruction (Smith et al, 2008). The evaluation of our results in patients submitted to retromolar or oropharyngeal tumor ablation and reconstruction showed a significant improvement of deglutition among those submitted to free flaps with a compromise of both oral and pharyngeal phases in the pectoralis major flap group. No significant difference in aspiration rate was demonstrated between the two groups (Bandeira et al, 2007).

In a direct comparison of swallowing function among patients submitted to free or pedicled flaps, the type of reconstruction had no significant impact on resumption of oral feeding. The significant factor for functional swallowing was defect location, with lateral defects having a significant better prognosis than central defects (Schache et al, 2009). When is the focus is shifted to speech, a direct comparison of the RFFF and the pectoralis major pedicled flap show a distinctive advantage of the free flap. Also, intraoral dehiscence rate for the pectoralis major flap was significantly higher than that of the RFFF (O'Neill et al, 2010).

In a cross-sectional study, a direct comparison between chemoradiation and primary surgery with microsurgical flap reconstruction was performed. The study included 49 patients and they used UoW - QoL modules c30+hn35 to compare the functional outcomes between the two groups. The majority of ICF categories failed to demonstrate any significant difference between the two groups but a trend toward better overall life quality was suggested in the surgical group (Tshierner et al, 2011). This article demonstrates that operative and non-operative management of oral cancer patients have similar functional outcomes.

When compared to the pectoralis major pedicled flap, the free flap possesses a major advantage in functional outcomes also outside the swallowing and speech domains. In a retrospective review of 100 patients among 491 eligible, speeds, shoulder function and mood were significantly better in patients submitted to free flaps (Hsing et al, 2011). The use of free flaps after salvage surgery in patients originally treated by radiotherapy or chemoradiation has significant worse functional outcomes than after initial surgery followed by adjuvant treatment. In a series of 72 patients, most patients (56 %) required enteral tube feeding on a definitive basis (Kostrzewa et al, 2010).

5. Risk factors and complications of free flap oral reconstruction

Patients submitted to free flap reconstruction might present in the post-operative period complications related to the ablative procedure, the reconstruction and its clinical conditions. Our major objective here is to discuss the complications related to the flap itself. In a review of 150 patients, female gender and operative time longer than 10 hours were significant predictors of major surgical complications (Rosenberg et al, 2009). In an analysis of 796 consecutive patients, two hundred thirty-nine patients (30 %) had a complication demanding lengthening of hospital stay or reoperation. Smoking, ASA score, and low preoperative hemoglobin levels were significant predictors of perioperative morbidity and the two last ones also for surgical complications (Patel et al, 2010).

Infections are a major concern after microsurgical reconstruction. By definition, oral surgeries are contaminated and therefore are already at a higher infection risk. In an analyis of 276 patients submitted to free flap reconstruction, one hundred and twelve patients

(40.6 %) had post-operative surgical-site infection. Duration of surgery and ASA (American Society of Anesthesiologists) score were significant factors for local and neck infection (Karakida et al, 2010). In our experience, surgical site infections were the most frequent post-operative complication, occurring in 94 patients (15.54 %). In two cases (0.33%), patients presented with infection at the donor site.

Although controversial, previous radiotherapy with or without chemotherapy is implicated in wound complications after oral cancer surgery (Sassler et al, 1995). Remodeling of the extracellular matrix and expression of transforming growth factor beta (1) were significantly different in patients submitted to previous irradiation and this factor alone was significant for flap success or failure (Lee & Thiele, 2010). In this setting, the transfer of healthy tissue with a reliable blood supply is of major significance for improving healing. The impact of radiotherapy on flap success rate seems to be negligible (Kruse et al, 2010). The addition of chemotherapy to radiotherapy in the adjuvant treatment doesn't have a significant impact on the success rate, with results comparable to that after radiotherapy alone (Kostrzewa et al, 2010).

In an analysis of 2372 free flaps for head and neck reonstruction, a major prognotic factor for flap loss was secondary reconstruction. The survival rate in primary reconstructions was 93.9 % compared to only 88.7 % in the secondary reconstruction setting ($p<0.05$). Posible factors to explain this difference include higher infection rate, delayed wound healing and depleted vessel neck (Nakatusuka et al, 2003). Thrombosis of the vascular anastomosis, although rare, is a significant complication and may lead to flap loss. In a recent review of multiple centers in the Netherlands, no single protocol for pharmacological thrombosis prevention could be defined. The authors emphasize the role of preoperative smoke cessation and careful vascular handling during surgery with an individualized postoperative treatment based on risk profile (Brands et al, 2009).

6. References

Agra IMG, Carvalho AL, Ulbrich FS, Campos OD, Martins EP, Magrin J & Kowalski LP. (2006). Prognostic factors in salvage surgery for recurrent oral and oropharyngeal cancer. *Head Neck*, Vol. 28, No. 2, (February 2006), pp. 107-113, ISSN 1043-3074.

Andrades P, Bohannon IA, Baranano CF, Wax MK & Rosenthal E. (2009). Indications and outcomes of double free flaps in head and neck reconstruction. *Microsurgery*, Vol. 29, No. 3, (March 2009), pp. 171-177, ISSN 1098-2752.

Archontaki M, Athanasiou A, Stavrianos SD, Korkolis DP, Faratzis G, Papadopoulou F, Kokkalis G & Rapidis AD. (2010). Functional results of speech and swallowing after oral microvascular free flap reconstruction. *European Archives of Otolaryngology Head and Neck Surgery*, Vol. 267, Nr. 11, (November 2010), pp. 1771-1777, ISSN 1434-4726

Ariyan S. (1979). The pectoralis major myocutaneous flap: a versatile flap for reconstruction in the head and neck. *Plastic Reconstrutive Surgery*, Vol. 63, No. 1, (January 1979), pp. 73-81, ISSN 0032-1052.

Ariyan S. (1979). Further experiences with the pectoralis major myocutaneous flap for the immediate repair defects from excisions of head and neck cancers. *Plastic Reconstructive Surgery*, Vol. 64, No. 5, (May 1979), pp. 605-612, ISSN 0032-1052.

Bakamjian VY. (1965). A two-stage method for pharyngo-esophageal reconstruction with a primary pectoral skin flap. *Plastic Reconstrutive Surgery*, Vol. 36, No. , (August 1965), pp. 173-184, ISSN 0032-1052.

Bandeira AKC, Tomazelli MFGG, do Vale-Prodomo LP, Vartanian JG, Faria JCM, Rodrigues ML, Kowalski LP, Carrara-de Angelis E. (2007) Analysis of swallowing after retromolar or oropharynx resection and reconstruction with myocutaneous or microvascular free flaps. *Applied Cancer Research*, Vol 27, No. 1, (January 2007), pp. 23-29, ISSN 1980-5578

Beausung ES, Ang EE, Lipa JE, Irish JC, Brown DH, Gullane PJ, Neligan PC. (2003). Microvascular free tissue transfer in elderly patients: the Toronto experience. *Head Neck*, Vol. 25, No. 7, (July 2003), pp. 549-553, ISSN 1043-3074.

Boruk M, Chernobilsky B, Rosenfeld RM & Har-El G. (2005). Age as a prognostic factor for complications of major head and neck surgery. *Archives of Otolaryngology Head and Neck Surgery*, Vol. 131, No. 7, (July 2005), pp. 605-609, ISSN 0886-4470.

Bozek A, Poissonnet G, Chamorey E, Laout C, Vallicioni J, Demard F, Peyrade F, Follana P, Bensadoun RJ, Benezery K, Tharial J, Marcy PY, Sudada A & Dassonville O. (2009). Radical ablative surgery and radial forearm free flap (RFFF) reconstruction for patients with oral and oropharyngeal cancer: postoperative outcomes and oncologic and functional results. *Acta Otolaryngologica*, Vol. 129, No. 6, (June 2009), pp. 681-687, ISSN 0001-6489.

Brands MT, van den Bosch SC, Dieleman FJ, Bergé SJ & Merkx MA. (2009). Prevention of thrombosis after microvascular tissue transfer in the head and neck. A review of the literature and the state of affairs in Dutch Head and Neck Cancer Centers. *International Journal of Oral and Maxillofacial Surgery*, Vol. 39, No. 2, (February 2010), pp. 101-106, ISSN 0901-5027.

Brennan JA, Cummings CW. (1999). Controversy in the management of tumors of the oral cavity. In:. *Comprehensive Management of Head and Neck Tumors*. Thawley SE, Panje WR, Batsakis JG, Lindberg RD (editors), pgs 733-735. WB Saunders ISBN: 0-7216-5582-3, Philadelphia - USA.

Bridger AG, O'Brien CJ & Lee KK. (1994). Advanced patient age should should not preclude the use of free-flap reconstruction for head and neck cancer. *American Journal of Surgery*, Vol. 168, No. 5, (November 1994), pp. 425-428, ISSN 0002-9610.

Brown L, Rieger JM, Harris J & Seikaly H. (2010). A longitudinal study of functional outcomes after surgical resection and microvascular reconstruction for oral cancer: tongue mobility and swallowing function. *Journal of Oral and Maxillofacial Surgery*, Vol. 68, No. 11, (November 2010), pp. 2690-2700, ISSN 0901-5027

Bussu F, Salgarello M, Adesi LB, Rigante M, Parrilla C, Guidi ML, Paludetti G & Almadori G. (2011). Oral cavity defect reconstruction using anterolateral thigh free flaps. *B-ENT*, Vol. 7, No. 1, (January 2011), pp. 19-25, ISSN 1781-782X

Camaioni A, Loreti A, Damiani V, Bellioni M, Passali FM & Viti C. (2008). Anterolateral thigh cutaneous flap vs radial forearm free-falp in oral and oropharyngeal reconstruction: an analysis of 48 flaps. *Acta Otorhinolaryngologica Italica*, Vol. 28, No. 1, (February 2008), pp. 7-12, ISSN 0392-100X.

Cho KJ, Joo YH, Sun DI & Kim MS. (2011). Perioperative clinical factors affecting volume changes of reconstructed flaps in head and neck cancer patients: free versus regional flaps. *European Archives of Otolaryngology Head and Neck Surgery*, Vol. 268, No. 7, (July 2011), pp. 1061-1065, ISSN 1434-4726.

de Vicente JC, de Villalaín L, Torre A & Peña I. (2008). Microvascular free tissue transfer for tongue reconstruction after hemiglossectomy: a functional assessment of radial forearm versus anterolateral thigh flap. *Journal of Oral and Maxillofacial Surgery*, Vol 66, No. 11, (November 2008), pp. 2270-2275, ISSN 0901-5027.

de Vicente JC, Rodríguez-Santamarta T, Rosado P, Peña I, de Villalaín L. Survival after free flap reconstruction in patients with advanced oral squamous cell carcinoma. *Journal of Oral and Maxillofacial Surgery* 2011 Jun 17 [Epub ahead of print] DOI 10.1016/j.joms.2011.02.202, ISSN 0901-5027.

Ersoy B, Sönnez A & Bayramiçli M. (2011) Sternocleidomastoid region restoration with lateral hemisoleus incorporated in free fibular flap for reconstruction of radical neck dissection and hemimandibulectomy. *Microsurgery* Vol. 31, No. 5, (May 2011), pp. 401-403, ISSN 1098-2752.

Faria JCM, Scopel GP, Rodrigues ML, Kowalski LP, Ferreira MC. (2007). The versatility of the free lateral arm flap in head and neck soft tisue reconstruction: analysis of 210 cases. *Journal of Plastic, Reconstructive and Aesthetic Surgery*, Vol. 61, No. 2, (February 2007), pp. 172-179, ISSN 1748-6815.

Fujioka M, Masuda K, Imamura Y. Fattys tissue atrophy if free flap used for head and neck reconstruction. *Microsurgery* Vol. 31, No. 1, (January 2011), pp. 32-35, ISSN 1098-2752.

Gal TJ & Futran ND. (2002). Outcomes research in head and neck reconstruction. *Facial Plastic Surgery* 2002, Vol. 18, No. 2, (April 2002), pp. 113-7, ISSN 0736-6825.

Hanasono MM, Weinstock YE & Yu P (2008). Reconstruction of extensive head and neck defects with multiple simultaneous free flaps. *Plastic Reconstructive Surgery*, Vol. 122, No. 6, (December 2008), pp. 1739-1746, ISSN 0032-1052.

Hanasono MM, Friel, MT, Klem C, Hsu PW, Robb GL, Weber RS, Roberts DB & Chang DW. (2009). Impact of reconstructive microsurgery in patients with advanced oral cavity cancers. *Head Neck*, Vol. 31, No. 10, (October 2009), pp. 1289-1296, ISSN 1043-3074.

Hartl DM, Dauchy S, Escande C, Bretagne E, Janot F & Kolb F. (2009). Quality of life after free-flap tongue reconstruction. *Journal of Laryngology and Otology*, Vol. 123, No. 5, (May 2009), pp. 550-554, ISSN 0022-2151.

Hsing CY, Wong YK, Wang CP, Wang CC, Jiang RS, Chen FJ, Liu SA. (2011). Comparison between free flap and pectoralis major pedicled flap for reconstruction in oral cavity cancer patients -- quality of life analysis. *Oral Oncology* Vol. 47, No. 6, (June 2011), pp. 522-527, ISSN 1368-8375.

Jacobson MC, Franssen E, Fliss DM, Birt D & Gilbert RW. (1995). Free forearm flap in oral reconstruction. *Archives of Otolaryngology Head and Neck Surgery*, Vol. 121, No. 9, (Steptember 1995), pp. 959-964, ISSN 0886-4470.

Karakida K, Aoki T, Ota Y, Yamaaki H, Otsuru M, Takahashi M, Sakamoto H & Miyasaka M. (2010). Analysis of risk factors for surgical-site infections in 276 oral cancer surgeries with microvascular free-flap reconstructions at a single university hospital. *Journal of Infection and Chemotherapy*, Vol. 16, No. 5, (October 2010), pp. 334-339, ISSN 1341-321X.

Karvonen-Gutierrez CA, Ronis DL, Fowler KE, Terrell JE, Gruber SB & Duffy SA. Quality of life scores predict survival among patients with head and neck cancer. *Journal of Clinical Oncology* 2008; 26, No. 16, (June 1, 2008), pp. 2754-2760, ISSN 0732-183X.

Kesting MR, Hölzle F, Wales C, Steinstraesser L, Wagenpfeil S, Mücke T, Rohleder NH, Wolff KD, Haler RJ. (2011). Microsurgical reconstruction of the oral cavity with free flaps from the anterolateral thigh and the radial forearm: a comparison of perioperative data from 161 cases. *Annals of Surgical Oncology*, Vol. 18, No. 7, pp. 1988-1994, (July 2011), ISSN 1068-9265.

Kostrzewa JP, Lancaster WP, Iseli TA, Desmond RA, Carroll WR & Rosenthal EL. Outcomes of salvage surgery with free flap reconstruction for recurrent oral and oropharyngeal cancer. *Laryngoscope* 2010; 120, No. 2, (February 2010): 267-272, ISSN 1531-4995.

Kruse AL, Luebbers HT, Grätz KW, Obwegeser JA. (2010). Factors influencing survival of free-flap in reconstruction for cancer of the head and neck: a literature review. *Mirosurgery* Vol. 30, No. 3, (March 2010), pp. 242=248, ISSN 1098-2752.

Lee S & Thiele C. factors associated with free flap complications after head and neck reconstruction and the molecular basis of fibrotic tissue rearrangement in preirradiated soft tissue. *Journal of Oral and Maxillofacial Surgery*, Vol. 68, No. 9, (September 2010), pp. 2169-2178, ISSN 1531-5053.

Loewen IJ, Boliek CA, Harris J, Seikaly H & Rieger JM. (2010). Oral sensation and function: a comparison of patients with innervated radial forearm free flap reconstruction to healthy matched individuals. *Head Neck*, Vol. 32, No. 1, (January 2010), pp. 85-95, ISSN 1043-3074.

López-Arcas JM, Arias J, Del Castillo JL, Burgueño M, Navarro I, Móran MJ, Chamorro M & Martorelli V. The fibula osteomyocutaneous flap for mandible reconstruction: a 15-year experience. *Journal of Oral and Maxillofacial Surgery* 2010; Vol. 68, No. 10, (Ocotber 2010), pp. 2377-2384, ISSN 0278-2391.

Marchetti C, Pizzigallo A, Cipriani R, Campobassi A & Badiali G. Does microvascular free flap reconstruction in oral squamous cell carcinoma improve patient survival? *Otolaryngology - Head and Neck Surg* 2008; 139 (6), (June 2008), pp. 775-780, ISSN 0194-5998.

McGregor IA. The temporal flap in intra-oral cancer: its uses in repairing the post-excisional defect. *British Journal of Plastic Surgery* 1963; 16: 10, (October 1963), pp. 318-335, ISSN 0007-1226.

Mücke T, Wolff KD, Wagenpfeil S, Mitchell DA & Hölzle. F. Immediate microsurgical reconstruction after tumor ablation predicts survival among patients with head and neck carcinoma. *Annals of Surgical Oncology* 2010; 17, No. 1, (January 2010), 287-295, ISSN 1068-9265.

Nakatsuka T, Harii K, Asato H, Takushima A, Ebihara S, Kimata Y, Yamada A, Ueda K & Ichioka S. Analytic review of 2372 fre flap transfers for head and neck reconstruction following cancer resection. *Journal of Reconstructive Microsurgery* 2003; 19, No. 6, pp. 363-368, ISSN 0743-684X.

O,Brien BM, Morrison WA, Ishida H, MacLeod AM & Gilbert A. (1974). Free flap transfers with microvascular anastomoses. *British Journal of Plastic Surgery*, Vol. 27, No. 3, (July 1974), pp. 220-230, ISSN 0007-1226.

O'Connell DA, Rieger J, Harris JR, Dziegielewski P, Zalmanowitz J, Sytsanko A, Li S, Wolfaart J, Hart RD & Seikaly H. Swallowing function in patients with base of tongue cancers treated with primary surgery and reconstructed with a modified radial forearm free flap. *Archives of Otolaryngology - Head and Neck Surgery* 2008; 134, No. 8, (August 2008), pp. 857-864, ISSN 0886-4470.

O'Neill JP, Shine N, Eadie PA, Beausang E, &Timon C. (2010). Free tissue transfer versus pedicled flap reconstruction of head and neck malignancy defects. *Irish Journal of Medical Sciences*, Vol. 179, No. 3, (September 2010), pp. 337-343, ISSN 0021-1265.

Pagedar, NA & Gilbert, RW. (2009). Principles of head and neck reconstruction. In: *Principles and practice of head and neck surgery and oncology*. Montgonomery PQ, Evans PHR & Gullane PJ. (editors). Informa UK, pp. 527-540, England.

Patel RS, McCluskey SA, Goldstein DP, Minkovich L, Irish JC, Brown DH, Gullane PJ, Lipa JE & Gilbert RW. (2010). Clinicopathologic and thrapeutic risk factors for perioperative complications and prolonged hospital stay in free flap reconstruction of the head and neck. *Head Neck*, Vol. 32, No. , pp. 1345-1353, ISSN 1043-3074.

Podrecca S, Salvatori P, Squadrelli Saraceno M, Fallahdar D, Calabrese L, Cantù G & Molinari R. (2006) Review of 346 patients with free-flap reconstruction following head and neck surgery for neoplasm. *Journal of Plastic, Reconstructive and Aesthetic Surgery*, Vol. 59, No. 2, (February 2006), pp.122-129, ISSN 1748-6815..

Rizvi TA, Rashid M, Ahmed B, Haq EU, Sarwar SU, Zia-ul-Islam M & Tamimy MS. (2009). Quality of life assessment in patients with locally advanced head and neck malignancy after ablative surgery and reconstruction with microvascular free flaps. *Journal of the College of Physicians and Surgeons - Pakistan*, Vol. 19, No. 2, (February 2009), pp. 108-112, ISSN 1681-7168.

Rodrigues ML, Faria JCM, Köhler HF, Kowalski LP. Retalhos ântero-lateral da coxa e reto abdominal em grandes reconstruções tridimensionais em cabeça e pescoço. (2006). *Revista Brasileira de Cirurgia de Cabeça e Pescoço*, Vol. 35, No. 4, (October 2006), pp. 244-248, (2006) ISSN 0100-2171

Rodrigues ML, Faria JCM, Kohler HF, Kowalski LP. Comparação entre os rtalhos microcirúrgicos antebraquial e lateral do braço em reconstruções de boca e orofaringe. (2007). *Revista Brasileira de Cirurgia de cabeça e Pescoço*, Vol. 36, No. 2, (Abril 2007), pp. 126-129 (). ISSN 0100-2171.

Rodrigues ML, Köhler HF, Magrin J, Bressan A, Faria JCMF & Kowalski LP. (2011). Which oral cancer patients benefit the most from microsurgical reconstruction? *European Journal of Plastic Surgery* 2011;, Vol. 34, No. 2, (April 2011), pp. 75-80, ISSN 0930-343X.

Rodrigues ML, Köhler HF, Faria JCM, Ikeda MK, Vartanian JG & Kowalski LP. (20090. Reconstruction after extended orbital exanteration using a fronto-lateral flap. *International Journal of Oral and Maxillofacial Surgery* 2009; Vol. 38, No. 8, (August 2009), pp. 850-854, ISSN 0901-5027.

Rosenberg AJ, van Cann EM, van der Bilt A, Koole R & van ES RJ. (2009). A prospective study on prognostic factors for free-flap reconstructions of head and neck defects. *International Journal of Oral and Maxillofacial Surgery*, Vol. 38, No. 6, (June 2009), pp. 666-670, ISSN 0901-5027.

Sassler AM, Esclamado RM & Wolf GT. (1995). Surgery after organ preservation therapy. Analysis of wound complications. *Archives of Otolaryngology Head and Neck Surgery*, Vol. 121, No. 2, (February 1995), pp. 162-165, ISSN 0886-4470.

Schache AG, Lieger O, Rogers P, Kelly A, Newman L & Kalavrezos N. (2009). Predictors of swallowing outcome in patients treated with surgery and radiotherapy for advanced oral and oropharyngeal cancer. *Oral Oncology*, Vol. 45, No. 9, (Setember 2009), pp. 803-808, ISSN: 1368-8375.

Sabesan T, Ramchandani PL & Ilankovan V. (2008) Sensory recovery in noninnevated free flap in oral and oropharyngeal reconstruction. *International Journal of Oral and Maxillofacial Surgery*, Vol. 37, No. 9, (September 2008), pp. 819-823, ISSN 0901-5027.

Seidenberg B, Rosenak S, Hurwitt ES & Som ML. (1959). Immediate reconstruction of the cervical esophagus by a revascularized isolated jejunal segment. *Annals of Surgery*, Vol. 149, No. 2, (February 1959), pp. 162-171, ISSN 0148-7043.

Smith JE, Suh JD, Erman A, Nabili V, Chhetri DK & Blackwell KE. (2008) Risk factors predicting aspiration after free flap reconstruction of oral cavity and oropharyngeal defects. *Archives of Otolaryngology - Head and Neck Surgery* 2008; 134, No. 11, (November 2008), pp. 1205-1208, ISSN 0886-4470.

Thankapaan K, Kuriakose MA, Chatni SS, Sharan R, Trivedi NP, Vijayaraghavan S, Sharma M & Iyer S. (2011) Lateral arm flap for oral tongue reconstruction: an analysis of surgical details, morbidity, and functional and aesthetic outcome. *Annals of Plastic Surgery*, Vol. 66, No. 3, (March 2011), pp. 261-266, ISSN 0148-7043.

Villaret AB, Cappiello J, Piazza C, Pedruzzi B & Nicolai P. (2008) Quality of life in patients treated for cancer of the oral cavity requiring reconstruction: a prospective study. *Acta Otorhinolaryngologica Italica*, Vol. 28, No. 3, (June 2008), pp. 120-125, ISSN 0392-100X.

Virgin FW, Iseli TA, Iseli CE, Sunde J, Carroll WR, Manuson JS & Rosenthal EL. (2010) Functional outcomes of fibula and osteocutaneous forearm free flap reconstruction for segmental mandibular defects. *Laryngoscope*, Vol. 120, No. 4, (April 2010), pp. 663-7, ISSN 0023-852X

Vos JD &Burkey BB. (2004) Functional outcomes after free flap reconstruction of the upper aerodigestive tract. *Current Opinion in Otolaryngology Head and Neck Surgery*, Vol.12, No. 4, (August 2004), pp. 305-310, ISSN 1068-9508.

Vries JPM, Acosta R, Soutar DS & Webster MHC. (1996) Recovery of sensation in the radial forearm free flap in oral reconstruction. *Plastic Reconstructive Surgery*, Vol 98, No. 4, (September 1996), pp. 649-656, ISSN 0032-1052.

Yoleri L, Mavioglu H. (2000) Total tongue reconstruction with free functional gracilis muscle transplantation: a technical note and review of the literature. *Annals of Plastic Surgery*, Vol. 45, No. 2, (August 2000), pp. 181-186, ISSN 0148-7043.

13

Management of Early-Stage Tongue Cancer

Kiyoto Shiga, Katsunori Katagiri,
Ayako Nakanome, Takenori Ogawa and Toshimitsu Kobayashi
Department of Otolaryngology-Head and Neck Surgery, Tohoku University Hospital, Japan

1. Introduction

In general, tongue cancer is usually treated surgically and additional therapy is carried out if patients have advanced cancers. Although surgical treatment is performed at the early stage of tongue cancer, still some problems emerge, such as late cervical lymph node metastasis and elective neck dissection. We previously recommended elective neck dissection for patients with T2 tongue cancers (Tateda et al., 2000). However, the range of tumor sizes that would require elective neck dissection remains to be determined.

Between 2001 and 2005, a total of 43 patients with oral tongue cancers were treated at Tohoku University Hospital. As for our patients with T2 N0 cancer, the pathological examination results revealed that 3 (43%) of the 7 patients who underwent elective neck dissection (late T2) had a lymph node metastasis. On the other hand, 4 of the 6 patients who did not undergo elective neck dissection in the first surgery (early T2) had a recurrence at the neck. In total, 7 (54%) of the 13 patients who were found to have T2 N0 tongue cancers developed lymph node metastases after the initial treatment. When there was a regional recurrence, salvage therapies were conducted. However, 3 of the 4 patients with early T2 who had a regional recurrence died of the disease. These data indicate that elective neck dissection should be considered for treating patients with T2 N0 tongue cancer to improve the poor prognoses associated with not undergoing elective neck dissection. We also investigated the relationship between nodal metastasis and tumor diameter and depth of tumor invasion. There was a significant difference between the frequency of the nodal metastasis in the patients with tumors less than 4 mm in depth and that in patients with tumors greater than 4 mm in depth, indicating that the depth of the tumor invasion is a critical factor for lymph node metastasis (Shiga et al., 2007).

Since 2005, we had been treating patients with T2 N0 tongue cancers by surgical removal of the tumor, that is, partial glossectomy and elective neck dissection. The improvement of the treatment results and the prognoses of the patients with early-stage oral tongue cancers are described and discussed.

2. Background

Tongue cancer is the most common type of oral cancer worldwide, and the majority of cases are defined as early cancer lesions. Because a standardized treatment strategy has not yet been developed, various therapies such as surgery, brachytherapy, chemotherapy, and radiation therapy are chosen to treat patients with tongue cancers in different hospitals. In our hospital, tongue cancer is usually treated surgically and additional therapy is conducted for patients with advanced clinical stage diseases. Elective neck dissection as a treatment for patients with early-stage oral tongue cancers and clinically normal necks remains a controversial issue (Haddadin et al., 1999; Hughes et al., 1993; Keski-Santti et al., 2006; O'Brien et al., 1986; Veness et al., 2005; Yuen et al., 1997). Several reports have described the results of immediate elective neck dissection versus delayed elective neck dissection, that is, performing the surgery after the patient is observed or watched to have developed of early-stage N0 tongue cancers, and it has been reported that the survival rate of "watched" patients was worse than that of patients having elective neck dissection (Cunningham et al., 1986; Ho et al., 1992; Lydiatt et al., 1993; Persky and Lagmay, 1999; Yuen et al 1997).

There have been several reports about histopathological parameters that predict neck metastasis of tongue cancer. Among these parameters, tumor thickness and depth of invasion have been studied and have often been documented (Asakage et al., 1998; Brown et al., 1989; Byers et al., 1998; Fukano et al., 1997; Jones et al., 1992; Lim et al., 2004; Rasgon et al., 1989; Sparano et al., 2004; Spiro et al., 1986). However, indications for elective neck dissection according to tumor thickness or depth of invasion have not yet been previously reported. Perhaps this is because of the clinical difficulty in accurately measuring tumor thickness and depth of invasion before the initial treatment.

We investigated the size of tongue cancers that require neck dissection. In our study from 2001 through 2005, the patients with N0 tumors smaller than 30 mm in diameter (T1 and early T2) underwent only partial glossectomy. The patients with N0 tumors larger than 30 mm in diameter (late T2) underwent partial glossectomy and elective neck dissection. As described in the following discussion, the patients with early T2 tumor had poorer outcomes because they had regional recurrences and distant metastases. In our study after 2005, the patients with T2 N0 tumors underwent partial glossectomy and elective neck dissection and showed remarkably better prognoses.

In addition, our results indicated that tumor thickness is a critical indicator of cervical lymph node metastasis in patients with T1 or T2 tongue cancers because a significant difference was observed even in our small number of patients.

3. 2001 series

3.1 Patients and methods

Between November 2001 and June 2005, 43 patients with tongue carcinomas were treated at the Tohoku University Hospital. None of the patients had distant metastasis at the time of first admission to the hospital. The tumors were defined according to the TNM classification by clinical examination, and computed tomographic (CT) scan and/or magnetic resonance imaging (MRI) findings. There were 8 patients with T1 N0 tumors (stage I) and 13 patients with T2 N0 tumors (stage II). There were 26 male and 17 female patients. The median patient age was 59 years (range, 24–86 years). All but 1 of the patients were found to have squamous cell carcinomas by histopathological examination. One patient with a T1 N0 tumor had a verrucous carcinoma of the tongue.

In our hospital, the initial treatment for early-stage tongue cancer is surgical resection of the primary tumor, that is, partial glossectomy with or without neck dissection. The neck dissection conducted for the patients with late T2 N0 tumors was supraomohyoid neck dissection (SOND). If a recurrent tumor was found in the neck after the surgery in the patients who did not undergo neck dissection at the first surgery, a neck dissection was conducted if possible. If a surgical resection was not possible, the patients were treated mainly by radiation therapy. If distant metastases were found, the patients were treated mainly by chemotherapy by using Docetaxel, cisplatin, and 5-fluorouracil.

The statistical analyses of the data were performed by the chi-square test and the Student *t* test. All the follow-up data were updated at the end of May 2006. The survival curves of the patients were calculated using the Kaplan–Meier method based on the first day of the patients' admission to the hospital. The survival curves were subjected to a log-rank test and the generalized Wilcoxon test.

3.2 Results

The characteristics and the outcomes of the patients with T1 N0 tumors were evaluated. One patient had a recurrent tumor in the ipsilateral neck (rN1) and underwent modified radical neck dissection. The other 9 patients with T1 N0 tumors had not encountered any recurrent tumors. The characteristics and the outcomes of the patients with T2 N0 tumors were also evaluated. One patient had a recurrent tumor in the neck (N3), which was not resectable. Although the patient underwent chemoradiation therapy, the neck tumor was not controlled by the therapy, and the patient died of the disease 11 months after the first treatment. Another patient also had a recurrent neck tumor (rN2a), and she underwent radical neck dissection 7 months after the first surgery. Although her neck tumor was completely resected and she had no recurrence, she had multiple lung metastases and died 19 months after the first treatment. However, another patient also had a recurrent neck tumor (rN2b), and he underwent radical neck dissection 12 months after the first surgery. Although his neck tumor was completely resected and he had no recurrence, he had multiple brain metastases and died of the disease 25 months after the first treatment. At 40 months, as determined by the Kaplan–Meier analysis, the disease-free survival rates of the patients with T1 N0 tumors and the patients with T2 N0 tumors were 100% and 60%, respectively (Shiga et al., 2007). There were no significant differences in survival rates between these 2 groups.

The depth of invasion of the tumors and their diameters were analyzed according to the existence of lymph node metastases. The analysis included all the patients with T1 or T2 tumors (n = 15 and 15, respectively). The diameters of the tumors ranged from 7 to 38 mm (mean, 23 mm) for the tumors without lymph node metastases, whereas they ranged from 15 to 35 mm (mean, 27 mm) for the tumors with lymph node metastases. There was no significant difference in diameter between these two groups. The depths of the tumors ranged from 1 to 17 mm (mean, 7.0 mm) for tumors without lymph node metastases, whereas they ranged from 4 to 22 mm (mean, 10.3 mm) for tumors with lymph node metastases. The shortest depth of tumor invasion that led to lymph node metastasis was 4 mm, and no lymph node metastases were observed in the patients whose tumors were shorter than 4 mm in depth of invasion. There was a significant difference between the frequencies of nodal metastasis in the patients with tumors less than 4 mm thick and those of the patients with tumors greater than 4 mm thick (p = 0.013). There was no significant difference in the frequencies of lymph node metastasis between the groups according to age, sex, or histopathological differentiation of squamous cell carcinoma, except for depth of invasion.

4. 2005 series

4.1 Patients and methods

Between July 2005 and June 2010, 75 patients with tongue carcinomas were treated at the Tohoku University Hospital. One patient had distant metastasis at the time of first admission to the hospital. Table 1 shows the TN classification of the patients with T1 and T2 tumors at the time of initial treatment. The tumors were defined according to the TNM classification by clinical examination, CT scan and/or MRI findings, and ^{18}F-fluorodeoxy glucose-positron emission tomography (FDG-PET). There were 16 patients with T1 N0 tumors (stage I) and 20 patients with T2 N0 tumors (stage II). There were 49 male and 26 female patients. The mean and median patient ages were 60.3 and 62 years, respectively (range, 24-86 years). All of the patients were found to have squamous cell carcinomas by histopathological examination.

	N0	N1	N2a	N2b	N2c	N3	
T1	16	1	0	0	0	0	17
T2	20	6	0	6	1	0	33
	36	7	0	6	1	0	50

Table 1. TN classification of the patients with T1 and T2 tongue cancers.

The treatment strategy was the same as that described previously except for the T2 N0 tumors. All of the patients who initially had T2 N0 tongue cancer underwent partial glossectomy and elective neck dissection.

The statistical analyses of the data were performed by the chi-square test and the Student *t* test. All the follow-up data were updated at the end of July 2011. The survival curves of the patients were calculated using the Kaplan-Meier method based on the first day of the patient's admission to the hospital. The survival curves were subjected to a log-rank test and the generalized Wilcoxon test.

4.2 Results

The characteristics and the outcome of the patients with T2 N0 tumors are summarized in Table 2. Four patients (patients 5, 7, 11, and 12) had lymph node metastases, which were revealed by the pathological examination results after the initial surgery. Patient 5 died of lung cancer 7 months after the surgery. Patient 7 had a local recurrence 4 months after the first surgery, and he hoped to receive brachytherapy in another hospital. Patient 16 had local recurrence, and resurgery was conducted. However, she died of lung and liver metastases 7 months after the second surgery. Patient 20 had recurrent neck tumors, but she did not see doctors until the tumor was unresectable. She was provided with the best supportive care. The follow-up data of the patients during the period 2021–2005 were updated at the end of July 2011, and the disease-free survival curves of the patients were calculated by Kaplan–Meier analysis. The disease-free survival rates at 60 months of the patients with T2 N0 tumors during the period of 2001–2005 and those during the period of 2005–2010 were 71.6% and 86.7%, respectively (Figure 1). There were no significant differences in disease-free survival rates between these 2 groups.

	Age	Gender	cTN	pTN	Differen-tiation	Diameter (mm)	Depth (mm)	Outcome
1	56	M	T2N0		MOD	26	7	NER
2	55	M	T2N0		*	*	*	NER
3	70	M	T2N0		WELL	38	18	NER
4	33	M	T2N0		WELL	27	9	NER
5	75	M	T2N0	T2N2b	MOD	*	10	7M, DND (lung cancer)
6	84	M	T2N0		WELL	30	8	NER
7	31	M	T2N0	T2N1	WELL	28	11	4M, local rec
8	68	M	T2N0		WELL	35	15	NER
9	73	F	T2N0		WELL	38	11	NER
10	28	M	T2N0		MOD	23	4	NER
11	75	M	T2N0	T2N1	POOR	39	15	NER
12	62	M	T2N0	T2N1	WELL	21	5	NER
13	59	M	T2N0		WELL	25	1	NER
14	61	M	T2N0		WELL	21	6	NER
15	24	M	T2N0		WELL	37	9	NER
16	58	F	T2N0		POOR	23	12	6M, local rec, surgery, 15M,DOD (lung & liver meta)
17	80	M	T2N0		WELL	23	6	NER
18	65	M	T2N0		MOD	25	5	NER
19	42	M	T2N0		MOD	26	8	NER
20	74	F	T2N0		WELL	36	15	18M, DOD (regional rec)

WELL, well differentiated squamous cell carcinoma; MOD, moderately differentiated squamous cell carcinoma; Poor, poorly differentiated squamous cell carcinoma; NER, no evidence of recurrence; DND, died not of disease; DOD, died of disease; M, months: rec, recurrence; meta, metastases. The asterisk indicates not determined. All patients underwent supraomohyoid neck dissection at surgery.

Table 2. Clinical features of patients with T2N0 tongue cancers.

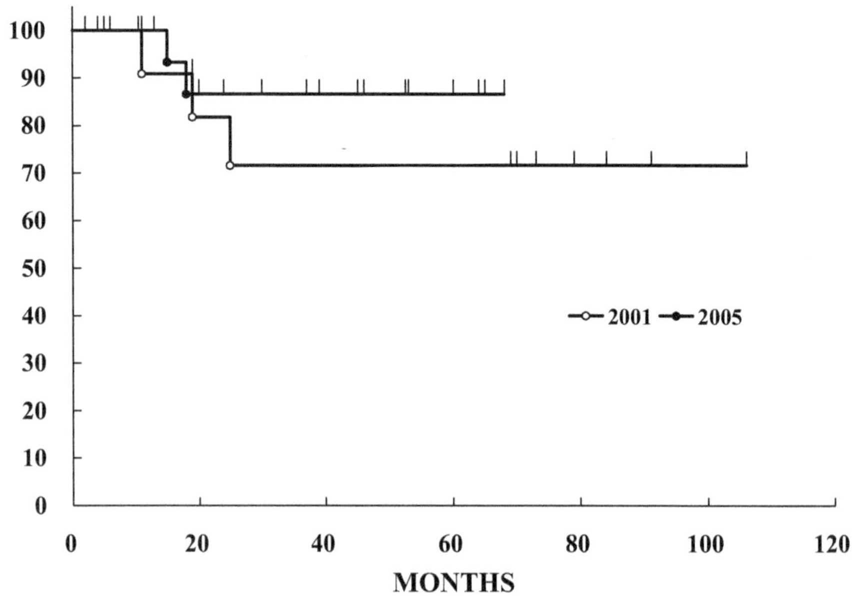

Fig. 1. Disease-free survival curve of the patients with T2 N0 tongue cancers. *Open circle*, the patients treated from 2001 to 2005; *closed circle*, the patients treated from 2005 to 2010.

5. Discussion - Management of early-stage oral tongue cancer

As for our T2 N0 cases between 2001 and 2005, the pathological examination results revealed that 3 (43%) of the 7 patients who underwent elective neck dissection (late T2) had a lymph node metastasis. On the other hand, 4 (67%) of the 6 patients who did not undergo elective neck dissection at the first surgery (early T2) had a recurrence at the neck. In total, 7 (54%) of the 13 patients who were initially found to have clinical T2 N0 tongue cancers had lymph node metastases at the time of initial treatment or afterwards. When the patients with T1 N0 and T2 N0 tumors were included, 5 (36%) of the 14 patients who did not undergo elective neck dissection at the time of the first surgery (T1 N0 + early T2 N0) had recurrences at the neck. This regional recurrence rate was as high as that reported previously (Cunningham et al., 1986; Haddadin et al., 1999; Ho et al., 1992; Keski-Santti et al., 2006; Yuen et al., 1997). When there was a regional recurrence, salvage therapies, such as neck dissection and/or radiation, and chemotherapy were conducted. Three of the 4 patients with early T2 cancer who had a regional recurrence died of the disease. The reasons for their deaths were uncontrolled regional recurrence, lung metastasis, and brain metastasis. These results indicated a poor survival rate of the patients with T2 N0 cancer in our 2001–2005 series, indicating that elective neck dissection is necessary for a good outcome in patients with T2 N0 tongue cancers. At this time, we concluded that elective neck dissection was necessary for the patients with clinical T2 N0 tumors because of the unexpectedly high incidences of regional lymph node metastases and the very poor prognoses of the patients with early T2 tumors.

In contrast to the patients with T2 N0 tumors during the period between 2001 and 2005, the recurrence of the tumors were observed in only 3 of the 20 patients with clinical T2 N0 tongue cancers in our 2005–2010 series. Two of them had a local recurrence after the initial treatment, and the other patient had a regional recurrence. The pathological examination results revealed that 20% (4 of the 20 patients) of the cases initially diagnosed as clinical T2 N0 tongue cancer had lymph node metastases, and this rate was lower than that of the cases in our 2001–2005 series. We assumed that one of the reasons why the frequencies of lymph node metastasis found by pathological examination of the surgical specimens were reduced was the introduction of the use of FDG-PET in the initial diagnostic examination of the patients with tongue cancers. We experienced some cases that were diagnosed as T2 N2c M0 tongue cancer and treated by surgery, with no lymph node metastasis found in the specimens. Although in some cases, overdiagnosis in the patients were obvious, in most of the cases, lymph node metastases were detected accurately by FDG-PET imaging. It should be revealed that accurate diagnosis is made by several modalities, such as CT scan, MRI, ultrasonography, and FDG-PET, by using these modalities effectively.

We conclude that elective neck dissection is necessary for patients with T2 N0 tumors because of the unexpectedly high frequency of regional lymph node metastases of T2 N0 tumors and the very poor prognoses of patients with early T2 tumors who did not undergo elective neck dissection.

As described in previous studies, the focus was on tumor thickness and depth of invasion as histopathological parameters that predict neck metastases of tongue cancers. There have been studies well documented in several literatures (Asakage et al 1998; Brown et al 1989; Byers et al 1998; Fukano et al 1997; Jones et al 1992; Lim et al 2004; Rasgon et al 1989; Sparano et al 2004; Spiro et al., 1986). However, indications for elective neck dissection according to tumor thickness or depth of invasion have not been previously reported. Perhaps this is because of the clinical difficulty in accurately measuring tumor thickness and depth of invasion before the initial treatment. Indeed, as a significant difference was observed even in our small number of patients, tumor thickness is a critical indicator of cervical lymph node metastasis in patients with T1 or T2 tongue cancers. There were some probes engineered using ultrasound sonography to detect tumors in oral cavities (Kodama et al., 2010; Yuen et al., 2008). We think these new modalities of ultrasound sonography and MRI findings are the powerful tools for detecting tumor thickness or depth of invasion of the tumors in the oral cavity. Investigating tumor thickness or depth of invasion before surgery, we could appropriately indicate surgery for patients with N0 tongue cancers. If the tumor is thick or invasion is deep, we must conduct elective neck dissection for the patients, even for those with T1 N0 tongue cancers.

6. Conclusion

Elective neck dissection is needed for patients with T2 N0 tongue cancers to reduce the rate of recurrence and improve the prognosis of the patients. At the same time, accurate diagnosis of the lymph node metastasis of the patients by several modalities including FDG-PET should be made to reduce the rate of misdiagnosis. Depth of the invasion of the tumor is a critical marker for the lymph node metastasis of patients with tongue cancers.

7. References

Asakage, T., Yokose, T., Mukai, K., Tsugane, S., Tsubono, Y., Asai, M., & Ebihara, S. (1998). Tumor thickness predicts cervical metastasis in patients with stage I/II carcinoma of the tongue. *Cancer*, Vol. 82, No. 8, (April 1998), pp. 1443-1448, ISSN 1097-0142

Brown, B., Barnes, L., Mazariegos, J., Taylor, F., Johnson, J., & Wagner, R.L. (1989). Prognostic factors in mobile tongue and floor of mouth carcinoma. *Cancer*, Vol. 64, No. 6, (September 1989), pp. 1195-1202, ISSN 1097-0142

Byers, R.M., El-Naggar, A.K., Lee, Y.Y., Rao, B., Fornage, B., Terry, N.H., Sample, D., Hankins, P., Smith, T.L., & Wolf, P.J. (1998). Can we detect or predict the presence of occult nodal metastases in patients with squamous cell carcinoma of the oral tongue? *Head & Neck*, Vol. 20, No. 2, (March 1998), pp. 138-144, ISSN 1097-0347

Cunningham, M.J., Johnson, J.T., Myers, E.N., Schramm, V.L. Jr., & Thearle, P.B. (1986). Cervical lymph node metastasis after local excision of early squamous cell carcinoma of the oral cavity. *American Journal of Surgery*, Vol. 152, No. 4, (October 1986), pp. 361-366, ISSN 0002-9610.

Fukano, H., Matsuura, H., Hasegawa, Y., & Nakamura, S. (1997). Depth of invasion as a predictive factor for cervical lymph node metastasis in tongue carcinoma. *Head & Neck*, Vol. 19, No. 3, (May 1997), pp. 205-210, ISSN 1097-0347

Haddadin, K.J., Souter, D.S., Oliver, R.J., Webster, M.H., Robertson, A.G., & MacDonald, D.G. (1999). Improved survival for patients with clinically T1/T2, N0 tongue tumors undergoing a prophylactic neck dissection. *Head & Neck*, Vol. 21, No. 6, (September 1999), pp. 517-525, ISSN 1097-0347

Ho, C.M., Lam, K.H., Wei, W.I., Lau S.K., & Lam, L.K. (1992). Occult lymph node metastasis in small oral tongue cancers. *Head & Neck*, Vol. 14, No. 5, (September-October 1992), pp. 359-363, ISSN 1097-0347

Hughes, C.J., Gallo, O., Spiro, R.H., & Shah, J.P. (1993). Management of occult neck metastases in oral cavity squamous cell carcinoma. *American Journal of Surgery*, Vol. 166, No. 4, (October 1993), pp. 380-383, ISSN 0002-9610

Jones, K.R., Lodge-Rigal, R.D., Reddick, R.L., Tudor, G.E., & Shockley, W.W. (1992). Prognostic factors in the recurrence of stage I and II squamous cell cancer of the oral cavity. *Archives of Otolaryngology – Head & Neck Surgery*, Vol. 118, No. 5, (May 1992), pp. 483-485, ISSN 0886-4470

Keski-Santti, H., Atula, T., Tornwall, J., Koivunen, P., & Makitie A. (2006). Elective neck treatment versus observation in patients with T1/T2 N0 squamous cell carcinoma of oral tongue. *Oral Oncology*, Vol. 42, No. 1, (January 2006), pp. 96-101, ISSN 1368-8375

Kodama, M., Khanal, A., Habu, M., Iwanaga, K., Yoshioka, I., Tanaka, T., Morimoto, Y., & Tominaga, K. (2010). Ultrasonography for intraoperative determination of tumor thickness and resection margin in tongue carcinomas. *Journal of Oral and Maxillofacial Surgery*, Vol. 68, No. 8, (August 2010), pp. 1746-1752, ISSN 0278-2391

Lim, S.C., Zhang, S., Ishii, G., Endoh, Y., Kodama, K., Miyamoto, S., Hayashi, R., Ebihara, S., Cho, J.S., & Ochiai, A. (2004). Predictive markers for late cervical metastasis in stage I and II invasive squamous cell carcinoma of the oral tongue. *Clinical Cancer Research*, Vol. 10, No. 1, (January 2004), pp. 166-172, ISSN 1078-0432

Lydiatt, D.D., Robbins, K.T., Byers R.M., & Wolf, P.F. (1993). Treatment of stage I and II oral tongue cancer. *Head & Neck*, Vol. 15, No. 4, (July-August 1993), pp. 308-312, ISSN 1097-0347

O'Brien, C.J., Lahr, C.J., Soong, S.J., Gandour, M.J., Jones, J.M., Urist, M.M., & Maddox, W.A. (1986). Surgical treatment of early-stage carcinoma of the oral tongue—would adjuvant treatment be beneficial? *Head & Neck Surgery*, Vol. 8, No. 6, (July-August 1986), pp. 401-408, ISSN 0148-6403.

Persky, M.S., & Lagmay, V.M. (1999). Treatment of the clinically negative neck in oral squamous cell carcinoma. *Laryngoscope*, Vol. 109, No. 1, (July 1999), pp. 1160-1164, ISSN 1531-4995.

Rasgon, B.M., Cruz, R.M., Hilsinger, R.L. Jr., & Sawicki, J.E. (1989) Relationship of lymph-node metastasis to histopathologic appearance in oral cavity and oropharyngeal carcinoma: a case series and literature review. *Laryngoscope*, Vol. 99, No. 11, (November 1989), pp. 1103-1110, ISSN 1531-4995

Shiga, K., Ogawa, T., Sagai, S., Kato, K.,& Kobayashi, T. (2007) Management of the patients with early stage oral tongue cancers. *The Tohoku Journal of Experimental Medicine*, Vol. 212, No. 4, (August 2007), pp. 389-396, ISSN 0040-8727

Sparano, A., Weinstein, G., Chalian, A, Yodul, M., & Weber, R. (2004). Multivariate predictors of occult neck metastasis in early oral tongue cancer. *Otolaryngology – Head & Neck Surgery*, Vol. 131, No. 4, (October 2004), pp. 472-476, ISSN 0886-4470

Spiro, R.H., Huvos, A.G., Wong, G.Y., Spiro, J.D., Gnecco, C.A., & Strong, E.W. (1986). Predictive value of tumor thickness in squamous cell carcinoma confined to the tongue and floor of the mouth. *American Journal of Surgery*, Vol. 152, No. 4, (October 1986), pp. 345-350, ISSN 0002-9610

Tateda, M., Shiga, K., Saijo, S., & Yokoyama, J. (2000). A clinical study of oral tongue cancer. *The Tohoku Journal of Experimental Medicine*, Vol. 192, No. 1, (September 2000), pp. 49-59, ISSN 0040-8727

Veness, M.J., Morgan, G.J., Sathiyaseelan, Y., & Gebski, V. (2005). Anterior tongue cancer and the incidence of cervical lymph node metastases with increasing tumor thickness: should elective treatment to the neck be standard practice in all patients? *ANZ Journal of Surgery*, Vol. 75, No. 3, (March 2005), pp. 101-105, ISSN 1445-1433

Yuen, A.P., Wei, W.I., Wong, Y.M., & Tang, K.C. (1997). Elective neck dissection versus observation in the treatment of early oral tongue carcinoma. *Head & Neck*, Vol. 19, No. 7, (October 1997), pp. 583-588, ISSN 1097-0347

Yuen, A.P.O., Ng, R.W.M., Lam, P.K.Y., & Ho, A. (2008). Preoperative measurement of tumor thickness of oral tongue carcinoma with intraoral ultrasonography. *Head & Neck*, Vol. 30, No. 2, (February 2008), pp. 230-234, ISSN 1097-0347

14

Blood Groups and Oral Lesions Diagnostics

Carlos Campi, Livia Escovich, Liliana Racca,
Amelia Racca, Carlos Cotorruelo and Claudia Biondi
National University of Rosario
Argentina

1. Introduction

Cancer incidence in humans has gradually increased over the last century. Surgical, radio, chemotherapeutic and biological treatments have experienced important advances, with concomitant reduction in the morbidity associated with the radical surgical practices of the past. The term "oral cancer" includes a diverse group of tumors arising from the oral cavity (Khalili, 2008). Usually included are cancers of the lip, tongue, pharynx, and oral cavity. The World Health Organization (WHO) reported oral cancer as having one of the highest mortality ratios amongst all malignancies (Parkin et al., 2000). Although oral cancer is rare and attracts little attention, it is more common than Hodgkin's disease tumours of brain, liver, bone, thyroid gland, stomach, ovaries, or cancer of the cervix. It ranks 12th among all cancers (Jemal et al., 2002). The vast majority of malignant neoplasms in the mouth are squamous cell carcinomas. Oral cancer incidence and mortality rates vary widely across the world. Mortality rate is an important tool that provides implicit information about incidence, diagnosis stage, solving capacity of health services, available technology and health programs to be applied. Although globally oral cancer represents an incidence of 3% (males) and 2% (females) of all malignant neoplasm, it has one of the lowest survival rates – 50 percent, within a five-year period (Greenlee et al., 2001).

It is important to diagnose oral cancer in its early stages, since the management of small and localized tumors involves less morbidity and mortality than more advanced-stage disease, where treatment must be more aggressive. Indeed, the stage in which the disease is diagnosed is directly correlated to long-term survival. (Onizawa et al., 2003). It is generally accepted that when diagnosed in its early stages, a favorable prognosis is expected, with a survival rate exceeding 90% at the 5-year follow-up. However, reviewing the literature exposes a less optimistic picture, because lymph node metastases seem to occur in 5% to 20% of cases (Regev et al., 1992, Khalili, 2008). However, in practice many malignancies are diagnosed and treated in advanced stages and/or once the patients have already experienced symptoms causing them to seek medical help. This explains the great interest in improving multidisciplinary therapies, and particularly in establishing more reliable techniques for diagnosing and prognosis of the illness (Miller & Kearney N, 2001).

The membrane, which defines the extent of the cell, is not only a physical boundary but also has many specific functions, among which is the capacity to react with other cells and the intracellular matrix (Ebnet & Vestweber, 1999, Hascall, 2000). Carbohydrates are structures found on the cell surface bound to either lipid or protein embedded in the membrane.

Changes in the carbohydrate structure of these cell-surface glycolipids and glycoproteins have been demonstrated during development, during cell maturation in adult tissue, and in relationship to malignant development.

Biochemical and molecular genetic studies have contributed to our molecular knowledge of blood group-associated molecules in the past few years (Dabelsteen, 1996, Fenderson et al., Fukuda, 2002, 1986, Hakomori, 1999, 2002, 2003, Le Pendu *et al.*, 2001). Among the 30 blood group systems presently identified, almost all have a molecular basis and present investigations are oriented towards the analysis of genetic polymorphisms, tissue-specific expression and structure-function relationships. Antigens defined by carbohydrate structures, among which ABO, Hh, Lewis and Secretor are the main representative species, are indirect gene products (Hakomori *et al.*, 1967). They are synthesized by Golgi-resident glycosyltransferases, which are the direct products of the blood group genes. Cell-surface carbohydrates are built up in a stepwise fashion when monosaccharides are tranferred from their sugar nucleotide derivatives to appropriate acceptors. Each particular type of transfer is catalyzed by a unique specific glycosyltransferase. In tumors, changes in glycosylation are found in both glycolipids and glycoproteins (Hakomori, 1999; Le Pendu *et al.*, 2001). Most studies have dealt with alteration of carbohydrates at the cell surface. However, several recent studies have shown that altered glycosylation plays a major role in most aspects of the malignant phenotype, including signal transduction and apoptosis. These studies have recently been reviewed (Hakomori, 2002; Hakomori & Handa, 2002, Dabelsteen & Gao, 2004). Historical studies associating the Lewis system antigens and/or ABH system secretory antigens with disease are varied and generally inconclusive. Critical analysis of these studies reveals that in many instances the serology is inadequate, mainly as a result of unappreciated difficulties in accurately phenotyping diseased individuals (Svensson, 2000).

Before a detailed account of the immunochemistry and genetics is presented, a brief summary will be given in order to orient the general reader. The A and B antigens were originally detected on erythrocytes by means of isoagglutinins in the serum of persons lacking these determinants. These antigens are synthesized from a common intermediate, H substance, by addition of a single sugar to the non reducing end of H oligosaccharide chains, and the immunologic reactivity of the H antigen is markedly decreased by the additional sugar. Group O erythrocytes and the saliva of group O secretors contain the H antigen. Even though the O antigen does not exist, the designation group O erythrocytes have been retained for historical reasons. The blood group H antigen is an oligosaccharide molecule whose expression is normally restricted to the surfaces of human erythrocytes and a variety of epithelial cells, including those that line the gastrointestinal, urinary, and respiratory tracts (Larsen et al. 1990). The H antigen is a fucosylated structure of the form Fucal-2Galf3-, whose expression is determined by GDP-L-fucose:P-D-galactoside 2-a-L-fucosyltransferases [a(1,2)Frs; EC 2.4.1.69]. These enzymes catalyze a transglycosylation reaction between their sugar nucleotide substrate GDP-L-fucose and oligosaccharide acceptor substrates with terminal type I (Gal81-3GlcNAc-) or type II (Gal, 81-4GlcNAc-) moieties. The secretor status is defined by the presence of H type 1 antigen in body secretions such as milk and saliva. H type 1 antigen belongs to both the Lewis and the ABO(H) histo-blood-group systems and is expressed in erythrocyte membranes and in several epithelial tissues, namely the gastricmucosa, the upper respiratory tract and the lower genito-urinary tract. Approximately 75 per cent of white persons secrete glycoproteins containing the same A, B or H antigens present on their erythrocytes (Moreno et al., 2009).

The Lewis antigens, Le^a and Le^b, are also found on erythrocytes and glycoproteins. These antigens appear on the same glycoproteins as the ABH determinants, but their synthesis is regulated by the independent gene *Le*. The operation of these independent genes on a common substrate results in a complex phenotypic interaction (Henry et al., 1995).

It is well established that the large array of functions that a tumour cell has to fulfill to settle as a metastasis in a distant organ requires cooperative activities between the tumour and the surrounding tissue and that several classes of molecules are involved, such as cell-cell and cell-matrix adhesion molecules and matrix degrading enzymes, to name only a few. Cell adhesion molecules are found on the surfaces of all cells, where they bind to extracellular matrix molecules or to receptors on other cells. Cell adhesion is critical in the dynamic processes necessary for tissue morphogenesis in development and the maintenance of complex differentiated tissues in adult organisms. Adhesion molecules have originally been thought to be essential for the formation of multicellular organisms and to tether cells to the extracellular matrix or to neighbouring cells (Marhaba & Zöller, 2004). CDD44 is the major human cell surface receptor for hyaluronate and functions in a diverse range of physiological processes. CD44 may play a role in stimulating *in vivo* aggressiveness of tumors through hyaluronate-rich stroma (Hudson et al., 1996). Expression of CD44 has been described to correlate with metastasis formation in various tumors, although evidence in oral cavity cancers is inconclusive.

2. ABO antigens

Although the ABO blood group antigens were initially identified as erythrocyte substances with a significance mainly ascribed to serology, it soon became clear that these antigens were found on most epithelial cells and in secretions (Landsteiner, 1900). These ABH antigens are carbohydrate antigens which in epithelia are expressed in a highly regulated way that correlates with the pattern of epithelial differentiation and with cell maturation (Ravn & Dabelsteen, 2000).

Profound changes in expression have been documented during epithelial cell migration in wound healing and in pathological processes such as malignant development, including oral carcinoma (Dabelsteen, 1996, Dabelsteen et al., 1998, Hakomori, 1996, Le Pendu et al., 2001). Tumor progression is often associated with altered glycosylation of the cell-surface proteins and lipids (Hakomori, 1996). The peripheral parts of these cell-surface glycoconjugates often carries many of the target molecules that reside in blood are also present in oral fluids, albeit at lower concentrations. Oral fluids are, however, relatively easy and safe to collect without the need for specialized equipment and training. Thus, oral fluids provide convenient samples for medical diagnostics, carbohydrate structures related to the ABO and Lewis blood-group antigens. The expression of histo-blood-group antigens in normal human tissues is dependent on the type of differentiation of the epithelium. In most human carcinomas, including oral carcinoma, a significant event is the decreased expression of histo-blood-group antigens A and B (Hakomori, 1999). The mechanisms of aberrant expression of blood-group antigens are not clear in all cases (Hamokori & Handa 2002, Le Pendu et al., 2001, Gao 2004a, 2004b). A relative down-regulation of the glycosyltransferase that is involved in the biosynthesis of A and B antigens is seen in oral carcinomas in association with tumor development (Hakomori, 1999, Le Pendu et al., 2001). However, several recent studies have shown that altered glycosylation plays a major role in most aspects of the malignant phenotype, including signal transduction and apoptosis. Studies of associations between various cancers and the ABO blood groups have shown elevated relative risks for some categories of disease (Campi et al., 2007, Khalil, 2008).

To investigate the association of expression of ABH antigens and oral cancer, we conducted a study of premalignant lesions and diagnosed malignant tumors. The patients analyzed in this study presented to the Stomatology Department of The Odontology Faculty of the National University of Rosario, Argentina during two years. In total 132 subjects were examined, half of whom suffered from oral pre-cancerous and cancerous lesions, while the other half were the control group (benign lesions: mucosceles, papiloma, etc). All of them were subjected to clinical oral examinations. In the group of patients with oral pre-cancerous and cancerous lesions (experimental group), a pathohistological examination of the oral mucosa was performed (Biondi et al., 2008).

All biopsies were fixed in 4% buffered formaldehyde, paraffin embedded, sectioned at 4μm, and stained with hematoxilyn and eosin. Sections (4 μm) from the tumor biopsies were placed on gelatine-coated slides. Sections were deparaffinized in xylene and brought to water through graded ethanol (100%).

2.1 Specific red cell adherence test

Specific red cell adherence test was performed on paraffin embedded sections to detect the intensity of isoantigens A, B and H (O) on the epithelial cell surface by a three layer sandwich technique, as described in (Vengelen-Tyler, V. 2002, Strauchen et al., 1980). Commercially available Anti A, Anti B, and Anti AB antisera from Span Diagnostic Limited and *Ulex europaeus* lectin (Anti H) were used. Slides of 4-5 micron section were deparaffinized and brought to water, immersed in Tris buffered saline 0.05 M (pH 7.4) for 30 minutes, covered with isologous antisera according to patients' blood group, and incubated for one hour with Anti- A, -B and -O antisera in a moist chamber at room temperature. The slides were then dipped in Tris buffered saline three times with occasional stirring to remove the unreacted antisera. A few drops of 2-5% isologous indicator RBC's suspension were added to the sections and incubated for 20 minutes in group A or B and one hour for group O. The slides were inverted over a support in a petridish containing Tris buffered saline such that the undersurface of the slide just touched the solution, and kept for five minutes to settle unreacted RBCs down. The slides were observed under low power magnification and photographed immediately.

Normal tissues containing blood group antigens, endothelium of blood vessels and RBCs acted as inbuilt positive controls, and adipose tissues acted as inbuilt negative controls.

In the present study the isoantigenicity of the epithelium was graded according to degree of adherence of indicator RBCs as strongly positive adherence (++++) to negative adherence (-). Intermediate levels were graded as + for 25% of adherence, ++ for 50% of adherence, and +++ for 75% of adherence.

The immunoadherence reaction to tissue sections using antibodies and red blood cells showed a significant loss of A, B or H antigens related to the stage of tumor development and the histological grade of malignancy (Table 1).

In the tissue sections studied, the endothelium of blood vessels was reactive with the erythrocytes (positive control), and adipose tissues did not react with the red blood cells (negative controls). Loss of A, B, and H antigens from the surface of red blood cells was observed in patients with oral malignancy (89,4%), while the other 10,6% conserved the ABH expression. 39.4 % of the benign lesions which were diagnosed anatomophatologically lost the antigenic reactivity.

	PRECANCEROUS CANCEROUS	BENIGN LESIONS
Parcial or total deletion	59	26
Antigenic conservation	7	40

Table 1. Expression of the ABH antigens in fixed tissue sections of oral lesions

Blood-group antigens can be present on key receptors controlling cell proliferation, adhesion, and motility, such as epidermal growth factor receptor, integrins, cadherins, and CD44 (Gao et al., 2004). The expression patterns of these various receptors differ according to the type of normal epithelium and the type of cancer, and therefore the role of ABH antigens in the biology of human cancers may also vary. The function of the expression of ABO antigens in normal stratified oral epithelium is unclear.

In routine diagnostic histopathology, classification of tumor type is based on the histological appearance of the most differentiated parts of the tumor. The prognosis of the tumor, on the other hand, is based partly on properties within the less differentiated parts. In most cases, the degree of differentiation is determined by cellular and tissue morphology and by the ability of the cells to synthesize certain specific products such as keratin and mucins. It has previously been demonstrated that the expression of cell surface carbohydrates in oral stratified epithelium is related to cell differentiation (Ravn & Dabelsteen, 1999). Most studies have dealt with alteration of carbohydrates at the cell surface.

The results we obtained have demonstrated that the patients examined showing benign lesions expressed the ABH antigens in the tissues analyzed but there were significant differences in the experimental group (Fig.1, 2). We also found a higher intensity of oral disease in the group with total ABH deletion, and the occurrence of epithelial dysplasia was most frequently found in this group. Within the most invasive tumors sites, a deletion of ABH reactivity correlated significantly with the stage of tumor development and histological malignancy grade.

In the sections studied, the endothelium of blood vessels was reactive with the erythrocytes (positive control) and adipose tissues did not react with the red blood cells (negative controls).

We used the loss of the expression of ABH antigens as a marker of differentiation.

As the expression of these antigens can be detected by monoclonal antibodies, they are a better objective marker of differentiation than the more commonly used subjective histological assessment. The presence or absence of blood group antigens has been used to predict the clinical course of patients with superficial transitional cell carcinoma of the bladder (Foresto et al., 2000). The red-cell adherence test has been the most widely accepted method of antigen determination, but this technique has inherent weaknesses. Recently, the immunoperoxidase assay has been used to detect antigens on tumor cells. We compared patients using the red-cell adherence and immunoperoxidase methods on adjacent micro cut sections. The red-cell adherence and immunoperoxidase methods performed similarly (89%) when assessing the presence or absence of antigen (Boileau et al., 1985).

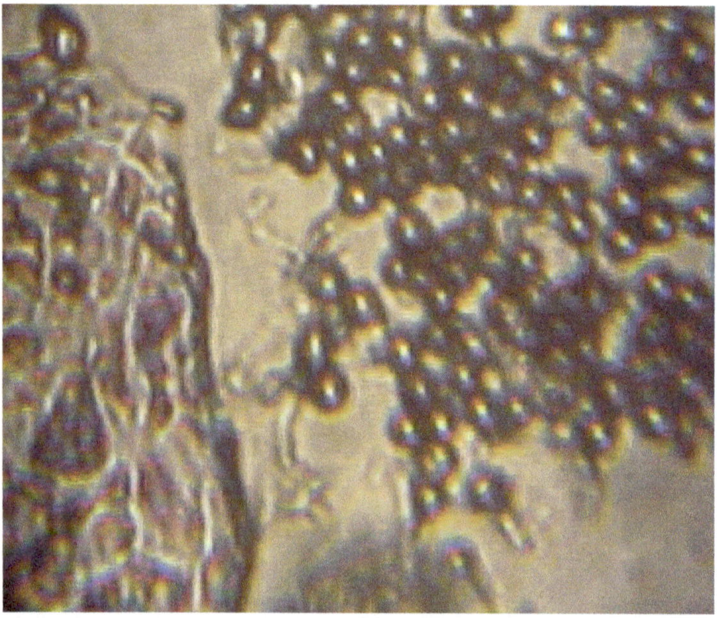

Fig. 1. Cancerous lesion: non inmunoadherence of red blood cells

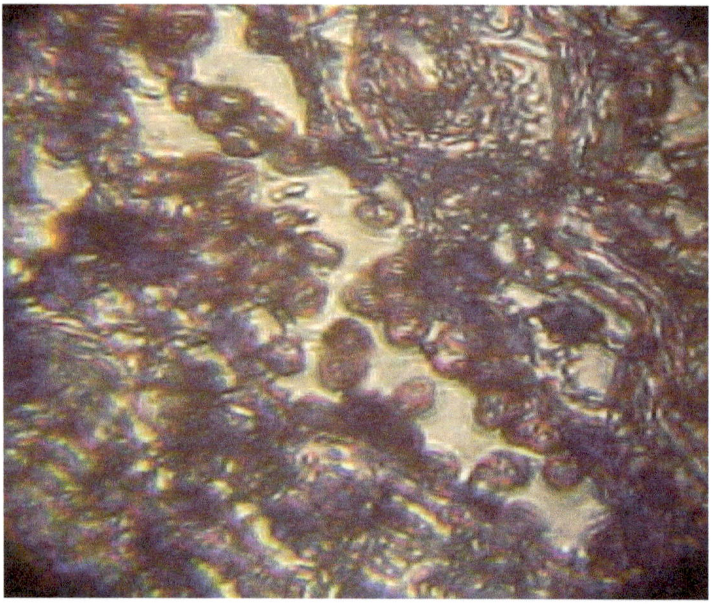

Fig. 2. Oral benign lesion: inmunoadherence of red blood cells to the tissue

Oral cancer often develops clinically as a two stage process, the first step being the appearance of a potentially malignant lesion and the second step the development of carcinoma. Leukoplakia and erythroplakia are clinical changes in the oral mucosa regarded as potentially malignant lesions (Gao et al., 2004). It is generally accepted that tumors are composed of heterogeneous cell populations with different biological behaviors. To obtain optimal prognostic information about the tumor, therefore, the entire tumor cell population should be studied. Despite the somewhat non representative nature of the biopsy material, it was possible to show that loss of ABH antigens was associated with the spread of tumor (stage). This could be of diagnostic and prognostic value.

Immunohistochemical studies of oral squamous cell carcinomas have shown loss of expression of A or B antigens in more than 80% of cases, all of which showed concomitant loss of A/B transferase (Gao et al., 2004a, 2004b). Studies of potentially malignant lesions have shown loss of A/B antigen in most lesions with epithelial dysplasia and in half of the lesions clinically. In the normal oral cavity, keratinized epithelium in the palate or gingiva shows little or no expression of A or B blood group antigen. Since a change from a non-keratinized to a keratinized differentiation pattern is a characteristic of many oral carcinomas and potentially malignant lesions, the lack of expression of blood-group antigens in such lesions could be due to a change in the differentiation pattern of the epithelium (Ravn & Dabelsteen, 2000, Dabelsteen et al., 1975). Other study has showed that the sequential expression of antigen is lost in carcinomas but retained in lesions with epithelial dysplasia and in lesions which clinically and histologically are regarded as benign. It also showed that although the sequential expression of carbohydrate antigens are retained in lesions with epithelial dysplasia, these lesions differ from normal and benign lesions due to an extended distribution of one of the carbohydrate structures (Dabelsteen et al, 1988). Some findings have also demonstrated that malignant development in stratified oral epithelium is associated with aberrant glycosylation of cellular glycoconjugates and that there are differences between premalignant lesions and carcinomas which may prove to be of diagnostic significance (Dabelsteen et al, 1988).

3. Secretor status and Lewis histo-blood group antigens

Although the ABO blood group antigens were initially identified, by Landsteiner, as erythrocyte substances with a significance mainly ascribed to serology, it soon became clear that these antigens were found on most epithelial cells and in secretions. Today the molecular and genetic basis of the ABH and Lewis systems and the associated secretory phenotypes has been resolved (Kelly 1995). The secretor gene (*FUT2*) codes for an α(1,2)fucosyltransferase that determines the ABH secretor status and influences the Lewis phenotype of an individual. The secretor status is defined by the presence of H type 1 antigen in body secretions such as milk and saliva H type 1 antigen belongs to both the Lewis and the ABO(H) histo-blood-group systems and is expressed in erythrocyte membranes and in several epithelial tissues, namely the gastricmucosa, the upper respiratory tract and the lower genito-urinary tract (Torrado, et al., 2000). Although the synthesis of H type 1 antigen is dependent on the sequential action of several glycosyltransferases, the secretor enzyme (FUT2), an *a*-1,2-fucosyltransferase, is responsible for the transfer of fucose in an *a*-1,2 linkage to form the terminal H type 1 structure (Oriol et al., 1986) .

The Lewis histo-blood group antigens Lewis a (Le^a) and Lewis b (Le^b) are carbohydrate structures that form epitopes on glycolipids and glycoproteins (Nishihara et al., 1994). Two independent genes determine the Lewis phenotype; the Lewis gene (*Le* and *le*), and the secretor gene (*Se* and *se*). Conventional Lewis blood grouping is difficult (e.g., in cancer patients and pregnant women) because of the presence of nongenuine Lewis negative individuals (Ørntoft, et al., 1991). The secretor status in Lewis-negative individuals is currently determined by a labor-intensive hemagglutination inhibition technique that uses heatinactivated saliva. In Lewis positive individuals, the secretor status is deduced from the Lewis phenotype: i.e.: Le(a-b+) individuals are secretors, and Le(a+b-) individuals are nonsecretors (Nishihara et al., 1994). The ABO blood group antigens are among the well-known fucosylated glycans. The expression of them is regulated by several glycosyltransferases that add monosaccharides to a precursor molecule in a sequential fashion (Mandel et al., 1992). The α(l,2) fucosyltransferase that forms the H antigen, an essential precursor of the A and B antigens, plays a regulatory role in the tissue expression of the ABO antigens.

The expression and secretion of ABO antigens in epithelial cells are controlled by secretortype α(l,2)fucosyltransferase activity, known as the Secretor (Se) transferase (*FUT2* gene product) (Narimatsu et al., 1996). Several different polymorphisms are known in the *FUT2* gene, some called as silent mutations, while others as to non-functional enzymes. Homozygous individuals with non-functional enzymes are termed non-secretors (se_/_). About 20% of individuals are non secretors who fail to express the ABO antigen in saliva. On the other hand, heterozygous individuals carrying one functional allele, have secretion similar to the wild-type. These are termed secretors (Se) (Narimatsu et al., 1996, Koda, et al., 1997).

Tumor progression is often associated with altered glycosylation of the cell-surface proteins and lipids. The peripheral part of these cell-surface glycoconjugates often carries carbohydrate structures related to the ABO and Lewis blood-group antigens. We analyzed the *FUT2* gene and Se status in patients with oral lesions (benign, pre-cancerous and cancerous lesions) in order to determine whether these factors could be a marker risk of oral cancer. In total 178 subjects were examined, half of whom suffered from oral lesions (benign, pre-cancerous and cancerous), while the other half were the healthy control group. All of them were subjected to clinical oral examinations and standard evaluation tests in order to establish the secretor status of their saliva (agglutination inhibition technique (Vengelen-Tyler, 2002). In the group of patients with oral benign, pre-cancerous and cancerous lesions (experimental group), a pathohistological examination of the oral mucosa was performed.

Patients with benign oral lesions showed hyperplasia caused by diverse agents such as infectious, inflammatory, traumatic, hormonal, and drugs. The premalignant lesions included leukoplakia and lichen planus. The malignant lesions studied were squamous cell carcinoma.

Appropriate informed consent was obtained from all subjects and all procedures were performed according to the ethical standards established by the University of Rosario.

Saline erythrocyte suspensions were used for serological studies. The Lewis phenotypes of fresh blood samples were determined by a hemagglutination method (Vengelen-Tyler, 2002), using anti-Le^a and anti-Le^b monoclonal antibodies. In order to establish the secretor status we analyzed their saliva by the agglutination inhibition technique.

3.1 Inhibition test for secretor status

Two or 3 ml of saliva were collected into wide mouthed tubes. In order to eliminate the mucine protein they were treated with thermal shocks. They were then centrifuged and the supernatants were transferred to clean test tubes and placed in a boiling water bath for 10 minutes to inactivate salivary enzymes. To 1 drop of appropriately diluted blood grouping reagent (anti-A, anti-B, or *Ulex europaeus* lectin) we added 1 drop of the patient's saliva. After incubation for 10 minutes at room temperature, we added 2 drops of 2% to 5% saline suspension of washed indicator red cells. Then, the tube was incubated for further 30 minutes and centrifuged in order to macroscopically inspect for agglutination. Agglutination of indicator cells by antibody in tubes containing saliva indicates that the saliva does not contain the corresponding antigen (non-secretor status). Failure of known antibody to agglutinate indicator cells after incubation with saliva indicates that the saliva contains the corresponding antigen (secretor status).

3.2 Molecular studies

3.2.1 DNA isolation

Genomic DNA was isolated from saliva samples. We designed a protocol for DNA extraction from these samples. They were subjected to thermal shock by successive freezing and thawing and centrifuged to work with the cell button. We used the technique CTAB-DTAB (dodecyltrimethylammoniumbromide/ cetyltrimethylammoniumbromide) adding CTAB directly without the addition of TE buffer (Yamamoto et al., 1990, Henry et al., 1995). The DNA concentration was measured spectrophotometrically at 260 nm and diluted in sterile water to a concentration of 100 ng per μL.

3.2.2 G428A polymorphism

The DNA samples were analyzed by ASO-PCR (allele specific oligonucleotid - polymerase chain reaction) with specific primers (Operon Lab) for G428 allele and the wild type allele of *FUT2* gene (Table 2). A fragment of 132 bp was amplified as described by Henry et al. (Henry et al., 1995), except for the annealing temperature modifications. According to gradient of PCR the Tm of the primers chosen was 66°C. The PCR products (132 bp) were analyzed in 2 % agarose gel containing ethidium bromide. The categorical data were examined with a X^2 test, and the ORs were calculated as measure of association.

Primers	Tm	Sequence	Specificity
FUT2-Se-428-s	68,8 °C	5'-CCGGTACCCCTGCTCGTG-3'	Se (direct)
FUT2-se-428-f	66,6 °C	5'-ACCGGTACCCCTGCTCGTA-3'	se (direct)
FUT2-all-523-as	66,7 °C	5'-CCGGCTCCCGTTCACCTG-3'	Non specific (reverse)

Table 2. Sequence of primers for the analysis of the G428A mutation

In our population the nonsense mutation (428 G-A) in the *FUT2* gene is the most frequent polymorphism. We studied the possible association between the 428 G-A in the *FUT2* gene and oral disease progression. The genotyping revealed that 18 (20.5%) of the 89 blood donors were found to be non-secretors (se_/_) and 79.5 % of the healthy individuals studied presented the Se gene *(FUT 2)* that governs the secretion of water-soluble ABH antigens into saliva (control group). These secreted antigens can be demonstrated in saliva by agglutination inhibition tests with ABH antisera and molecular biology through analysis of the *FUT 2* gene. In contrast, twenty-eight patients (58%) with oral pre-cancerous and cancerous lesions were non secretors, OR = 2.43; CI 95% (1.03; 5.71) (p= 0.0407) (Table 3). We found a higher intensity of oral disease in the non-secretor group, and epithelial dysplasia was found exclusively in this group.

	Benign Lesions (mucoceles, papilloma, etc)	**Pre-cancerous + Cancerous**
***FUT2* -Se (Secretor Status)**	26	20
***FUT2* -se (Non Secretor Status)**	15	28

Table 3. Secretor status in patients with oral lesions

The molecular analysis showed that 48.31% of patients was homozygous for the G428A mutation (the mutation present in the 2 alleles), while the other patients were homozygous for the secretor status (none of them presented the allele G428A), or heterozygous secretor (1 allele presented with the mutation G428A) (Fig. 3).

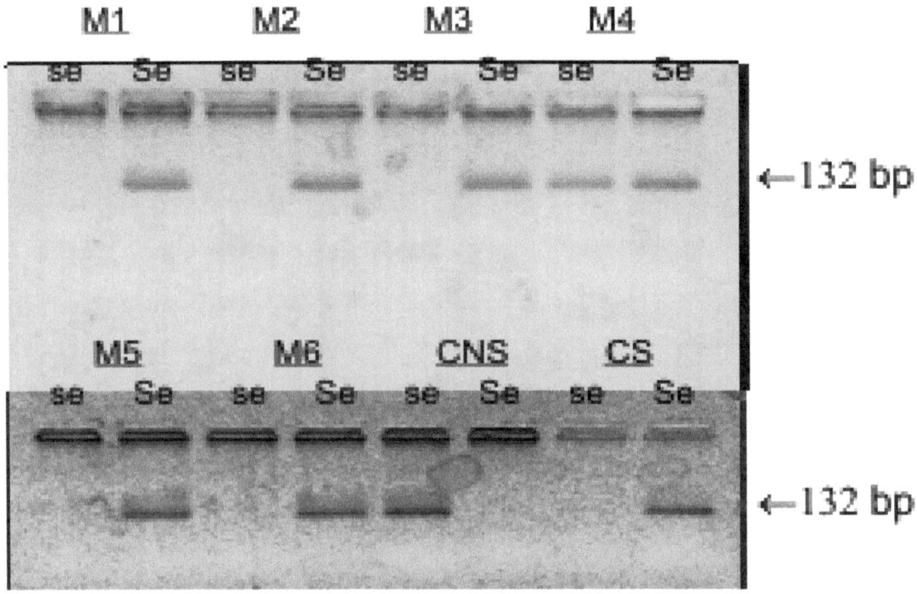

Fig. 3. The agarose gel shows the PCR products of 132 bp for the M1-M6 samples. Each sample was analysed for the wild type allele (Se) and for G428A allele (se) and was run together with secretor control (CS) and non-secretor control (CNS).

The secretor status is defined by the presence of H type 1 antigen in body secretions such as milk and saliva. H type 1 antigen belongs to both the Lewis and the ABO (H) histo-blood-group systems and it is expressed in erythrocyte membranes and in several epithelial tissues. The secretor enzyme (FUT2), an *α*-1,2-fucosyltransferase, is responsible for the fucose transfer in an *α*-1,2 linkage to form the terminal H type 1 structure. The cell-surface fucosylated oligosacharides participate in several biological processes, such as embryogenesis, tissue differentiation, tumour metastasis, inflammation and bacterial adhesion (Dabelsteen, 2004). About 20% of the Caucasian population is non-secretor. Several disease correlations have been linked to non-secretor status. In general, being non-secretor results in several disadvantages regarding metabolism and immune function (Campi et al., 2007, Le Pendu et al., 2001, Daniels, 2007).

Our results have demonstrated that most of the individuals examined in the healthy group were secretor (have the *FUT2* gene) (79.5 %) and there were significant difference between secretors and non-secretors in the experimental group. We have also found a higher intensity of oral disease in the non-secretor group, and the occurrence of epithelial dysplasia was mostly found in the non-secretor group. This study evaluated the association between oral lesions and polymorphisms of the *Se* genes. We found that oral pre-cancerous and cancerous lesions were increased among individuals with non secretor status and nonsense mutation 428G→A (Trp143→stop) (58.33%). We found 20 patients diagnosed histopathologically as malignant lesions despite the secretory status. We also observed that the red cell Lewis antigen reactivity does appear to be associated with the secretor status in the saliva, a conclusion supported by the observation that some individuals with Le(a-b+) red cells show reactivity of ABH antigens in their secretions and they have the *FUT2* gene.

The studies of patients with premalignant and malignant oral lesions, in which non-secretor status predominates, appear to be an associated risk marker for the development of oral cancer. Leukoplakia and erythroplakia are clinical changes in the oral mucosa regarded as potentially malignant lesions (Clausen et al., 1994, Hakomori, 1999). Certain histopathological changes may indicate a malignant potential in a lesion. However, the presence of such changes is not a reliable predictor of malignant transformation, and their absence does not mean that the patient is out of risk of developing a tumour (Gao et al., 2004b).

Although the relationship between epithelial dysplasia in a leukoplakia and malignant transformation of the lesion is debatable, many workers consider that the finding of epithelial dysplasia indicates a higher likelihood to develop malignancy. It is, however, more probable that the antigen changes found in the dysplastic lesions are associated with other factors, such as cell movement and growth rate, rather than malignancy per se (Dabelsteen, et al., 1975).

Our study evaluated the association between oral lesions and polymorphisms of the *Se* genes and secretor status. We found that oral pre-cancerous and cancerous were increased among individuals with non-secretor status and nonsense mutation 428G→A (Trp143→stop). We also demonstrated that the Le (a+b-) antigen expression was present in the population showing greater risk. The studies of patients with pre malignant and malignant oral lesions, in which non-secretor status predominates, show that this status appears to be an associated risk marker for the development for oral cancer.

4. CD44

CD44 is a transmembrane glycoprotein that binds hyaluronan, extracellular matrix proteins and growth factors. Alternative splicing of a single gene generates a family of splice variants (CD44vl-10) in addition to the standard isoform. Cell adhesion molecules are essential for maintaining the stable structure of stratified squamous epithelium. In normal epithelium, keratinocytes are attached to each other and to the underlying basement membrane. Cell adhesion, however, must be dynamic to facilitate the mobility and turnover of cells. In dynamic situations, keratinocytes alter their cell-cell and cell-ECM interactions by virtue of altered expression and function of cell adhesion molecules. The expression of cell adhesion molecules is normally tightly regulated-forming, persisting, or declining in an ordered fashion. This allows for controlled cell proliferation, mobility, differentiation, and survival. Many of these processes are misregulated in malignant tumours, and it has been shown that many of the characteristics of tumour cells are attributable to the aberrant expression or function of cell adhesion molecules. However, multiple CD44 isoforms are expressed by normal stratified squamous epithelia, such as the epidermis and the lining of the oral cavity (Hudson et al., 1996).

The neoplastic transformation of normal epithelial cells to metastatic tumour cells is a complex process involving a number of alterations in the expression of genes implicated in cell proliferation, cell adhesion and cell migration. Tumour progression is the process by which tumour cells acquire malignant properties, such as progressive growth, invasion and metastasis (Nowell, 1986). One of the genes involved in these processes is *CD44* which appears to be one of the most promising candidates as a cancer diagnosis marker (Otavia, et al., 2001). Several studies have provided evidence that the expression of CD44 is specifically altered in many types of tumours. They show aberrant expression and processing of CD44 transcripts and cell surface expression of CD44 appears to change profoundly during tumour metastasis, particularly during the progression of various carcinomas (Assimakopoulos et al., 2002). Numerous studies based on immunohistochemical analyses of paraffin-embedded or frozen tissue sections using different monoclonal antibodies to CD44 isoforms and molecular biological techniques have provided evidence that in many types of tumours there is overexpression of CD44 isoforms.

We investigate by confocal microscopy, the expression of CD44 protein in epithelial cells obtained from saliva samples from patients with oral lesions. We studied 28 patients with various oral lesions (benign, pre-cancerous and cancerous), and a control group (n = 32) who had no alterations. We worked with saliva samples subjected to thermal shock and washed with phosphate buffered saline. They were concentrated by centrifugation. Then 10^6 cells were incubated with anti-CD44 antibody suitable dilution for 30 min at room temperature. After washing with phosphate buffered saline, it was incubated with secondary antibody labeled with allophycocyanin (APC). Parallel internal controls were processed for each sample. The different cell suspensions were washed with phosphate buffered saline and observed by confocal microscopy (Nikon C1) using 639 nm red laser. The results obtained showed fluorescence corresponding to the presence of CD44 protein in samples from patients diagnosed with cancer and precancer. A higher intensity was observed in individuals with a pathological diagnosis of squamous cell carcinoma (Fig 4). In contrast, samples from patients with benign lesions showed no fluorescence images as samples of the control group (Fig. 5). These findings indicate that overexpression of CD44 molecule analyzed could be considered as a marker of risk in individuals with oral lesions.

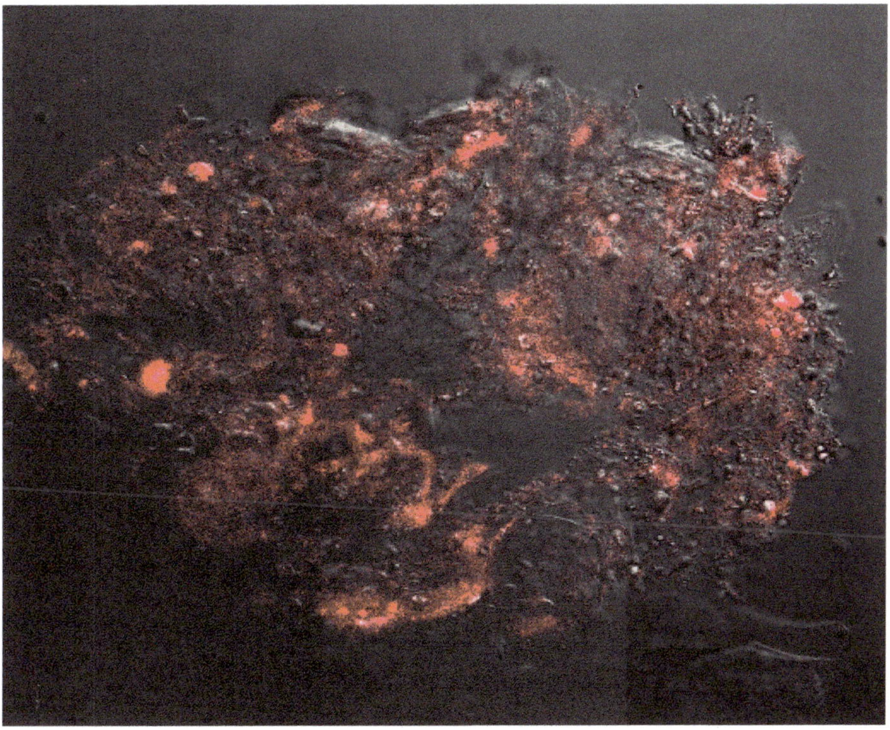

Fig. 4. Image of squamous carcinoma cells obtained by confocal microscopy. The over expression of CD44 protein is noted by the red fluorescence observed on cell membranes and in cytoplasms.

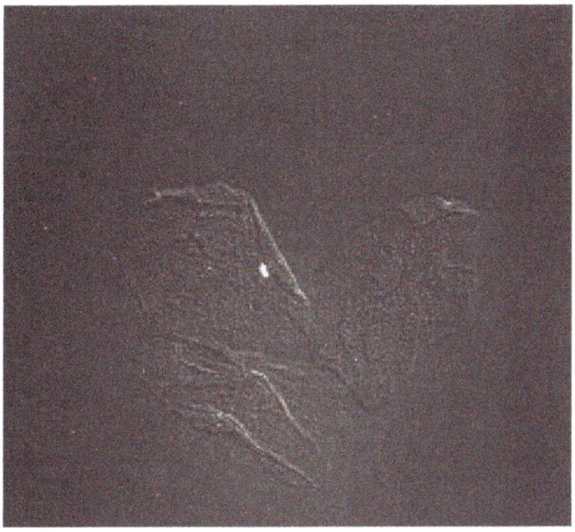

Fig. 5. Image of benign lesions cells obtained by confocal microscopy. No red fluorescence is observed indicating the absence of CD44 protein expression.

Studies on early premalignant lesions and on early stage malignancies of several types of common tumours, such as breast, bladder and colon, have reported increased CD44 isoform expression and aberrant CD44 transcript processing, but also a marked heterogeneity in the pattern of expression within the tumour. These specific alterations in CD44 expression become clear and distinct with tumour progression, with higher expression levels achieved in invasive and metastatic tumour cells. Several mechanisms, based on the properties of CD44 as the major hyaluronan CD44 in squamous cell carcinomas receptor and as a signal transmitter and growth presenting molecule, have been proposed to explain the role of elevated CD44 expression during tumour development and progression (Knudson, 1998).

5. Conclusion

Clinical examination and histopathological studies of biopsied material are the classical and the most accepted diagnostic methods used for precancerous and cancerous oral lesions. While conventional oral examination may be useful in the discovery of some oral lesions, it does not identify all potentially premalignant and/or malignant lesions.

It has been shown that leukoplakias from patients who subsequently developed malignancy all demonstrated loss of expression of histo-blood group antigen in the lesions that preceded the carcinomas. This may indicate that the change in expression of A/B antigen is an early event in the malignant development process.

We propose that areas of SRCA-test negative epithelium are closely related to invasive carcinomas and may be their precursor lesions. However, as it is generally accepted that cancer cells must undergo a whole series of changes to become metastatic, it is remarkable the degree of expression of a single carbohydrate structure was significantly correlated with aggressive clinical behaviour of the tumour. It is therefore possible that further prognostic information can be obtained by detecting a group of other related carbohydrate structures at the cancer cell membranes.

Our findings also demonstrate that the Se genotypes affect the risk of developing malignant oral disease defined by the secretor status. The study also evaluated the association between oral lesions and polymorphisms of the *Se* genes. We found that oral pre-cancerous and cancerous lesions were increased among individuals with non secretor status and nonsense mutation 428G→A (Trp143→stop).

Thus, we think that CD44 might be a good candidate as a predictor of prognosis in this group of cancers. However, a larger series with clinical follow-up and study of other biological markers of tumor progression is needed to determine whether it is an independent prognostic factor or not.

In summary, our results indicate that at the same time as the morphological changes that occur during the process of oral carcinogenesis, another series of events occurs. Further follow-up studies are required to clarify the role of predictive markers of risk in precursor lesions of oral cancer

6. References

Assimakopoulos, D.; Kolettas, E.; Patrikakos, G.& Evangelou, A. (2002). The role of CD44 in the development and prognosis of head and neck squamous cell carcinomas. *Histol Histopathol*, Vol. 17, N° 4, (October 2002), pp. 1269-1281, ISSN 0213-3911

Biondi, C.; Campi, C.; Escovich, L.; Racca, A.; García Borrás, S.; Cotorruelo, C. (2008). Loss of A, B, and H antigens in oral cancer. *Inmunología,* Vol. 27, N° 3 (April 2008). pp. 127-131, ISSN 0213-9626

Boileau, M.; Cowles, R.; Schmidt, K. & Schmidt, W. (1985). Comparison of specific red-cell adherence and immunoperoxidase staining techniques for ABO(H) blood-group cell-surface antigens on superficial transitional cell carcinoma of the bladder. *J Surg Oncol,* Vol. 30, Nª2, (October 1985), pp. 72-79, ISSN 0022-4790

Campi, C.; Escovich, L.; Valdés, V.; García-Borrás, S.; Racca L.; Racca, A.; Cotorruelo, C. & Biondi, C. (2007). Secretor status and ABH antigens expression in patients with oral lesions. *Med Oral Patol Oral Cir Bucal,* Vol. 12, pp. E431-E434. ISSN 1698-6946

Dabelsteen, E.; Roed-Petersen, B. & Pindborg, J. (1975). Loss of epithelial blood group antigens A and B in oral premalignant lesions. *Acta Pathol Microbiol Scand (A),* Vol. 83, N° 3, (My 1975), pp. 292-300, ISSN 0903-4641

Dabelsteen E (1996). Cell surface carbohydrates as prognostic markers in human carcinomas. *J Pathol,* Vol. 179, N° 4, (August 1996), pp.358-369, ISSN 1096-9896

Dabelsteen, E. & Gao,S. (2004). ABO Blood-group Antigens in Oral Cancer. *J Dent Res,* Vol. 84, N° 1, (June 2004), pp. 21-28, ISSN 0022-0345

Dabelsteen, E.; Gron, B.; Mandel, U. & Mackenzie, I. (1998). Altered expression of epithelial cell surface glyco- 19 conjugates and intermediate filaments at the margins of mucosal wounds. *J Invest Dermatol,* Vol. 111, pp. 592–597, ISSN 0022-202X

Daniels G. (2007). Functions of red cell surface proteins. *Vox Sang,* Vol. 93, N° 4, (November 2007), 331-340, ISSN 1423-0410

Ebnet, K. & Vestweber, D. (1999). Molecular mechanisms that control leukocyte extravasation: the selectins and the chemokines. *Histochem Cell Biol,* Vol. 112, N° 1, (July 1999), pp.1-23, ISSN 0948-6143

Fenderson, B.; Holmes, E.; Fukushi, Y. & Hakomori, S. (1986). Coordinate expression of X and Y haptens during murine embryogenesis. *Developmental Biology,* Vol. 114, N° 1, (March 1986), pp. 12-21, ISSN 0012-1606

Foresto, P.; Biondi, C.; Racca, L.; Brufman, A.;. Yaber, F.; Solís, E.; Provenzal, O. & Valverde, J. (2000). Glicosilación anormal de antígenos ABH solubles en patoloías tumorales del tracto urinario. *Archivos Españoles de Urología.,* Vol.53, N° 3, pp. 196-199, ISSN N° 0004-0614

Fukuda M (2002). Roles of mucin-type O-glycans in cell adhesion. *Biochim Biophys Acta,* Vol. 1573, N° 3, pp. 394-405, ISSN 0304-4165

Gao, S.; Bennett, E.; Reibel, J.; Chen, X.; Christensen, E.; Krogdahl, A. & Dabelsteen, E. (2004a). Histo-blood group ABO antigen in oral potentially malignant lesions and squamous cell carcinoma—genotypic and phenotypic characterization. *APMIS,* Vol. 112, N° 1, (January 2004), pp. 11-20, ISSN 1600-0463

Gao, S.; Worm, J.; Guldberg, P.; Eiberg, H.; Krogdahl, A. & Liu, C. (2004b). Genetic and epigenetic alterations of the blood group *ABO* gene in oral squamous cell carcinoma. *Int J Cancer,* Vol. 109, N° 2, pp, 230-237, ISSN 1097-0215

Greenlee, R.; Hill-Harmon, M.; Murray, T. & Thun M. (2001). Cancer statistics. *CA Cancer J Clin,* Vol. 51, pp. 15–36, ISSN 0007-9235

Hakomori, S.; Koscielak, J.; Bloch, K. & Jeanloz R. (1967). Immunologic relationship between blood group substances and a fucose-containing glycolipid of human adenocarcinoma. *J Immunol,* Vol. 98, N° 1 (January 1967), pp. 31-38, ISSN 0022-1767

Hakomori S. (1996). Tumor malignancy defined by aberrant glycosylation and sphingo(glyco) lipid metabolism. *Cancer Res*, Vol. 56, pp. 5309–5318, ISSN 0008-5472

Hakomori S (1999). Antigen structure and genetic basis of histo-blood groups A, B and O: their changes associated with human cancer. *Biochim Biophys Act,*. Vol. 1473, N° 1, (December 1999). pp. 247-266, ISSN 0304-4165

Hakomori, S. (2002). Glycosylation defining cancer malignancy: new wine in an old bottle. *Proc Natl Acad Sci USA*, Vol. 99, N° 19, (August 2002), pp. 10231-10233, ISSN 0027-8424

Hakomori S (2003). Structure, organization, and function of glycosphingolipids in membrane. *Curr Opin Hematol*, Vol. 10, N°1, (January 2003), pp. 16-24, ISSN 1065-6251

Hakomori, S. & Handa K. (2002). Glycosphingolipid-dependent cross-talk between glycosynapses interfacing tumor cells with their host cells: essential basis to define tumor malignancy. *FEBS Lett*, Vol. 531, N° 1, (September 2002), pp. 88-92, ISSN 0014-5793

Hascall VC (2000). Hyaluronan, a common thread. *Glycoconjugate Journal*, Vol. 17, N° 7-9, (July 2000), pp. 607-616, ISSN 0282-0080

Henry, S.; Oriol, R.; Samuelsson, B. (1995). Lewis histo-blood group system and associated secretory phenotypes. *Vox Sang*. Vol. 69, pp. 166-82, ISSN 1423-0410

Hudson, D.; Speight, P. & Watt, F. (1996). Altered expression of CD44 isoforms in squamous-cell carcinomas and cell lines derived from them. *Int J Cancer*, Vol. 66, N° 1, (May 1996), pp. 457-463, ISSN 1097-0215

Jemal, A.; Thomas, A.; Murray, T & Thun, M. (2002). Cancer statistics, 2002. *CA Cancer J Clin*, Vol.52. N° 1, (Jan-Feb 2002), pp. 23-47, ISSN 0007-9235

Kelly, R.; Rouquier, S.; Giorgi, D.; Lennon, G. & Lowe I. (1995) Sequence and expression of a candidate for the human secretor blood group α(1,2)fucosyltransferase gene (FUT2). Homozygosity for an enzyme-inactivating nonsense mutation commonly correlates with the non-secretor phenotype. *J Biol Chem*. Vol. 270, N° 9, pp. 4640-4649, ISSN 0021-9258

Khalili, J. (2008). Oral cancer: risk factors, prevention and diagnostic. *Experimental Oncology*, Vol. 30, N°4, pp. 259–264, ISSN 1812-9269

Knudson, W. (1998). The role of CD44 as a cell surface hyaluronan receptor during tumour invasion of connective tissue. *Front. Biosci.*, Vol. 3, pp. d604-d615, ISSN 1093-9946

Koda, Y.; Soejima, M.; Wang, B. & Kimura, H. (1997). Structure and expression of the gene encoding secretor-type galactoside 2-alpha-Lfucosyltransferase (FUT2). *Eur J Biochem* Vol. 246, N° 3, pp. 750-755, ISSN 00142956

Koda, Y.; Tachida, H.; Soejima, M.; Takenaka, O. & Kimura H. (2000). Ancient origin of the null allele se(428) of the human ABO-secretor locus (FUT2). *J Mol Evol*, Vol. 50, N° 3, pp.:243–248, ISNN 0022-2844

Landsteiner, K. (1900). Zur Kenntnis der antifermentativen, lytischen und agglutinierenden Wirkungen des Blutserums und der Lymphe. *Zbl Bakterial* , Vol. 27, pp. 357–62.

Le Pendu, J. ; Marionneau, S.; Cailleau-Thomas, A.; Rocher, J.; Moullac-Vaidye, B. & Clement M. (2001). ABH and Lewis histo-blood group antigens in cancer. *APMIS*, Vol. 109, N° 1, (January 2001), pp.9-31, ISSN 1600-0463

Mandel, U.; Langkilde, N.; Ørntoft T.; Hamilton Therkildsen, M.; Karkov, J.; Reibel, J.; White, T.; Clausen, H. & Dabelsteen, E. (1992). Expression of histo-blood group A/B gene defined glycosyltransferases in normal and malignant epithelia: correlation with A/B carbohydrate expression. *Int J Cancer,* Vol. 52, N° 1, (August 1992), pp. 7-12, ISSN 1097-0215

Marhaba, R. & Zöller, M. (2004). CD44 in cancer progression: adhesion, migration and growth regulation. *J Mol Histol.* Vol. 35, N° 3, (March 2004), pp. 211-31, ISSN 1567-2379

Miller, M. & Kearney, N. (2001). Oral care for patients with cancer: a review of the literature. *Cancer Nursing,* Vol. 24, N° 4, (August 2001), pp.:241-254, ISSN 0162-220X

Mollison, P.; Emgelfriet, C. & Contreras P. (1997). *Blood Transfusion en Clinical Medicine.* 11th Ed.. Blackwell Scientific Publications. Oxford, ISBN-13: 978-0-632-06454-0

Moreno, A.; Campi, C.; Escovich, L.; García Borrás, S.; Racca, L.; Racca, A.; Cotorruelo, C. & Biondi. C. (2009). Analysis of the *FUT2* gene and Secretor status in patients with oral lesions. *Inmunología.* Vol. 28, N° 3, pp. 131-134, ISSN 0213-9626

Narimatsu, H.; Iwasaki, H.; Nishihara, S.; Kimura, H.; Kudo, T., Yamauchi, Y. & Hirohashi, S. (1996). Genetic evidence for the Lewis enzyme, which synthesizes type-1 Lewis antigens in colon tissue, and intracellular localization of the enzyme. *Cancer Res,* Vol. 56, N° 2, (January 1996), pp. 330–338, ISSN 0008-5472

Nishihara, S.; Narimatsu, H.; Iwasaki, H.; Yazawa, S.; Akamatsu, S.; Ando, T. & Seno T. (1994). Molecular genetic analysis of the human Lewis histo-blood group system. *J Biol Chem* , Vol. 269, pp. 29271–29278, , ISSN 0021-9258

Oriol, R., Le Pendu, J. and Mollicone, R. (1986). Genetics of ABO, H, Lewis, X and related antigens. *Vox. Sang.* Vol. 51, pp. 161–171, ISSN 1423-0410

Onizawa, K.; Nishihara, K.; Yamagata, K.; Yusa, H., Yanagawa, T. & Yoshida, H. (2003). Factors associated with diagnostic delay of oral squamous cell carcinoma. *Oral Oncoly,* Vol. 39, N° 8 (April 2003), pp.781-788, ISSN 1368-8375

Ørntoft, T.; Holmes, E.; Johnson, P.; Hakomori, S. & Clausen, H. (1991). Differential tissue expression of the Lewis blood group antigens: enzymatic, immunohistologic, and immunochemical evidence for Lewis a and b antigen expression in Le(a2b2) individuals. *Blood,* Vol. 77, pp.:1389–1396, ISSN 0006-4971

Otavia, L.; Caballero, .L.; de Souza, S.; Bretani, R.& Simpson A. (2001). Alternative spliced transcripts as cancer markers. *Dis. Markers,* Vol. 17, N° 2, pp. 67-75, ISSN 0278-0240

Parkin, M.; Bray, F.; Ferlay, J & Pisani, P. (2001). Estimating the world cancer burden: Globocan 2000. *Int J Cancer,* Vol. 94, N° 2, (July 2001), pp. 153–156, ISSN 1097-0215

Ravn, V, & Dabelsteen, E. (2000). Tissue distribution of histo-blood group antigens. *APMIS,* Vol. 108, N° 1, (January 2000), pp. 1–28, ISSN 1600-0463

Regev E, Zeltser R, Lustmann J. (1992).Lip carcinoma in renal allograft recipient with long-term immunosuppressive therapy. *Oral Surg.* Vol. 73, N° 4, (April 1992), pp. 412-414, ISSN 1079-2104

Strauchen, J.; Bergman, S. & Hanson, T. (1980). Expression of A and B Tissue Isoantigens in benign and malignant lesions of the Breast. *Cancer;* Vo. 45, N° 8, pp. 2149-2155, ISSN 0008-543X

Svensson, L.;. Petersson,A. & Henry, S. (2000). Secretor genotyping for A385T, G428A, C571T, C628T, 685delTGG,G849A, and other mutations from a single PCR. *Transfusion,* Vol. 40, N° 7, (July 2000), pp. 856-860, ISSN 1537-2995

Wang, B.; Akiyama, K.; Jia, J. & Kimura, H. (1994). Measuring type 1 and type 2 antigens in human saliva by immunoassay using artificial antigens as standard substances. *Forensic Sci. Int.* Vol. 67, Nº 1, (June 1994), pp 1-8, ISSN 0379-0738

Yamamoto, F. (1995). Molecular genetics of ABO histo-blood groups. *Vox sanguinis*. Vol. 69, Nº 1, (July 1995), pp. 1-7, ISNN 1423-0410

Yamamoto, F.; Clausen, H.; White, T.; Marken, J. & Hakomori, S. (1990). Molecular genetic basis of the histo-blood group ABO system. *Nature*, Vol. 345, (May 1990), pp. 229–33 ISSN 0028-0836

15

Functional Biomarkers of Oral Cancer

Masumi Tsuda and Yusuke Ohba
Laboratory of Pathophysiology and Signal Transduction
Hokkaido University Graduate School of Medicine
Japan

1. Introduction

Oral squamous cell carcinoma (OSCC) is the most common head and neck cancers, and rank as one of the top ten cancers worldwide. More worrying is that the incidence of oral cancer appears to be increasing in many parts of the world. OSCC is characterized by a high degree of local invasiveness and a high rate of metastasis to the cervical lymph nodes. Survival of patients with OSCC has not improved in the last 40 years, despite recent advances in surgical procedures and the availability of new chemotherapeutic agents. In addition, surgical resection results in significant functional and cosmetic defects; therefore, it is important to develop conservative therapeutics, whereupon identification of markers representing OSCC aggressiveness would be worthwhile to decide the most suitable treatment for each patient from therapeutic options.

Given that the head and neck region is an environment challenged by a large variety of insults, including pathogens, foods, and chemicals, the relationship between cancer cells and inflammatory stroma might be of particular importance for arising malignancies there. The microenvironment plays a critical role in tumor initiation and progression, and may provide attractive therapeutic targets. In fact, it affects not only tumor growth, invasion, and metastasis, but also drug metabolism and accessibility; hence the role of stromal elements has been extensively investigated at a molecular level. Although host-tumor interactions are two-way communications between cancer cells and stroma; however, knowledge about the cancer cell properties specifically evoked in the microenvironment is still limited.

In this review, we provide an overview of the literatures regarding "functional biomarkers" of OSCCs, introduce our recent discovery of the *in vivo*-specific maker, and discuss significance of these factors in diagnostic and clinical implication.

2. Cellular biomarkers in OSCC

Major cellular biomarkers correlated with the clinical outcome of OSCC have been reported, which were refined with a focus on the relationship between prognostic or survival parameters of OSCC patients and their expression levels, mainly using immunohistochemistry (Oliveira & Ribeiro-Silva, 2011). The biomarkers could be classified into five groups based on their biological functions: 1) cell cycle progression and proliferation; 2) tumor suppression and apoptosis; 3) hypoxia; 4) angiogenesis; and 5) cell adhesion and matrix degradation.

2.1 Cell cycle progression and proliferation biomarkers

Several biomarkers belonging to this group have been identified: a family of epidermal growth factor receptors (EGFRs); cyclin D1; cyclin B1; Ki-67; proliferating cell nuclear antigen (PCNA); and Akt1. The EGFR family includes four members: HER-1 (EGFR, ErbB1), HER-2 (neu/ErbB2), HER-3 (ErbB3), and HER-4 (ErbB4). EGFR activation, as its name indicates, can augment the malignant potential of epithelial cells (LaCasse et al., 2008), and the overexpression correlates with poor prognosis in OSCC patients (Agra et al., 2008; Laimer et al., 2007; Silva et al., 2008, 2009). Cyclin proteins are key regulators of cell cycle progression. Cyclin D1 amplification is frequently detected as molecular alterations in OSCC and other head and neck cancers (Yu et al., 2005). There is a significant association between the combined expression of EGFR, cyclin D1, and p53 and an unfavorable overall survival in OSCC patients (Shiraki et al., 2005). Cyclin B1 is useful in predicting occult cervical lymph-node metastasis in OSCC (Harada et al., 2006). Ki-67 and PCNA are well-established cell proliferation markers, and Ki-67 expression increases sharply in early OSCC, but significantly decreases during disease progression (Derka et al., 2006), while that of PCNA was not significantly associated with the survival (Kim et al., 2007; Lim et al., 2005; Myoung et al., 2006). Akt plays a pivotal role in cell survival and proliferation. Overexpression of Akt is a significant indicator for predicting poor prognosis in OSCC patients (Lim et al., 2005).

2.2 Tumor suppression and apoptosis biomarkers

Five subsets of biomarkers were identified in this group: p53/p63, p21/p27, Bcl-2 family members, the retinoblastoma (Rb) protein, and Survivin. The tumor suppressor p53 is one of the most studied biomarkers in OSCC, as well as in other malignancies. The high expression of p53 is especially detected at advanced stages of carcinogenesis, and is also associated with a poor prognosis (Oliveira et al, 2007a, 2007b, 2008), while the clinical significance of that of p63, a p53 homologue, remains controversial (Oliveira et al., 2007a, 2007b; Lo Muzio et al., 2005a, 2007). Mutation of p53 occurs in 50% of OSCC cases (Ogden et al., 1992, 1996), which might be pertinent to consequent overexpression of this molecule. $p21^{waf1/cip1}$ and $p27^{Kip1}$ play an important function in regulating cell cycle progression through the inhibitory action on cyclin-dependent kinases. There are controversial findings concerning the clinical outcome of $p21^{waf1/cip1}$-positive OSCCs (Fillies et al., 2007; Nemes et al., 2005), whereas no significant association between $p27^{Kip1}$ expression and OSCC prognosis has been identified (Fillies et al., 2007). Bcl-2 family members include both anti- and pro-apoptotic proteins, and thereby regulate apoptosis either positively or negatively through their balance (Camisasca et al., 2009). The survival rate of patients with Bcl-2-negative and Bax-positive OSCC tumors was significantly higher than those with other expression profiles of these molecules (Kato et al., 2008; Zhang et al., 2009). The Rb pathway plays a crucial role in regulating cell cycle progression. OSCCs lacking Rb indeed display aggressiveness with the poor prognosis (Soni et al., 2005). Survivin is an inhibitor of apoptosis and overexpressed in most of OSCCs, indicating a potential biomarker of aggressiveness and invasiveness (Lippert et al., 2007; Lo Muzio et al., 2005b).

2.3 Hypoxia biomarkers

Four hypoxia-related biomarkers have been reported as putative prognostic parameters: hypoxia inducible factor 1α (HIF-1α); carbonic anhydrase IX (CA IX); glucose transporter 1 (GLUT-1); and erythropoietin receptor (EPOR). In hypoxic environments, stabilized HIF-1α induces the transactivation of more than 70 genes, including vascular endothelial growth factor (VEGF), involved in hypoxia adaptation and/or reversion (Fillies et al., 2005; Liu et al., 2008). The diffuse overexpression of HIF-1α had been associated with a good prognosis in OSCC patients (Fillies et al., 2005), whereas recently the opposite evidences have been reported (Lin et al., 2008; Liu et al., 2008). The latter finding might be supported by the ability of HIF-1α in inducing VEGF and promoting invasive phenotypes. Indeed, HIF family members are implicated in epithelial mesenchymal transition (EMT) of cancer cells (Yang MH., 2008). CA IX, a member of HIF-1-dependent CA family, is a transmembrane glycoprotein involved in pH homeostasis (Sakata et al., 2008). Overexpression of CA IX has been shown to significantly associate with recurrence and worse survival in OSCC patients (Choi et al., 2008). GLUT is also regulated via the HIF-1 pathway, mediates cellular glucose uptake, and namely represents as an endogenous marker of hypoxia (Kunkel et al., 2007). There is evidence that GLUT-1 is associated with aggressiveness in OSCC (Jonathan et al., 2006). Erythropoietin (EPO) is a glycoprotein hormone and synthesized in the kidneys in response to hypoxemia, and OSCC has been known to express its cognate receptor EPOR (Arcasoy et al., 2005). High expression of EPOR can be associated with a significantly worse prognosis in patients with oral tongue squamous cell carcinoma (Roh et al., 2009).

2.4 Angiogenesis biomarkers

Four angiogenic biomarkers were identified as possible prognostic parameters: VEGF; endoglin (CD105); CD34; and Eph receptor tyrosine kinases. VEGF functions mainly as an angiogenic cytokine that promotes proliferation, differentiation, and migration of vascular endothelial cells. Therefore, it should be ideally discussed in the section of humoral factors, but we would like to state here due to the importance of its intracellular transcriptional regulation by HIF-1. The patients with VEGF-positive tumors have significantly poor survival (Chien et al., 2006; Shao et al., 2008). Despite the established role of VEGF for angiogenesis, a recent study showed that an anti-VEGF antibody failed to interrupt the connection between OSCC and endothelial cells (Yamada et al., 2011); hence VEGF functions in tumor progression, other than angiogenesis, have yet to be determined. CD105, a regulatory component of the TGF-β receptor complex, can modulate angiogenesis. High expression of CD105 in primary OSCC may identify patients at risk of the recurrence with worse prognosis (Chuang et al., 2006). In addition, the existence of penetrating vessels within tumor nests, endothelial cells of which can be visualized by CD34 staining, was significantly associated with risk of cervical lymph node metastasis (Kademani et al., 2009). The Eph receptors and their membrane-anchored ephrin ligands can stimulate invasive behavior in a tumor through a cell-cell communication system capable of bi-directional signaling, thereby promoting a more aggressive and metastatic phenotype (Campbell et al., 2008; Wimmer-Kleikamp et al., 2005). High expression of EphA2 was associated with a poor survival in tongue SCC patients (Shao et al., 2008).

Category (section no.) / *Pathways* (section no.) / Biomarker	Status	Cellular/clinical characteristics
Cellular Biomarker (2)		
Cell cycle promotion and proliferation (2.1)		
EGFR	overexpression	poor prognosis
Cyclin D1	amplification	unfavorable overall survival
Cyclin B1	overexpression in cytoplasm	cervical lymph node metastasis
Ki-67	increase (early), decrease (late)	poor overall survival
PCNA	positive	no significant association on survival
Akt	overexpression	poor prognosis
Tumor suppression and apoptosis (2.2)		
p53	overexpression, mutation	poor prognosis
p63	positive	controversial
p21	overexpression	controversial
p27	overexpression	no significant association on survival
Bcl-2	negative	higher survival
Bax	positive	higher survival
Rb	loss	malignant conversion, poor prognosis
survivin	overexpression	aggressive and invasive
Hypoxia (2.3)		
HIF-1α	diffuse overexpression	good prognosis or controversial
CA IX	overexpression	recurrence with worse survival
GLUT-1	high expression	metastasis, worse overall survival
EPOR	high expression	worse prognosis
Angiogenesis (2.4)		
VEGF	positive	poor prognosis
CD105	high expression	recurrence with worse prognosis
CD34	positive within tumor nests	cervical lymph node metastasis
Eph A2	high expression	poor survival
Cell adhesion and matrix degradation (2.5)		
MMP-7,-9, -13, -14	positive	poor prognosis
CD44	irregular cytoplasmic staining	poor overall survival
E-cadherin	downregulation	EMT, worse prognosis
N-cadherin	upregulation	EMT
β- and γ-catenin	positive	poor prognosis
versican	overexpression in stroma	unfavorable outcome
Humoral Biomarker (3)		
Parathyroid hormone-related protein (3.1)		
PTHrP	high expression	malignant conversion
Endothelins and their receptors (3.2)		
Endothelins (ETs)	overexpression	tumor growth and progression
ET_AR, ET_BR	overexpression	tumor growth and progression
Inflammatory Cytokines and Chemokines (3.3)		
Interleukin (IL)-6	high expression	tolerance to immune system
IL-8	high expression	controversial
TNF-α	high expression	controversial
CXCL13	high expression	tumor development and progression
***In vivo* specific Biomarker (4)**		
Receptor activator of NF-κB ligand		
RANKL	high expression *in vivo*	tumor development and progression

Table 1. Molecular biomarkers and its correlation with cellular or clinical characteristics.

2.5 Cell adhesion and matrix degradation biomarkers

Five classes of matrix degradation- and cell adhesion-related molecules were identified as putative prognostic biomarkers associated with OSCC: matrix metalloproteinases (MMPs), CD44, cadherins, catenins, and versican. The MMPs are a family of proteases, highly expressed by invasive tumor cells and the adjacent stroma, and essential for ECM degradation (de Vicente et al., 2005). Of over 20 known members of MMPs, expression of MMP-7, -9, -13, and -14 (MT1-MMP) were significantly associated with poor prognosis of OSCC patients (De Vicente et al., 2005, 2007; Luukkaa et al., 2006). The CD44 family is widely expressed transmembrane glycoproteins that bind to hyaluronic acid, growth factors, and ECM proteins, regulating cell migration and adhesion (Georgolios et al., 2006). In contrast to strong membranous staining in normal squamous cell epithelium, the irregular cytoplasmic staining of CD44 in OSCC has been shown to correlates with poor disease-free and overall survivals (Kosunen et al., 2007). Cadherins are a family of transmembrane glycoproteins involved in cell-cell adhesion (Munoz-Guerra et al., 2005). In most epithelial cells, the intracellular domain of E-cadherin binds to catenins, forming the cadherin-catenin complex involved in the intracellular transduction of cell-to-cell contact signals. The reduced expression of E-cadherin, frequently concomitant with N-cadherin upregulation, leads to loss of cell-cell adhesion and acquisition of the mesenchymal phenotype (i.e. EMT), which plays an important role in tumor invasion and dissemination (Lyons et al., 2007). Accordingly, a decrease in the expression of β- and γ-catenins can also predict poor prognosis of OSCC (Ueda et al., 2006). Versican is a major proteoglycan of the ECMs, and its overexpression was observed in diverse tumors. This molecule plays an essential role in tumor growth by repressing cell adhesion, stimulating cell proliferation and migration, and regulating angiogenesis (Rahmani et al., 2006). High stromal versican expression in OSCC specimens is an independent predictor for an unfavorable prognosis (Pukkila et al., 2007).

3. Humoral biomarkers in OSCC

Given that the significance of the microenvironment for OSCC initiation and/or promotion has been shown, as mentioned above, humoral factors that correlate with clinical features would be of particular important. VEGF may serve as a prototype molecule bridging between cancer cells and stromal component, namely endothelial cells as described (see 2.4). In this section, humoral biomarkers are enumerated irrespective of their source and their mode of action, para- or autocrine.

3.1 Parathyroid hormone-related protein (PTHrP)

PTHrP was originally identified as a major factor responsible for humoral hypercalcemia in malignancies (Burtis et al., 1990), and acts as a stimulator of osteoclastic bone resorption (Liao & McCauley, 2006). Therefore, plasma PTHrP level can be a predictor of existence of bone metastatic lesions in a wide range of tumors. PTHrP produced by cancer cells promotes malignant conversion (increased cell proliferation, survival, adhesion, migration, and invasion) of breast, colon, and prostate cancers (Shen et al., 2004), as well as OSCC (Nomura et al., 2007). Because OSCC expresses the PTH/PTHrP receptor PTH1R, its mechanism of action is in a paracrine or autocrine manner (Yamada et al., 2008). It is noteworthy that the expression level of PTHrP is regulated by downstream signaling of EGFR, another class of biomarker for malignant potential of OSCC (see 2.1). In addition, a recently developed, rapid screening system identifies PTHrP as one of the validated predictors for OSCC (Ziober et al., 2006).

3.2 Endothelins and their receptors as biomarkers in OSCC

Hoffmann et al. recently reported novel functional biomarkers in OSCC, endothelin (ET) and its receptor, which are overexpressed in OSCC (Hoffmann et al., 2010). ETs comprise a family of three small peptides: ET-1, ET-2, and ET-3 (Yanagisawa et al, 1988; Levin, 1995). ET-1 is expressed primarily in endothelial cells, and ET-2 is in the kidneys and the intestine, whereas ET-3 is found mainly in the brain (Levin, 1995). ETs exert their effects by binding to cell-surface receptors, namely ET-A (ET_AR) and ET-B (ET_BR). Both receptors belong to the G-protein-coupled receptor super-family (Levin, 1995; Kusserow et al., 2004; Motte et al, 2006; Bhalla et al., 2009). ET_AR binds ET-1 with 10-times greater affinity than ET-3, whereas ET_BR binds all three ETs with similar affinity. In general, most ET-1 functions are therefore mediated by interaction with ET_AR (Guise et al., 2003).

ET-1, ET_AR, and ET_BR are overexpressed in OSCC, in which ET-1 acts as a survival factor to induce proliferation via ET_AR and ET_BR (Awano et al., 2006). Schmidt et al. demonstrated a significant elevation in the levels of ET-1 in HSC-3 cells (Schmidt et al, 2007), a lineage obtained from human OSCC. ET_AR activation by ET-1 largely contributes to tumor growth and progression through induction of cell proliferation, survival, angiogenesis, and metastatic spread, thus indicating that ET_AR antagonism might improve cancer treatment (Rosano et al., 2006; Nelson et al, 2003). ET-1 can also modulate tumor angiogenesis through induction of VEGF, which is accounted for by an increase in HIF-1α level by ET_AR activation (Bagnato et al, 2002). Besides their anti-angiogenic effect, ET receptor antagonists can also prevent the production of MMPs from macrophages (Grimshaw, 2007). Taken together, it is tempting to infer that blocking ET receptors, especially ET_AR, might be a useful alternative as an adjuvant treatment of OSCC. Nevertheless, whether ET antagonists provide significant clinical benefit for patients with OSCC is a vital and controversial issue. In several clinical trials of metastatic castration-resistant prostate cancer patients, atrasentan, a competitive inhibitor of ET-1, did not improve the primary or secondary endpoint (Carducci, 2007; Nelson, 2008). Similar results have been obtained in other studies using a different ET antagonist zibotentan. Therefore, results of adequate, long-term clinical trials for OSCC are awaited.

3.3 Inflammatory cytokines and chemokines

Given the specific property of the oral cavity that is always challenged by a large variety of insults, including pathogens, foods, and chemicals, chronic inflammation and its molecular components such as cytokines or chemokines would be particular important for the development and progression of OSCC. In fact, several cytokines and chemokines are identified as biomarker of OSCC.

Interleukin (IL)-6 and IL-8 have been implicated as potential biomarkers for OSCC. (St John et al., 2004). When these cytokines are expressed together with VEGF, OSCC has been shown to acquire resistance in a manner dependent on immune effectors (Teruel et al., 2008). In addition, the concentration of saliva IL-6 in OSCC patients are significantly higher than that of control group, whereas results regarding IL-8 and tumor necrosis factor-α are controversial (SahebJamee et al., 2008).

Chemokines are also implicated in tumor progression and metastasis of OSCC (Krieg & Boyman, 2008). More recently, gene expression profiling studies implicated chemokine ligand-13 (CXCL13) in OSCC tumor development and progression (Ziober et al., 2006). CXCL13 (BCA-1) that binds monogamously to the CXCR5 receptor was originally discovered to facilitate B-cell chemotaxis (Legler et al., 1998). CXCL13 can upregulate receptor activator of NF-κB ligand (RANKL), a member of the tumor necrosis factor family critical for osteoclastogenesis (Hsu et al., 1999), through activation of c-Jun N terminus kinase and nuclear factor of activated T cells (NFAT)-4, implicating CXCL13 as a potential biomarker to predict OSCC bone invasion or osteolysis (Yuvaraj et al., 2009).

4. *In vivo*-specific biomarkers — Lessons from RANKL

Survival of patients with OSCC has not improved over the past few decades, despite recent advances in the treatments. One of the fundamental factors explaining the poor outcome is that a great proportion of oral cancers are diagnosed at advanced stages. In addition, surgical resection results in significant functional and cosmetic defects. Therefore, it is important to develop biomarkers for early diagnosis, as well as for the prediction of disease progression and/or aggressiveness to decide the most suitable treatment for each patient from therapeutic options. These facts have prompted molecular exploration for novel markers, and indeed lead to the discovery of manifold biomarkers, as described in the previous sections.

Meanwhile, if a marker were functional in tumorigenesis, aggressiveness, or progression, it can be a plausible therapeutic target. As far as now, most markers have been identified because of their high expression in tumor tissues, evaluated by immunohistochemistry, and the significance are evaluated by comparison with clinical course of the patients, followed by functional analysis *in vitro*. However, given the specific feature of the oral cavity that is an environment challenged by a large variety of insults, including pathogens, foods, and chemicals, the molecules exert their functions *in vivo* would be more preferable.

We have recently identified the osteoclastic cytokine RANKL as a marker for invasive and aggressive OSCC with its molecular function as an EMT and angiogenesis inducer (Yamada et al., 2011). Of particular interest is that both RANKL expression and function solely depend on the microenvironment; neither its high expression nor function, as the EMT inducer could not be reproduced *in vitro*. In other word, it is not necessarily enough to explore molecular functions only using *in vitro* settings. In the latter part of this review, we highlight the story of how RANKL is characterized as an *in vivo*-specific biomarker with the experimental procedures used, so that such attractive and valuable candidates for biomarker would not be abandoned because of the absence of *in vitro*-experimental evidence, as hypothesized

4.1 High expression of RANKL in *in vivo* OSCC but not in cell lines

We initially probed bone invasion-related factors in OSCC, and indeed reported that PTHrP is expressed in OSCC and enhances the malignant potential of OSCC (Yamada et al., 2008). We therefore hypothesized that PTHrP induces the expression of RANKL in a manner analogous to osteoblasts (Leibbrandt & Penninger, 2008; Mundy, 2002; Roodman, 2004), and examined the expression of RANKL mRNA and protein by quantitative RT-PCR and immunohistochemistry, respectively, in 20 human OSCC samples, including those in the tongue and the gingiva. In all cases, high expression (from 6 to 123-fold) was observed compared to human control gingival fibroblast (Figure 1A), and the expression level of RANKL was positively correlated with the histological grading of differentiation and invasive histological architecture based on Yamamoto-Kohama classification (Yamamoto et al., 1983). In addition, abundant RANKL protein was observed in atypical cancer cells diffusely invaded into surrounding tissues. Nevertheless, none of the tested OSCC cell lines displayed such abundant RANKL expression as that observed *in vivo*. In particular, cell lines established from poorly differentiated SCC with aggressive invasiveness failed to do so. These results raise the possibility that the RANKL expression level in cell lines is repressed under culture conditions, and RANKL is a microenvironment-induced cytokine *in vivo*, of which expression is implicated in progression and biological malignancies of OSCC.

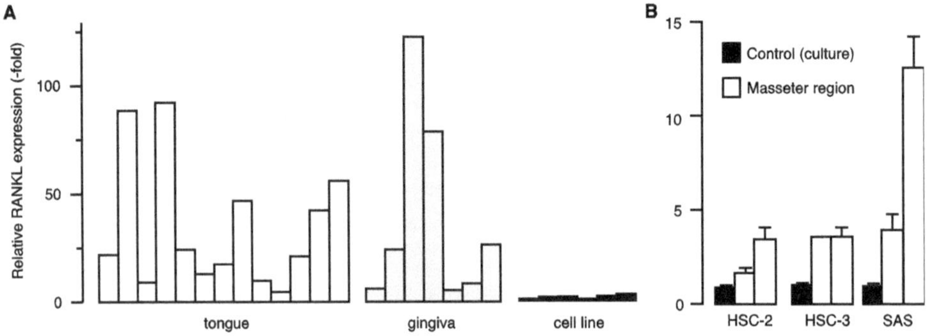

Fig. 1. High RANKL expression *in vivo*. (A) mRNA levels in human OSCC specimens of tongue and gingival cancers and OSCC cell lines were evaluated by quantitative PCR. (B) Cells of OSCC cell lines were inoculated into nude mice and allowed to form tumor. The mRNA level in each sample was determined by quantitative PCR.

4.2 Environment-dependent expression of RANKL

To test the aforementioned hypothesis, several OSCC cell lines were inoculated into the masseter muscles of mice, one of the most established sites for an oral cancer orthotopic model (Cui et al., 2005; Nomura et al., 2007; Suda et al., 1997). As expected, RANKL expression was dramatically augmented at both mRNA and protein levels compared to those in cultured cells (Figure 1B). Moreover, the higher RANKL expression levels are observed in poorly differentiated, invasive SCC, in accordance with our clinicopathological findings.

To assess the contribution of the oral environment to RANKL expression and subsequent tumor formation, HSC-3 cells, a OSCC cell line that formed tumors most efficiently in the orthotopic model, were also injected into the muscle of hindlimbs. This region was selected in analogy to the orthotopic site (intramuscular), as well as by its anatomical location far from the oral cavity. Tumors formed in the hindlimbs were significantly smaller than those in the masseter region (Figure 2A and B). In parallel with their tumor weight, RANKL could be detected in the masseter region tumors, but not in the hindlimb ones (Figure 2C). Thus, RANKL expression requires the orthotopic environment and correlates with tumor formation ability. Moreover, masseter region tumors, but not hindlimb ones, displayed the histological pattern of poorly differentiated squamous cell carcinoma (Figure 2D).

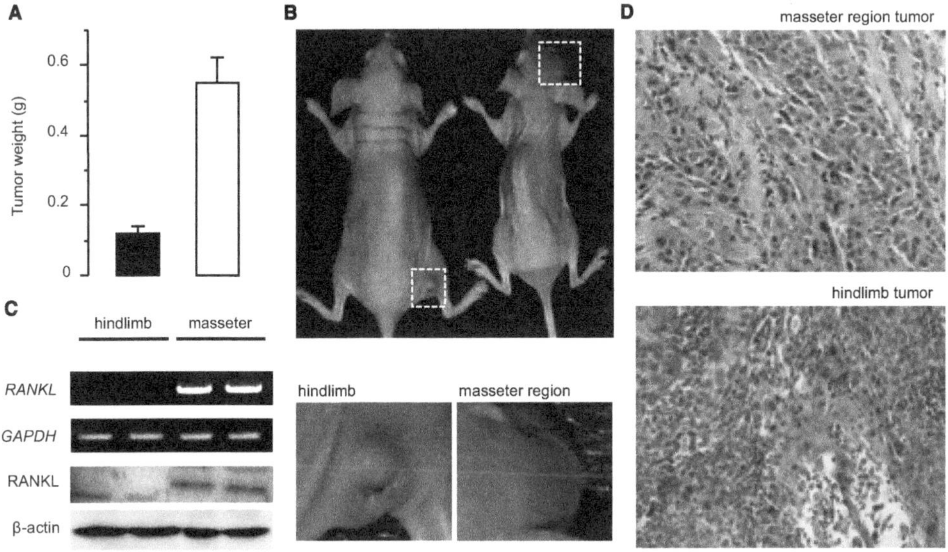

Fig. 2. Environment-dependent expression of RANKL. The OSCC cell line HSC-3 cells were injected into the masseter or hindlimb region of the mice. After 28 days, the formed tumors were weighted (A) and photographed (B). Expression levels of RANKL mRNA and protein in the tumors were analyzed by quantitative RT-PCR and immunoblotting, respectively (C). Histology of the tumors are also shown (D).

4.3 RANKL expression accelerates tumor malignancy

To further verify the role for RANKL in OSCC tumor formation, we established HSC-3 cell lines that stably express RANKL, and injected them into the mouse hindlimbs. RANKL-expressing cells achieved efficient tumor formation in the hindlimbs, whereas control cells failed to form sizable tumors, similar to parental cells as described above (Figure 3A-C). These results together demonstrate that RANKL expression, which ordinarily depends on the oral environment, possesses the potential of inducing OSCC formation. By HE staining, it was revealed that RANKL-expressing, hindlimb-injected tumors exhibited more poorly differentiated and invasive characters than control tumors, consistent with the results observed in human specimens.

4.4 RANKL induces epithelial-mesenchymal transition (EMT)

Immunohistochemical analysis also revealed that E-cadherin was disappeared from the cell-to-cell contact sites in tumors formed by RANKL-expressing cells, whereas control tumors displayed typical E-cadherin pattern (Figure 3D). Moreover, in response to E-cadherin disappearance from the plasma membrane, intense staining for N-cadherin was observed in the tumor cell cytoplasm in RANKL-expressing tumors. These findings raise the possibility that RANKL promotes loss of epithelial character, i.e. evokes EMT, a fundamental process during tumor development and progression (Yang J & Weinberg, 2008).

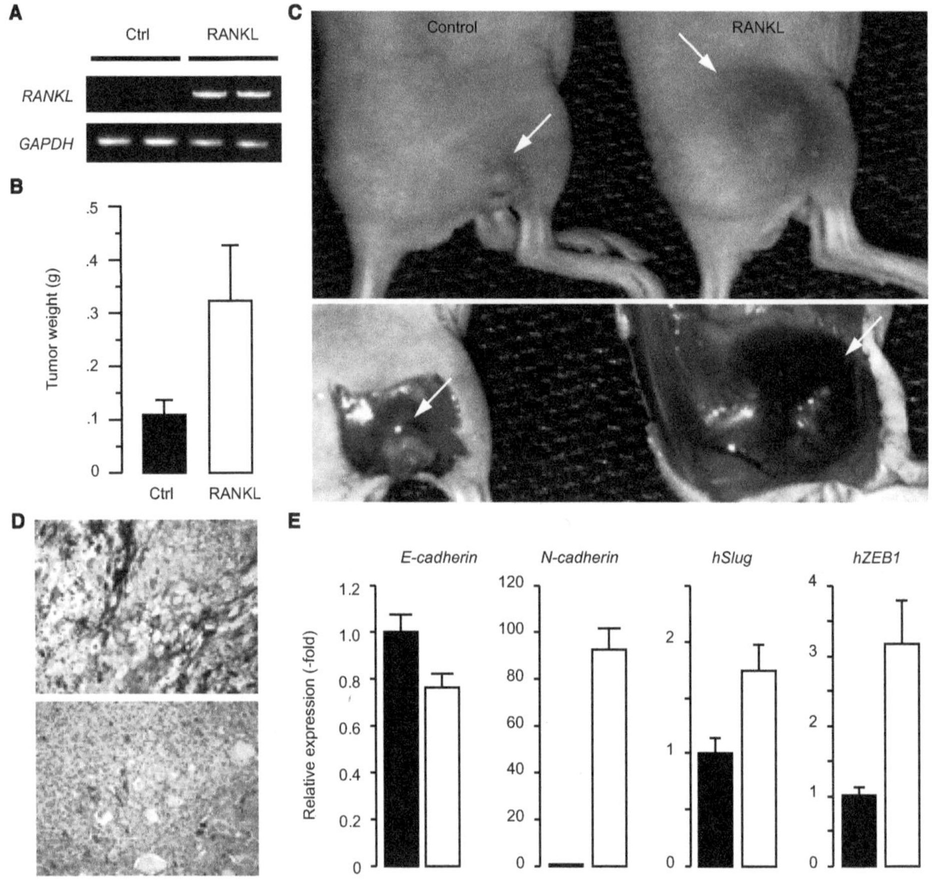

Fig. 3. OSCC tumor formation in hindlimb is facilitated by RANKL. Control (Ctrl) and RANKL-expressing cells (RANKL) were injected into hindlimb muscles and, after 28 days, the tumors were weighed (B), and photographed (C). RANKL mRNA in the tumors was examined by RT-PCR (A). The sections from the control (upper panel) and RANKL-expressing (lower) tumors were subjected to immunohistochemistry using an antibody against E-cadherin (D). mRNA levels of E-adhetin, N-cadherin, Slug, and ZEB1 were also analyzed by quantitative PCR (E).

To test whether RANKL-expressing tumors in fact underwent EMT, we evaluated the expression levels of E-cadherin, N-cadherin, and several transcription factors implicated in EMT (Gotzmann et al., 2004). Indeed, expression of E-cadherin was significantly decreased in RANKL-expressing tumor cells. Accordingly, N-cadherin expression was dramatically upregulated in tumor tissues expressing RANKL. Therefore, these results confirmed that cadherin switching from E-cadherin to N-cadherin occurs in tumors expressing RANKL. Of transcription factors implicated in inducing EMT including Slug, Snail, Twist, and ZEB1, Slug and ZEB1 were upregulated in RANKL-expressing tumors (Figure 3E). However, we could note no differences in their expression *in vitro*. Moreover, notwithstanding the dramatic increment in tumor formation of RANKL-expressing cells in the hindlimbs, there are no significant differences in *in vitro* proliferation, motility, and invasiveness between RANKL-expressing and control cell lines. Thus, RANKL functions, in addition to its expression, are also in a manner dependent on *in vivo*.

4.5 Significance of RANKL as an *in vivo*-specific biomarker

Beyond its cell autonomous function, RANKL possesses ability to promote tumor angiogenesis, to our surprise, in a manner independent of VEGF. RANKL-expressing tumors were grossly rich in blood vessels, and immunohistochemical analysis using an antibody against CD31, a well-established marker for endothelial cells, revealed that RANKL-expressing tumors harbor significantly more abundant tumor microvessels than control tumors. Interestingly, this angiogenic potency was hampered in the presence of osteoprotegerin (OPG), a RANKL decoy receptor that inhibits RANK-RANKL signaling, whereas neutralization of VEGF using an anti-VEGF antibody failed to do so. These results together demonstrate that RANKL promotes tumor angiogenesis in a manner dependent on its cognate receptor RANK, as reported previously (Kim et al., 2002), but independent of VEGF.

One of the most serious clinical concerns accompanying OSCC is a high potential for local invasion, frequently targeting the adjacent bone. To conquer this, radical and surgical procedures have been enforced; however, the patients suffering from the deprivation of fundamental functions, including mastication and vocalization. Our findings may resolve this longstanding issue in OSCC; the recognition of RANKL and its relevant signaling as potential targets for conservative therapy will enable us to hamper the tumorigenesis and invasion by cutting the connection between OSCC and the tumor microenvironment.

In addition to the conventional molecular targeted therapy (i.e. small compounds and humanized antibodies), RANKL may constitute a better candidate for cancer immunotherapy. Several tumor antigens such as cancer-testis antigens provide specific targets for cancer cells due to their restricted expression patterns (Maio et al., 2003; Nicholaou et al., 2006; Suri, 2006). However, in the case that these molecules are not essential for cancer cell survival, the cells can escape the challenge of the immune system by reducing the expression of the antigens. Since the expression of RANKL in response to the microenvironment is critical for OSCC progression, we strongly propose RANKL-RANK signaling as being central to the conservative, multimodal treatment for this disease.

5. Conclusion

In summary, we have overviewed biomarkers with a particular focus on ones, functions of which are relevant to OSCC development, progression and its malignant potential. As we disclose, *in vivo* "functional biomarkers" such as RANKL would be of particular importance for both diagnosis and therapy of this disease.

The mechanism underlying the microenvironment-specific RANKL expression remains to be addressed. Given that the head and neck regions including the oral cavity are always challenged by every pathogen, the involvement of inflammatory responses might be indispensable for OSCC tumor initiation and progression (Allen et al., 2007; Choi & Myers, 2008; Ferris & Grandis, 2007; Lin et al., 2002; Pries et al., 2006). In addition, this region is also abundant in a range of growth factors that contribute to malignant conversion of OSCC through activating diverse cancer-related signaling pathways (Yamada et al., 2008; Nagano

& Saya, 2004; Ponta et al., 2003; Todd & Wong, 1999). We thus explored RANKL-inducing agents from a wide range of growth factors as well as inflammatory cytokines; however, failed to identify it so far. CXCL13 can certainly upregulate RANKL (Yuvaraj et al., 2009), albeit less efficiently compared to the upregulation observed *in vivo* (unpublished result). In the future, we believe that through our observations and the unveiling of remaining associated issues, the establishment of more rational, potent anti-cancer therapy with consideration of the communication between cancer cells and their respective microenvironment will eventually be accomplished.

6. Acknowledgment

We thank Tamaki Yamada for performing overall experiments; Tomomi Takahashi for pathological assistance; Yasunori Totsuka and Masanobu Shindoh for critical discussion, Jun-ichi Hamada, Masahiko Takahata, Takuya Watanabe, Hiroshi Takayanagi, and Jun-ichi Miyazaki for providing materials; Noriko Toyoda for technical assistance; and all members of our laboratories for helpful discussion. This study was supported in part by Grants-in-Aid from the Ministry of Education, Culture, Sports, Sciences, and Technology, from Japan Society for Promotion of Sciences, and grants from the Japan Science and Technology Agency, Akiyama Foundation, and Mochida Memorial Foundation for Medical and Pharmaceutical Research.

7. References

Agra IM, Carvalho AL, Pinto CA, Martins EP, Filho JG, Soares FA, Kowalski LP. (2008). Biological markers and prognostic in recurrent oral cancer after salvage surgery. *Arch Otolaryngol Head Neck Surg,* 134, 743–749.

Allen CT, Ricker JL, Chen Z, Van Waes C. (2007). Role of activated nuclear factor-kappaB in the pathogenesis and therapy of squamous cell carcinoma of the head and neck. *Head Neck,* 29, 959-971.

Arcasoy MO, Amin K, Chou SC, Haroon ZA, Varia M, Raleigh JA. (2005). Erythropoietin and erythropoietin receptor expression in head and neck cancer: relationship to tumor hypoxia. *Clin Cancer Res,* 11, 20–27.

Awano S, Dawson LA, Hunter AR, Turner AJ, Usmani BA. (2006). Endothelin system in oral squamous carcinoma cells: Specific siRNA targeting of ECE-1 blocks cell proliferation. *Int J Cancer,* 118, 1645–1652.

Bagnato A, Spinella F. (2002). Emerging role of endothelin-1 in tumor angiogenesis. *TRENDS Endocrinol Metabol,* 14(1), 44–50.

Bhalla A, Haque S, Taylor I, Winslet M, Loizidou M. (2009). Endothelin receptor antagonism and cancer. *Eur J Clin Invest,* 39(S2), 74–77.

Burtis WJ, Brady TG, Orloff JJ, Ersbak JB, Warrell Jr. RP, Olson BR, Wu TL, Mitnick ME, Broadus AE, Stewart AF. (1990). Immunochemical characterization of circulating parathyroid hormone-related protein in patients with humoral hypercalcemia of cancer. *N Engl J Med,* 322, 1106–1112.

Camisasca DR, Honorato J, Bernardo V, da Silva LE, da Fonseca EC, de Faria PA, Dias FL, Lourenc¸o Sde Q. (2009). Expression of Bcl-2 family proteins and associated clinicopathologic factors predict survival outcome in patients with oral squamous cell carcinoma. *Oral Oncol,* 45, 225–233.

Campbell TN, Robbins SM. (2008). The Eph receptor/ephrin system: an emerging player in the invasion game. *Curr Issues Mol Biol*, 10, 61–66.

Carducci MA, Saad F, Abrahamsson PA, Dearnaley DP, Schulman CC, North SA, Sleep DJ, Isaacson JD, Nelson JB. (2007). A phase 3 randomized controlled trial of the efficacy and safety of atrasentan in men with metastatic hormone-refractory prostate cancer. *Cancer*, 110, 1959–1966.

Chien CY, Su CY, Hwang CF, Chuang HC, Chen CM, Huang CC. (2006). High expressions of CD105 and VEGF in early oral cancer predict potential cervical metastasis. *J Surg Oncol*, 94, 413–417.

Choi S, Myers JN. (2008). Molecular pathogenesis of oral squamous cell carcinoma: implications for therapy. *J Dent Res*, 87, 14-32.

Choi SW, Kim JY, Park JY, Cha IH, Kim J, Lee S. (2008). Expression of carbonic anhydrase IX is associated with postoperative recurrence and poor prognostic in surgically treated oral squamous cell carcinoma. *Hum Pathol*, 39, 1317–1322.

Chuang HC, Su CY, Huang HY, Chien CY, Chen CM, Huang CC. (2006). High expression expression of CD105 as a prognostic predictor of early tongue cancer. *Laryngoscope*, 116, 1175–1179.

Cui N, Nomura T, Noma H, Yokoo K, Takagi R, Hashimoto S, Okamoto M, Sato M, Yu G, Guo C, Shibahala T. (2005). Effect of YM529 on a model of mandibular invasion by oral squamous cell carcinoma in mice. *Clin Cancer Res*, 11, 2713-2719.

Derka S, Vairaktaris E, Papakosta V Vassiliou S, Acil Y, Vylliotis A, Spyridonidou S, Lazaris AC, Mourouzis C, Kokkori A, Moulavasili P, Perrea D, Donta I, Yapijakis C, Patsouris E. (2006). Cell proliferation and apoptosis culminate in early stages of oral oncogenesis. *Oral Oncol*, 42, 540–550.

de Vicente JC, Fresno MF, Villalain L, Vega JA, Herna´ndez Vallejo G. (2005). Expression and clinical significance of matrix metalloproteinase-2 and matrix metalloproteinase-9 in oral squamous cell carcinoma. *Oral Oncol*, 41, 283–293.

de Vicente JC, Lequerica-Ferna´ndez P, Santamarı´a J, Fresno MF. (2007). Expression of MMP-7 and MT1-MMP in oral squamous cell carcinoma as predictive indicator for tumor invasion and prognosis. *J Oral Pathol Med*, 36, 415–424.

Ferris RL, Grandis JR. (2007). NF-kappaB gene signatures and p53 mutations in head and neck squamous cell carcinoma. *Clin Cancer Res*, 13, 5663-5664.

Fillies T, Werkmeister R, van Diest PJ, Brandt B, Joos U, Buerger H. (2005). HIF1-alpha overexpression indicates a good prognostic in early stage squamous cell carcinomas of the oral floor. *BMC Cancer*, 5, 84.

Fillies T, Woltering M, Brandt B, Van Diest JP, Werkmeister R, Joos U, Buerger H. (2007). Cell cycle regulating proteins p21 and p27 in prognostic of oral squamous cell carcinomas. *Oncol Rep*, 17, 355–359.

Georgolios A, Batistatou A, Charalabopoulos A, Manolopoulos L, Charalabopoulos K. (2006). The role of CD44 adhesion molecule in oral cavity cancer. *Exp Oncol*, 28, 94–98.

Gotzmann J, Mikula M, Eger A, Schulte-Hermann R, Foisner R, Beug H, Mikulits W. (2004). Molecular aspects of epithelial cell plasticity: implications for local tumor invasion and metastasis. *Mutat Res*, 566, 9-20.

Grimshaw MJ. (2007). Endothelins and hypoxia-inducible factor in cancer. *Endocr Relat Cancer*, 14, 233–244.

Guise TA, Yin JJ, Mohammad KS. (2003). Role of endothelin-1 in osteoblastic bone metastases. *Cancer*, 97(S3), 779–784.

Harada H, Omura K, Nakajima Y, Hasegawa S, Mogi S. (2006). Cyclin B1 is useful to predict occult cervical lymph node metastases in tongue carcinoma. *J Exp Clin Cancer Res*, 25(3), 351–356.

Hoffmann RR, Yurgel LS, Campos MM. (2010). Endothelins and their receptors as biological markers for oral cancer. *Oral Oncology*, 46, 644-647.

Hsu H, Lacey DL, Dunstan CR, Solovyev I, Colombero A, Timms E, Tan HL, Elliott G, Kelley MJ, Sarosi I, Wang L, Xia XZ, Elliott R, Chiu L, Black T, Scully S, Capparelli C, Morony S, Shimamoto G, Bass MB, Boyle WJ. (1999). Tumor necrosis factor receptor family member RANK mediates osteoclast differentiation and activation induced by osteoprotegerin ligand. *Proc Natl Acad Sci USA*, 96, 3540–3545.

Jonathan RA, Wijffels KI, Peeters W, de Wilde PC, Marres HA, Merkx MA, Oosterwijk E, van der Kogel AJ, Kaanders JH. (2006). The prognostic value of endogenous hypoxia-related markers for head and neck squamous cell carcinomas treated with ARCON. *Radiother Oncol*, 79, 288–297.

Kademani D, Lewis JT, Lamb DH, Rallis DJ, Harrington JR. (2009). Angiogenesis and CD34 expression as a predictor of recurrence in oral squamous cell carcinoma. *J Oral Maxillofac Surg*, 67, 1800-1805.

Kato K, Kawashiri S, Yoshizawa K, Kitahara H, Yamamoto E. (2008). Apoptosisassociated markers and clinical outcome in human oral squamous cell carcinomas. *J Oral Pathol Med*, 37, 364–371.

Kim SJ, Shin HJ, Jung KY, Baek SK, Shin BK, Choi J, Kim BS, Shin SW, Kim YH, Kim JS, Oosterwijk E. (2007). Prognostic value of carbonic anhydrase IX and Ki-67 expression in squamous cell carcinoma of the tongue. *Jpn J Clin Oncol*, 37, 812–819.

Kim YM, Lee YM, Kim HS, Kim JD, Choi Y, Kim KW, Lee SY, Kwon YG. (2002). TNF-related activation-induced cytokine (TRANCE) induces angiogenesis through the activation of Src and phospholipase C (PLC) in human endothelial cells. *J Biol Chem*, 277, 6799-6805.

Kosunen A, Pirinen R, Ropponen K, Pukkila M, Kellokoski J, Virtaniemi J, Sironen R, Juhola M, Kumpulainen E, Johansson R, Nuutinen J, Kosma VM. (2007). CD44 expression and its relationship with MMP-9, clinicopathological factors and survival in oral squamous cell carcinoma. *Oral Oncol*, 43, 51–59.

Krieg C & Boyman O. (2008). The role of chemokines in cancer immune surveillance by the adaptive immune system. *Semin Cancer Biol*, 19, 76–83.

Kunkel M, Moergel M, Stockinger M, Jeong JH, Fritz G, Lehr HA, Whiteside TL. (2007). Overexpression of GLUT-1 is associated with resistance to radiotherapy and adverse prognostic in squamous cell carcinoma of the oral cavity. *Oral Oncol*, 43, 796–803.

Kusserow H, Unger T. (2004). Vasoacitive peptides, their receptors and drug development. *Basic Clin Pharmacol Toxicol*, 94, 5–12.

LaCasse EC, Mahoney DJ, Cheung HH, Plenchette S, Baird S, Korneluk RG. (2008). IAP-targeted therapies for cancer. *Oncogene*, 27, 6252–6275.

Laimer K, Spizzo G, Gastl G, Obrist P, Brunhuber T, Fong D, Barbieri V, Jank S, Doppler W, Rasse M, Norer B. (2007). High EGFR expression predicts poor prognostic in patients with squamous cell carcinoma of the oral cavity and oropharynx: a TMA-based immunohistochemical analysis. *Oral Oncol*, 43, 193–198.

Leibbrandt A, Penninger JM. (2008). RANK/RANKL: regulators of immune responses and bone physiology. *Ann N Y Acad Sci*, 1143, 123-150.

Legler DF, Loetscher M, Roos RS, Clark-Lewis I, Baggiolini M, Moser B. (1998). B cell-attracting chemokine 1, a human CXC chemokine expressed in lymphoid tissues, selectively attracts B lymphocytes via BLR1/CXCR5. *J Exp Med*, 187, 655–660.

Levin ER. Endothelins. (1995). *N Eng J Med*, 333, 356–363.

Liao J & McCauley LK. (2006). Skeletal metastasis: Established and emerging roles of parathyroid hormone related protein (PTHrP). *Cancer Metastasis Rev*, 25, 559–571.

Lim J, Kim JH, Paeng JY, Kim MJ, Hong SD, Lee JI, Hong SP. (2005). Prognostic value of activated Akt expression in oral squamous cell carcinoma. *J Clin Pathol*, 58, 1199–1205.

Lin DT, Subbaramaiah K, Shah JP, Dannenberg AJ, Boyle JO. (2002). Cyclooxygenase-2: a novel molecular target for the prevention and treatment of head and neck cancer. *Head Neck*, 24, 792-799.

Lin PY, Yu CH, Wang JT, Chen HH, Cheng SJ, Kuo MY, Chiang CP. (2008). Expression of hypoxia-inducible factor-1 alpha is significantly associated with the progression and prognostic of oral squamous cell carcinomas in Taiwan. *J Oral Pathol Med*, 37, 18–25.

Lippert BM, Knauer SK, Fetz V, Mann W, Stauber RH. (2007). Dynamic Survivin in head and neck cancer: molecular mechanism and therapeutic potential. *Int J Cancer*, 121, 1169–1174.

Liu SY, Chang LC, Pan LF, Hung YJ, Lee CH, Shieh YS. (2008). Clinicopathologic significance of tumor cell-lined vessel and microenvironment in oral squamous cell carcinoma. *Oral Oncol*, 44, 277–285.

Lo Muzio L, Santarelli A, Caltabiano R, Rubini C, Pieramici T, Trevisiol L, Carinci F, Leonardi R, De Lillo A, Lanzafame S, Bufo P, Piattelli A. (2005a). p63 overexpression associates with poor prognostic in head and neck squamous cell carcinoma. *Hum Pathol*, 36, 187–194.

Lo Muzio L, Farina A, Rubini C, Pezzetti F, Stabellini G, Laino G, Santarelli A, Pannone G, Bufo P, de Lillo A, Carinci F. (2005b). Survivin as prognostic factor in squamous cell carcinoma of the oral cavity. *Cancer Lett*, 225, 27–33.

Lo Muzio L, Campisi G, Farina A, Rubini C, Pastore L, Giannone N, Colella G, Leonardi R, Carinci F. (2007). Effect of p63 expression on survival in oral squamous cell carcinoma. *Cancer Invest*, 25, 464–469.

Luukkaa M, Vihinen P, Kronqvist P, Vahlberg T, Pyrho¨nen S, Ka¨ha¨ ri VM, Gre´nman R. (2006). Association between high collagenase-3 expression levels and poor prognostic in patients with head and neck cancer. *Head Neck*, 28, 225–234.

Lyons AJ, Jones J. (2007). Cell adhesion molecules, the extracellular matrix and oral squamous carcinoma. *Int J Oral Maxillofac Surg*, 36, 671–679.

Maio M, Coral S, Fratta E, Altomonte M, Sigalotti L. (2003). Epigenetic targets for immune intervention in human malignancies. *Oncogene*, 22, 6484-6488.

Motte S, Mcentee K, Naeije R. (2006). Endothelin receptor antagonists. *Pharmacol Ther*, 110, 386–414.

Mundy GR. (2002). Metastasis to bone: causes, consequences and therapeutic opportunities. *Nat Rev Cancer*, 2, 584-593.

Muñoz-Guerra MF, Marazuela EG, Ferna´ndez-Contreras ME, Gamallo C. (2005). P-cadherin expression reduced in squamous cell carcinoma of the oral cavity: an indicator of poor prognosis. *Cancer*, 103, 960–969.

Myoung H, Kim MJ, Lee JH, Ok YJ, Paeng JY, Yun PY. (2006). Correlation of proliferative markers (Ki-67 and PCNA) with survival and lymph node metastasis in oral squamous cell carcinoma: a clinical and histopathological analysis of 113 patients. *Int J Oral Maxillofac Surg*, 35, 1005–1010.

Nagano O, Saya H. (2004). Mechanism and biological significance of CD44 cleavage. *Cancer Sci*, 95, 930-935.

Nelson J, Bagnato A, Battistini B, Nisen P. (2003). The endothelin axis: emerging role in cancer. *Nat Rev Cancer*, 3(2), 110–116.

Nelson JB, Love W, Chin JL, Saad F, Schulman CC, Sleep DJ, Qian J, Steinberg J, & Carducci M. (2008). Phase 3, randomized, controlled trial of atrasentan in patients with nonmetastatic, hormone-refractory prostate cancer. *Cancer*, 113, 2478- 2487.

Nemes JA, Nemes Z, Ma´rton IJ. (2005). p21WAF1/CIP1 expression is a marker of poor prognostic in oral squamous cell carcinoma. *J Oral Pathol Med*, 34, 274–279.

Nicholaou T, Ebert L, Davis ID, Robson N, Klein O, Maraskovsky E, Chen W, Cebon J. (2006). Directions in the immune targeting of cancer: lessons learned from the cancer-testis Ag NY-ESO-1. *Immunol Cell Biol*, 84, 303-317.

Nomura T, Shibahara T, Katakura A, Matsubara S, Takano N. (2007). Establishment of a murine model of bone invasion by oral squamous cell carcinoma. *Oral Oncol*, 43, 257-262.

Oliveira LR, Ribeiro-Silva A, Zucoloto S. (2007a). Prognostic impact of p53 and p63 immunoexpression in oral squamous cell carcinoma. *J Oral Pathol Med*, 36, 191–197.

Oliveira LR, Ribeiro-Silva A, Zucoloto S. (2007b). Prognostic significance of p53 and p63 immunolocalisation in primary and matched lymph node metastasis in oral squamous cell carcinoma. *Acta Histochem*, 109, 388–396.

Oliveira LR, Ribeiro-Silva A, Costa JP, Simo˜es AL, Matteo MA, Zucoloto S. (2008). Prognostic factors and survival analysis in a sample of oral squamous cell carcinoma patients. *Oral Surg Oral Med Oral Pathol Oral Radiol Endod*, 106, 685–695.

Oliveira LR, Ribeiro-Silva A. (2011). Prognostic significance of immunohistochemical biomarkers in oral squamous cell carcinoma. *Int J Oral Maxillofac Surg*, 40, 298-307.

Ogden GR, Cowpe JG, Green M. (1992). Cytobrush and wooden spatula for oral exfoliative cytology. A comparison. *Acta Cytol*, 36, 706–710.

Ogden GR, Leigh I, Chisholm DM, Cowpe JG, Lane EB. (1996). Exfoliative cytology of normal oral mucosa. Assessing the basal cell keratin phenotype. *Acta Cytol*, 40, 933–936.

Ponta H, Sherman L, Herrlich PA. (2003). CD44: from adhesion molecules to signalling regulators. *Nat Rev Mol Cell Biol*, 4, 33-45.

Pries R, Nitsch S, Wollenberg B. (2006). Role of cytokines in head and neck squamous cell carcinoma. *Expert Rev Anticancer Ther*, 6, 1195-1203.

Pukkila M, Kosunen A, Ropponen K, Virtaniemi J, Kellokoski J, Kumpulainen E, Pirinen R, Nuutinen J, Johansson R, Kosma VM. (2007). High stromal versican expression predicts unfavourable outcome in oral squamous cell carcinoma. *J Clin Pathol*, 60, 267–272.

Rahmani M, Wong BW, Ang L, Cheung CC, Carthy JM, Walinski H, McManus BM. (2006). Versican: signaling to transcriptional control pathways. *Can J Physiol Pharmacol*, 84, 777–792.

Roh JL, Cho KJ, Kwon GY, Ryu CH, Chang HW, Choi SH, Nam SY, Kim SY. (2009). The prognostic value of hypoxia markers in T2-staged oral tongue cancer. *Oral Oncol*, 45, 63–68.

Roodman GD. (2004). Mechanisms of bone metastasis. *N Engl J Med*, 350, 1655-1664.

Rosano` L, Spinella F, Di Castro V, Decandia S, Nicotra MR, Natali PG, Bagnato A. (2006). Endothelin-1 is required during epithelial to mesenchymal transition in ovarian cancer progression. *Exp Biol Med*, 231, 1128–1131.

SahebJamee M, Eslami M, AtarbashiMoghadam F, Sarafnejad A. (2008). Salivary concentration of TNFalpha, IL1 alpha, IL6, and IL8 in oral squamous cell carcinoma. *Med Oral Patol Oral Cir Bucal*, 13, E292-295.

Sakata K, Someya M, Nagakura H, Nakata K, Oouchi A, Takagi M, Hareyama M. (2008). Brachytherapy for oral tongue cancer: an analysis of treatment results with various biological markers. *Jpn J Clin Oncol*, 38, 402–407.

Schmidt BL, Pickering V, Liu S, Quang P, Dolan J, Connelly ST, Jordan RC. (2007). Peripheral endothelin-A receptor antagonism attenuates carcinoma-induced pain. *Eur J Pain*, 11, 406–414.

Shao Z, Zhang WF, Chen XM, Shang ZJ. (2008). Expression of EphA2 and VEGF in squamous cell carcinoma of the tongue: correlation with the angiogenesis and clinical outcome. *Oral Oncol*, 44, 1110–1117.

Shen X, Qian L, Falzon M. (2004). PTH-related protein enhances MCF-7 breast cancer cell adhesion, migration, and invasion via an intracrine pathway. *Exp Cell Res*, 294, 420–433.

Shiraki M, Odajima T, Ikeda T, Sasaki A, Satoh M,Yamaguchi A,Noguchi M, Nagai I, Hiratsuka H. (2005). Combined expression of p53, cyclin D1 and epidermal growth factor receptor improves estimation of prognostic in curatively resected oral cancer. *Mod Pathol*, 18, 1482–1489.

Silva SD, Perez DE, Alves FA, Nishimoto IN, Pinto CA, Kowalski LP, Graner E. (2008). ErbB2 and fatty acid synthase (FAS) expression in 102 squamous cell carcinomas of the tongue: correlation with clinical outcomes. *Oral Oncol*, 44, 484–490.

Silva SD, Cunha IW, Nishimoto IN, Soares FA, Carraro DM, Kowalski LP, Graner E. (2009). Clinicopathological significance of ubiquitin-specific protease 2a (USP2a), fatty acid synthase (FASN), and ErbB2 expression in oral squamous cell carcinomas. *Oral Oncol*, 45, e134–e139.

Soni S, Kaur J, Kumar A, Chakravarti N, Mathur M, Bahadur S, Shukla NK, Deo SV, Ralhan R. (2005). Alterations of rb pathway components are frequent events in patients with oral epithelial dysplasia and predict clinical outcome in patients with squamous cell carcinoma. *Oncology*, 68, 314–325.

St John MA, Li Y, Zhou X, Denny P, Ho CM, Montemagno C, Shi W, Qi F, Wu B, Sinha U, Jordan R, Wolinsky L, Park NH, Liu H, Abemayor E, & Wong DT. (2004). Interleukin 6 and interleukin 8 as potential biomarkers for oral cavity and oropharyngeal squamous cell carcinoma. *Arch Otolaryngol Head Neck Surg*, 130, 929-935.

Suda T, Jimi E, Nakamura I, Takahashi N. (1997). Role of 1 alpha,25-dihydroxyvitamin D3 in osteoclast differentiation and function. *Methods Enzymol*, 282, 223-235.

Suri A (2006): Cancer testis antigens--their importance in immunotherapy and in the early detection of cancer. *Expert Opin Biol Ther*, 6, 379-389.

Teruel A, Romero M, Cacalano NA, Head C, Jewett A. (2008). Potential contribution of naïve immune effectors to oral tumor resistance: role in synergistic induction of VEGF, IL-6, and IL-8 secretion. *Cancer Immunol Immunother*, 57, 359-366.

Todd R, Wong DT. (1999). Epidermal growth factor receptor (EGFR) biology and human oral cancer. *Histol Histopathol*, 14, 491-500.

Ueda G, Sunakawa H, Nakamori K, Shinya T, Tsuhako W, Tamura Y, Kosugi T, Sato N, Ogi K, Hiratsuka H. (2006). Aberrant expression of beta- and gamma-catenin is an independent prognostic marker in oral squamous cell carcinoma. *Int J Oral Maxillofac Surg*, 35, 356–361.

Wimmer-Kleikamp SH, Lackmann M. (2005). Eph-modulated cell morphology, adhesion and motility in carcinogenesis. *IUBMB Life*, 57, 421–431.

Yamada T, Tsuda M, Ohba Y, Kawaguchi H, Totsuka Y, Shindoh M. (2008). PTHrP promotes malignancy of human oral cancer cell downstream of the EGFR signaling. *Biochem Biophys Res Commun*, 368, 575-581.

Yamada T, Tsuda M, Takahashi T, Totsuka Y, Shindoh M, Ohba Y. (2011). RANKL expression specifically observed *in vivo* promotes epithelial mesenchymal transition and tumor progression. *Am J Pathol*, 178, 2846-2857.

Yamamoto E, Kohama G, Sunakawa H, Iwai M, Hiratsuka H. (1983). Mode of invasion, bleomycin sensitivity, and clinical course in squamous cell carcinoma of the oral cavity. *Cancer*, 51, 2175-2180.

Yanagisawa M, Kurihara H, Kimura S, Tomobe Y, Kobayashi M, Mitsui Y, Yazaki Y, Goto K, Masaki T. (1988). A novel potent vasoconstrictor peptide produced by vascular endothelial cells. *Nature*, 332, 411–415.

Yang MH, Wu MZ, Chiou SH, Chen PM, Chang SY, Liu CJ, Teng SC, Wu KJ. (2008). Direct regulation of TWIST by HIF-1alpha promotes metastasis. *Nat Cell Biol*, 10, 295-305.

Yang J, Weinberg RA. (2008). Epithelial-mesenchymal transition: at the crossroads of development and tumor metastasis. *Dev Cell*, 14, 818-829.

Yuvaraj S, Griffin AC, Sundaram K, Kirkwood KL, Norris JS, Reddy SV. (2009). A Novel Function of CXCL13 to Stimulate RANK Ligand Expression in Oral Squamous Cell Carcinoma Cells. *Mol Cancer Res*, 7, 1399–1407

Yu Z, Weinberger PM, Haffty BG, Sasaki C, Zerillo C, Joe J, Kowalski D, Dziura J, Camp RL, Rimm DL, Psyrri A. (2005). Cyclin d1 is a valuable prognostic marker in oropharyngeal squamous cell carcinoma. *Clin Cancer Res*, 11, 1160–1166.

Zhang M, Zhang P, Zhang C, Sun J, Wang L, Li J, Tian Z, Chen W. (2009). Prognostic significance of Bcl-2 and Bax protein expression in the patients with oral squamous cell carcinoma. *J Oral Pathol Med*, 38, 307–313.

Ziober AF, Patel KR, Alawi F, Gimotty F, Weber RS, Feldman MM, Chalian AA, Weinstein GS, Hunt J, Ziober BL. (2006). Identification of a Gene Signature for Rapid Screening of Oral Squamous Cell Carcinoma. *Clin Cancer Res*, 12, 5960-5971.

Part 3

Molecular Pathogenesis

16

Epigenetic Profiling of Oral Cancer

A. Santoro[1,2], G. Pannone[1], S. Papagerakis[5],
R. Serpico[3], A. Guida[3], L. Lo Muzio[4] and P. Bufo[1]
[1]Department of Surgical Sciences,
Section of Pathological Anatomy and Cytopathology, University of Foggia, Foggia,
[2]Department of Surgical Sciences,
Institute of Pathological Anatomy, University of Bari, Bari,
[3]Department of Oral Pathology, Orthodontics and Oral Surgery,
Second University of Napoli, Napoli,
[4]Department of Surgical Sciences, Section of Oral Pathology,
University of Foggia, Foggia,
[5]Department of Otolaryngology – Head and Neck Surgery and Oncology,
Medical School University of Michigan Ann Arbor, Ann Arbor, MI,
[1,2,3,4]Italy
[5]USA

1. Introduction

Oral squamous cell carcinoma (OSCC) is the most common type of oral neoplasm, accounting for over 90% of all mouth malignancies and 38% of head and neck tumors. Worldwide, OSCC is the eighth most common human cancer, with more than 500,000 new cases being diagnosed every year. Surprisingly, the number of annual deaths for this disease has practically not changed in the last 30 years (Funk, G.F.; Karnell, L.H., 2002).

This is because invasive surgical treatments (involving both oral cavity and neck) are still the only effective way to treat OSCC; thus detection in early stages could dramatically improve cure rates and quality of life by minimizing invasive surgery (Scully, C., 1995). To improve diagnosis and prevention, researchers have spent considerable effort to understand which genetic and/or environmental changes may be related to this tumor. Although environmental risk factors associated with development of oral cancer have been sufficiently understood (smoking, alcohol, betel, diet, living habits, etc.), knowledge of the genetic bases in oral carcinogenesis is still a challenging task. OSCC is a result of multiple genes alterations, which are modulated by individual predisposing conditions and environmental influences. Furthermore, in the last ten years a new category of non-genetic events able to modify gene expression has been massively investigated: the so called 'epigenetic phenomena' (Bird, A., 2007).

Epigenetic factors are non-genetic phenomena which interfere with genes expression. Such modifications pass on successive generations of cells, even if there is no mutation in corresponding genes. Epigenetic events are linked with carcinogenesis when one or more oncogenes/tumour suppressors are directly or indirectly affected such that their expression and function may be permanently altered (Feinberg, A.P., 2001)

Cellular aging, risk factors and, as recently discovered, chronic inflammation via mediators, such as IL-6, may be potential inducers of epigenetic alterations in oral mucosa cells. It is a general belief that these alterations would accumulate in the normal-appearing mucosa while carcinogenesis is in progress, or before any tumor lesion is detected.

Three major types of such epigenetic mechanism are currently known: DNA hyper-methylation, histone code changes and RNA interference.

1.1 DNA hyper-methylation

Methylation is the biochemical addition of a methyl group(-CH3) to a molecule. In cellular biology, this refers to methylation of DNA, RNA and proteins. Protein methylation has been extensively studied recently and it is an essential post-translational modification that affects its function. RNA methylation is less understood and it probably plays a role in message stability. DNA methylation is the only normally occurring modification of DNA from bacteria to humans, although it plays a different role in eukaryotes and in prokaryotes (Baylin, S.B.; Herman, J.G., 2000)

In mammals, methylation physiologically affects cytosine bases incorporated into DNA, primarily when it is followed by a guánosine (hence it is defined as Cytosine-phospho-Guanosine or CpG methylation). CpG sites are distributed unevenly in the genome. They are rare in 99% of the human genome, and most of these CpG sites are modified by methylation. It follows that about 1% of the genome consists of CpG rich areas, typically 500-2000 base pairs long, and are named CpG islands. About half of all CpG islands corresponds to transcription start sites and promoters of expressed genes, while non-promoter associated CpG islands are less well understood and can be methylated in normal tissues. About half of all genes has CpG islands in their promoters. Most promoter-associated CpG islands are free of methylation, regardless of the expression state of the associated gene. Genes that do not have CpG islands in their promoters show different patterns of methylation; some rare CpG sites are typically methylated in their transcription start areas when the gene is inactive, and un-methylated when the gene is active, but non-CpG island methylation does not prevent gene expression; it can be reversed quickly upon gene activation and may serve primarily to regulate the degree of acute gene activation by transcription factors. DNA hyper-methylation in promoter-associated CpG islands is considered the same way as proper genetic modification for its ability to influence genes expression. A switch from un-methylated to methylated CpG islands was first demonstrated on the inactive X-chromosome in women in the rare instances when a cell needs mono-allelic expression for normal function, and then in about 100 genes that are imprinted (Mono-allelic expression based on parental origin). DNA hyper-methylation is now regarded as an epigenetic mechanism of gene silencing in mammals. The DNA-methyltransferase enzymes (DNMT1, DNMT3a and DNMT3b) are essential to establish and preserve normal patterns of DNA methylation, and are helped in this function by other proteins, such as DNMT3L (Robertson, K.D., 2001). Hyper-methylation role in oral carcinogenesis will be treated in the second section of this chapter.

1.2 Histone code changes

In eukaryotic cells, DNA is wrapped around an octameric histone core to form the nucleosome, the fundamental subunit of chromatin. Many residues in the histone proteins are subject to reversible post-translational modifications, emerging as important epigenetic mediators of gene expression changes. There are numerous possible modifications of histone tails which regulate genes expression, such as acetylation, methylation, ubiquitylation and phosphorylation. Histone methylation, mediated by histone methyltransferases (HMTs), can have either positive or negative effects on gene expression. Increase in histone acetylation generally correlates with gene activation, and results from the dynamic interplay between histone acetyltransferases (HATs) and histone deacetylases (HDACs). Furthermore, histone modifications play an important role in chromosome structure, and silencing marks are enriched at silenced loci, such as imprinted genes, suggesting that they play a role there as well. The ultimate mediators of histone methylation associated gene silencing appear to be proteins that bind specific modified histone and recruit effector protein complexes. Among these, the ones which seems to play a significant role in carcinogenesis belongs to ING protein family. The ING proteins (ING 1-5) are involved in cell cycle, apoptosis and senescence. The ING family emerged as putative tumor suppressor gene (TSG), and its major mechanism of activity entails the conserved plant homeodomain (PHD), which binds to histones in a methylation-sensitive pathway, e.g. binding histone H3 tri-methylated on lysine 4 (H3K4me3), suggesting that ING proteins may contribute to the maintenance of the epigenetic code. Furthermore, ING family members contain nuclear localization signals and N-terminal sequences, which play an important role in the interaction with histone acetyltransferase (HAT) and histone deacetyltransferase (HDAC). Although ING proteins have the same PHD motif, the variation in the N-terminal dictates the differences in the suppressive ability of ING in various tumors. ING proteins are involved in transcriptional regulation of genes, such as the p53-inducible gene p21. In cancer cells, INGs mRNA levels are often lost or suppressed but their genes are rarely mutated; indeed, the inactivation of the normal function is achieved through allelic loss of genomic regions containing the ING gene, alteration in the ING promoter region, variation of mRNA splicing efficacy or reduced mRNA stability. It is most probably a combination of these aberrant mechanisms that resulted in reduced levels of ING protein. Furthermore, the mechanism of suppression of ING expression may be related to the abnormally high methylation levels of the ING gene promoter, which have been related to low transcript levels. Recently, the potential roles of ING proteins as prognostic biomarkers, detector of aggressive behavior of tumors as well as predictive factor of chemo-radiotherapy response, have been hypothesized. Emerging evidence on the function of ING and related regulatory mechanisms strongly points to ING as a candidate TSG and therefore a potential target in the molecular therapy of some types of cancer (Gunduz, M.; Demircan, K., 2009; Gunduz, M.; Gunduz, E.; Rivera, R.S., 2008). Being research on INGs in its early stages, this topic will not be treated in this chapter.

1.3 RNA interference (RNAi)

In 2006, Andrew Fire and Craig C. Mello shared the Nobel Prize in Physiology or Medicine for their work on RNA interference in the nematode worm *C. elegans*, which they published in 1998 (Fire, A.; Xu, S., 1998).

RNA interference (**RNAi**) is a system involved in controlling gene activation in living cells. Two types of small RNA molecules - microRNA (miRNA) and small interfering RNA (siRNA) - are considered as key mechanisms related to RNA interference. The scientific community considers RNA interference the breakthrough biological discovery of the decade with the potential to change how diseases are treated. Being RNAi machinery in every cell and any gene a potential target, any disease caused by or greatly exacerbated by the expression of a dominant gene can in principle be treated by RNAi. This means that the list of potential indications is long. Diseases that are intractable or poorly responsive to current therapy include cancer, neurodegenerative disease, viral infection, and macular degeneration, and these are indeed the most sudied disease models (Dykxhoorn, D.M.; Palliser, D., 2006). In this chapter we discuss the possible role of siRNa and miRNA in oral cancer.

- **Small interfering RNAs** (**siRNA**), sometimes referred to as **short interfering RNAs** or **silencing RNAs**, represent a class of double-stranded RNA molecules, 20-25 nucleotides in length, that play a notable role in the RNA interference (RNAi) pathway, where it interferes with the expression of a specific gene, but also in RNAi-related pathways as well as in antiviral mechanism or in shaping the chromatin structure of a genome. siRNAs were first discovered by David Baulcombe's group at the Sainsbury Laboratory in Norwich, England, as part of post-transcriptional gene silencing (PTGS) in plants. The group published their findings in *Science* in a paper titled "A species of small antisense RNA in post-transcriptional gene silencing in plants"(Hamilton, A.; Baulcombe, D., 1999). Shortly thereafter, in 2001, synthetic siRNAs were shown to be able to induce RNAi in mammalian cells by Thomas Tuschl, and colleagues in a paper published in *Nature* (Elbashir, S.; Harborth, J., 2001). This discovery led to a surge in interest in harnessing siRNA for biomedical research and drug development. It is expected that in some situations turning off or knocking down the activity of a gene with an siRNA could produce a therapeutic benefit. However, applying RNAi via siRNAs to living animals, especially humans, poses many challenges. Under experiments, siRNAs show different effectiveness in different cell types in a manner as yet poorly understood. Anyway, the effectiveness of gene silencing achieved with siRNA surpasses what has been possible in the past using other small nucleic acids, such as antisense oligonucleotides or ribozymes. In a head-to-head comparison, expression of siRNAs knocked down genes fold about 100–1000 times more efficiently than antisense oligonucleotides. The high efficiency may be related to the fact that one siRNA can be used over and over to guide the cleavage of many mRNAs. The high efficiency may also be due to protection of the active component of the siRNA (the antisense or guide strand) from digestion by endogenous RNases. Local siRNA administration has shown benefit in small animal models involving the lung, vagina, subcutaneous tissue, muscle, eye and central nervous system (Dykxhoorn D.M.; Palliser, D., 2006). Although siRNA are emerging as targeted cancer therapeutics inhibiting tumor-specific proteins or pathways, they have not totally eliminated the problem of toxicity. In fact, siRNA therapeutics are hindered by poor intracellular uptake, limited blood stability and non-specific immune stimulation. To address these problems, ligand-targeted, sterically stabilized nanoparticles have been adapted for siRNA. Intravenous administration into tumor-bearing mice gave selective tumor uptake, siRNA sequence-specific inhibition of protein expression within the tumor and inhibition of both tumor angiogenesis and growth rate. The results suggest achievement of two levels of targeting: tumor tissue selective delivery via the nanoparticle ligand and gene pathway selectivity via the siRNA oligonucleotide. This opens the door for better targeted therapy with both tissue and gene selectivity. (Schiffelers, R.M.; Ansari A., 2004). Results of phase I studies of the first two therapeutic RNAi trials (indicated for age-related macular degeneration, aka AMD), reported at the end of 2005, indicated that siRNAs are well tolerated and have suitable pharmacokinetic properties (Tansey, B., 2006). Other trials have indicated that Ebola-targeted siRNAs may be effective as post-exposure prophylaxis in humans, with 100% of non-human primates surviving a lethal dose of Zaire Ebolavirus, the most lethal strain (Geisbert, T.W.; Lee, A.C.H., 2010). The emerging siRNAs role in oral carcinogenesis will be treated in the third section of this chapter.

- **Micro-RNAs (miRNAs),** first identified in Caenorhabditis elegans in 1993, are small non-coding RNAs, which play an essential role in modifying genes expression. They are composed of 20–22 nucleotides, typically excised from 60–110 nucleotide foldback RNA precursor structures (Kim V.N. & Nam, J.W, 2006; Pasquinelli, A.E., Hunter, S., 2005). miRNAs seem to be implied in regulation of one third of the genes present in the human genome. Hundreds of miRNAs are expressed in eukaryotic cytoplasm, where they effect their action by mediation on RNA transcript cleavage and/or regulation of translation quote (Bentwich, I.; Avniel, A., 2005; Berezikov, E.; Guryev, V., 2005).

Since 2000, miRNAs have been investigated en mass and their mechanism of production and mode of action have been well characterized. The biogenesis of miRNAs involves a complex protein system, including members of the Argonaute family, Polymerase-II-dependent transcription and the RNase IIIs Drosha and Dicer (Lee, Y.; Ahn, C., 2003; Bartel, D.P.,2004). In particular, miRNAs are transcribed by RNA polymerase II or RNA polymerase III as a part of an intron of mRNA or as an independent gene unit; then, initially transcribed miRNAs, which can be several hundred to thousands of nucleotides long, are cleaved into a <100 nucleotide stem-loop structure by a type III RNase, named Drosha (Bernstein, E.; Caudy, A.A., 2001).

These pre-miRNAs are then exported from the nucleus to the cytoplasm by exportin 5 (Kim, V.N., 2004), and once there, the pre-miRNAs undergo another round of cleavage by Dicer, another type III RNase. The fully cleavage process results in miRNAs approximately 18 to 24 nucleotides long. These mature miRNAs- which are usually named "miR X", being x a cardinal number - are bound by a protein complex, called RNA-induced silencing complex (RISC). This active miRNA-RISC complex binds to target mRNAs based on sequence homology between the miRNA and the mRNA. Typically, the miRNA blocks mRNA translation and/or leads to mRNA degradation. Because miRNAs bind with imperfect complementary to target mRNAs, it is estimated that one miRNA is capable of binding >100 different mRNAs with different binding efficiencies. The number of human miRNAs is in excess of 450, twice as many as initial calculations indicated and more than 1,000 predicted miRNA genes are awaiting experimental confirmation.With about 1,000 miRNAs expected to be present in the human genome, it is postulated that ~30% of all mRNAs are post-transcriptionally regulated by miRNAs. Hence they are considered to play important roles in cell growth, differentiation, apoptosis, stress response, immune response, and glucose secretion. It has recently been proved that miRNAs are differentially expressed in cancer cells compared with normal cells, and it seems that miRNAs cluster (changing their number in the order of ten to hundreds)can characterize different types of solid and haematopoietic tumor cells more accurately than mRNA, suggesting that there is a link between miRNAs and cancer and that miRNAs can be used to detect cancerous/precancerous condition. miRNAs located in genomic regions amplified in cancers (such as the *miR-17–92* cluster) function as oncogenes, whereas miRNAs located in portions of chromosomes deleted in cancers (such as the *miR-15a–miR-16-1* cluster) function as tumour suppressors (Kent, O.A. & Mendell, J.T., 2006; Gregory, R.I. & Shiekhattar, R., 2005). The genomic abnormalities found to influence the activity of miRNAs are represented by chromosomal rearrangements, genomic amplifications or deletions and mutation and also by epigenetic silencing (Kozaki, K.; Imoto, I., 2008).

Abnormal expression of mature miRNAs or of their precursor have important consequences for the expression of various protein-coding genes involved in malignant transformation if compared with the corresponding normal tissues, and can be found by various genome-wide techniques (including different microarray platforms or bead-based flow cytometry) (Calin, G. A. *et al.*, 2004). It has been stated that miRNA expression fingerprints correlate with clinical and biological characteristics of tumors, including tissue type, tumor origin, differentiation, aggression and response to therapy .(Lu, J. *et al.*, 2005). Volinia, S. *et al.*, 2006). Germline sequence abnormalities were identified in microRNA (miRNA) genes or transcripts , and in targeted sequences in messenger RNAs (mRNAs) that interact with miRNAs. This fact seems to partially explain familiar predisposition to cancer (He, H. *et al.*, 2005). Finally, miRNAs should efficaciously affect and improve cancer diagnosis and prognosis types. The miRNAs role in oral carcinogenesis will be treated in the third section of this chapter.

2. Gene promoters hyper-methylation

Hyper-methylation of cytosine base in CpG islands of gene promoters is an epigenetic phenomenon able to down regulate the expression of genes. When an oncogene expression is influenced, this phenomenon is directly linked with carcinogenesis (Kulkarni, V. & Saranath, D., 2004).

In oral district, many genes are considered to cause OSCC if their methylation status is altered. Among the considerably high amount of investigated genes, only the significant ones in oral cancer will be considered.

2.1 Inhibitors of canonical WNT-pathway

WNT proteins are a large family of secreted glycoproteins activating at least three signalling pathways: the canonical WNT-pathway or WNT-ß-catenin, the non-canonical WNT pathway or planar cell polarity (PCP) and WNT-Ca2+ pathway (Cadigan, K.M. & Nusse, R., 1997).

The canonical pathway operates by stabilizing ß-catenin. The stabilization of ß-catenin in the canonical pathway translates a WNT signal into the transient transcription of T-cell factor/lymphocyte enhancer factor (TCF/LEF) family of transcription factors to stimulate the expression of target genes; the process results in initiating cellular proliferation. The main receptor of secreted WNT proteins at plasma-membrane is the protein Frizzled (Fz), but other Fz co-receptors are required for proper WNT signalling, such as low-density lipoprotein receptor-related proteins (LRP-5 or LRP-6). WNT-inhibitors may be classified into two types: a) the ones that interfere with WNT activity by binding to LRP-5and LRP-6, including Dickkopf (DKK)proteins, and b) the ones that interact directly with WNT proteins, including secreted Frizzled related proteins (SFRPs) and WNT inhibitory factor -1 (WIF-1). DKK proteins interact with the co-receptors LRP-5/6 and inhibit signalling by disrupting the binding of LRP-6 to the WNT/Fz ligand-receptor complex (Aguilera, O.; Muñoz, A., 2007).

SFRPs, a family of highly conserved glycoproteins, share structural similarities with the Frizzled receptor family of proteins and antagonize the WNT pathway at the level of receptor-ligand binding (Bovolenta, P.; Rodriguez, J., 2006; Rattner, A.; Hsieh, J.C., 1997). Thus, they play a crucial role in cell proliferation and differentiation, epithelial-mesenchymal communication and embryogenesis (Bafico, A.; Gazit, A., 1999).

WIF-1 is a secreted inhibitor of WNT signalling and its expression results in cell growth inhibition via G1 (Tang, Y.; Simoneau, A.R., 2009). Mechanisms of WIF-1-induced G1 arrest include (a) SKP2(SKP2 gene contains two TCF/LEF-1 consensus binding sites within the promoter) down-regulation leading to p27/Kip-1 accumulation and (b) c-myc down-regulation releasingp21/WAF-1 transcription. Chronic activation of WNT can be caused by loss of WNT inhibitors through epigenetic silencing. Although disregulation of the WNT-ß-catenin pathway is a frequent event in several human cancers (Clevers, H., 2006; Giles, R.H.; van Es, J.H., 2003), its potential implications in oral cancer has been investigated in only a few works. SFRP1 promoter is hypermethylated in 24% cases of OSCC according to Sogabe et al. (Sogabe, Y.; Suzuki, H., 2008), while Pannone et al. found it was statistically significant less methylated in OSCC than in healthy mucosa; according to Pannone et al., other genes as SFRP2, 4, 5, WIF1 and DKK2 are statistically significant hyper-methylated in OSCC if compared to healthy mucosa (Pannone, G.; Bufo, P., 2010). Sogabe et al. (Sogabe, Y.; Suzuki, H., 2008) also found that SFRP2 and 5 were hyper-methylated in 36% and 16% of tumoral cases respectively.

2.2 Tumor-suppressor genes

A tumor suppressor gene is a gene encoding for a protein which functions include avoiding atypical transformation of cell population, preventing cancer development, protecting a cell from the inauspicious path to cancer. Mechanisms by which a tumor suppressor protein effects its function can be very different: controlling cell cycle genes - including oncogenes -, controlling/repairing mismatches in DNAs duplication, initiate apoptosis in case of cellular atypia, allowing cell adhesion to prevent tumor cells dissociation. Inactivation of several tumor-suppressor genes has been attributed to aberrant hyper-methylation of their promoter regions. E-cadherin, p16, p15, hMLH1, MGMT and many others are well-known tumor-suppressor genes, that are considered to be widely inactivated by methylation in cancers (Muthusamy, V.; Nobuo, T., 2003).

E-cadherin, a member of the cadherin superfamily, is a calcium-dependent homotypic epithelial cell-cell adhesion glycoprotein (Figure 1). E-cadherin is located on the surface of normal epithelial cells and decrease of E-cadherin expression has been found in cancers. It has been postulated that the loss of this protein, facilitates tumor cell dissociation and metastasis. Diminished E-cadherin expression has been documented in association with the acquisition of invasiveness in vitro and poor prognosis in many carcinomas. E-cadherin promoter hyper-methylation, in oral squamous cell carcinomas, is one of the most investigated phenomenon (Chen, Q.; Lipkina, G., 2004). In OSCC epigenetic hyper-methylation occurs in 35-85% cases; only in very rare cases the difference of E-cadherin promoter hyper-methylation between carcinoma and healthy mucosa is not statistically significant. Supic et al. found that hyper-methylated E-cadherin OSCC patients had a worse survival (p= 0,039), and according to Chang et al. recurrent OSCCs compared to primary tumors are more hyper-methylated and the difference is statistically significant (Chang, H.W.; Chow, V.; 2002).

Yet, it has been found by de Moraes et al. and Yeh et al. that promoter hyper-methylation is not related to E-cadherin expression (according to de Moraes et al. in some cases this ratio may be even inverse) (de Moraes, R.V.; Oliveira, D.T., 2008; Yeh, K.T.; Shih, M.C., 2002).

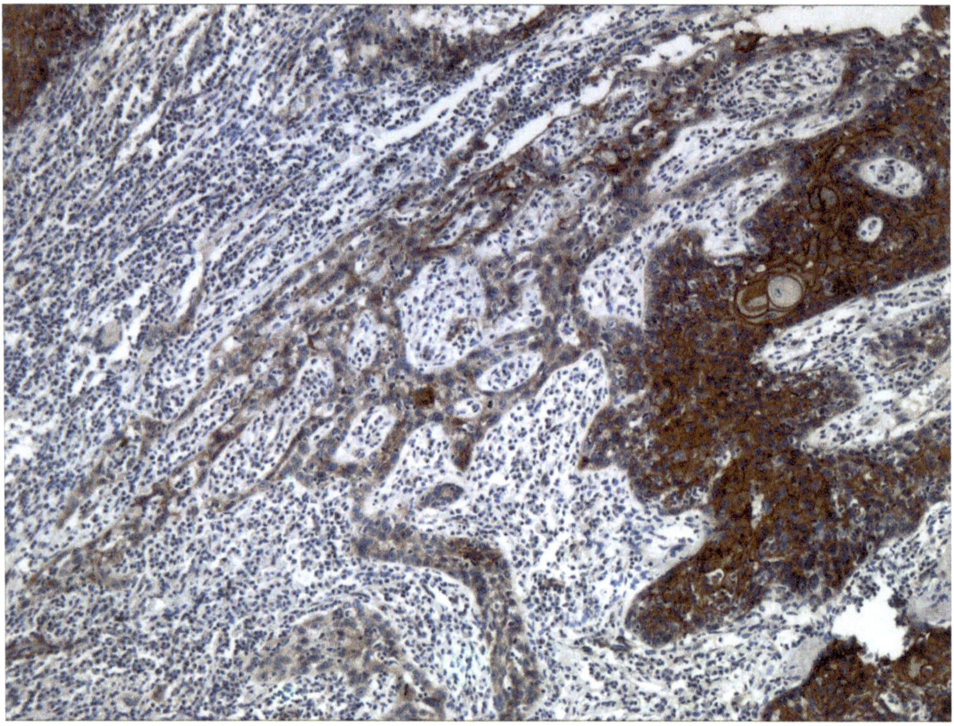

Fig. 1. **Immunohistochemical expression of E-cadherin in oral cancer. (LSAB-HRP-, nuclear counterstaining with haematoxylin, original magnification x1 00).** In this representative case of moderately differentiated oral cancer, superficial neoplastic cells keep membranous protein expression. In the deeply infiltrating neoplastic cells E-cadherin lose membranous staining and assume cytoplasmic positivities.

p16 is a cycline-dependent kinase (CDKN2A) inhibitor involved in regulation of the cell cycle by cyclin D–Rb pathway, which control is virtually lost in all tumors. This tumor suppressor protein is one of the INK4 class members of cell-cycle inhibitors. The expression of p16 retains Rb-family proteins in a hypo-phosphorylated state, which promotes the binding of E2F to achieve G1 cell-cycle arrest. In OSCC, p16 promoter is hyper-methylated in 23-86,8% cases (Huang, M.J.; Yeh, K.T., 2002; Liu, H.W.; Hu, B.Q., 2005; Merlo, A.; Herman, J.G., 1995). Moreover, Hall et al. found that 57% of pre-malignant lesions with hyper-methylated p16 underwent malignant transformation, while non-p16-hypermethylated pre-malignant lesions evolved into cancer in 1% cases (Hall, G.L.; Shaw, R.J., 2008) .

When a difference between metastatic-non metastatic OSCC was investigated, p16 promoter was more hyper-methylated in metastatic OSCCs than in non-metastatic ones and the difference wsa statistically significant. Dong et al. found an high correlation between promoter hyper-methylation and un-expression of p16 (Dong, Y.Y.; Wang, J., 2006).

Adjacent to p16 gene lies the p15 gene, also called CDKN2B gene. Takeshima et al. reported that its promoter is never methylated in healthy epithelial cells, while it shows a certain degree of hyper-methylation in OSCC (Takeshima, M.; Saitoh, M., 2008), also confirmed by Viswanathan et al. (Viswanathan, M.; Tsuchida, N., 2003).

DNA mismatch repair (MMR) is a system for recognizing and repairing mistakes, arisen during DNA replication and recombination, as well as repairing some forms of DNA damage. It is apparent how bad function/low expression of proteins involved in these mechanisms is strictly related to cancer. Among all the genes involved in this system, hMLH1 and hMSH2 promoter hyper-methylation have been investigated to understand their potential role in oral carcinogenesis (González-Ramírez, I.; Ramírez-Amador, V., 2010). hMLH1, the human homolog of bacterial Mut L, is involved in mismatch repair (Veigl, M.L.; Kasturi, L., 1998). hMLH1 promoter is hyper-methylated in 0-76% oral squamous cell carcinoma cases. When protein expression was investigated, it was found unexpressed in 32-36% only among hyper-methylated cases. Czerniski et al. reported that in their experience 100% of patients with multiple oral malignancies showed hyper-methylation in hMLH1 or hMSH2 compared with 31.5% of single tumor patients, although often hyper-methylated cells expressed these 2 proteins anyway. They concluded that hMLH1 and hMSH2 might be related with predisposition to develop multiple oral malignancies (Czerninski, R.; Krichevsky, S., 2009).

DAPK Death-associated protein kinase (DAPK) is a calmodulin-regulated serine/threonine kinase and possesses apoptotic and tumor-suppressive functions. Although it is unclear whether DAPK elicits apoptosis-independent activity to suppress tumor progression, it has been hypothesized that it may affect its apoptotic function to suppress tumor progression by regulating cell polarity during migration. Supic et al. reported that DAPK promoter methylation is higher in OSCC mucosa than in healthy control in a statistically significant way, and that its presence on surgical margins is an independent prognostic factor for overall survival (Supić, G.; Kozomara, R., 2009). Promoter hyper-methylation of DAPK gene detected in surgical margins may be a useful molecular marker to explain the poor survival of some OSCC patients.

MGM is the gene involved in repairing methylated guanosine residues due to alkylated carcinogens. Alkylating agents are known to be carcinogenic because of the formation of O6-alkylguanine from alkylation of the O6 position of DNA and they are responsible for malignant transformation and mutations. O6-methylguanine-DNAmethyltransferase (MGMT) plays a role in the mechanism of resistance to alkylating agents by repairing O6-alkylguanineby, removing the alkyl group and restoring guanine (Rosas, S.L.; Koch, W., 2001). Aberrant promoter hyper-methylation of MGMT in OSCC has been found in 12,2-73,7% cases and widely considered related to oral carcinogenesis (Kato, K.; Hara, A., 2006; Kordi-Tamandani, D.M.; Moazeni-Roodi, A.K., 2010; Taioli, E.;Ragin, C., 2009).

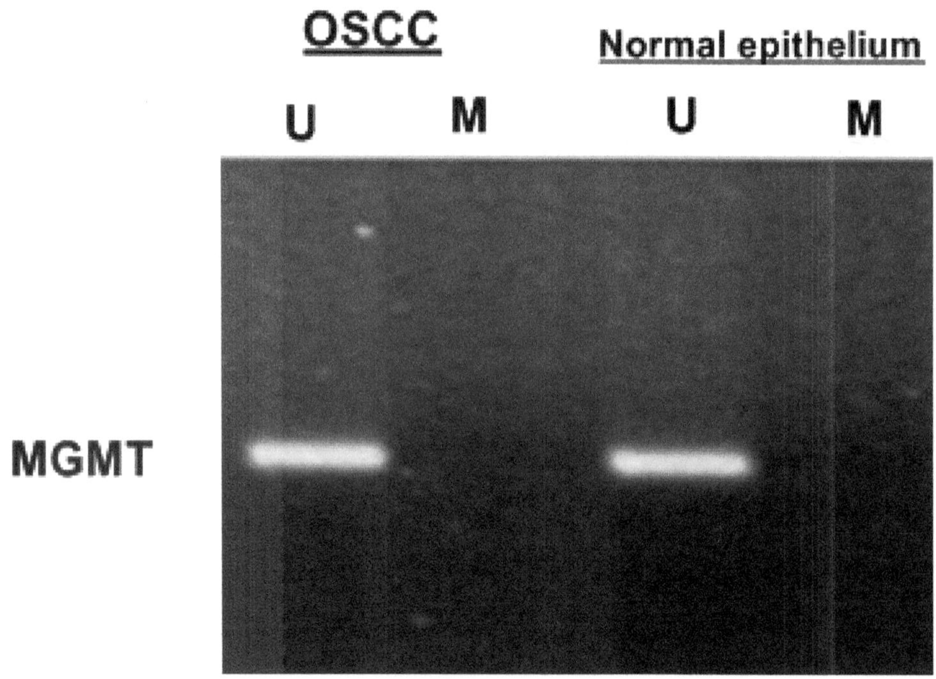

Fig. 2. **Promoter methylation status of MGMT in OSCC.**
In our study MGMT represents a frequently un-methylated gene. M, Methylated DNA; U, un-methylated DNA. Methylation specific (MSP) PCR technique, performed on formalin-fixed, paraffin-embedded tumor and control samples.
To test the integrity of isolated DNA the wide housekeeping haemoglobin gene was amplified by PCR and visualized by gel electrophoresis for both control and pathological samples. The DNA quantity was evaluated by a Nano Drop Spectrophotometer (CELBIO). Sodium bisulfite modification of 100μg DNA for each sample was also performed. All methylation-specific PCRs were optimized to detect >5% methylated substrate in each sample. Each experiment was performed in triplicate.

RUNX3 (Runt-related transcription factor 3) is a protein member of the runt domain-containing family of transcription factors. This protein interacts with a high amount of enhancers and promoters, either activating or suppressing transcription, and with other transcription factors. It functions as a tumor suppressor, and, in some cancers, the gene is frequently deleted or transcriptionally silenced. Gao et al. reported that RUNX3 gene and protein were under-expressed in OSCCs due to promoter hyper-methylation, with frequent protein delocalization. The study showed how both down-regulation of protein expression and protein mislocalization were correlated with the differentiation grades in OSCCs. They consider RUNX3 a useful diagnostic marker and a potential therapeutic target for OSCC, playing an important role in oral carcinogenesis (Gao, F.; Huang, C., 2009). On the other hand, de Freitas Cordeiro-Silva et al. reported a not-statistically-significant hyper-methylation of RUNX3 gene in oral neoplastic mucosa (de Freitas Cordeiro-Silva, M.; Oliveira, Z.F., 2011).

Other tumor suppressor genes that have been found significantly hyper-methyated in oral cancer are: Deleted in Colon Cancer (DCC, encoding a transmembrane protein with structural similarity to neural cell adhesion molecule), Ras association domain-containing protein 1(RASSF1, a protein similar to RAS effector protein) (Tran, T.N.; Liu, Y., 2005), Kinesin-like protein 1A (KIF1A, a member of kinesines superfamily), Nidogen-2 and Homeobox protein Hox-A9 (NID2 and HOXA9, involved in cellular differentiation and apoptosis) (Guerrero-Preston, R.; Soudry, E., 2011), Endothelin receptor type B (EDNRB, a member of endothelin receptors family).

2.3 Retinoids

Retinoids, analogues of retinol (vitamin A) have been widely tried in the prevention of oral squamous cell cancer, and as a cure for its precancerous lesions. In pre-clinical studies, retinoids have been shown to suppress carcinogenesis in a variety of epithelial tissues, including skin, oral mucosa, trachea, prostate, lung, bladder and mammary glands (Shao, Z.; Shen, Z., 1995; Lotan, Y.; Xu, X.C., 2000; Xu, X.C.; Sozzi, G., 1997). Many of the effects of retinoids result from modulation of gene expression by at least 2 distinct classes of nuclear receptor: retinoic acid receptors (RAR-a, b and g) and retinoid X receptors (RXR-a, b and g), belonging to the steroid/thyroid hormone superfamily, even if the mechanisms underlying these clinically significant anti-carcinogenic activities are not completely understood. Defects in retinoid receptor structure, expression and function have been detected in various types of cancer cell *in vitro* and *in vivo* (Gebert, J.F.; Moghal, N., 1991; Geisen, C.; Denk, C., 1997).

These defects may enhance cancer development by interfering with retinoid signaling, thereby abrogating the putative physiological anti-carcinogenic effects of natural retinoids (Lotan, R., 1996). Reduction in RARb mRNA has been observed in several malignant tumors (Caliaro, M.J.; Marmouget, C., 1994; Rochaix, P.; Monteil-Onteniente, S., 1998) and in oral malignant-premalignant lesions (Chakravarti, N.; Mathur, M., 2001; Xu, X.C.; Ro, J.Y., 1994). Rar-beta 2 promoter hyper-methylation was investigated by Youssef et al. and found in 66% of OSCC cases (p=0,002 if compared to healthy mucosa) (Youssef, E.M.; Lotan, D., 2004).

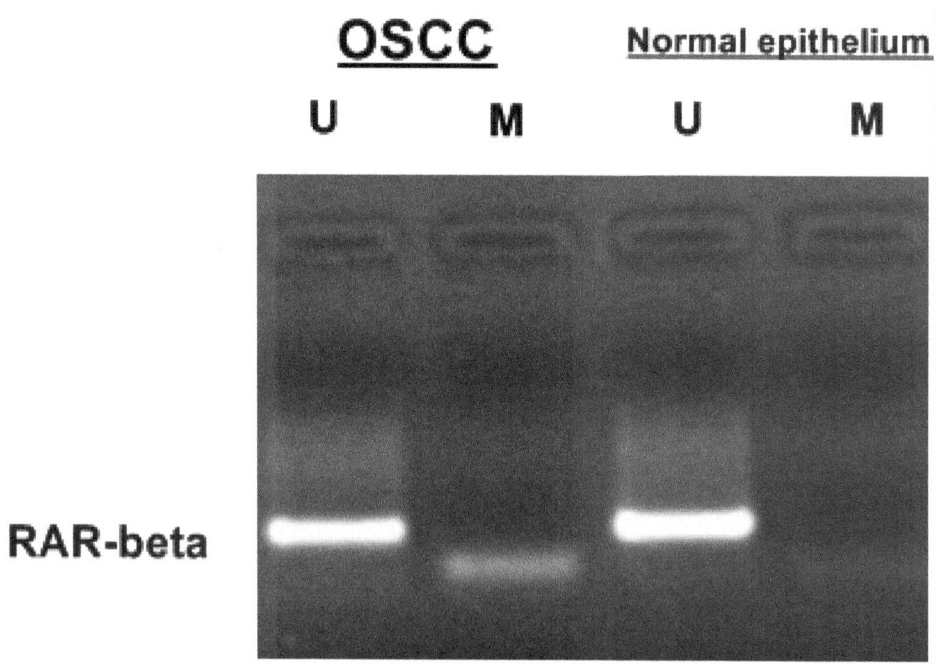

Fig. 3. **Promoter methylation status of RAR-beta in OSCC.**
A representative case of OSCC with methylated promoter of RAR-beta. M, Methylated DNA; U, un-methylated DNA. Methylation specific (MSP) PCR technique, performed on formalin-fixed, paraffin-embedded tumor and control samples.
To test the integrity of isolated DNA the wide housekeeping haemoglobin gene was amplified by PCR and visualized by gel electrophoresis for both control and pathological samples. The DNA quantity was evaluated by a Nano Drop Spectrophotometer (CELBIO). Sodium bisulfite modification of 100µg DNA for each sample was also performed. All methylation-specific PCRs were optimized to detect >5% methylated substrate in each sample. Each experiment was performed in triplicate. In our study RAR-beta represents a frequently un-methylated gene in cancer. In this figure we reported a representative OSCC with methylated promoter of RAR-beta.

Finally, it seems appropriate to conclude this section by reporting synthetically our experimental data. In our laboratory we have analysed, in a series of primary OSCCs with matched normal oral mucosa, the methylation status of a panel of genes, including some of the above mentioned ones and in particular: hMLH1, MGMT, and RAR-beta-2, in order to define an epigenetic fingerprint of the oral cancer (unpublished data). This study would integrate our first results, obtained in a previous published work on methylation status of WNT pathway inhibitors in oral cancer (Pannone, G., *et al.*, 2010). Thirty-seven cases of formalin-fixed, paraffin-embedded OSCC with relative controls of normal oral epithelium were analysed by methylation specific PCR (MSP). Also in this work we have observed different frequencies of gene methylation (Table 1). Characteristically, and in addition to the literature reported data, we have noted that also the healthy oral mucosa shows a methylated background. In our study population the most frequently methylated gene in cancer was represented by hMLH1(53%), although higher levels of methylation were found in control oral mucosa. RAR-beta-2 (Figure 3) and MGMT (Figure 2) promoter hyper-methylation was found in both cases only in 13.5% of OSCCs, but more frequently in healthy oral mucosa (respectively, 28.5% and 23% of studied cases). Therefore, for all genes, logistic multiple regression was performed, in order to verify the association between methylation status of gene promoter (covariates) and presence of cancer (response variable). The Wald test confirmed the statistical significance for RAR-beta-2 (p=0.044; CI at 95%).

Similarly to other reviewed and here commented works, this study highlights the importance of epigenetic silencing, showing that a panel of genes may be useful in clinical practice separating normal oral epithelia from the cancerous ones if their DNAs were analysed by methylation specific PCR technique.

All these results not only shed light on a molecular mechanism contributing to OSCC tumorigenesis, but also suggest that employing of an epigenetic fingerprint, together with the classical histo-pathological parameters, may improve the current diagnostic tools, but also contribute indirectly to therapeutics as predictor of choice for the correct clinical management of oral neoplastic and pre-neoplastic lesions.

Variables	**Methylation frequency in OSCC (n.37)**	**Methylation frequency in oral mucosa (n.20)**
hMLH1	*56%*	*61%*
MGMT	*13.5%*	*23%*
RAR-b	*13.5%*	*28.5%*

Table 1. **Methylation frequencies in our representative series of OSCCs.**
Table summarizes data referring to our MSP analysis in oral cancer.

3. RNA interference (siRNA and miRNA)

Cancer is a multi-factorial disease that requires inactivation of tumour-suppressor genes and activation of proto-oncogenes. DNA sequences of these genes are transcribed to mRNA, which is finally translated into functionally aberrant proteins. This may depend on genetic and non-genetic changes, eventually induced by external factor risks. In this frame, RNA is not a 'passive intermediate product' between DNA and proteins. The expression of genes is also dependent on RNA-based mechanisms, including nonsense-mediated decay, alternative splicing, RNA editing, and in particular siRNA and micro-RNAs (miRNAs).

3.1 siRNA

Therapeutic use of some siRNAs has been tested in oral cancer both in vivo and in vitro. Some studies correlate siRNA trasfection with OSCC pathogenesis and other features like metastasis, vascular invasion, angiogenesis and cell proliferation. Muramatsu T and Saitoh M (Muramatsu, T.; Saitoh, M., 2008) have studied the expression of syndecan-1 in some oral cancer cell lines (HSC2, HSC3, HSC4, Ca9-22, SAS, KB and BSC-OF) and tested whether transfection of an siRNA against human syndecan-1 affected the malignant potential of these cells. Syndecan-1 is a prognostic factor in various types of tumors, suggesting its correlation with malignancy and metastasis. Quantitative real-time RT-PCR (QRT-PCR) was carried out and showed that syndecan-1 was expressed in Ca9-22 cells and that it was significantly higher (> 10-fold) than in the other oral cancer cell lines. Transfection of syndecan-1 siRNA was carried out on Ca9-22 cells, which increased their growth rate and their invasive ability.

Nadarajah Vigneswaran and Jean Wu have utilized small interference RNAs (siRNA) to silence cystatin M gene expression in a metastatic oral cancer cell line (MDA-686Ln) expressing high levels of cystatin M, a well known inhibitor of lysosomal cysteine proteinases. By quantitative real-time RT-PCR and Western blotting authors showed that siRNAs were effective in suppressing cystatin M expression by > 50% at both mRNA and protein levels Cystatin M inhibition significantly increased the enzymatic activities of some lysosomal enzymes both in the media and intracellularly. MDA-686Ln cells treated with siRNA also demonstrated markedly increased proliferation rate, in vitro motility and invasiveness. (Vigneswaran, N.; Wu, J., 2006).

Reduced expression of p27 is frequently observed in various cancers including oral squamous cell carcinoma and is due to an enhancement of its ubiquitination, by S phase kinase-interacting protein 2 (Skp2), an F box protein. Overexpression of Skp2 was frequently found in oral squamous cell carcinoma and inversely correlated with p27 expression. Yasusei Kudo and Shojiro Kitajima investigated if small interfering RNA (siRNA)-mediated gene silencing of Skp2 can be employed in order to inhibit p27 down-regulation in oral squamous cell carcinoma. They proved that Skp2 siRNA transfection decreased Skp2 protein and induced the accumulation of p27 protein in oral squamous cell carcinoma cells, interestingly with an important inhibition of the neoplastic cell proliferation both *in vitro* and *in vivo*. These findings suggest that siRNA-mediated gene silencing of Skp2 can be a novel modality of cancer gene therapy for suppression of p27 down-regulation (Yasusei Kudo; Shojiro Kitajima, 2005).

Human telomerase RNA (hTR) and human telomerase reverse transcriptase (hTERT) are considered effective molecular targets for current anticancer therapy. Y Li and M Li investigated the therapeutic effects of targeting and reducing Human telomerase (hTR) and human telomerase reverse transcriptase (hTERT) individually or in combination by recombinant adenovirus-delivered small interfering RNA (siRNA) in oral squamous cell carcinoma (OSCC) Tca8113. The levels of hTR mRNA, hTERT mRNA, hTERT protein and telomerase activity in Tca8113 cells human were heavily reduced, demonstrating that the siRNA-expressing recombinant adenoviruses were an effective anticancer tool for treatment of OSCC.. Furthermore, the mechanism of this anticancer effect in OSCC was not only related to the inhibition of cell proliferation and the induction of cell apoptosis, but might also involve the inhibition of tumor angiogenesis of solely targeting hTR was more direct and efficient, compared with the effect of targeting hTR and hTERT in combination, or hTERT exclusively (Li,Y.;, Li, M., 2011).

Finally, ongoing experimental studies are proving the attractiveness and the efficacy of siRNAs as a modern and innovative genetic engineering method.

3.2 miRNA

miRNAs based mechanisms of gene expression regulation could constitute one or more epigenetic steps involved in cancer development (Lu, J.; Getz, G.; 2005). The expression pattern of miRNAs are usually altered in many cancers and appear to be tumor and tissue specific. Several variations of miRNA expression have been identified in oral squamous cell carcinoma tissues/cell lines, and even their plasmatic/salivary levels, when compared to the corresponding normal controls (Gomes, C.C.; Gomez, R.S., 2008).

On these bases, therapeutic use of some miRNAs has been tested in vitro. In addition, there are some profiling studies that correlate miRNA expression profiles with OSCC pathogenesis and other features like metastasis, chemo-resistance, prognosis, vascular invasion, alcohol, HPV positivity (Jiang, J.; Lee, E.J., 2005).

3.2.1 Alteration in intracellular, plasmatic, salivary levels

miRNA function regulating gene expression by binding mRNAs and causing degradation of the transcription product or blocking its translation. Therefore, if this process affects tumor suppressor genes o proto-oncogenes, miRNAs may have a key role in carcinogenesis and, potentially, in cancer therapy.

Indeed, in the last ten years the biggest research effort has been put to find out if there were a significant change in miRNA quantity in OSCC tissues, so that we could have used miRNAs as hallmark for early diagnosis; for the same reason, significant changes of miRNAs quantity in OSCC patients have been investigated in serum and saliva. Of the approximately 100 miRNAs identified in OSCC cells, researchers have discovered alteration of cytoplasmic levels only in a small amount, and, among these, in a few cases the meaning of this change is known. Most of the investigated miRNAs show an increase in OSCC cells: miR 21, 24, 31, 155, 181, 184, 211, 345, 375 (Chang, K.W.; Liu, C.J., 2008)

Among these, high level of miR 21, by down-regulating TPM1, PTEN and PDC4, seems to be related to high tumor invasion and poor prognosis (Li, J.; Huang, H., 2009; Reis, P.P.; Tomenson, M., 2010).

Mechanism of function of miRNAs 24 and 181 is known too, targeting the first the RNA binding protein "dead end 1" (DND1) and therefore influencing CDKN1B, and the latter influencing K-RAS expression (Liu, X; Wang, A., 2010; Lin, S.C.; Liu, C.J., 2010; Shin, K.H.; Bae, S.D., 2011). Furthermore, some miRNAs (31, 184) showed high plasmatic level in OSCC, decreasing dramatically after tumor excision (Liu, C.J.; Kao, S.Y., 2010). On the other hand, miRNAs let-7b, 26, 100, 107, 124, 125, 133, 138, 139, 200, 375 decrease in cancer. Decreased cytoplasmic levels of miRNA 124 have been related to a loss of intergrin beta-1 (ITGB1) expression (Hunt, S.; Jones, A.V., 2010); let-7b under-expression causes an over-expression of "Dicer", an RNAase III endonuclease required for RNA maturation, resulting in increased cell proliferation (Jakymiw, A.; Patel, R.S., 2010).

In saliva, approximately 50 RNAs have been found; among these, miR 125 and 200 showed a statistically significant lower level in OSCC patients. (Lo, W.L.; Yu, C.C., 2011).

3.2.2 Precancerous lesions and risk factors

Some miRNAs have been put in relation with risk factors, chemo-resistance, and malignant progression of lesions. In a very few cases, we know biomolecular basis of this phenomenon.

Cerivigne et al. quantified miR expression changes in leukoplakia and same-site OSCC in 43 sequential progressive samples from 12 patients and four non-progressive leukoplakias from four different patients, and identified a miR signature associated with progression (Cerivigne, N.K.; Reis, P.P., 2009),

These findings were also validated using quantitative RT-PCR in an independent cohort of 52 progressive dysplasias and OSCCs, and five non-progressive dysplasias. The result of the study was that global miR expression profiles distinguished progressive leukoplakia/OSCC from non-progressive leukoplakias/normal tissues. miR-21, miR-181b and miR-345 expressions were consistently increased and associated with increases in lesion severity during progression. They concluded that over-expression of miR-21, miR-181b and miR-345 could play a role in malignant transformation.

Lajer et al. characterized the expression of miRNAs in clinically sampled oral and pharyngeal squamous cell carcinoma (OSCC and PSCC) to describe the influence of HPV, analyzing 51 patients with OSCC/PSCC and 40 control patients with microarray method. HPV positive OSCC patients revealed perturbations of 21 miRNAs, most significantly miR-127-3p and miR363. They concluded that the influence of HPV on miRNA could help understanding the distinct clinical behavior of HPV-infected tumors (Lajer, C.B.; Nielsen, F.C., 2011).

Wald A.I et al. stated that miRNAs differentially expressed in the presence of HPV-16 might provide biomarkers for SCCHN (Squamous cell carcinoma of head and Neck) and identify cellular pathways targeted by the virus (Wald, A.I.; Hoskins, E.E., 2010). Some Authors showed that the miRNAs miR-363, miR-33, and miR-497 were up-regulated, whereas miR-155, miR-181a, miR-181b, miR-29a, miR-218, miR-222, miR-221, and miR-142-5p were down-regulated in HPV-positive cells compared to both HPV-negative SCCHN and normal oral keratinocytes (Liu, X.; Yu, J., 2009).

Moreover, HPV-16 E6 oncogene altered miRNA expression in human foreskin keratinocytes (HFKs) and in an HPV-16-positive cell line with E6 knockdown using siRNA.

Finally, Avissar et al. reported that, in oral and pharyngeal squamous cell carcinoma patients, expression of miR-375 has been shown to increase with alcohol consumption. This shows further damage caused by alcohol, in addition to the many ones already known (Avissar, M.; McClean, M.D., 2009).

3.2.3 New expectations of treatment

Due to their capacity to regulate gene expression, miRNAs may contribute to improve treatment by both representing a new chemotherapy drug both helping to understand mechanisms of resistance to already existing chemotherapy drugs or radiotherapy (Wu, B.H.; Xiong, X.P., 2011).

Researches on therapeutic use of miRNAs are in vitro studies of inhibition of OSCC cell growth after regulating one or more miRNAs expression. Wong et al. report that inhibition of miR-184 could reduce cell proliferation rate and/or induce apoptosis in tongue SCC cell lines, by down-regulation of c-Myc (Wong, T.S.; Ho, W.K., 2009; Wong, T.S.; Liu, X.B., 2008). Henson et al. found that transfecting cells with exogenous miR-125b and miR-100, which are down-regulated in OSCC tumors and cell lines, significantly reduced cell proliferation and modified the expression of target and non-target genes, including some genes that are overexpressed in radio-resistant OSCC cells. They concluded that the down-regulation of miR-125b and miR-100 in OSCC could play a role in the development and/or progression of disease and may contribute to the loss of sensitivity to ionizing radiation (Henson, B.J.; Bhattacharjee, S., 2009).

Finally, miRNAs may play a role in resistance to cisplatinum chemotherapy (Yu, Z.W.; Zhong, L.P., 2010). Yu et al. demonstrated that inducing let-7a miRNA proliferation in head and neck cancer cell lines could significantly inhibit the *stemness* signature and the chemo-resistant abilities (Yu, C.C.; Chen, Y.W., 2010).

The development of modified miRNA molecules with longer *in vivo* half lives and efficiency, such as the locked nucleic acid (LNA)-modified oligonucleotides, the anti-miRNA oligo nucleotides (AMOs) and the 'antagomirs' is the first step towards bringing these fundamental research advances into medical practice (Orom, U.A., Kauppinen, S., 2006; Weiler, J., Hunziker, J., 2005). Upcoming *in vivo* experiments of miRNA transgenics and knockouts will offer valuable information about safety and efficacy.

4. Meaning of epigenetic and future perspectives

With an annual incidence worldwide of over 500 000 cases, oral squamous cell carcinoma is the eighth most common malignancy today. This epithelial cancer is characterized by the poor outcome, with the surgical margin status as a relevant prognostic factor associated with local recurrence and poor survival. Screening and early detection are believed to decrease both morbidity and mortality associated with OSCC because, unlike many other anatomic sites, oral cavity pre-malignant lesions are often visible upon clinical examination. Oral carcinogenesis is a multi-factorial process involving numerous genetic processes that can alter the function of oncogenes, tumor suppressor genes, and other related molecules. The resulting anomalies can increase the production of growth factors and the number of cell surface receptors, and/or increase transcription or intracellular messenger factor levels. These changes can cause a loss of tumor suppressor activity and give rise to malignant cell phenotypes, able to increase cellular proliferation, weakening cell cohesion, causing local infiltration and metastasis.

Epigenetic phenomena are non-genetic event able to cause modification in gene expression. Such modifications may be passed on successive generations of cells. Under these bases, if one or more oncogenes are directly or indirectly affected by epigenetic changes, malignant cell transformation may occur, because these alterations pass on successive generations of cells, even if there is no mutation in correspondent genes (Esteller, M.; Corn, P.G., 2001).

Cellular aging, risk factors and, as recently discovered, condition of chronic inflammation via mediators such as IL-6 may be potential inducers of epigenetic alterations in oral mucosa cells (Gasche, J.A.; Hoffmann, J., 2011).

We have seen that, among the three possible epigenetic phenomena - DNA hyper-methylation, histone code changes and RNA interference, hyper-methylation and miRNAs are the most investigated, and for that reason best understood.

About gene promoter hyper-methylation, p16 and E-cadherin are the most investigated genes, generally statistically significantly hyper-methylated in OSCC. Hall et al. found, in one of the most interesting study, an high correlation between malignant transformation and p16 promoter methylation status (Hall, G.L.; Shaw, R.J., 2008).

As for p16, E-cadherin is highly methylated in malignant lesions but it has not been found, when investigated, a correlation between methylation status and protein expression - in some cases hyper-methylation led to a protein hyper-expression. Inhibitors of WNT pathway methylation promoter status were investigated in a few works, only SFRP 2, 4, 5, DKK2 and WIF 1 were found to be statistically significantly hyper-methylated if compared to healthy tissue. SFRP 1 promoter is less methylated in OSCC according to Pannone et al. hMLH1 promoter methylation investigation produced heterogeneous results (from 0 to 76%) (Pannone, G.; Bufo, P., 2010); still, it is interesting to notice that, in hyper-methylated OSCC, protein expression was reduced in about 30% cases only. MGMT and Rar-beta-2 are generally found hyper-methylated in OSCC. Researches on other genes, such as DCC, RASSF1, KIF1A, NID2, HOXA9 and EDNRB showed promising results, proving that there is still much to investigate (Ogi, K.; Toyota, M., 2002).

What emerges from a critical review of literature data is that methylation status of oncogenes promoters does not seem a valid parameter to predict oncoprotein expression. On the other hand, a methylation profile variation in dysplastic cells cannot be denied. Hyper-methylation of oncogenes promoters in oral mucosa cells emerges as a warning light of ongoing/occurred malignant transformation, concurring to outline a "molecular fingerprint" which can be very helpful in malignancies diagnosis. Still, another most interesting application of epigenetics could be the upstaging of surgical margins. Some works show that the histologically negative surgical margins of OSCC exhibits frequent aberrant DNA methylation changes for number of many cancer-related genes (Sinha, P.; Bahadur, S., 2009). Revealing promoter hyper-methylation present in negative margins could be an useful molecular marker for the poor overall survival (Supic, G.; Kozomara, R., 2011). Surgical excision of the entire affected oral mucosa is not feasible, but the inclusion of more rigorous treatment and more intensive surveillance during follow-up in patients with methylation changes detected in surgical margins may provide an enhanced overall survival.

It is apparent that further studies on larger patients groups and additional quantitative/qualitative validation are needed to understand which one(s) is/are the most significant gene(s).

The analyses of miRNA expression profiles have been found to be useful in the classification and diagnosis of some human tumors (Liu, X.; Chen, Z., 2009). Although the causes of miRNA mis-expression in cancer cells is not understood, it is interesting to note that, in cancer cells, some overexpressed oncogenic miRNAs are located in amplified genomic regions, whereas the down-regulated suppressor miRNAs are located in deleted genomic regions. Over-expression of oncogenic miRNA may reduce protein products of tumor-suppressor genes. On the other hand, loss of tumor-suppressor miRNA expression may cause elevated levels of oncogenic protein. One or both of these alterations could represent new targets for cancer diagnosis and treatment in the future. The demonstration that miRNA expression is related to stage of some tumours may also be a useful tool for prognosis analysis, and it should be evaluated in OSCC staging. In recent years, since researchers have focused on epigenetic alterations in OSCC cells, the emergence of miRNA knowledge and its potential action create new perspectives in understanding cell transformation. The discovery of miRNA, 20-22 nucleotide-long members of the non-coding RNA family, adds another layer of gene regulation that is altered as cancer develops. They may be present as intergenic transcription units or found in the intronic sequences of protein-coding genes. More than 1,000 of these sequences have been identified until now, and functional studies have identified that miRNAs act as conventional tumor suppressors or as oncogenes, and affect both translation and stability of target mRNA. Most of them are negative regulators of gene expression and have fundamental roles in biologic processes with this function being deregulated as cancer develops, but still, there is much more to understand.

Since distinct miRNA expression profiles vary between OSCC and healthy mucosa, analysis of miRNA expression profiles offers an opportunity for early-stage diagnosis of OSCC, showing a high sensitivity and specificity to classify OSCC. Also, some individual miRNAs have been suggested to be putative specific biomarkers for OSCC diagnosis and prognosis, such as aberrantly over-expressed miR21 (Cervigne, N.K.; Reis, P.P., 2009),. In addition, miRNAs seem to hold significant potential as diagnostic tools to detect metastatic disease.

Some miRNAs have been linked with risk factors, chemo-resistance, and malignant progression of lesions (Kumar, M.S.; Lu, J., 2007). In a very few cases, we know biomolecular basis of this phenomena. A small number of miRNAs have been revealed to have profound prognostic values in determining the survival of patients with OSCC. By multivariate analyses, miR-21 expression is proposed as an independent predictor of poor survival for patients with OSCC. Different studies support the idea of a strong association of high expression level of miR21 and significantly decreased 5-year survival in patients with OSCC. Over-expression of miR-21, miR-181b and miR-345 could play a role in malignant transformation (Cervigne, N.K.; Reis, P.P., 2009).

HPV-positive oral-oropharyngeal SCCs appear as a distinct entity, different from HPV-negative tumors. There is a strong prevalence in younger patients without sex predilection. Up to 20% of these cancers develops in patients without traditional risk factors, i.e. smoking and alcohol abuse. Conversely, their risk factors include young age at first intercourse, promiscuity, and history of genital warts in men and number of sexual partners in women. As positive personal history of oral–genital and oral–anal sexual contacts (during which the HPV infection may be transmitted to the oral cavity) increases the risk for HPV-positive HNSCCs, they may be regarded as a sexually transmitted disease. It is assumed that long-lasting oral HPV infection, which prevalence increases after the onset of sexual activity, precedes the development of HPV-positive HNSCC for about 10 years. In addition, these tumors seem to berelated to immune-suppression. HPV positive OSCC patients revealed perturbations of 21 miRNAs, most significantly miR-127-3p and miR363. It has been hypothesized that the influence of HPV on miRNA could help understanding the distinct clinical behavior of HPV-infected tumors (Liu, X.; Yu, J., 2009). . In oral and pharyngeal squamous cell carcinoma patients, over-expression of miR375 has been put in relation with alcohol consumption. This shows further damage caused by alcohol, in addition to the many ones we already know(Avissar, M.; McClean, M.D., 2009). .

Moreover, low expression levels of miR205 was found to significantly correlate with loco-regional relapse of OSCC, independent of disease severity at diagnosis and treatment, and miRNA expression level seems to change with different malignancy grades and reflect the risk of OPL16 or the biological characteristics of OSCC such as the metastatic potential and chemo-sensitivity or chemo-resistance (Shiiba M.; Uzawa K., 2010).

An increasing amount of studies show that miRNAs circulate stably in body fluids, with different expression pattern in blood and saliva, of healthy and cancer patients. Most of investigated miRNAs show an increase in OSCC cells: miR 21, 24, 31, 155, 181, 184, 211, 345, 375. On the other hand,miRNAs let-7b, 26, 100, 107, 124, 125, 133, 138, 139, 200, 375 seem decreased in OSCC cells (Henson, B.J.; Bhattacharjee, S., 2009; Liu, X.; Jiang, L, 2009).

Elevated levels of miRNA in plasma (31, 184) have been detected in OSCC patients compared with case controlled individuals. Indeed, some miRNAs showed high plasmatic level in OSCC, decreasing dramatically after tumor excision. Saliva, easy to collect, is an ideal medium for clinical applications. About 50 miRNAs were revealed to be present in both whole saliva and supernatant saliva of patients with OSCC; among these, miR 125 and 200 showed a statistically significant lower level in OSCC patients versus healthy controls. Another study showed that over-expressed miR31 was also detectable in the saliva of OSCC patients. These circulating miRNAs seem to be released from the OSCC tissues into the bloodstream, causing the remarkable reduction of plasmatic miRNAs in patients after surgical excision of the tumor All these data support the view that circulating miRNAs could be used as non-invasive and powerful OSCC biomarkers (Liu, C.J.; Kao, S.Y., 2010).

Due to their ability to regulate gene expression, miRNAs may contribute to improve treatment by both representing a new chemotherapy drug both helping to understand mechanisms of resistance to already existing chemotherapy drugs or radiotherapy.

We need further evidence to understand miRNAs role as either oncogenes or tumor suppressors regulating key genes, involved in the initiation and progression of human cancer. If this role would be definitively proved, this would provide the rational basis for miRNA-based cancer therapy. Up-regulating the expression of tumor suppressive miRNAs at low levels in OSCC as well as inhibiting the expression of oncogenic miRNAs over-expressed is the effective approach for the therapeutic purpose. Inhibition of miR184 could reduce cell proliferation rate and/or induce apoptosis in tongue SCC cell lines, by down-regulation of c-Myc (Liu, C.J.; Kao, S.Y., 2010). It has been found that transfecting cells with exogenous miR125b and miR100, which are down-regulated in OSCC tumor and cell lines, significantly reduce cell proliferation and modified the expression of target and non-target genes, including some that are over-expressed in radio-resistant OSCC cells. Some Authors concluded that the down-regulation of miR 125b and miR100 in OSCC could play a role in the development and/or progression of disease and may contribute to the loss of sensitivity to ionizing radiation (Henson, B.J.; Bhattacharjee, S., 2009; Lo, W.L.; Yu, C.C., 2011; Wong, T.S.; Ho, W.K., 2009; Wong, T.S.; Liu, X.B., 2008).

Finally, miRNA may play another role in resistance to cisplatinum chemotherapy. It has been demonstrated that inducing let-7a miRNA proliferation in head and neck cancer cell lines could considerably inhibit the *stemness* signature and the chemo-resistant abilities (Yu, Z.W.; Zhong, L.P., 2010; Yu, C.C.; Chen, Y.W., 2010).

However, at present, it is still a big challenge to design a specific and efficient drug delivery system for miRNA-based drugs.

The discovery of miRNAs provides new insights into the pathogenesis and progression of OSCC, which was thought to be a disease characterized exclusively by alterations in oncogenic and tumor suppressive protein-coding genes. A number of aberrantly expressed miRNAs have been verified either as oncogenes or tumor-suppressors, participating in various biological processes of OSCC, including proliferation, apoptosis, metastasis and chemoresistance. In addition, these mis-expressed miRNAs have been proved to have potential as diagnostic and prognostic tools. Furthermore, the role of miRNAs in cancers makes it possible to design miRNA-based therapy for OSCC. Although still little is known in this field, compelling evidence gives exciting promises that miRNAs will improve the management of OSCC in the near future. Further studies are needed to generate additional information about tumour-suppressor miRNAs and oncogenic miRNAs involved in OSCC pathogenesis, including oral pre-malignancies transformation (Clague, J.; Lippman, S.M., 2010).

5. Summary

The purpose of this chapter was to review the current state of knowledge of the genetic /epigenetic alterations that are specifically observed in oral mucosal pre-malignancy and cancer. The ultimate goal of research on OSCC is to identify the specific candidate biomarkers that would have optimal predictive capacity in identification of those dysplastic lesions most likely to progress to OSCC over time, pointer towards the right therapy, help to better define surgical margins.

Taking a critical look, we must highlight how carcinogenesis is a complex phenomenon, involving a wide pool of genes which expression can be modified by an astonishing amount of factors. On the other hand, an epigenetic methylation/histonic/miRNA profile variation in dysplastic cells cannot be denied. These changes in oral mucosa cells emerge as a warning light of ongoing/occurred malignant transformation, concurring to outline a "molecular fingerprint" which can be very helpful in malignancies diagnosis. It appears that the best way to understand hyper-methylation phenomenon role in carcinogenesis should not be exclusively investigating its frequency in OSCC cells - always comparing results to healthy mucosa from OSCC patients and healthy mucosa from healthy patients, but also monitoring pre-malignant oral lesions, establishing a correlation between this epigenetic event and malignant transformation.

6. References

Aguilera, O.; Muñoz, A.; Esteller, M. & Fraga, M.F.(2007). Epigenetic alterations of the WNT/beta-catenin pathway in human disease. *Endocr Metab Immune Disord Drug Targets*, Vol. 7,pp 13-21

Avissar, M.; McClean, M.D.; Kelsey, K.T. & Marsit, C.J. (2009). MicroRNA expression in head and neck cancer associates with alcohol consumption and survival. *Carcinogenesis*, Vol. 30, No. 12, (December 2009), pp 2059-63

Bafico, A.; Gazit, A.; Pramila, T.; Finch, P.W.; Yaniv, A. & Aaronson S.A. (1999). Interaction of frizzled related protein (FRP) with WNT ligands and the frizzled receptor suggests alternative mechanisms for FRP inhibition of WNT signalling. *J Biol Chem* Vol. 274, pp 16180-16187

Bartel, D. P. (2004) MicroRNAs: genomics, biogenesis mechanism, and function. *Cell,* Vol. 116, pp. 281–297

Baylin, S.B.; Herman, J.G. (2000).DNA hypermethylation in tumorigenesis. *Trends Genet*, Vol. 16, pp168 -73

Bentwich, I.; Avniel, A.; Karov, Y.; Aharonov, R.; Gilad, S.; Barad, O.; Barzilai, A.; Einat, P.; Einav, U.; Meiri, E.; Sharon, E.; Spector, Y. & Bentwich, Z. (2005). Identification of hundreds of conserved and non conserved human microRNAs. *Nat Genet*, Vol. 37, pp766–70

Berezikov, E.; Guryev, V.; van de Belt, J.; Wienholds, E.; Plasterk, R.H. &Cuppen, E. (2005). Phylogenetic shadowingand computational identification of human micro-RNA genes. *Cell*, Vol. 120, pp21–4

Bernstein, E.; Caudy, A.A.; Hammond, S.M. & Hannon, G.J. (2001). Role for a bidentate ribonuclease in the initiation step of RNA interference. *Nature*, Vol. 409, pp 363–6

Bird, A. (2007). Perceptions of epigenetics. *Nature*, Vol. 447, No. 7143, pp 396–398

Bovolenta, P.; Rodriguez, J. &Esteve, P. (2006). Frizzled/RIK mediated signalling in axon guidance. *Development*, Vol.133, pp 4399-4408

Cadigan, K.M. & Nusse, R.(1997) WNT signalling: a common theme in animal development. *Genes Dev*, Vol. 11, pp 3286-3305

Caliaro, M.J.; Marmouget, C.; Guichard, S.; Mazars, P.; Valette, A.; Moisand, A.; Bugat, R. & Jozan, S. (1994). Response of four human ovarian carcinoma cell lines to all-trans retinoic acid: relationship with induction of differentiation and retinoic acid receptor expression. *Int J Cancer*, Vol. 56, pp 743–748

Calin, G. A. (2004). MicroRNA profiling reveals distinct signatures in B cell chronic lymphocytic leukemias. *Proc Natl Acad Sci USA*, Vol. 101, pp 11755–11760

Cervigne, N.K.; Reis, P.P.; Machado, J.; Sadikovic, B.; Bradley, G.; Galloni, N.N.; Pintilie, M.; Jurisica, I.; Perez-Ordonez, B.; Gilbert, R.; Gullane, P.; Irish, J.& Kamel-Reid, S. (2009). Identification of a microRNA signature associated with progression of leukoplakia to oral carcinoma. *Hum Mol Genet*, Vol. 18, No.24, (December 2009), pp 4818-29

Chakravarti, N.; Mathur, M.; Bahadur, S.; Shukla, N.K.; Rochette-Egly, C. & Ralhan, R. (2001). Expression of RARa and RARb in human oral potentially malignant and neoplastic lesions. *Int. J. Cancer*, Vol. 91, pp27–31

Chang, H.W.; Chow, V.; Lam, K.Y.; Wei, W.I. & Yuen, A. (2002). Loss of E-cadherin expression resulting from promoter hypermethylation in oral tongue carcinoma and its prognostic significance. *Cancer*, Vol. 94, No. 2, pp 386-92

Chang, K.W.; Liu, C.J.; Chu, T.H.; Cheng, H.W.; Hung, P.S.; Hu, W.Y& Lin, S.C. (2008)Association between high miR-211 microRNA expression and the poor prognosis of oral carcinoma. *J Dent Res*, Vol. 87, No. 11, (November 2008), 1063-8

Chen, Q.; Lipkina, G.; Song, Q. & Kramer, R.H. (2004). Promoter methylation regulates cadherin switching in squamous cell carcinoma. *Biochem Biophys Res Commun*, Vol. 315, No. 4, (March 2004), pp 850-6

Clague,J.; Lippman, S.M.; Yang, H.; Hildebrandt, M.A.; Ye, Y.; Lee, J.J. & Wu, X. (2010).Genetic variation in MicroRNA genes and risk of oral premalignant lesions. *Mol Carcinog*, Vol. 49, No. 2, (February 2010), 183-9 pp

Clevers, H. (2006). WNT/beta-catenin signalling in development and disease. *Cell*, Vol. 127, pp 469-480

Czerninski, R.; Krichevsky, S.; Ashhab, Y.; Gazit, D.; Patel, V. & Ben-Yehuda, D. (2009). Promoter hypermethylation of mismatch repair genes, hMLH1 and hMSH2 in oral squamous cell carcinoma. *Oral Dis.*, Vol. 15, No. 3, (April 2009), pp206-13

de Freitas Cordeiro-Silva, M.; Oliveira, Z.F.; de Podestá, J.R.; Gouvea, S.A.; Von Zeidler, S.V. & Louro, I.D.; Methylation analysis of cancer-related genes in non-neoplastic cells from patients with oral squamous cell carcinoma. *Mol Biol Rep*, Epub ahead of print, March 2011

de Moraes, R.V.; Oliveira, D.T.; Landman, G.; de Carvalho, F.; Caballero, O.; Nonogaki, S.;Nishimoto, I. & Kowalski, L.P. (2008).E-cadherin abnormalities resulting from CPG methylation promoter in metastatic and non metastatic oral cancer. *Head Neck.*, Vol. 30, No. 1, (January 2008), pp 85-92

Dong, Y.Y.; Wang, J.; Dong, F.S.; Wang, X.; Li, H.X. & Gu, H.T. (2006).The relationship between methylation of p16 INK 4/CDKN2 gene in promoter region and progress of squamous cell carcinoma of buccal mucosa. *Zhonghua Kou QiangYiXue Za Zhi*, Vol. 41, No. 5, (May 2006), pp 297-8

Dykxhoorn, D. M.; Palliser D. & Lieberman, J (2006). The silent treatment: siRNAs as small molecule drugs. *Gene Therapy*, Vol. 13, pp 541-552

Dykxhoorn, D.M.; Palliser, D. & Lieberman, J (2006). The silent treatment: siRNAs as small molecule drugs. *Gene Therapy*, Vol. 13, pp 541-552.

Elbashir, S.; Harborth, J.; Lendeckel, W.; Yalcin, A.; Weber, K. & Tuschl, T. (2001). Duplexes of 21-nucleotide RNAs mediate RNA interference in cultured mammalian cells. *Nature*, Vol. 411, no. 6836, pp. 494–988

Esteller, M.; Corn, P.G.; Baylin, S.B. & Herman, J.G. (2001). A gene hypermethylation profile of human cancer. *Cancer Res*, Vol. 61, pp 3225–9

Feinberg, A.P. (2001) Cancer epigenetics takes center stage. *Proc Natl Acad SciUSA*, Vol. 98, pp 392–4

Fire, A.; Xu, S.; Montgomery, M.; Kostas, S.; Driver, S. & Mello, C. (1998). Potent and specific genetic interference by double-stranded RNA in *Caenorhabditis elegans*. *Nature*, Vol. 391, No. 6669, pp 806–11

Funk, G.F.; Karnell, L.H.; Robinson, R.A.; Zhen, W.K.; Trask, D.K. & Hoffman, H.T.(2002).Presentation, treatment, and outcome of oral cavity cancer: a National Cancer Data Base report. *Head Neck*, Vol. 24, pp165–80

Gao, F.; Huang, C.; Lin, M.; Wang, Z.;Shen, J.; Zhang, H.; Jiang, L. & Chen, Q. (2008)Frequent inactivation of RUNX3 by promoter hypermethylation and protein mislocalization in oral squamous cell carcinomas. *J Cancer Res Clin Oncol*, Vol.135, No. 5, May 2009, pp739-47.

Gasche, J.A.; Hoffmann, J.; Boland, C.R.& Goel, A. (2011).Interleukin-6 promotes tumorigenesis by altering DNA methylation in oral cancer cells.*Int J Cancer*, Vol. 129, No. 5 (September 2011), pp1053-63

Gebert, J.F.; Moghal, N.; Frangioni, J.V.; Sugarbaker, D.J. & Neel, B.G. (1991) High frequency of retinoic acid beta abnormalities in human lung cancer. *Oncogene*, Vol. 6, pp 1859 -1868

Geisen, C.; Denk, C.; Gremm, B.; Baust, C.; Karger, A.;Bollag, W. &Schwarz, E. (1997). High-level expression of the retinoic acid receptor beta gene in normal cells of the uterine cervix is regulated by the retinoic acid receptor alpha and is abnormally down-regulated in cervical carcinoma cells. *Cancer Res*, Vol. 57, pp 1460 -1467

Giles, R.H.; van Es, J.H. & Clevers, H. (2003). Caught up in a WNT storm: WNT signalling in cancer. *Biochim Biophys Acta* Vol. 1653: pp 1-24

Gomes, C.C.; Gomez, R.S. (2008). MicroRNA and oral cancer: Future perspectives.*Oral Oncology*, Vol. 44,pp 910- 914

González-Ramírez, I.; Ramírez-Amador, V.; Irigoyen-Camacho, M.E.; Sánchez-Pérez, Y.; Anaya-Saavedra, G.; Granados-García, M.; García-Vázquez, F. & García-Cuellar, C.M. (2010). hMLH1 promoter methylation is an early event in oral cancer. *Oral Oncol.*, Vol. 47, No. 1,(January 2011), pp22-6

Gregory, R. I. & Shiekhattar, R. (2005). MicroRNA biogenesis and cancer. *Cancer Res*, Vol. 65, pp 3509–3512

Guerrero-Preston, R.; Soudry, E.; Acero, J.; Orera, M.; Moreno-López, L.; Macía-Colón, G.; Jaffe, A.; Berdasco, M.; Ili-Gangas, C.; Brebi-Mieville, P.; Fu, Y.; Engstrom, C.; Irizarry, R.A.; Esteller, M.; Westra, W.; Koch, W.; Califano, J. & Sidransky, D. (2011). NID2 and HOXA9 Promoter Hypermethylation as Biomarkers for Prevention and Early Detection in Oral Cavity Squamous Cell Carcinoma Tissues and Saliva. *Cancer Prev Res (Phila)*, Vol. 4, No. 7, (July 2011), pp1061-72

Gunduz, M.; Demircan, K.; Gunduz, E.; Katase, N.; Tamamura, R. & Nagatsuka, H. (2009) Potential usage of ING family members in cancer diagnostics and molecular therapy. *Curr Drug Targets*, Vol. 10, No. 5, (May 2009), 465-76

Gunduz, M.; Gunduz, E.; Rivera, R.S. & Nagatsuka, H. (2008).The inhibitor of growth (ING) gene family: potential role in cancer therapy. *Curr Cancer Drug Targets*, Vol. 8, No. 4, (June 2008), 275-84

Hall, G.L.; Shaw, R.J.; Field, E.A.; Rogers, S.N.; Sutton, D.N.; Woolgar, J.A.; Lowe, D.; Liloglou, T.; Field, J.K. & Risk, J.M. (2008) p16 Promoter methylation is a potential predictor of malignant transformation in oral epithelial dysplasia. *Cancer Epidemiol Biomarkers Prev.*, Vol. 17, No. 8, (August 2008), pp 2174-9

Hamilton, A. & Baulcombe, D. (1999). A species of small antisense RNA in posttranscriptional gene silencing in plants. *Science*, Vol. 286, no. 5441, pp 950–2

He, H. (2005). The role of microRNA genes in papillary thyroid carcinoma. *Proc Natl Acad Sci USA*, Vol. 102, pp 19075–19080

Henson, B.J.; Bhattacharjee, S.; O'Dee, D.M.; Feingold, E. & Gollin, S.M.(2009)Decreased expression of miR-125b and miR-100 in oral cancer cells contributes to malignancy. *Genes Chromosomes Cancer*, Vol. 48, No. 7, (July 2009), 569-82

Huang, M.J.; Yeh, K.T.; Shih, H.C.; Wang, Y.F.; Lin, T.H.; Chang, J.Y.; Shih, M.C. & Chang, J.G. (2002).The correlation between CpG methylation and protein expression of P16 in oral squamous cell carcinomas. *Int J Mol Med*, Vol. 10, No.5, (November2002), pp 551-4

Hunt, S.; Jones, A.V.; Hinsley, E.E.; Whawell, S.A. & Lambert, D.W. (2010).MicroRNA-124 suppresses oral squamous cell carcinoma motility by targeting ITGB1. *FEBS Lett*, Vol. 585,No. 1, (January 2011), pp187-92

Jakymiw, A.; Patel, R.S.; Deming, N.; Bhattacharyya, I.; Shah, P.; Lamont, R.J.; Stewart, C.M.; Cohen, D.M. & Chan, E.K. (2010). Overexpression of dicer as a result of reduced let-7 MicroRNA levels contributes to increased cell proliferation of oral cancer cells. *Genes Chromosomes Cancer*. Vol. 49, No. 6, (June 2010), pp549-59

Jiang, J.; Lee, E.J.; Gusev, Y. & Schmittgen, T.D. (2005). Realtime expression profiling of microRNA precursors in human cancer cell lines. *Nucleic Acids Res*, Vol. 33, pp 5394–403

Kato, K.; Hara, A.; Kuno, T.; Mori, H.; Yamashita, T.; Toida, M. & Shibata, T. (2006). Aberrant promoter hypermethylation of p16 and MGMT genes in oral squamous cell carcinomas and the surrounding normal mucosa. *J Cancer Res ClinOncol*, Vol. 132, No. 11, (June 2006), pp735-43

Kent, O.A. & Mendell, J.T. (2006). A small piece in the cancer puzzle: microRNAs as tumor suppressors and oncogenes. *Oncogene*, Vol. 25, pp 6188–96

Kim, V. N. & Nam, J. W. (2006) Genomics of microRNA. *Trends Genet*, Vol.22, pp 165–173

Kim, V.N. (2004). MicroRNA precursors in motion: exportin-5 mediates their nuclear export. *Trends Cell Biol*, Vol. 14, pp156–9

Kordi-Tamandani, D.M.; Moazeni-Roodi, A.K.; Rigi-Ladiz, M.A.; Hashemi, M.; Birjandian, E. &Torkamanzehi, A. (2010). Promoter hypermethylation and expression profile of MGMT and CDH1 genes in oral cavity cancer. *Arch Oral Biol*, Vol. 55, No. 10, (October 2010), pp809-14

Kozaki, K.; Imoto, I.; Mogi, S.;Omura, K. & Inazawa, J. (2008) Exploration of tumorsuppressive microRNAs silenced by DNA hypermethylation in oral cancer.*Cancer Res*, Vol. 68, No. 7, pp 2094–105

Kudo, Y.; Kitajima, S.; Ogawa, I.; Kitagawa, M.; Miyauchi, M. & Takata, T. (2005). Small interfering RNA targeting of S phase kinase–interacting protein 2 inhibits cell growth of oral cancer cells by inhibiting p27 degradation. *Mol Cancer Ther*, Vol. 4, (March 2005); p 471

Kulkarni, V. & Saranath, D. (2004) Concurrent hypermethylation of multiple regulatory genes in chewing tobacco associated oral squamous cell carcinomas and adjacent normal tissues. *Oral Oncol.*, Vol. 40, No.2,(February 2004), pp 145-53

Kumar, M.S.; Lu, J.; Mercer, K.L.; Golub, T.R. & Jacks, T. (2007) Impaired microRNA processing enhances cellular transformation and tumorigenesis. *Nat Genet*, Vol. 39, pp673–7

Lajer, C.B.; Nielsen, F.C.;Friis-Hansen, L.; Norrild, B.; Borup, R.; Garnæs, E.; Rossing, M.; Specht, L.; Therkildsen, M.H.;Nauntofte, B.; Dabelsteen, S. & von Buchwald, C. (2011).Different miRNA signatures of oral and pharyngeal squamous cell carcinomas: a prospective translational study. *Br J Cancer*, Vol. 104, No. 5, (March 2011), pp830-40

Lee, Y.; Ahn, C.; Han, J.; Choi, H.; Kim, J.; Yim, J.; Lee, J.; Provost, P.; Rådmark, O.; Kim, S. & Kim, V.N. (2003). The nuclear RNaseIII Drosha initiates microRNA processing. *Nature*, Vol. 425, pp415–9

Li, J.; Huang, H.; Sun, L.; Yang, M.; Pan, C.; Chen, W.; Wu, D.; Lin, Z.; Zeng, C.; Yao, Y.; Zhang, P. & Song, E. (2009).MiR-21 indicates poor prognosis in tongue squamous cell carcinomas as an apoptosis inhibitor. *Clin Cancer Res*, Vol. 15, No. 12, (June 2009), pp3998-4008

Li, Y.; Li, M.; Yao, G.; Geng, N.; Xie, Y.; Feng, Y.; Zhang, P.; Kong, X.; Xue, J.; Cheng, S.; Zhou, J. & Xiao L. (2011). Telomerase inhibition strategies by siRNAs against either hTR or hTERT in oral squamous cell carcinoma. *Cancer Gene Therapy*, Vol. 18, (May 2011), pp 318-325

Lin, S.C.; Liu, C.J.; Lin, J.A.; Chiang, W.F.; Hung, P.S. & Chang, K.W. (2010).miR-24 up-regulation in oral carcinoma: positive association from clinical and in vitro analysis. *Oral Oncol*, Vol. 46, No. 3, (March 2010), pp204-8

Liu, C.J.; Kao, S.Y.; Tu, H.F.; Tsai, M.M.; Chang, K.W. & Lin, S.C. (2010) Increase of microRNA miR-31 level in plasma could be a potential marker of oral cancer. *Oral Dis*, Vol. 16, No. 4, (May 2010), pp360-4

Liu, H.W.; Hu, B.Q. & Cao, C.F. (2005). The p16 methylation in oral leukoplakia and oral squamous cell carcinoma. *Zhonghua Kou Qiang Yi XueZaZhi*. Vol. 40, No. 2, (March 2005), pp 94-7

Liu, X.; Chen, Z.; Yu, J.; Xia, J. & Zhou, X. (2009). MicroRNA profiling and head and neck cancer. *Comp Funct Genomics*, Epub,(June 2009)

Liu, X.; Jiang, L.; Wang, A.; Yu, J.; Shi, F. & Zhou, X. (2009). MicroRNA-138 suppresses invasion and promotes apoptosis in head and neck squamous cell carcinoma cell lines. *Cancer Lett*, Vol. 286, no.2, pp 217–22

Liu, X.; Yu, J.; Jiang, L.; Wang, A.; Shi, F.; Ye, H. & Zhou, X. (2009). MicroRNA-222 regulates cell invasion by targeting matrix metalloproteinase 1 (MMP1) and manganese superoxide dismutase 2 (SOD2) in tongue squamous cell carcinoma cell lines. *Cancer Genomics Proteomics*, Vol. 6, No. 3, pp 131–9

Liu, X; Wang, A.; Heidbreder, C.E.; Jiang, L.; Yu,J.; Kolokythas, A.; Huang, L.; Dai, Y. & Zhou, X. (2010).MicroRNA-24 targeting RNA-binding protein DND1 in tongue squamous cell carcinoma. *FEBS Lett*, Vol. 584, No. 18, (September 2010), pp4115-20

Lo, W.L.; Yu, C.C.; Chiou, G.Y.; Chen, Y.W.; Huang, P.I.; Chien, C.S.; Tseng, L.M.; Chu, P.Y.; Lu, K.H.; Chang, K.W.; Kao, S.Y. & Chiou, S.H. (2011). MicroRNA-200c attenuates tumour growth and metastasis of presumptive head and neck squamous cell carcinoma stem cells. *J Pathol*, Vol. 223, No. 4, (March 2011), pp482-95

Lotan, R. (1996). Retinoids in cancer chemoprevention. *FASEB J*, Vol. 10, pp 1031–1039

Lotan, Y.;Xu, X.C.; Shalev, M.; Lotan, R.; Williams, R.; Wheeler, T.W.; Thompson, T.C. & Kadmon, D. (2000). Differential expression of nuclear retinoid receptors in normal and malignant prostates. *J Clin Oncol*, Vol. 18, pp 116 –121

Lu, J. (2005). MicroRNA expression profiles classify human cancers. *Nature* Vol. 435, pp 834–838

Lu, J.; Getz, G.; Miska, E.A.; Alvarez-Saavedra, E.; Lamb, J.; Peck, D.; Sweet-Cordero, A.; Ebert, B.L.; Mak, R.H.; Ferrando, A.A.; Downing, J.R.; Jacks, T.; Horvitz, H.R. & Golub, T.R. (2005). MicroRNA expression profiles classify human cancers. *Nature*, Vol. 435, pp834–8

Merlo, A.; Herman, J.G.; Mao, L.; Lee, D.J.; Gabrielson, E.; Burger, P.C.;Baylin, S.B. & Sidransky, D. (1995). 5-CpG island methylation is associated with transcriptional silencing of the tumour suppressor p16/CDKN2/MTS1 in human cancers. *Nat Med*,Vol.1, pp686 -92

Muramatsu, T.; Saitoh, M.; Ro, Y.; Uekusa, T.; Iwamura, E.; Ohta, K.; Kohno, Y.; Abiko, Y. & Shimono, M. (2008). Inhibition of syndecan-1 expression and function in oral cancer cells) Oncol Rep. Vol. 20, No. 6, pp 1353-7

Muthusamy, V.; Nobuo, T. & Govindaswamy S. (2003). Promoter hypermethylation profile of tumor-associated genes p16, p15, hmlh1, mgmt and e-cadherin in oral squamous cell carcinoma. *Int. J. Cancer*,Vol. 105, pp41–46

Ogi, K.; Toyota, M.; Ohe-Toyota, M.; Tanaka, N.; Noguchi, M.; Sonoda, T.; Kohama, G. & Tokino, T. (2002).Aberrant methylation of multiple genes and clinicopathological features in oral squamous cell carcinoma. *ClinCancer Res.*, Vol. 8, No. 10, (October 2002), pp 3164-71.

Pannone, G.; Bufo, P.; Santoro, A.; Franco, R.; Aquino, G; Longo, F.; Botti, G.; Serpico, R.; Cafarelli, B.; Abbruzzese, A.; Caraglia, M.; Papagerakis, S. & Lo Muzio, L. (2010). WNT pathway in oral cancer: epigenetic inactivation of WNT-inhibitors. *OncolRep*,Vol. 24, No.4,(October 2010), pp1035-41

Pasquinelli, A. E.; Hunter, S. & Bracht, J. (2005). MicroRNAs: a developing story. *Curr Opin Genet Dev*, Vol. 15, pp 200–205

Rattner, A.; Hsieh, J.C.; Smallwood, P.M.; Gilbert, D.J.; Copeland, N.G.; Jenkins N.A. & Nathans, J. (1997): A family of secreted proteins contains homology to the cysteine-rich ligand-binding domain of frizzled receptors. *Proc Natl Acad Sci USA*, Vol. 94, pp 2859-2863

Reis, P.P.; Tomenson, M.; Cervigne, N.K.; Machado, J.; Jurisica, I.; Pintilie, M.; Sukhai, M.A.; Perez-Ordonez, B.; Grénman, R.; Gilbert, R.W.; Gullane, P.J.; Irish, J.C. & Kamel-Reid, S. (2010) Programmed cell death 4 loss increases tumor cell invasion and is regulated by miR-21 in oral squamous cell carcinoma. *Mol Cancer*, Vol. 10, No. 9, (September 2010), p 238

Robertson, K.D. (2001). DNA methylation, methyltransferases, and cancer. *Oncogene*, Vol. 20, pp 3139 -55

Rochaix, P.; Monteil-Onteniente, S.; Rochette-Egly, C.; Caratero, C.; Voigt, J.J. & Jozan, S. (1998). Reduced expression of retinoic acid receptor beta protein (RAR beta) in human papillary thyroid carcinoma: immunohistochemical and western blot study. *Histopathology*, Vol. 33, pp 337–343

Rosas, S.L.; Koch, W.; da Costa Carvalho, M.G.; Wu, L.; Califano, J.;Westra, W.; Jen, J. & Sidransky, D. (2001).Promoter hypermethylation patterns of p16, O6-methylguanine-DNA-methyltransferase, and death-associated protein kinase in tumors and saliva of head and neck cancer patients. *Cancer Res.*,Vol. 61, No. 3, (February 2001), 939-42

Schiffelers, R.M.; Ansari, A.; Xu, J.; Zhou, Q.; Tang, Q.; Storm, G. & Mole, G siRNA therapy by tumor selective delivery with ligand-targeted sterically stabilized nanoparticle. *Oxford JournalsCancer*, 2004. Life Sciences, Nucleic Acids Research,Volume32, Issue19

Scully, C. (1995). Oral precancer: preventive and medical approaches to management. *Oral Oncol*, Vol.31B, pp16 -26

Shao, Z.; Shen, Z.& Fontana, J.A. (1995). Expression of the retinoic acid nuclear receptors and retinoid X receptor gene in human breast cancer. *Chung Hua Chung Liu TsaChih*, Vol. 17, pp 425– 428

Shiiba M., Uzawa K. and Tanzawa H. MicroRNAs in Head and Neck Squamous Cell Carcinoma (HNSCC) and Oral Squamous Cell Carcinoma (OSCC)(2010). *Cancers.*, *2*, 653-669

Shin, K.H.; Bae, S.D.; Hong, H.S.; Kim, R.H.; Kang, M.K. & Park, N.H. (2011).miR-181a shows tumor suppressive effect against oral squamous cell carcinoma cells by downregulating K-ras. *Biochem Biophys Res Commun*. Vol. 404, No. 4, (January 2011), pp896-902

Sinha, P.;Bahadur, S.; Thakar, A.; Matta, A.; Macha, M.; Ralhan, R. & Gupta, S.D. (2009). Significance of promoter hypermethylation of p16 gene for margin assessment in carcinoma tongue. *Head Neck.*, Vol. 31, No. 11, (November 2009), pp 1423-30

Sogabe, Y.; Suzuki, H.; Toyota, M.; Ogi, K.; Imai, T.; Nojima, M.; Sasaki, Y.; Hiratsuka, H. & Tokino, T. (2008) Epigenetic inactivation of SFRP genes in oral squamous cell carcinoma. *Int J Oncol*, Vol. 32, No. 6, (June 2008), pp 1253-61

Supić, G.; Kozomara, R.; Branković-Magić, M.; ović, N. & Magić, Z. (2009). Gene hypermethylation in tumor tissue of advanced oral squamous cell carcinoma patients. *Oral Oncol.*, Vol. 45, No. 12,(December 2009), pp 1051-7

Supic, G.; Kozomara, R.; Jovic, N.; Zeljic, K. & Magic, Z. (2011). Prognostic significance of tumor-related genes hypermethylation detected in cancer-free surgical margins of oral squamous cell carcinomas. *Oral Oncol*, Vol47, No. 8, (August 2011), pp 702-8

Taioli, E.;Ragin, C.; Wang, X.H.; Chen, J.; Langevin, S.M.; Brown, A.R.; Gollin, S.M.; Garte, S. & Sobol, R.W. (2009).Recurrence in oral and pharyngeal cancer is associated with quantitative MGMT promoter methylation.*BMC Cancer*, Vol. 6, No. 9, (October 2009), pp 354

Takeshima, M.; Saitoh, M.; Kusano, K.; Nagayasu, H.; Kurashige, Y.; Malsantha, M.; Arakawa, T.; Takuma, T.; Chiba, I.; Kaku, T.; Shibata, T. &Abiko, Y. (2008). High frequency of hypermethylation of p14, p15 and p16 in oral pre-cancerous lesions associated with betel-quid chewing in Sri Lanka. *J Oral Pathol Med*, Vol. 37, No. 8, September 2008, pp475-9

Tang, Y.;Simoneau, A.R.; Liao, W.X.;Yi, G.; Hope, C.; Liu, F.; Li, S.;Xie, J.; Holcombe, R.F.;Jurnak, F.A.;Mercola, D.; Hoang, B.H. &Zi, X. (2009). WIF-1, a WNT pathway inhibitor, regulates SKP2 and c-myc expression leading to G1 arrest and growth inhibition of human invasive urinary bladder cancer cells. *Mol Cancer Ther*, Vol. 8, pp 458-468

Tansey, B. (2006). Macular degeneration treatment interferes with RNA messages. *San Francisco Chronicle*, 11 August 2006.

Tran, T.N.; Liu, Y.; Takagi, M.; Yamaguchi, A. & Fujii, H. (2005). Frequent promoter hypermethylation of RASSF1A and p16INK4a and infrequent allelic loss other than 9p21 in betel-associated oral carcinoma in a Vietnamese non-smoking/non-drinking female population. *J Oral Pathol Med*, Vol. 34, No. 3,(March 2005),pp150-6

Veigl, M.L.; Kasturi, L.; Olechnowicz, J.; Ma, A.; Lutterbaugh, J.D.; Periasamy, S.; Li, G.M.; Drummond, J.; Modrich, P.L.; Sedwick, W.D. & Markowitz, S.D. (1998). Biallelic inactivation of hMLH11 by epigenetic mechanism causing human MSI cancers. *Proc Natl Acad Sci USA*, Vol. 95, pp8698 -702

Vigneswaran, N.; Wu, J.; Nagaraj, N.; James, R.; Zeeuwen, P. & Zacharias, W. (2006). Silencing of cystatin M in metastatic oral cancer cell line MDA-686Ln by siRNA increases cysteine proteinases and legumain activities, cell proliferation and in vitro invasion. *Life Sciences*, Vol. 78, no. 8, (January 2006), pp 898-907

Viswanathan, M.; Tsuchida, N. & Shanmugam, G. (2003)Promoter hypermethylation profile of tumor-associated genes p16, p15, hMLH1, MGMT and E-cadherin in oral squamous cell carcinoma. *Int J Cancer*, Vol. 105, No. 1, (May 2003), pp41-6

Volinia, S. (2006). A microRNA expression signature of human solid tumors define cancer gene targets. *Proc Natl Acad Sci USA*, Vol. 103, pp 2257–2261

Wald, A.I.; Hoskins, E.E.; Wells, S.I.; Ferris, R.L. & Khan S.A. (2010). Alteration of microRNA profiles in squamous cell carcinoma of the head and neck cell lines by human papillomavirus). *Head Neck*, Vol. 33, no. 4, pp 504-12

Wong, T.S.; Ho, W.K.; Chan, J.Y.; Ng, R.W. & Wei, W.I. (2009)Mature miR-184 and squamous cell carcinoma of the tongue. *Scientific World Journal*, Vol. 15, No. 9, (February 2009), 130-2

Wong, T.S.; Liu, X.B.; Wong, B.Y.; Ng, R.W.; Yuen, A.P. & Wei, W.I. (2008).Mature miR-184 as Potential Oncogenic microRNA of Squamous Cell Carcinoma of Tongue. *Clin Cancer Res*, Vol. 14, No. 9, (May 2008), pp 2588-92

Wu, B.H.; Xiong, X.P.; Jia, J. & Zhang, W.F. (2011). MicroRNAs: New actors in the oral cancer scene.*Oral Oncology*, Vol. 47, pp 314–319

Xu, X.C.; Ro, J.Y.; Lee, J.S.; Shin, D.M.; Hong, W.K. & Lotan, R. (1994). Differential expression of nuclear retinoid receptors in normal, premalignant and malignant head and neck tissues. *Cancer Res*, Vol. 54, pp 3280 -3287

Xu, X.C.; Sozzi, G.; Lee, J.S.; Lee, J.J.; Pastorino, U.; Pilotti, S.;Kurie, J.M.; Hong, W.K. & Lotan, R. (1997). Suppression of retinoic acid receptor B in non-small cell lung cancer in vivo implications for lung cancer development. *J Nat Cancer Inst*, Vol. 89, pp624–629

Yeh, K.T.; Shih, M.C.; Lin, T.H.; Chen, J.C.; Chang, J.Y.; Kao, C.F.; Lin, K.L. & Chang, J.G. (2002).The correlation between CpG methylation on promoter and protein expression of E-cadherin in oral squamous cell carcinoma. *Anticancer Res.*, Vol. 22, No. 6C, (November-December 2002), pp 3971-5

Youssef, E.M.; Lotan, D.; Issa, J.P.; Wakasa, K.; Fan, Y.H.; Mao, L.; Hassan, K.; Feng, L.; Lee, J.J.; Lippman, S.M.; Hong, W.K. & Lotan, R.(2004). Hypermethylation of the retinoic acid receptor-beta(2) gene in head and neck carcinogenesis. *Clin Cancer Res*, Vol. 10, No. 5, (March 2004), pp 1733-42

Yu, C.C.; Chen, Y.W.; Chiou, G.Y.; Tsai, L.L.; Huang, P.I.; Chang, C.Y.; Tseng, L.M.; Chiou, S.H.; Yen, S.H.; Chou, M.Y.; Chu, P.Y. & Lo, W.L. (2010). MicroRNA let-7a represses chemoresistance and tumourigenicity in head and neck cancer via stem-like properties ablation. *Oral Oncol*, Vol. 47, No.3, (March 2011), pp202-10.

Yu, Z.W.; Zhong, L.P.; Ji,T.; Zhang, P.; Chen, W.T. & Zhang, C.P. (2010). MicroRNAs contribute to the chemoresistance of cisplatin in tongue squamous cell carcinoma lines. *Oral Oncol*, Vol. 46, No. 4, pp 317–22

17

Reduced Expression of Syndecan-1 in Oral Cancer

Takashi Muramatsu[1,2,3]
[1]*Oral Health Science Center hrc8,*
[2]*Department of Pathology,*
[3]*Department of Clinical Pathophysiology*
Tokyo Dental College, Chiba,
Japan

1. Introduction

The syndecan family is composed of four closely related proteins (syndecan-1–4) encoded by four different genes. Syndecan-1 binds cells via its heparan sulfate chains to a variety of components of the interstitial matrix, including types I, III and V collagen, fibrillar collagen, fibronectin and tenascin. In previous studies it has been noted that expression of syndecan-1 correlates with malignancy in various tissues including uterine cervix and esophagus. Several reports on head and neck carcinoma have suggested that reduced expression of syndecan-1 is associated with the prognosis of such neoplasms. Anatomical location may influence the expression of syndecan-1 in squamous cell carcinoma (SCC), since previous studies examined this type of cancer in various tissue sites of the oral cavity. Also, previous reports evaluated the immunohistochemical positive ratio ignoring patterns of expression; nevertheless, immunoreaction to syndecan-1 was located only at the cell membranes, and not in the cytoplasm. No study has shown whether or not syndecan-1 is associated with mode of invasion, although invasion correlates to malignant behavior and prognosis.

We investigated syndecan-1 immunoreactivity in primary SCC arising exclusively from the tongue, and the relationship between expression pattern of immunoreactivity and various clinico-pathological parameters was analyzed. Forty-three cases of SCC arising in lateral border of tongue were investigated. From the immunohistochemical staining pattern, the cases were divided into two groups based on expression of syndecan-1 at the supra-peripheral cells of the tumor nest: Group A, completely or mainly positive; Group B, sporadically positive or negative. Most poorly differentiated SCC cases were classified into Group B (81.8%). The number of Group B cases in T1–2 was different from that in T3–4. The number of cases where syndecan-1 expression was reduced was much greater in T3–4, and represented the majority of Group B (86.7%). More than 80% of Grade 4D cases were in Group B (83.3%) based on the Yamamoto–Kohama criteria. These results indicate that reduction of syndecan-1 correlates to histological grading, tumor size and mode of invasion in tongue SCC.

We also investigated the expression of syndecan-1 in oral cancer cell lines and tested whether transfection of an siRNA against human syndecan-1 affected the malignant potential of these cells. Seven different human oral cancer cell lines (HSC2, HSC3, HSC4, Ca9-22, SAS, KB and BSC-OF) were used. In order to examine syndecan-1 function, siRNA was transfected into the cells, after which the cell growth rate and invasive ability were evaluated. QRT-PCR showed that syndecan-1 was expressed in Ca9-22 cells and that it was significantly higher (>10-fold) than in the other oral cancer cell lines. Transfection of syndecan-1 siRNA was carried out on Ca9-22 cells, which increased their growth rate 1.4-fold above controls. The invasive ability of Ca9-22 cells treated with syndecan-1 siRNA was significantly higher (2-fold; n=5) than the controls. These results suggest that syndecan-1 directly contributes to the growth and invasive ability of these cells.

1.1 Syndecan

Cell surface adhesion receptors bind cells to their extracellular matrix and couple such interactions with intercellular signaling mechanisms. It is apparent that alternations in cell adhesion can influence almost every stage of cellular transformation. The development of malignant epithelial neoplasm is associated with disruption of cell-to-cell and cell-to-matrix adhesion.

Syndecans are family of heparan sulfate proteoglycan receptors that are thought to participate in both cell-to-cell and cell-to-matrix adhesion. The syndecans are composed of a core protein, to which sulphated and unbranched carbohydrate chains, glyosaminoglycans, are covalently attached. The core proteins contain an extracellular, a transmembrane and an intracellular domain, and their amino acid sequances are homologous, especially between the two last domains. The syndecans interact with extracellular matrix components, other cell surface components, and growth factors, including basic fibroblast growth factor (Hayashi *et al.*, 1987; Inki *et al.*, 1991). The syndecan family is composed of four closely related proteins; syndecan-1, syndecan-2 (fibroglycan), syndecan-3 (N-syndecan), and syndecan-4 (amphiglycan, ryudocan); encoded by four different genes. Syndecan-1 consists of a 310 amino acid long core protein in human, and is an 85-92 kDa type I integral membrane proteoglycan and binds cells via its heparan sulfate chains to a variety of components of the interstitial matrix, including types I, III and V collagen, fibrillar collagen, fibronectin and tenascin. The syndecan-1 also contains chondroitin sulfacte. The syndecan-1 is thought to function as a matrix receptor that transduces information between the extracellular matrix and the inside of the cell (Inki *et al.*, 1994; Sanderson *et al.*, 1992). Syndecan-1 is expressed in distinct differentiation stages of normal lymphoid cells. During lymphocyte differentiation, syndecan-1 is expressed only when and where lymphoid cells interact with type I collagen (Sanderson *et al.*, 1989)., thus it occurs on the cell surface of B cells in the pre-B-cells stage and immature B cells, but is absent from matured B cells, and re-appears on plasma cells (Sebestyen *et al.*, 1999). Sydecan-1 may mediate the adhesion of lymphoid cells to bone marrow matrix and to the interstitial matrix of peripheral lymphoid organs. The most abundant expression of syndecan-1 in the adult organism is found in stratified squamous epithelia, such as epidermis, oral mucosa and vagina. Syndecan-1 is found on basolateral surfaces of the epithelial cells, endothelial ells of sprouting capillaries and embryonic condensing mesenchymal cells (David *et al.*, 1993; Sanderson *et al.*, 1989). In normal tongue tissue, the basal, supra-basal and lower prickle cell layers of the epithelium were immunohistochemically positive for syndecan-1, and positive reactions were usually distinct on the cell surfaces (Figure 1a, 1b). The cell membrane facing the basement membrane was essentially negative for syndecan-1 staining. The upper prickle cell and superficial layer of the epithelium lacked syndecan-1 reactivity. However, obvious matrix ligands for syndecan-1 are not found within these tissues. Therefore, syndecan-1 may have different functions in stratified epithelia.

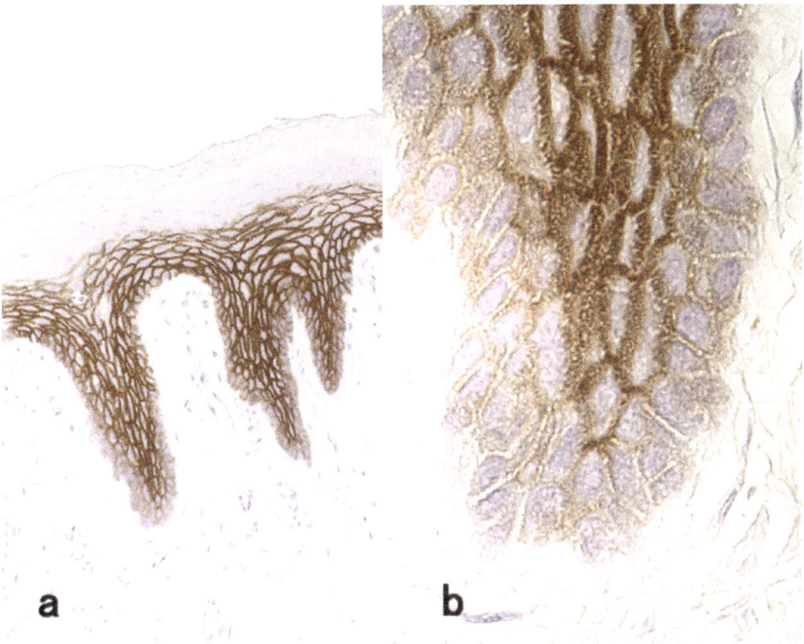

Fig. 1. Immunohistochemical expression pattern of syndecan-1 in normal tongue epithelium. (a) Syndecan-1 expression in the normal tongue. In normal tissues, the basal, suprabasal and lower prickle cell layers of the epithelia are positive for syndecan-1. (b) Higher magnification of (a). The cell membrane facing the basement membrane is essentially negative for syndecan-1. The upper prickle cell and superficial layers of the epithelia lacked syndecan-1 reactivity.

Intracellular tail of syndecan seems to combine the cytoskeleton and cellular components, and the extracellular part of the molecule seems to bind different ligands. Presumably, syndecan-1 plays an important role in cellular functions such as proliferation, cell-to-matrix and cell-to-cell adhesion (Gattei *et al.*, 1999). Interaction of cells and extracellular matrix is important in the maintenance of normal cell architecture and growth, but is especially highlighted during embryonic development involving morphogenetic interactions between different cell types. The expression of syndecan-1 is developmentally highly regulated in a fashion which suggests that syndecan-1 is one of the molecules that participate in reciprocal morphogenetic interactions during embryonic development (Vainio *et al.*, 1991). During mouse tooth development, syndecan-1 is induced by primitive dental epithelium in condensed mesenchyme, but later disappears and becomes localized again in the epithelial cells (Thesleff *et al.*, 1996). Although there have been many investigations, the function of syndecan isbeen still largely unknown.

1.2 Syndecan-1 in cancer

In previous studies it has been noted that reduced expression of syndecan-1 correlates to malignancy in various tissues including uterine cervix (Inki *et al.*, 1994; Rintala *et al.*, 1999), endometrium (Miturski *et al.*, 1998), esophagus (Mikami *et al.*, 2001), breast (Barbareschi *et al.*, 2003), lung (Anttonen *et al.*, 2001), kidney (Gokden *et al.*, 2006), liver (Charni *et al.*, 2009), multiple myeloma (Sebestyen *et al.*, 1999). These earlier reports showed that syndecan-1 expression was reduced during malignant transformation of various epithelia (Inki and Jalkanen, 1996). Syndencan-1 was also lost rapidly by myeloma cells entering into apoptosis, thus syndecan-1 is a marker of viable myeloma cells (Jourdan *et al.*, 1998). Many immunohistochemical studies have demonstrated absent or decreased expression of syndecan-1 in many kinds of carcinomas with more aggressive characteristics (Fujiya *et al.*, 2001; Inki *et al.*, 1994; Kumar-Singh *et al.*, 1998; Matsumoto *et al.*, 1997; Stanley *et al.*, 1999; Toyoshima *et al.*, 2001; Wiksten *et al.*, 2000; Wiksten *et al.*, 2001). There are several reports on syndecan-1 expression in head and neck carcinoma (Anttonen *et al.*, 1999; Inki *et al.*, 1994; Kurokawa *et al.*, 2003; Kurokawa *et al.*, 2006; Muramatsu *et al.*, 2008; Ro *et al.*, 2006). However, head and neck carcinoma includes oral, nasal, laryngeal and esophageal carcinomas, and investigation of syndecan-1 expression in oral cancer has been limited.

1.3 Syndecan-1 in oral cancer

Oral cancer is the fifth most common type of cancer in the world. Despite modern intervention, the 5-year survival rate for this disease has improved only marginally over the past decade and recurrent disease is observed in 50% of patients (Greenlee *et al.*, 2001). Survival curves of oral cancer patients have plateaued over the past two decades and remain among the worst of all cancer sites (Takes *et al.*, 1997). Recent studies in this field have focused on the development of specific markers that reflect the biological properties of tumors and have use in early detection, disease monitoring and determining the prognosis of patients with oral cancer (Alevizos *et al.*, 2001; Le *et al.*, 2003; Macabeo-Ong *et al.*, 2003).

Syndecan-1 has been reported to be a prognostic factor for tumor progression and survival in various types of malignant tumors, which suggests a close correlation of syndecan-1 expression with malignancy and metastasis (Inki *et al.*, 1994; Kurokawa *et al.*, 2006). In general, transformed cells are often characterized by an abundant secretion of syndecan-1, which results in metastasis formation (Senger *et al.*, 1983; Senger and Perruzzi, 1985). Earlier studies associated syndecan-1 levels with prognosis and have suggested syndecan-1 as a candidate biomarker for the malignant potential of head and neck tumors.

It has been reported that a marked down-regulation of syndecan-1 expression is associated with dysplastic change in the oral epithelium. Kurokawa *et al.* (2003) also found a significant correlation between the down-regulation of syndecan-1 expression and the grade of oral epithelial dysplasia. Down-regulation has also been reported in SCCs of the head and neck compared to expression in the corresponding normal epithelium (Soukka *et al.*, 2000), suggesting that syndecan-1 was a useful marker for evaluating pre-malignant lesions of the head and neck region. In head and neck tumors,

Soukka *et al.* (2000) reported that 65% of oral SCC cases showed negative or weak staining for syndecan-1, of which 35% were totally negative. In our study, 36 of the 72 cases (50%) were negative or weakly intense for syndecan-1 expression. Inki *et al.* (1991) and Soukka *et al.* (2000) reported that intermediate and strong positive staining for syndecan-1 was localized on cell surfaces, especially in cell–cell contact sites. Moreover, Inki *et al.*(1994) demonstrated that syndecan-1 expression was associated with tumor size and histological grade, and tumors with a poor histological grade expressed syndecan-1 at lower levels.

These earlier reports point to reduction of syndecan-1 expression as being a biomarker in head and neck cancer. However, evaluation is different in various studies. For example, anatomical location may influence the expression of syndecan-1 in SCC, since previous studies examined this type of cancer in various tissue sites of the oral cavity such as tongue, maxillary gingiva, mandibular gingiva, oral floor, and buccal mucosa. Also, previous reports evaluated the immunohistochemical positive ratio ignoring patterns of expression; nevertheless, immunoreaction to syndecan-1 was located only at the cell membranes, and not in the cytoplasm.

1.4 Reduction pattern of syndecan-1 in oral cancer

As mentioned above, previous reports evaluated the immunohistochemical positive ratio ignoring patterns of expression. Evaluations of immunohistochemical findings were only reported as negative, weakly positive or positive in previous studies (Kurokawa *et al.*, 2006; Soukka *et al.*, 2000), and the positive ratio was employed frequently as an evaluation of the immunostaining (Anttonen *et al.*, 1999; Inki *et al.*, 1994). Nevertheless, immunoreaction to syndecan-1 was located only at the cell membranes, and not in the cytoplasm of the tumor cells. The evaluation method shown in these earlier reports was vague and not objective. Ro *et al.* (2006)used a new method based on the pattern of immunostaining for syndecan-1. The method was focused on reduced patterns of syndecan-1 in the supra-peripheries, because recent studies had showed that reduction of syndecan-1 expression was associated with proliferative activity (Ki-67 expression)(Kurokawa *et al.*, 2003). Both Ki-67 and syndecan-1 are localized in cells of the supra-basal layer as well, and this was evaluated. This method is considered to be more objective and exact for evaluation than that used in previous studies, because it estimates immunoreactivity restricted to the supra-peripheries of the tumor nests.

From the patterns of immunohistochemical staining, the cases were divided into two groups according to the expression of syndecan-1 as follows. Group A: complete or mostly surround type. Syndecan-1-positive reactions were observed at the supra-peripheral cell layers of the tumor nest without break, or loss of syndecan-1 was seen at within 50% of the supra-peripheral cell layer of the tumor nest (Figure 2a-d). Group B: sporadic expression or negative type. Immunoreactions with syndecan-1 at the supra-peripheral cell layer of the tumor nests were sporadically reduced. Loss of syndecan-1 was seen in 50% or more of the cells (Figures 2e-h). In SCC, positive reactivity for syndecan-1 was usually detected at the supra-periphery of the tumor nests. We divided the cases into two groups according to their immunoreactivity, and the number of cases was 18 (41.8%) in Group A and 25 (58.2%) in Group B.

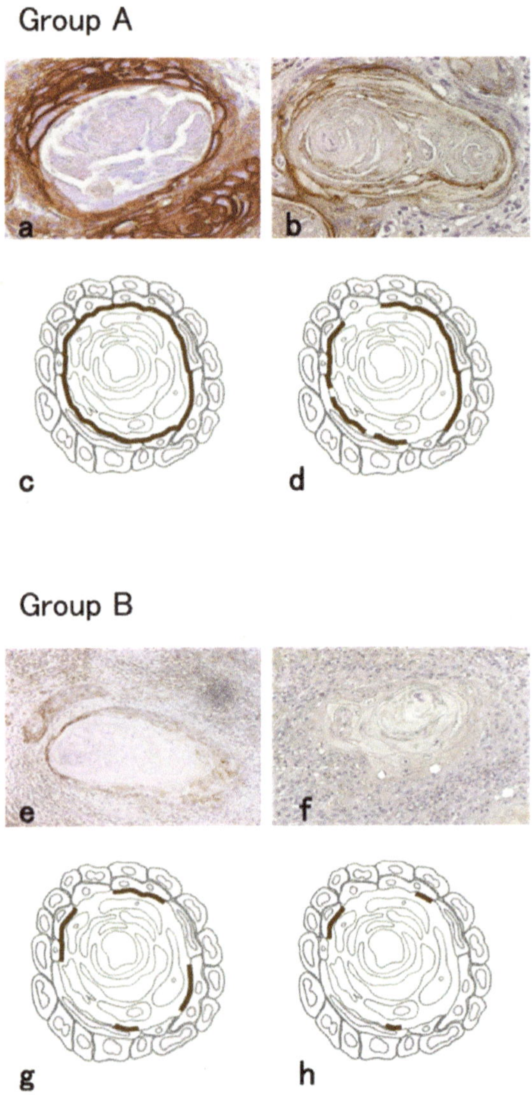

Fig. 2. Immunohistochemical expression pattern of syndecan-1 in SCC of the tongue. We divided pattern of immunohistochemical staining into 2 groups according to the expression of syndecan-1 at periphery of the tumor nest. Group A: Completely (a) or mostly (b) surrounded type. Staining surrounds the tumor nests without a break (a, c). Loss of syndecan-1 staining surrounding the tumor nests is found within 50% of the cells (b, d). Figure (c) and (d) are scheme of figure (a) and (b), respectively. Group B: Sporadically expression (e) or negative type (f). Loss of syndecan-1 surrounding the tumor nests is seen in 50% or more than of the cells (e-h). Syndecan-1 expression is weak (e) or completely negative (f). Figures (g) and (h) are scheme of figure (e) and (f), respectively.

1.5 Syndecan-1 expression and clinical parameters

Some investigators demonstrated that syndecan-1 immunoreactivity in primary SCC arising exclusively from the head and neck, especially from the oral cavity, and the relationship between expression pattern of immunoreactivity and various clinico-pathological parameters such as Tumor-Node-Metastasis (TNM) system and histological grading of the differentiation of SCC, was analyzed.

	Group A % (n)	Group B % (n)	
Histological grade			
well	50.0 (12)	50.0 (12)	N.S.
moderately	50.0 (4)	50.0 (4)	N.S.
poorly	18.2 (2)	81.8 (9)	*
Tumor size			
T1 - 2	57.1 (16)	42.9 (12)	N.S.
T3 - 4	13.3 (2)	86.7 (13)	*
Stage			
stage I - II	50.0 (7)	50.0 (7)	N.S.
stage III - IV	37.9 (11)	62.1 (18)	N.S.
Mode of invasion			
Grade 1	50.0 (1)	50.0 (1)	N.S.
Grade 2	54.5 (6)	45.4 (5)	N.S.
Grade 3	40.0 (6)	60.0 (9)	N.S.
Grade 4C	37.5 (3)	62.5 (5)	N.S.
Grade 4D	16.7 (1)	83.3 (5)	*
Invasion depth			
0 - 3 mm	27.3 (3)	72.7 (8)	*
3 - 6 mm	33.3 (5)	66.7 (10)	N.S.
6 - 9 mm	62.5 (5)	37.5 (3)	N.S.
9 mm -	50.0 (5)	50.0 (5)	N.S.
Lymph node metastasis			
pN0	35.7 (5)	64.3 (9)	N.S.
pN1	40.0 (4)	60.0 (6)	N.S.

N.S.: not siginificant
*: statistically significant ($p<0.01$)

Table 1. Correlation between reduction of syndecan-1 and clinicopathological parameters

Ro et al., (2006) investigated forty-three cases of SCC arising in lateral border of tongue **(Table 1)**. For histological grade, a reduction in syndecan-1 staining was apparent in poorly differentiated SCC (81.8%), while in well or moderately differentiated SCCs, there was no difference. Regarding tumor size, the number of sporadically positive or negative syndecan-1 cases in T1 or T2 SCC was different from that in T3 or T4. Reduction in syndecan-1 expression was dramatically greater in T3 and T4, and such cases represented the majority of negative syndecan-1 cases (86.7%). Concerning stage, the incidence of syndecan-1-negative cases in stages I and II was different from that in stages III and IV. Sixty-two percent of stages III and IV cases were in of negative syndecan-1 cases, suggesting that advanced SCC shows greatly reduced expression of syndecan-1. However, there was no correlation between reduction of syndecan-1 and depth of invasion or lymphatic metastasis. The results of the earlier studies (Inki *et al.*, 1994; Kurokawa *et al.*, 2006; Ro *et al.*, 2006) suggest that reduction of syndecan-1 expression is correlated with tumor size, histological grade and mode of invasion in SCC of tongue as well as other body sites (Anttonen *et al.*, 2001; Kumar-Singh *et al.*, 1998), but is not associated with lymph-node metastasis and depth of invasion, which are accurate predictors of clinical outcome. There has been controversy regarding the relationship between lymphatic metastasis and syndecan-1 expression. Anttonen *et al.* (1999) noted that strong syndecan-1 expression was associated with lack of lymph-node metastasis, but Inki *et al.* (1994) demonstrated that there was no association between syndecan-1 expression and the presence of cervical node metastasis, the results of the present study being in agreement with Inki *et al.* (1994). It is proposed that while syndecan-1 may be a useful candidate biomarker, it is not an accurate predictor of clinical outcome in SCC of tongue.

1.6 Syndecan-1 on oral SCC invasion

Oral cancer is characterized by a high degree of invasion into local tissues. The mode of invasion of the malignant tumor is an important factor in predicting prognosis, and has been studied in head and neck tumors in particular (Jakobsson *et al.*, 1973; Yamamoto *et al.*, 1983). Recent evidence suggests that cells present at the invasive tumor front of carcinomas have different molecular characteristics compared with those in superficial areas of the tumor, making the invasive front the most important area of the tumor for determining the prognosis (Bryne *et al.*, 1989; Bryne, 1991; Bryne *et al.*, 1992). Bryne *et al.* (1995) described a multiple-factor histological grading system of the invasive front of tumors of the head and neck: it consisted of the pattern of invasion, the degree of keratinization, nuclear polymorphism, and the host response. Kearsley and Thomas (1993) reported a strong correlation between total malignancy grading scores based on several pathological parameters and the prognosis in oral SCC. Kurokawa *et al.* (2006) evaluated the association between the loss of syndecan-1 expression and the histological grade of malignancy at the deep invasive front in oral SCC using the method of Bryne *et al.* (1992). and reported a statistically significant correlation between the down-regulation of syndecan-1 expression and prognosis, differentiation and pattern of invasion at the deep invasive front in oral SCC (Kurokawa *et al.*, 2006).

On the other hand, there has been reported classification on mode of invasion by Yamamoto *et al.* (1983), named as Yamamoto–Kohama's criteria **(Table 2)**. They have been widely utilized and considered useful for estimating risk factors (Yamamoto *et al.*, 1983). The Grade 4C oral SCC is charaterized by a cord-like, diffuse, deep invasion forming cord-shaped micro-tumor nests. Grade 4D oral SCC invades the deeper portion diffusely as a single cell or a few cells.

The study by Ro *et al.* (2006) employed Yamamoto-Kohama's mode-of-invasion criteria, and the correlation between mode of invasion and reduction of syndecan-1 expression was demonstrated by diffuse invading SCC having only faint expression of syndecan-1. More than 70% of Grades 4C and 4D were classified into syndecan-1 reduced or negative cases (71.4%) according to Yamamoto-Kohama's criteria. Expression of syndecan-1 has been known to suppress the level of matrix metalloproteinase (MMP)-9 and to inhibit cell invasion into type I collagen (Kaushal *et al.*, 1999; Liebersbach and Sanderson, 1994). Syndecan-1 is degraded by heparanase (Reiland *et al.*, 2004), and mode of invasion is associated with MMPs (P *et al.*, 2001) and heparanase activity (Ikebe *et al.*, 1999). These reports suggest that reduced expression of syndecan-1 is strongly associated with the mode of invasion.

Grade
1. Well-defined borderline
2. Cords, less marked borderline
3. Groups of cells, no distinct borderline
4. Diffuse invasion
4C: Cord-like type
4D: Widespread type

Yamamoto-Kohama's classification (1983)

Table 2. Histological grading of mode of invasion

2. Studies in oral cancer cells

Recent *in vitro* studies have indicated that syndecan-1 plays a role in inhibiting cell invasion and suppressing the growth of carcinoma cell lines (Ito *et al.*, 2003; Liebersbach and Sanderson, 1994; Liu *et al.*, 1998; Mali *et al.*, 1994).

Our earlier study showed that the reduction of immunoreactivity for syndecan-1 in oral SCC cells was associated with tumor size, suggesting that syndecan-1 contributes to their malignant behavior including changes in growth and invasive ability (Ro *et al.*, 2006). A reduction of syndecan-1 expression was associated with proliferative activity (Ki-67 expression) (Kurokawa *et al.*, 2003). Furthermore, Su et al reported that shedding of syndecan-1 by stromal fibroblasts stimulated the proliferation of human breast cancer cells via activation of FGF2 (Su *et al.*, 2007). However, expression levels and function(s) of syndecan-1 in oral cancers have not been clarified. Muramatsu *et al.*, (2008) investigated the expression of syndecan-1 in oral cancer cell lines and tested whether transfection of an siRNA against human syndecan-1 affected the malignant potential of these cells. Seven different human oral cancer cell lines (HSC2, HSC3, HSC4, Ca9-22, SAS, KB and BSC-OF) were used. In order to examine syndecan-1 function, siRNA was transfected into the cells, after which the cell growth rate and invasive ability were evaluated. To validate the high expression levels of syndecan-1 in human oral cancer cell lines, QRT-PCR was carried out. Based on the $\Delta\Delta$Ct relative to KB cells, the relative expression levels of syndecan-1 mRNA in oral carcinoma cell lines were calculated. Several cell lines showed expression of syndecan-1 at high levels. In particular, syndecan-1 was expressed in Ca9-22 cells at a higher level (13.2-fold) than in KB cells. Immunofluorescence analysis showed that positive reactions for syndecan-1 were observed strongly at the cell membrane of Ca9-22 cells, while diffuse faint dot reactions were seen in KB cells. Based on those QRT-PCR and immunofluorescence results, we used Ca9-22 cells as a model for high expression of syndecan-1 as a model cell line. In order to characterize the effects of syndecan-1 siRNA, we carried out QRT-PCR analysis using mRNAs from non-transfected (control) and from transfected Ca9-22 cells. After 48 h of incorporation, decreased expression (1/10-fold) of syndecan-1 was seen in the siRNA-transfected cells, suggesting that siRNA blocked syndecan-1 expression very efficiently in Ca9-22 cells. Cell growth. To examine whether syndecan-1 is associated with cell growth, the growth of siRNA-transfected cells and control cells was measured. Ca9-22 cells had increased growth after syndecan-1 siRNA transfection. The numbers of siRNA-transfected Ca9-22 cells and control cells at 48 h were 6.0×10^5 and 4.1×10^5, respectively and at 72 h were 11.8×10^5 and 8.0×10^5, respectively. The cell growth rate of control cells was lower than the siRNA-transfected cells at 48 and at 72 h, and were significantly different at both time points ($p<0.01$). Invasion assay. To examine the effect of syndecan-1 on the invasive ability of Ca9-22 cells, a Matrigel assay was used. The numbers of invasive siRNA-transfected and control Ca9-22 cells were 718.4 per mm^2 and 378.8 per mm^2 (average), respectively, which was significantly higher ($p<0.01$) **(Figure 3)**. Our results show that the reduction of syndecan-1 function by siRNA leads to higher levels of cell proliferation, which suggests that syndecan-1 is directly associated with cell proliferation. Furthermore, cell migration has been reported to influence invasiveness and to be an important factor in the incidence of metastasis.

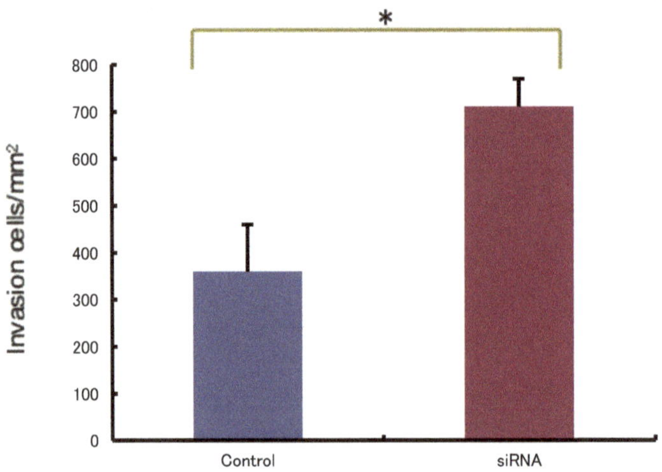

Fig. 3. Invasion assay.
The Matrigel assay was used to investigate the effects of syndecan-1 on the invasive ability of Ca9-22 cells. The number of invading cells was significantly higher in the siRNA-transfected group (* $P<0.01$).

Moreover, the invasive ability of tumors is closely related to the incidence of metastasis and the prognosis of the disease. As shown in previous studies, reduced expression of syndecan-1 correlates with metastasis of various tumors. There have been only a few studies that showed a correlation between syndecan-1 and invasion in oral cancers, but there has been no previous functional study of syndecan-1 using an oral cancer cell line. Therefore, we examined whether syndecan-1was associated with the invasive ability of Ca9-22 cells. Our results show that invasiveness increased when syndecan-1 function was blocked in siRNA-transfected Ca9-22 cells. The expression of syndecan-1 is known to suppress the level of matrix metalloproteinase (MMP)-9 and to inhibit cell invasion into type I collagen (Kaushal *et al.*, 1999; Liebersbach and Sanderson, 1994). Moreover, syndecan-1 can be degraded by heparanase (Reiland *et al.*, 2004), and invasion is associated with MMPs (O-Charoenrat *et al.*, 2001), and heparanase activities (Ikebe *et al.*, 1999). The syndecan-1 siRNA may induce MMPs and heparanase activity and thus reduce the expression of syndecan-1 in Ca9-22 cells.

3. Conclusion

The results of earlier studies, taken together with our studies, suggest that syndecan-1 is a candidate for being a useful biomarker, but is not an accurate predictor of clinical outcome in oral SCC, and directly contributes to the growth and invasive ability of oral cancer cells.

4. References

Alevizos I, Mahadevappa M, Zhang X, Ohyama H, Kohno Y, Posner M, Gallagher GT, Varvares M, Cohen D, Kim D, Kent R, Donoff RB, Todd R, Yung CM, Warrington JA, Wong DT (2001). Oral cancer in vivo gene expression profiling assisted by laser capture microdissection and microarray analysis. *Oncogene* 20(43):6196-204.

Anttonen A, Kajanti M, Heikkila P, Jalkanen M, Joensuu H (1999). Syndecan-1 expression has prognostic significance in head and neck carcinoma. *Br J Cancer* 79(3-4):558-64.

Anttonen A, Heikkila P, Kajanti M, Jalkanen M, Joensuu H (2001). High syndecan-1 expression is associated with favourable outcome in squamous cell lung carcinoma treated with radical surgery. *Lung Cancer* 32(3):297-305.

Barbareschi M, Maisonneuve P, Aldovini D, Cangi MG, Pecciarini L, Angelo Mauri F, Veronese S, Caffo O, Lucenti A, Palma PD, Galligioni E, Doglioni C (2003). High syndecan-1 expression in breast carcinoma is related to an aggressive phenotype and to poorer prognosis. *Cancer* 98(3):474-83.

Bryne M, Koppang HS, Lilleng R, Stene T, Bang G, Dabelsteen E (1989). New malignancy grading is a better prognostic indicator than Broders' grading in oral squamous cell carcinomas. *J Oral Pathol Med* 18(8):432-7.

Bryne M (1991). Prognostic value of various molecular and cellular features in oral squamous cell carcinomas: a review. *J Oral Pathol Med* 20(9):413-20.

Bryne M, Koppang HS, Lilleng R, Kjaerheim A (1992). Malignancy grading of the deep invasive margins of oral squamous cell carcinomas has high prognostic value. *J Pathol* 166(4):375-81.

Bryne M, Jenssen N, Boysen M (1995). Histological grading in the deep invasive front of T1 and T2 glottic squamous cell carcinomas has high prognostic value. *Virchows Arch* 427(3):277-81.

Charni F, Friand V, Haddad O, Hlawaty H, Martin L, Vassy R, Oudar O, Gattegno L, Charnaux N, Sutton A (2009). Syndecan-1 and syndecan-4 are involved in RANTES/CCL5-induced migration and invasion of human hepatoma cells. *Biochim Biophys Acta* 1790(10):1314-26.

David G, Bai XM, Van der Schueren B, Marynen P, Cassiman JJ, Van den Berghe H (1993). Spatial and temporal changes in the expression of fibroglycan (syndecan-2) during mouse embryonic development. *Development* 119(3):841-54.

Fujiya M, Watari J, Ashida T, Honda M, Tanabe H, Fujiki T, Saitoh Y, Kohgo Y (2001). Reduced expression of syndecan-1 affects metastatic potential and clinical outcome in patients with colorectal cancer. *Jpn J Cancer Res* 92(10):1074-81.

Gattei V, Godeas C, Degan M, Rossi FM, Aldinucci D, Pinto A (1999). Characterization of anti-CD138 monoclonal antibodies as tools for investigating the molecular polymorphism of syndecan-1 in human lymphoma cells. *Br J Haematol* 104(1):152-62.

Gokden N, Greene GF, Bayer-Garner IB, Spencer HJ, Sanderson RD, Gokden M (2006). Expression of CD138 (Syndecan-1) in renal cell carcinoma is reduced with increasing nuclear grade. *Appl Immunohistochem Mol Morphol* 14(2):173-7.

Greenlee RT, Hill-Harmon MB, Murray T, Thun M (2001). Cancer statistics, 2001. *CA Cancer J Clin* 51(1):15-36.

Hayashi K, Hayashi M, Jalkanen M, Firestone JH, Trelstad RL, Bernfield M (1987). Immunocytochemistry of cell surface heparan sulfate proteoglycan in mouse tissues. A light and electron microscopic study. *J Histochem Cytochem* 35(10):1079-88.

Ikebe T, Shinohara M, Takeuchi H, Beppu M, Kurahara S, Nakamura S, Shirasuna K (1999). Gelatinolytic activity of matrix metalloproteinase in tumor tissues correlates with the invasiveness of oral cancer. *Clin Exp Metastasis* 17(4):315-23.

Inki P, Stenback F, Talve L, Jalkanen M (1991). Immunohistochemical localization of syndecan in mouse skin tumors induced by UV irradiation. Loss of expression associated with malignant transformation. *Am J Pathol* 139(6):1333-40.

Inki P, Joensuu H, Grenman R, Klemi P, Jalkanen M (1994). Association between syndecan-1 expression and clinical outcome in squamous cell carcinoma of the head and neck. *Br J Cancer* 70(2):319-23.

Inki P, Jalkanen M (1996). The role of syndecan-1 in malignancies. *Ann Med* 28(1):63-7.

Ito Y, Yoshida H, Nakano K, Takamura Y, Miya A, Kobayashi K, Yokozawa T, Matsuzuka F, Matsuura N, Kuma K, Miyauchi A (2003). Syndecan-1 expression in thyroid carcinoma: stromal expression followed by epithelial expression is significantly correlated with dedifferentiation. *Histopathology* 43(2):157-64.

Jakobsson PA, Eneroth CM, Killander D, Moberger G, Martensson B (1973). Histologic classification and grading of malignancy in carcinoma of the larynx. *Acta Radiol Ther Phys Biol* 12(1):1-8.

Jourdan M, Ferlin M, Legouffe E, Horvathova M, Liautard J, Rossi JF, Wijdenes J, Brochier J, Klein B (1998). The myeloma cell antigen syndecan-1 is lost by apoptotic myeloma cells. *Br J Haematol* 100(4):637-46.

Kaushal GP, Xiong X, Athota AB, Rozypal TL, Sanderson RD, Kelly T (1999). Syndecan-1 expression suppresses the level of myeloma matrix metalloproteinase-9. *Br J Haematol* 104(2):365-73.

Kearsley JH, Thomas S (1993). Prognostic markers in cancers of the head and neck region. *Anticancer Drugs* 4(4):419-29.

Kumar-Singh S, Jacobs W, Dhaene K, Weyn B, Bogers J, Weyler J, Van Marck E (1998). Syndecan-1 expression in malignant mesothelioma: correlation with cell differentiation, WT1 expression, and clinical outcome. *J Pathol* 186(3):300-5.

Kurokawa H, Matsumoto S, Murata T, Yamashita Y, Tomoyose T, Zhang M, Fukuyama H, Takahashi T (2003). Immunohistochemical study of syndecan-1 down-regulation and the expression of p53 protein or Ki-67 antigen in oral leukoplakia with or without epithelial dysplasia. *J Oral Pathol Med* 32(9):513-21.

Kurokawa H, Zhang M, Matsumoto S, Yamashita Y, Tanaka T, Takamori K, Igawa K, Yoshida M, Fukuyama H, Takahashi T, Sakoda S (2006). Reduced syndecan-1 expression is correlated with the histological grade of malignancy at the deep invasive front in oral squamous cell carcinoma. *J Oral Pathol Med* 35(5):301-6.

Le QT, Sutphin PD, Raychaudhuri S, Yu SC, Terris DJ, Lin HS, Lum B, Pinto HA, Koong AC, Giaccia AJ (2003). Identification of osteopontin as a prognostic plasma marker for head and neck squamous cell carcinomas. *Clin Cancer Res* 9(1):59-67.

Liebersbach BF, Sanderson RD (1994). Expression of syndecan-1 inhibits cell invasion into type I collagen. *J Biol Chem* 269(31):20013-9.

Liu W, Litwack ED, Stanley MJ, Langford JK, Lander AD, Sanderson RD (1998). Heparan sulfate proteoglycans as adhesive and anti-invasive molecules. Syndecans and glypican have distinct functions. *J Biol Chem* 273(35):22825-32.

Macabeo-Ong M, Shiboski CH, Silverman S, Ginzinger DG, Dekker N, Wong DT, Jordan RC (2003). Quantitative analysis of cathepsin L mRNA and protein expression during oral cancer progression. *Oral Oncol* 39(7):638-47.

Mali M, Andtfolk H, Miettinen HM, Jalkanen M (1994). Suppression of tumor cell growth by syndecan-1 ectodomain. *J Biol Chem* 269(45):27795-8.

Matsumoto A, Ono M, Fujimoto Y, Gallo RL, Bernfield M, Kohgo Y (1997). Reduced expression of syndecan-1 in human hepatocellular carcinoma with high metastatic potential. *Int J Cancer* 74(5):482-91.

Mikami S, Ohashi K, Usui Y, Nemoto T, Katsube K, Yanagishita M, Nakajima M, Nakamura K, Koike M (2001). Loss of syndecan-1 and increased expression of heparanase in invasive esophageal carcinomas. *Jpn J Cancer Res* 92(10):1062-73.

Miturski R, Jalkanen M, Postawski K, Jakowicki J, Inki P (1998). Immunohistochemical expression of syndecan-1 in human endometrial cancer cells. *Int J Mol Med* 2(4):397-401.

Muramatsu T, Saitoh M, Ro Y, Uekusa T, Iwamura E, Ohta K, Kohno Y, Abiko Y, Shimono M (2008). Inhibition of syndecan-1 expression and function in oral cancer cells. *Oncol Rep* 20(6):1353-7.

O-Charoenrat P, Rhys-Evans PH, Eccles SA (2001). Expression of matrix metalloproteinases and their inhibitors correlates with invasion and metastasis in squamous cell carcinoma of the head and neck. *Arch Otolaryngol Head Neck Surg* 127(7):813-20.

Reiland J, Sanderson RD, Waguespack M, Barker SA, Long R, Carson DD, Marchetti D (2004). Heparanase degrades syndecan-1 and perlecan heparan sulfate: functional implications for tumor cell invasion. *J Biol Chem* 279(9):8047-55.

Rintala M, Inki P, Klemi P, Jalkanen M, Grenman S (1999). Association of syndecan-1 with tumor grade and histology in primary invasive cervical carcinoma. *Gynecol Oncol* 75(3):372-8.

Ro Y, Muramatsu T, Shima K, Yajima Y, Shibahara T, Noma H, Shimono M (2006). Correlation between reduction of syndecan-1 expression and clinico-pathological parameters in squamous cell carcinoma of tongue. *Int J Oral Maxillofac Surg* 35(3):252-7.

Sanderson RD, Lalor P, Bernfield M (1989). B lymphocytes express and lose syndecan at specific stages of differentiation. *Cell Regul* 1(1):27-35.

Sanderson RD, Hinkes MT, Bernfield M (1992). Syndecan-1, a cell-surface proteoglycan, changes in size and abundance when keratinocytes stratify. *J Invest Dermatol* 99(4):390-6.

Sebestyen A, Berczi L, Mihalik R, Paku S, Matolcsy A, Kopper L (1999). Syndecan-1 (CD138) expression in human non-Hodgkin lymphomas. *Br J Haematol* 104(2):412-9.

Senger DR, Asch BB, Smith BD, Perruzzi CA, Dvorak HF (1983). A secreted phosphoprotein marker for neoplastic transformation of both epithelial and fibroblastic cells. *Nature* 302(5910):714-5.

Senger DR, Perruzzi CA (1985). Secreted phosphoprotein markers for neoplastic transformation of human epithelial and fibroblastic cells. *Cancer Res* 45(11 Pt 2):5818-23.

Soukka T, Pohjola J, Inki P, Happonen RP (2000). Reduction of syndecan-1 expression is associated with dysplastic oral epithelium. *J Oral Pathol Med* 29(7):308-13.

Stanley MJ, Stanley MW, Sanderson RD, Zera R (1999). Syndecan-1 expression is induced in the stroma of infiltrating breast carcinoma. *Am J Clin Pathol* 112(3):377-83.

Su G, Blaine SA, Qiao D, Friedl A (2007). Shedding of syndecan-1 by stromal fibroblasts stimulates human breast cancer cell proliferation via FGF2 activation. *J Biol Chem* 282(20):14906-15.

Takes RP, Baatenburg de Jong RJ, Schuuring E, Hermans J, Vis AA, Litvinov SV, van Krieken JH (1997). Markers for assessment of nodal metastasis in laryngeal carcinoma. *Arch Otolaryngol Head Neck Surg* 123(4):412-9.

Thesleff I, Vaahtokari A, Vainio S, Jowett A (1996). Molecular mechanisms of cell and tissue interactions during early tooth development. *Anat Rec* 245(2):151-61.

Toyoshima E, Ohsaki Y, Nishigaki Y, Fujimoto Y, Kohgo Y, Kikuchi K (2001). Expression of syndecan-1 is common in human lung cancers independent of expression of epidermal growth factor receptor. *Lung Cancer* 31(2-3):193-202.

Vainio S, Jalkanen M, Vaahtokari A, Sahlberg C, Mali M, Bernfield M, Thesleff I (1991). Expression of syndecan gene is induced early, is transient, and correlates with changes in mesenchymal cell proliferation during tooth organogenesis. *Dev Biol* 147(2):322-33.

Wiksten JP, Lundin J, Nordling S, Kokkola A, Haglund C (2000). A prognostic value of syndecan-1 in gastric cancer. *Anticancer Res* 20(6D):4905-7.

Wiksten JP, Lundin J, Nordling S, Lundin M, Kokkola A, von Boguslawski K, Haglund C (2001). Epithelial and stromal syndecan-1 expression as predictor of outcome in patients with gastric cancer. *Int J Cancer* 95(1):1-6.

Yamamoto E, Kohama G, Sunakawa H, Iwai M, Hiratsuka H (1983). Mode of invasion, bleomycin sensitivity, and clinical course in squamous cell carcinoma of the oral cavity. *Cancer* 51(12):2175-80.

18

Model of Chromosomal Instability in Oral Carcinogenesis and Progression

Walter Giaretti
Biophysics and Cytometry Section, Department of Diagnostic Oncology, National Institute for Cancer Research, Genoa
Italy

1. Introduction

Epidemiologic and experimental evidence indicate that oral cancer originates and progresses with the contribution of carcinogen exposure, mainly from tobacco smoking (IARC, 1986, 2004). This is thought to contribute to DNA damage within the mucosa and, in particular, to subsequent gene mutations, chromosomal instability and aneuploidy, resulting in an increased risk of developing oral cancer. Accumulation of genetic/genomic aberrations over time leads to a multi-step process of carcinogenesis in which the functions of genes which control the cell cycle (proliferation and apoptosis), chromosome stability, angiogenesis, invasion and metastasis, become aberrant (Califano et al., 1996; Hanahan & Weinberg 2011; Martorell-Calatayud et al., 2009). Chromosomal aberrations in oral cancer are located, in particular, at 9p21, 17p13, 3q26, 11q13, 3p21, 14q32 (Forastiere et al., 2001; Gollin, 2001) corresponding to several putative tumor suppressor genes and oncogenes including p16 at 9p21 and TP53 at 17p13.

Studies aimed at elucidating the steps of transition between the oral precursor lesions and oral cancer and, in particular, the transition from visually normal appearing non-dysplastic oral mucosa to precursor lesions are potentially very informative. Such investigations address the theory of "field cancerization" (Slaughter et al., 1953) and its more recent genetic explanation (Braakhuis et al., 2003; Tabor et al., 2001). These studies have led to a genetic progression model of oral cancer (Braakhuis et al., 2004). A critical step in this model is the conversion of a patch, in which stem cells share genetic/genomic aberrations, into an expanding field in which many more aberrations occur and which sometimes becomes visible as leukoplakias and erythroplakias (Braakhuis et al., 2002; Reid et al., 1997; Van Houten et al., 2000). The role of chromosomal instability during the genesis and progression of oral cancer has clearly been indicated by several studies but still our understanding of the molecular mechanisms is relatively poor. Analyses were performed with the use of different techniques including loss of heterozygosity (Braakhuis et al., 2004; Bremmer et al., 2008; Graveland et al., 2011; Lydiatt et al., 1998; Mithani et al., 2007; Partridge et al., 1997; Tsantoulis et al., 2007), comparative genomic hybridization and gene expression array (Bremmer et al., 2008; Cha et al., 2011; Garnis et al., 2009; Liu et al., 2006, 2011; Smeets et al., 2009; Snijders et al., 2005; Squire et al., 2002;), in situ hybridization (Nees et al., 1993; Voravud et al., 1993), immunohistochemistry (Nees et al., 1993), multiplex ligation-dependent probe amplification (Bremmer et al., 2008; Cha et al., 2011; Liu et al., 2006), DNA image cytometry (Bremmer et al., 2008; Diwakar et al., 2005) and DNA flow cytometry (DNA FCM) (Donadini et al., 2010; Hemmer, 1990, 1997; Pentenero et al., 2009; Saito, 1998, 1991, 1995; Seoane et al., 1998). DNA FCM was often adopted as a useful technique for detecting the presence of DNA aneuploid sublines in several human predisposing and preneoplastic lesions such as Barrett's esophagus (Reid et al., 2000), ulcerative colitis (Rabinovitch et al., 1999; Risques et al., 2008), colorectal adenomas (Giaretti et al., 1994) and oral lesions (Donadini et al., 2010; Pentenero et al., 2009; Saito, 1998, 1991, 1995; Seoane et al., 1998).

2. High resolution DNA FCM of oral lesions and visually normal non-dysplastic mucosa

The DNA FCM data provided so far for the human oral precancerous lesions were mainly derived from paraffin-embedded material of dysplastic oral potentially malignant lesions (OPMLs). In order to better investigate early oral fields of carcinogenesis and to separate them from later progression steps, we have included the analysis of non-dysplastic "oral clinically normal appearing mucosa sited in OPML and OSCC distant fields within the same subsites" (ODFs; n = 122). In addition, we have analyzed multiple samples from OPMLs without and with dysplasia at histology, including also the lesion margins. OPMLs in our series of cases were clinically identified mainly as white lesions of the oral mucosa or leukoplakias (n = 235). Further, we analyzed, though in a relatively small number of cases, oral verrucous carcinomas (OVCs; n = 9) and oral squamous cell carcinomas (OSCCs; n = 32). In all cases the multiple samples were only from fresh/frozen material. Patients were recruited in three different medical centers: the Oral Medicine and Oral Oncology Section of the University of Turin, the Department of Otolaryngology, "S. Martino Hospital" in Genoa and the National Institute for Cancer Research in Genoa. Patient written consent was obtained in every case according to the Institutional Ethic Committees. Diagnosis in every case was obtained from the Pathology Departments of the same Institutions. In particular, the diagnosis of OPMLs, using both incisional biopsies and/or microbiopsies as previously detailed (Navone et al., 2008) was based on internationally accepted criteria with levels of diagnostic certainty C3-C4 (Van der Waal et al., 2009). The assessment of the degree of dysplasia was carried out by a specially trained pathologist according to the WHO guidelines (IARC, 2005). Tissue fragments were minced on Petri dishes using scalpels and collected in 2 ml detergent solution (0.1 M citric acid, 0.5% Tween-20) (Otto, 1994) and then submitted to mechanical disaggregation in a disposable 50 µm Medicon using a Medimachine (DAKO, Copenhagen, Denmark). Nuclei suspensions were obtained and filtered over a 50 µm nylon sieve (CellTrics, Partec GmbH, Muenster, Germany). An absolute count of the nuclei in suspension was performed by FCM (CyFlow® ML, Partec GmbH (Shapiro, 2003)) after 1 to 10 dilution in water. The final volume was calculated to obtain the concentration of 600,000 nuclei/ml. One volume (1/7 of the final volume) of detergent solution was first added followed by 10 min incubation and gentle shaking. Finally, 6 volumes (6/7 of the final volume) of staining solution (0.4 M Na2HPO4, 5 µM DAPI in water) were added. Samples were kept on dark for a minimum of 15 min incubation before filtering and FCM analysis. Excitation of DAPI was provided with an UV mercury lamp (HBO-100 W, Partec GmbH) and the emitted blue fluorescence was collected using a 435 nm long-pass filter. Measurements of DNA content histograms were performed with a high resolution DNA FCM (CyFlow® ML, PartecGmbH (Shapiro, 2003)) according to quality controls and analysis consensus criteria (Ormerod et al., 1998). Only samples with at least 2 separate G0–G1 peaks were considered DNA aneuploid. Sex specific human lymphocytes and "true oral normal mucosa" from healthy donors were used as DNA diploid controls. DNA Index (DI) values were evaluated as the ratio of the mean channel number of the DNA aneuploid G0–G1 peak to the mean channel number of the DNA diploid G0–G1 peak. Thus, DNA diploid and aneuploid sublines have values respectively DI =1 and DI ≠ 1. The CV values of the G0–G1 peaks for the DNA diploid normal mucosa samples from healthy donors were used as a measure of accuracy (DNA resolution): a mean CV= 1.88±0.26% was obtained by a Gaussian curve fitting method (FloMax Software 3.0b4 2001, Partec GmbH). The mean CV value using human lymphocytes from sex specific healthy donors was 1.2 ± 0.2%. Data collection, management and analyses were done using Microsoft Office Excel and the SPSS 16.0 software package (Apache Software Foundation, Chicago, IL, USA). The association between two variables in 2 x 2 contingency tables was evaluated with the Fisher exact test. A p-value < 0.05 was taken as statistically significant.

Table 1a shows the prevalence of DNA aneuploidy for 7 subgroups of oral mucosa/lesions: "true normal mucosa" from healthy donors (n = 36), non-dysplastic ODFs corresponding to OPMLs (n = 105), and OPMLs without (n = 208) and with dysplasia (n=27) were DNA aneuploid respectively in none of the cases, in 12/105 (11.4%), 37/208 (17.8%) and in 10/27 (37%). The samples relative to advanced cancer, respectively OVCs and OSCCs, were DNA aneuploid in 6/9 (66.7%) and 25/32 (78.1%) cases. ODFs corresponding to OSCCs were DNA aneuploid in 3/17 (17.6%) cases. Two or more DNA aneuploid sublines were detected in none of the ODFs, in 5/37 (13.5%) of the OPMLs without dysplasia, in 2/10 (20%) of the OPMLs with dysplasia. OVCs and OSCCs presented respectively multiple DNA aneuploid sublines in 2/6 (33.3%) and in 13/25 (52%) cases.

Oral mucosa/lesion groups	N. cases within groups	N. DNA aneuploid cases	One DNA aneuploid subline	Two or more DNA aneuploid sublines
"True normal mucosa" from healthy donors	36	0 (0%)	-	-
ODFs corresponding to OPMLs	105	12 (11.4%)	12 (100%)	0 (0%)
OPMLs without dysplasia	208	37 (17.8%)	32 (86.5%)	5 (13.5%)
OPMLs with dysplasia	27	10 (37.0%)	8 (80.0%)	2 (20.0%)
OVCs	9	6 (66.7%)	4 (66.7%)	2 (33.3%)
ODFs corresponding to OSCCs	17	3 (17.6%)	3 (100%)	0 (0%)
OSCCs	32	25 (78.1%)	12 (48.0%)	13 (52.0%)

Abbreviations: ODFs = non-dysplastic oral clinically normal appearing mucosa sited in OPML and OSCC distant fields within the same anatomical subsites; OPMLs = Oral Potentially Malignant Lesions (mainly leukoplakias); OVCs = Oral Verrucous Carcinomas; OSCCs = Oral Squamous Cell Carcinomas.

Table 1a. DNA aneuploidy by high resolution DNA FCM among 7 different groups of oral lesions and non-dysplastic normal appearing mucosa. The last 2 columns report the cases with single and multiple DNA aneuploid sublines.

All the DI aneuploid sublines (n = 126) were subdivided in 2 classes: DNA near-diploid (DI ≠ 1 and <1.4) and DNA high aneuploid (DI ≥1.4) (Table 1b). ODFs and OPMLs without dysplasia were characterized by near-diploid sublines respectively in 12/12 (100%) and in 38/43 (88.4%) of the cases. OVCs had a significantly higher frequency of DNA near-diploid aneuploid cases than OSCCs (respectively, 87.5% and 33.3%; p=0.006). In contrast, OPMLs with dysplasia and OSCCs had high aneuploid sublines respectively in 5 out of 12 (41.7%) and in 32 out of 48 (66.7%) of the cases. The prevalence of high aneuploidy in OPMLs with dysplasia was statistically significantly higher than in OPMLs without dysplasia (p = 0.03).

Oral mucosa/lesion groups	N. DNA aneuploid sublines	N. DNA near-diploid aneuploid sublines (DI≠1 and DI<1.4)	N. DNA high aneuploid sublines (DI≥1.4)
"True normal mucosa" from healthy donors	-	-	-
ODFs corresponding to OPMLs	12	12 (100%)	0 (0%)
OPMLs without dysplasia	43	38 (88.4%)	5 (11.6%)
OPMLs with dysplasia	12	7 (58.3%)	5 (41.7%)
OVCs	8	7 (87.5%)	1 (12.5%)
ODFs corresponding to OSCCs	3	2 (66.7%)	1 (33.3%)
OSCCs	48	16 (33.3%)	32 (66.7%)

Abbreviations: ODFs = non-dysplastic oral clinically normal appearing mucosa sited in OPML and OSCC distant fields within the same anatomical subsites; OPMLs = Oral Potentially Malignant Lesions (mainly leukoplakias); OVCs = Oral Verrucous Carcinomas; OSCCs = Oral Squamous Cell Carcinomas.

Table 1b. Presence of DNA near-diploid (DI≠1 and DI<1.4) and high aneuploid (DI≥1.4) sublines among 7 different groups of oral mucosa/lesions. DNA aneuploidy was measured by high resolution DNA FCM.

3. Discussion

The incidence of DNA aneuploidy by FCM reported in the literature ranges from about 10% to 40% for dysplastic OPMLs (Donadini et al. 2010; Pentenero et al. 2009; Saito et al., 1998, 1991, 1995; Seoane et al., 1998) and up to about 80% for OSCCs (Donadini et al., 2010; Pentenero et al. 2009; Hemmer, 1990, 1997). These values may strongly depend on the tissue material type (paraffin embedded or fresh-frozen) and DNA FCM resolution. In the present study, partly based on a previous data set that was already published (Donadini et al., 2010), we have performed FCM measurements at optimized conditions (fresh-frozen material, concentration of 600,000 nuclei/ml, DAPI staining in nuclei suspensions, UV incident light, the use of a dedicated instrument). Correspondingly, the CV values of the G0-G1 peaks of human normal control DNA diploid nuclei were commonly near 1%, while a minimum DNA change of 2.4% was detected (Figure 1). It is likely that DNA FCM at lower resolution and higher CV values would not allow separating DNA near-diploid aneuploid sublines with only slight DNA changes above/below DNA diploidy.

The present data set confirmed in a larger number of cases that, while "true normal oral mucosa" and human lymphocytes of healthy donors were DNA diploid in all cases, non-dysplastic "clinically normal appearing mucosa fields of the oral cavity" (ODFs) in patients with OPMLs already contained DNA aneuploid sublines in a subgroup of cases (12/105, 11%).

Moreover, it was found that OPMLs that could be clinically identified mainly as white lesions of the oral mucosa (leukoplakias) and classified without dysplasia at histology, contained already DNA aneuploid sublines in 37/208 (18%) of the cases. These data appear in agreement with the concept of field effect in oral carcinogenesis (Braakhuis et al., 2003; Bremmer et al., 2008; Leemans, 2011; Tabor et al., 2001; Van der Waal, 1997). The data obtained for the non-dysplastic OPMLs, in particular, were in agreement with previous literature reports including two studies from our group using an independent patient population (Donadini et al., 2010; Pentenero et al., 2009; Saito, 1995). These data were, however, in contrast with other studies, which did not detect DNA aneuploid sublines in such lesions (Kahn et al., 1992; Saito, 1998). The present study has additionally highlighted that ODFs and OPMLs without dysplasia were characterized by single near-diploid DNA aneuploid sublines. On the contrary, OPMLs with dysplasia contained high DNA aneuploid sublines (DI ≥1.4) in slightly less than half of the cases (42%). High DNA aneuploid sublines were predominant (67%) for the OSCCs, which were in addition characterized by the presence of multiple DNA aneuploid sublines in 52% of the DNA aneuploid cases. In contrast, OVCs were characterized by DNA near-diploid aneuploid sublines in 67% of the cases in agreement with previously published data (Pentenero et al., 2011). Overall, the present data support a previous model of aneuploidy genesis and evolution (Giaretti, 1994). Accordingly, a transition from DNA diploidy to near-diploid aneuploidy would be an early step of the natural history of OPMLs, while high DNA aneuploidy (likely to derive from the endoreduplication of a DNA hypo-diploid or hyper-diploid near-diploid cell) would frequently occur as a later event in OPMLs with dysplasia and OSCCs (Figure 1). From the clinical point of view, one can speculate that the detection of DNA content genomic aberrations in oral fields, which appear visually and histologically normal, and in OPMLs may have profound implications for improvement of the present patient management by identifying individuals at high risk to develop cancer (Brennan et al., 2007; Dakubo et al., 2007; Lodi et al., 2006).

Moreover, it is possible, though still unproved, that the OSCC group in which near-diploid aneuploid DIs remained "frozen" during time are at better prognosis compared to OSCCs with multiple DNA aneuploid sublines with high DNA aneuploidy. Interestingly, OVCs that were mainly characterized by DI values in the near-diploid region are known to be less aggressive and at better prognosis than OSCCs.

Clearly, what is still strongly needed in the model system of oral preneoplasia and neoplasia is a better understanding of the origin and dynamic evolution of chromosomal instability, chromosomal aberrations and aneuploidy (Albertson et al., 2003; Asteriti et al., 2010; Compton et al., 2011; Geigl et al., 2008; Giet et al., 2005; Kops et al., 2005; Lingen et al., 2011; Sieber et al., 2003; Suijkerbuijk & Kops, 2008; Thompson et al., 2010; Viet & Schmidt, 2010). In other models of cancer genesis and progression, like the colorectal adenoma-carcinoma sequence, the Barrett's esophagus and the ulcerative colitis transition to carcinoma, the role of APC and TP53 has been highlighted (Fodde et al., 2001; Giaretti et al., 2004; Rabinovitch et al., 2004). A role of TP53 in oral cancer chromosomal instability (Negrini et al., 2010) is also likely to occur due to different sources of TP53 inactivation including HPV infection in different sites of the oral cavity (Leemans, 2011; Klingelhutz et al., 2005; Tsantoulis et al., 2007). Studies that linked the genome-wide integrity analysis with gene expression profiles have provided powerful indications that chromosomal instability and aneuploidy massively deregulate the cellular transcriptome (Albertson et al., 2003). Future studies coupling both these techniques are likely to contribute to discover specific recurrent genomic aberrations, which encompass specific genes with a potential role in the genesis of chromosomal instability and aneuploidy. The functional consequences of specific DNA gains/losses are, however, not only involving oncogenes and tumor suppressor genes. More subtle and complex mechanisms are present since many aberrations span large chromosomal regions including normal genes, which coordinately and cooperatively may influence important cell functions as proliferation, differentiation, apoptosis and DNA repair.

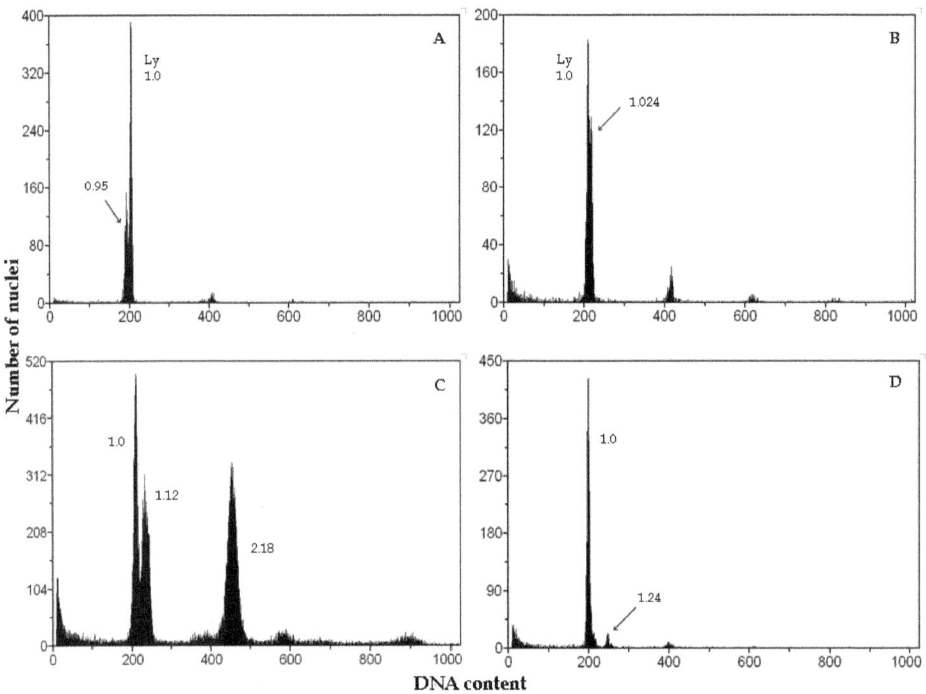

Fig. 1. Examples of DNA content histograms from oral fresh/frozen mucosa/lesions as obtained by low background and high resolution DNA FCM. A model of DNA aneuploidization and evolution.

Single DNA aneuploid sublines in the DNA near-diploid aneuploid region (DI≠1 and DI<1.4) are shown in A and B for two OPMLs. Sex specific human lymphocytes (Ly) and true normal mucosa of healthy donors were used as DNA diploid controls (DI=1.0). Multiple DNA aneuploid sublines for an OSCC with DI values respectively of 1.12 and 2.18 are shown in C. This example illustrates a model of DNA aneuploidisation as previously reported (Giaretti, 1994; Donadini et al., 2010). The key mechanism of DNA aneuploidisation appears related to a loss of symmetry of DNA content during an abnormal mitotic division in which the two daughter cells loose or gain respectively a small amount of DNA and generate DNA near-diploid aneuploid sublines (see examples A and B). A second step of DNA aneuploidy evolution appears to be due to the endoreduplication of the DNA near-diploid aneuploid cells sublines (see example C). The large G0-G1 subpopulation of cells with DI= 2.18 is characterized by a relatively large CV value (about 3% with respect to 2% of the G0-G1 DNA diploid peak), which is indicative of chromosomal instability and potential loss of DNA. The DI= 2.18 value of the high DNA aneuploid G0-G1 peak was likely originated from an initial DI value of 2.24 (twice as much of the original near-diploid DI=1.12) with the loss of 2.7% DNA.

An example of DNA histogram with a small G0-G1 DNA aneuploid peak (with 5% of the total number of nuclei in this case) and with DI= 1.24 is shown in D to illustrate that such a small percentage of DNA aneuploid nuclei can be sufficient to be detected by our high resolution and low background DNA FCM measurements. This approach was characterized by the use of fresh/frozen tissue material, nuclei suspensions at the fixed concentration of 600,000 nuclei/ml, DAPI staining and a dedicated FCM instrument (see details in the text; Donadini et al., 2010; Shapiro, 2003).

4. Acknowledgements

This study has been supported by "Compagnia di San Paolo - Programma Oncologia" and by Philip Morris International. Thanks are due, in particular, to A. Donadini, M. Maffei and P. Castagnola for critically reading the manuscript.

5. References

Albertson, D.G., Collins, C., McCormick, F. & Gray, J.W. (2003). Chromosome aberrations in solid tumors. *Nat. Genet.* 34, pp 369-376.

Asteriti, I.A., Rensen, W.M., Lindon, C., Lavia, P. & Guarguaglini, G. (2010). The Aurora-A/TPX2 complex: a novel oncogenic holoenzyme? *Biochim. Biophys. Acta.* 1806, pp 230-239.

Braakhuis, B.J., Tabor, M.P., Leemans, C.R., Van der Waal, I., Snow, G.B. & Brakenhoff, R.H. (2002). Second primary tumors and field cancerization in oral and oropharyngeal cancer: molecular techniques provide new insights and definitions. *Head Neck.* 24, pp 198-206.

Braakhuis, B.J., Tabor, M.P., Kummer, J.A., Leemans, C.R. & Brakenhoff, R.H. (2003). A genetic explanation of Slaughter's concept of field cancerization: evidence and clinical implications. *Cancer Res.* 63, pp 1727-1730.

Braakhuis, B.J., Leemans, C.R. & Brakenhoff, R.H. (2004). A genetic progression model of oral cancer: current evidence and clinical implications. *J. Oral Pathol. Med.* 33, pp 317-322 .

Bremmer, J.F., Braakhuis, B.J., Brink, A., Broeckaert, M.A., Belien, J.A., Meijer, G.A., Kuik, D.J., Leemans, C.R., Bloemena, E., Van der Waal, I. & Brakenhoff, R.H. (2008). Comparative evaluation of genetic assays to identify oral pre-cancerous fields. *J. Oral Pathol. Med.* 37, pp 599-606.

Brennan, M., Migliorati, C.A., Lockhart, P.B., Wray, D., Al-Hashimi, I., Axell, T., Bruce, A.J., Carpenter, W., Eisenberg, E., Epstein, J.B. , Holmstrup, P., Jontell, M., Nair, R., Sasser, H., Schifter, M., Silverman, B., Thongprasom, K., Thornhill, M., Warnakulasuriya, S. & Van der Waal, I. (2007). Management of oral epithelial dysplasia: a review. *Oral Surg. Oral Med. Oral Pathol. Oral Radiol. Endod.* 103 Suppl, S19 e11-12

Califano, J., van der Riet, P., Westra ,W. , Nawroz, H., Clayman, G., Piantadosi, S., Corio, R., Lee, D., Greenberg, B., Koch, W. & Sidransky, D. (1996). Genetic progression model for head and neck cancer: implications for field cancerization. *Cancer Res.* 56, pp 2488-2492.

Cha, J.D., Kim, H.J. & Cha, I.H.(2011). Genetic alterations in oral squamous cell carcinoma progression detected by combining array-based comparative genomic hybridization and multiplex ligation-dependent probe amplification. *Oral Surg Oral Med Oral Pathol Oral Radiol Endod.* 111(5), (2011 May), pp 594-607.

Compton D.A. (2011). Mechanisms of aneuploidy. *Curr Opin Cell Biol.* 23(1), (2011 Feb), pp 109-13.

Dakubo, G.D., Jakupciak, J.P., Birch-Machin, M.A. & Parr, R.L. (2007). Clinical implications and utility of field cancerization. *Cancer Cell. Int.* 7, 2.

Donadini, A., Maffei, M., Cavallero, A., Pentenero, M., Malacarne, D., Di Nallo, E., Truini, M., Navone, R., Mereu, P., Scala, M., Santelli, A., Gandolfo, S., & Giaretti, W. (2010). Oral cancer genesis and progression: DNA near-diploid aneuploidization and endoreduplication by high resolution flow cytometry. *Cell. Oncol.* 32, pp 373–383.

Fodde, R., Kuipers, J., Rosenberg, C., Smits, R., Kielman, M., Gaspar, C., van Es, J.H., Breukel, C., Wiegant, J., Giles, R.H. & Clevers, H. (2001). Mutations in the APC tumour suppressor gene cause chromosomal instability. *Nat. Cell Biol.* 3, pp 433-438 .

Forastiere, A., Koch, W., Trotti, A. & Sidransky, D. (2001). Head and neck cancer. *N. Engl. J. Med.* 345, pp 1890-1900.

Geigl, J.B., Obenauf, A.C., Schwarzbraun, T. & Speicher, M.R. (2008). Defining 'chromosomal instability'. *Trends Genet* .24(2), (2008 Feb), pp 64-9.

Giaretti, W. (1994). A model of DNA aneuploidization and evolution in colorectal cancer. *Lab. Invest.* 71, pp 904–910.

Giaretti, W., Venesio, T., Prevosto, C., Lombardo, F., Ceccarelli, J., Molinu, S. & Risio, M. (2004). Chromosomal instability and APC gene mutations in human sporadic colorectal adenomas. *J. Pathol.* 204, pp 193-199.

Giet, R., Petretti, C. & Prigent, C. (2005). Aurora kinases, aneuploidy and cancer, a coincidence or a real link? *Trends Cell Biol.* 15, pp 241-250.

Graveland, A.P., Golusinski, P.J., Buijze, M., Douma, R., Sons, N., Kuik, D.J., Bloemena, E., Leemans, C.R., Brakenhoff, R.H. & Braakhuis, B.J. (2011). Loss of heterozygosity at 9p and p53 immunopositivity in surgical margins predict local relapse in head and neck squamous cell carcinoma. *Int J Cancer.* 15,128(8),(2011 Apr), pp 1852-9.

Gollin, S.M. (2001) Chromosomal alterations in squamous cell carcinomas of the head and neck: window to the biology of disease. *Head Neck.* 23, pp 238-253.

Hanahan, D. & Weinberg, RA. (2011). Hallmarks of Cancer: The Next Generation. *Cell.* 144, pp 646-74

Hemmer, J. & Kreidler, J. (1990). Flow cytometric DNA ploidy analysis of squamous cell carcinoma of the oral cavity. Comparison with clinical staging and histologic grading. *Cancer.* 66, pp 317–320.

Hemmer, J., Thein, T. & Van Heerden, W.F. (1997). The value of DNA flow cytometry in predicting the development of lymph node metastasis and survival in patients with locally recurrent oral squamous cell carcinoma. *Cancer.* 79, pp 2309–2313.

International Agency for Research on Cancer (1986). *Tobacco smoking. IARC Monogr Eval Carcinog Risk Chem Hum.* 38, pp 35-394.

International Agency for Research on Cancer (2004). *Tobacco smoke and involuntary smoking, IARC Monogr Eval Carcinog Risk Chem Hum.* pp 1-1438.

International Agency for Research on Cancer (2005). *Pathology and Genetics of Head and Neck Tumours.. IARC Monogr Eval Carcinog Risk Chem Hum.*

Kahn, M.A., Dockter, M.E. & Hermann-Petrin, J.M. (1992). Flow cytometer analysis of oral premalignant lesions: a pilot study and review. *J. Oral Pathol. Med.* 21, pp 1–6.

Klingelhutz, A.J., Qian, Q., Phillips, S.L., Gourronc, F.A., Darbro, B.W. & Patil, S.R. (2005). Amplification of the chromosome 20q region is associated with expression of HPV-16 E7 in human airway and anogenital epithelial cells. *Virology.* 30,340(2), (2005 Sep), pp 237-44.

Kops, G.J., Weaver, B.A. & Cleveland, D.W. (2005). On the road to cancer: aneuploidy and the mitotic checkpoint. *Nat. Rev. Cancer.* 5, pp 773-785.

Leemans, C.R., Braakhuis, B.J., Brakenhoff, R.H. (2011). The molecular biology of head and neck cancer. *Nat Rev Cancer.* 11(1), (Jan 2011), pp 9-22.

Lingen, M.W., Pinto, A., Mendes, R.A., Franchini, R., Czerninski, R., Tilakaratne, W.M., Partridge, M., Peterson, D.E. & Woo, S.B. (2011). Genetics/epigenetics of oral premalignancy: current status and future research. *Oral Dis.* 17 Suppl 1, (2011 Apr), pp 7-22.

Liu, C.J., Lin, S.C., Chen, Y.J., Chang, K.M. & Chang, K.W.(2006). Array-comparative genomic hybridization to detect genome wide changes in microdissected primary and metastatic oral squamous cell carcinomas. *Mol Carcinog.* 45(10), (2006 Oct), pp 721-31.

Liu, W., Zheng, W., Xie, J., Zhang, B., Ma, W. & Chen, X. (2011). Identification of genes related to carcinogenesis of oral leukoplakia by oligo cancer microarray analysis. *Oncol Rep.*;26(1), (2011 Jul), pp 265-74.

Lodi, G., Sardella, A., Bez, C., Demarosi, F. & Carrassi, A. (2006). Interventions for treating oral leukoplakia. *Cochrane Database Syst. Rev.* CD001829.

Lydiatt, W.M., Anderson, P.E., Bazzana, T., Casale, M., Hughes, C.J., Huvos, A.G., Lydiatt, D.D. & Schantz, S.P. (1998). Molecular support for field cancerization in the head and neck. *Cancer.* 82, pp 1376-1380.

Martorell-Calatayud, A., Botella-Estrada, R., Bagan-Sebastian, O., Sanmartin-Jimenez, J.V. & Guillen-Barona, C. (2009). Oral leukoplakia: clinical, histopathologic, and molecular features and therapeutic approach. *Actas Dermosifiliogr.* 100, pp 669-684.

Mithani, S.K., Mydlarz, W.K., Grumbine, F.L., Smith, I.M. & Califano, J.A. (2007). Molecular genetics of premalignant oral lesions. *Oral Dis.* 13(2), (2007 Mar), pp 126-33.

Navone, R., Pentenero, M., Rostan, I., Burlo, P., Marsico, A., Broccoletti, R., Scully, C. & Gandolfo, S. (2008). Oral potentially malignant lesions: first-level micro-histological diagnosis from tissue fragments sampled in liquid-based diagnostic cytology. *J. Oral Pathol. Med.* 37, pp 358-363.

Nees, M., Homann, N., Discher, H., Andl, T., Enders, C., Herold-Mende, C., Schuhmann, A. & Bosch, F.X. (1993). Expression of mutated p53 occurs in tumor-distant epithelia of head and neck cancer patients: a possible molecular basis for the development of multiple tumors. *Cancer Res.* 53, pp 4189-4196.

Negrini, S., Gorgoulis, V.G. & Halazonetis, T.D. (2010). Genomic instability: an evolving hallmark of cancer. *Nat Rev Mol Cell Biol.* 11(3), (2010 Mar), pp 220-8.

Ormerod, M.G., Tribukait, B., & Giaretti, W. (1998). Consensus report of the task force on standardisation of DNA flow cytometry in clinical pathology. DNA Flow Cytometry Task Force of the European Society for Analytical Cellular Pathology, *Anal. Cell. Pathol.* 17, pp 103-110.

Otto, F.J. (1994). High-resolution analysis of nuclear DNA employing the fluorochrome DAPI, in *Methods Cell Biol.*, ASCB, pp. 211-217, Academic Press, San Diego.

Partridge, M., Emilion, G., Pateromichelakis, S., Phillips, E. & Langdon, J. (1997). Field cancerisation of the oral cavity: comparison of the spectrum of molecular alterations in cases presenting with both dysplastic and malignant lesions. *Oral Oncol.* 33(5), (1997 Sep),pp 332-7.

Pentenero, M., Giaretti, W., Navone, R., Demurtas, A., Rostan, I., Bertolusso, G., Broccoletti, R., Arduino, P.G, Malacarne, D. & Gandolfo, S. (2009). DNA aneuploidy and dysplasia in oral potentially malignant disorders: association with cigarette smoking and site. *Oral Oncol.* 45, pp 887–890.

Pentenero, M., Donadini, A., Di Nallo, E., Maffei, M., Marino, R., Familiari, U., Broccoletti, R., Castagnola, P., Gandolfo, S. & Giaretti, W. (2011). Distinctive chromosomal instability patterns in oral verrucous and squamous cell carcinomas detected by high-resolution DNA flow cytometry. *Cancer.* 117(22), pp 5052-7.

Rabinovitch, P.S., Dziadon, S., Brentnall, T.A., Emond, M.J., Crispin, D.A., Haggitt R.C. & Bronner, N.P. (1999). Pancolonic chromosomal instability precedes dysplasia and cancer in ulcerative colitis. *Cancer Res.* 59, pp 5148–5153.

Rabinovitch, P.S. (2004). Genomic instability and progression to cancer in two models of preneoplastic disease: Barrett's esophagus and ulcerative colitis. *Cell. Oncol.* 26, pp 210-211.

Reid, B.J., Levine, D.S., Longton, G., Blount, P.L. & Rabinovitch, P.S. (2000). Predictors of progression to cancer in Barrett's esophagus: baseline histology and flow cytometry identify low- and high-risk patient subsets, *Am. J. Gastroenterol.* 95, pp 1669–1676.

Reid, C.B., Snow, G.B., Brakenhoff, R.H. & Braakhuis, B.J. (1997). Biologic implications of genetic changes in head and neck squamous cell carcinogenesis. *Aust. N Z J Surg.* 67, pp 410-416.

Risques, R.A., Lai, L.A., Brentnall, T.A., Li, L., Feng, Z., Gallaher, J., Mandelson, M.T., Potter, J.D., Bronner, M.P. & Rabinovitch, P.S. (2008). Ulcerative colitis is a disease of accelerated colon aging: evidence from telomere attrition and DNA damage. *Gastroenterology* 135, pp 410–418.

Saito, T., Notani, K., Miura, H., Fukuda, H., Mizuno, S., Shindoh, M. & Amemiya, A. (1991). DNA analysis of oral leukoplakia by flow cytometry. *Int. J. Oral Maxillofac. Surg.* 20, pp 259-263.

Saito, T., Yamashita, T., Notani, K., Fukuda, H., Mizuno, S., Shindoh, M. & Amemiya, A. (1995). Flow cytometric analysis of nuclear DNA content in oral leukoplakia: relation to clinicopathologic findings. *Int. J. Oral Maxillofac. Surg.* 24, pp 44-47.

Saito, T., Mizuno, S., Notani, K., Fukuda, H., Kobayashi, I., Shindoh, M. & Kohgo, T. (1998). Flow cytometric analysis of cell cycle fractions in oral leukoplakia. *Int. J. Oral Maxillofac. Surg.* 27, pp 217–221.

Seoane, J., Bascones, A., Asenjo, J.A., Garcia-Pola, M. & Varela-Centelles, P.I. (1998). Flow cytometric analysis of nuclear DNA content in oral leukoplakia. *Clin. Otolaryngol. Allied. Sci.* 23, pp 136–140.

Shapiro, H.M. (2003). Partec GmbH, in: *Practical Flow Cytometry*, 4th edn, pp. 427–428, Wiley, Hoboken, New Jersey.

Sieber, O.M., Heinimann, K. & Tomlinson, I.P. (2003). Genomic instability : the engine of tumorigenesis? *Nat Rev Cancer.* 3(9), (2003 Sep), pp 701-8.

Slaughter, D.P., Southwick, H.W., Smejkal, W. (1953). Field cancerization in oral stratified squamous epithelium; clinical implications of multicentric origin. *Cancer* 6, pp 963-968.

Smeets, S.J., Brakenhoff, R.H., Ylstra, B., Van Wieringen, W.N., Van de Wiel, M.A., Leemans, C.R. & Braakhuis, BJ. (2009). Genetic classification of oral and oropharyngeal carcinomas identifies subgroups with a different prognosis. *Cell Oncol.* 31(4), pp 291-300.

Snijders, A.M., Schmidt, B.L., Fridlyand, J., Dekker, N., Pinkel, D., Jordan, R.C. & Albertson, D.G. (2005). Rare amplicons implicate frequent deregulation of cell fate specification pathways in oral squamous cell carcinoma. *Oncogene.* 16, 24(26), pp 4232-42.

Squire, J.A., Bayani, J., Luk, C., Unwin, L., Tokunaga, J., MacMillan, C., Irish, J., Brown, D., Gullane, P. & Kamel-Reid, S. (2002). Molecular cytogenetic analysis of head and neck squamous cell carcinoma: By comparative genomic hybridization, spectral karyotyping, and expression array analysis. *Head Neck.* 24(9), (2002 Sep), pp 874-87.

Suijkerbuijk, S.J. & Kops, G.J.(2008). Preventing aneuploidy: the contribution of mitotic checkpoint proteins. *Biochim Biophys Acta.* 1786(1), (2008 Sep), pp 24-31.

Tabor, M.P., Brakenhoff, R.H., van Houten, V.M., Kummer, J.A., Snel, M.H., Snijders, P.J., Snow, G.B., Leemans, C.R. & Braakhuis, B.J. (2001). Persistence of genetically altered fields in head and neck cancer patients: biological and clinical implications. *Clin. Cancer Res.* 7, pp 1523-1532.

Thompson, S.L., Bakhoum, S.F. & Compton, D.A. (2010). Mechanisms of chromosomal instability. *Curr Biol.* 23, 20(6), (2010 Mar), pp R285-95.

Tsantoulis, P.K., Kastrinakis, N.G., Tourvas, A.D., Laskaris, G. & Gorgoulis, V.G. (2007). Advances in the biology of oral cancer. *Oral Oncol.* 43(6), (2007 Jul), pp 523-34.

Van der Waal, I., Schepman, K.P., Van der Meij, E.H. & Smeele, L.E. (1997). Oral leukoplakia: a clinicopathological review. *Oral Oncol.* 33, pp 291–301.

Van der Waal, I. (2009). Potentially malignant disorders of the oral and oropharyngeal mucosa; terminology, classification and present concepts of management. *Oral Oncol.* 45, pp 317-323.

Van Houten, V.M., Tabor, M.P., Van den Brekel, M.W., Denkers, F., Wishaupt, R.G., Kummer, J.A., Snow, G.B. & Brakenhoff, R.H. (2000). Molecular assays for the diagnosis of minimal residual head-and-neck cancer: methods, reliability, pitfalls, and solutions. *Clin. Cancer Res.* 6, pp 3803-3816.

Viet, C.T. & Schmidt B.L. (2010). Understanding oral cancer in the genome era. *Head Neck.* 32(9), (2010 Sep), pp 1246-68.

Voravud, N., Shin, D.M., Ro, J.Y., Lee, J.S., Hong, W.K. & Hittelman, W.N. (1993). Increased polysomies of chromosomes 7 and 17 during head and neck multistage tumorigenesis. *Cancer Res.* 53, pp 2874-2883.

19

Expression of Metallothionein in Oral Cancer

Dziegiel Piotr, Pula Bartosz and Podhorska-Okolow Marzena
Department of Histology and Embryology, Wroclaw Medical University
Poland

1. Introduction

Metallothioneins (MTs) are ubiquitous proteins expressed in almost all organisms. MTs were isolated in 1957 for the first time from renal cortex as proteins responsible for binding cadmium (Margoshes & Valee, 1957, Coyle et al., 2002, Vasák et al., 2005). MTs are highly evolutionary conserved between species. Nevertheless, the role of these proteins has not been fully clarified yet and continues to generate interest among researchers. At present, several studies on MTs are focused on, their significance in the process of carcinogenesis, their potential prognostic value, and their involvement in resistance to cytostatic drugs.

1.1 MT structure and synthesis

MTs are low molecular weight of 6 -7 kDa proteins. The molecules of MT demonstrate a highly conserved amino acid sequence: the protein isolated from various organs of various animal species differ only insignificantly (Vasák et al., 2000). The molecule is formed by a single polypeptide chain of 61 to 68 amino acids, depending on the type. About 30% of MTs comprise of cystein residues while aromatic amino acids and histidine are absent. The cystein residues occur in typical tandem sequences of cys-aa1-cys, cys-aa1-aa2-cys, cys-cys, where aa1 and aa2 denotes amino acid other than cystein. The number and distribution of the sequences determine the tertiary structure, stability, and capability for binding metallic ions. The high number of cystein residues is a source of high content of thiol groups (-SH) through which metal ions are bound (Coyle et al., 2002). Their ability to bind heavy metals, such as zinc, copper, mercury, lead, nickel, iron and cadmium has been demonstrated in many studies. One MT molecule may bind up to seven ions of bivalent, and up to twelve ions of univalent metals (Palmiter et al., 1998). In the structure of MT two globular domains can be distinguished, α and β (Zangger et al., 2002). The C-terminal domain α comprises amino acids 31- 68 and binds four Cd ions while the N-terminal domain β, comprises amino acids 1 to 30 and captures three metal ions, including two Zn ions and one Cd ion. Within the MT molecule, the most pronounced antigenicity is shown by regions of the domain β (Dziegiel, 2004). MTs represent a non-uniform group of proteins. Analysis of their structure and function allowed distinction into four principal isoforms: MT-1, MT-2, MT-3 and MT-4 (Mididoddi et al., 1996). Isoforms MT-1 and MT-2 are well recognized and characterized because they are expressed almost in all tissues of the organism. The highest concentrations of these proteins were demonstrated in the kidney, liver, pancreas and intestine (Davis et al., 2000; Coyle et al., 2002). Expression of MT-3 and MT-4 isoforms is tissue specific and are present in the body in much lower amounts. MT-3 can be noted mainly in cerebral neurons of central nervous system (Hidalgo et al., 2001). The expression of MT-4 is restricted to stratified squamous epithelium of the skin and upper part of the alimentary tract (Quaife et al., 1994). MT are encoded by 17 genes, including 13 genes that code for MT-1, two for MT-2, and individual genes coding for MT-3 and MT-4. There are at least 10 MT genes which encode functional proteins: MT-1A, MT-1B, MT-1E, MT-1F, MT-1G, MT-1H, MT-1X, MT-2A, MT-3 and MT-4 (Palmiter et al., 1992; Quaife et al., 1994). In human, genes encoding for MTs are located on chromosome 16, within the 16q13 region (Mididoddi et al., 1996). MTs are intracellular proteins and their presence was demonstrated in the cytoplasm and in the cell nucleus (Bay et al., 2001). Their synthesis can be induced by several substances, such as heavy metals, hormones, cytokines, growth factors, organic compounds and free radicals (Samson et al., 1998; Haq et al., 2003; Ghoshal et al., 2001). The principal physiological factors, which induce MT synthesis are zinc ions (Zn^{2+}) which are bound by the transcription factor, MTF-1 (*metal response element-binding transcription factor*). The MTF-1 is a protein with domains of zinc finger structure, responsible for interaction with DNA. The MTF-1 binds to the MRE (*metal response element*) sequence within the MT gene promoter. Binding of MTF-1 to MRE initiates the process of MT gene transcription (Langmade et al., 2000; Otsuka et al., 2000; Saydam et al., 2002). The remaining metals (e.g. Pb^{2+}, Ni^{2+}, Fe^{2+}, Cd^{2+}, Bi^{2+}) initiate transcription of MT genes also with mediation of MRE but they are not bound by the MTF-1 transcription factor. They manifest a higher affinity to MT and they replace zinc ions from MT molecules. Released zinc ions are subsequently bound by MTF-1 (Mursta et al., 1999; Koizumi et al., 1999; Lichtlen et al., 2001). Similarly, oxygen free radicals could also replace zinc ions from MT molecule and in this way stimulate MT synthesis. Oxidation of MT by hydrogen peroxide (H_2O_2) leads to release of zinc ions (Andrews, 2000; Nguyen et al., 2003). MT synthesis could also be induced by other factors, such as glucocorticoids, which through glucocorticoid receptors (GR) bind to specific regulatory sequences, GRE (*glucocorticoid response element*) in the promoter region of MT genes (Davis et al., 2000; Hernández et al., 2000).

1.2 Effect of MT on cell proliferation and differentiation processes

MTs are thought to be engaged in the control of cell proliferation and differentiation (Schmidt et al., 1999). The metal binding properties of MT, including binding of zinc ions, allow MT to act as a zinc donor. The zinc-dependent enzymes play a crucial role in DNA replication, transcription and protein biosynthesis. Presumably, in this way MT could modulate the functional activity of many factors controlling the cell cycle (Ostrakhovitch et al. 2007). In the course of cell cycle the distribution of MT in the cell is changed from the cytoplasm to the nucleus, what may indicate the protein's involvement in DNA synthesis. In many studies an increased expression of MT both in the cell nucleus and in the cytoplasm was demonstrated in hepatocytes during liver regeneration, in kidneys undergoing compensatory growth following nephrectomy, and in rapidly growing parabasal cells of stratified squamous epithelium (Zalups et al., 1995; Ioachim et al., 1999; Cherian et al., 2006). The increased expression of MT, correlated to the augmented cell proliferation, was also observed in cells of various human tumours (Theocharis et al., 2004). In mitotically inactive cells (G0 phase) expression of MT can be detected in the cytoplasm while in dividing cells its activity becomes shifted to the nucleus. The high cytoplasmic expression of MT is observed at the end of G1 phase and at the G1/S threshold while the peak accumulation of MT in cell nucleus can be detected in phases S and G2 (Cherian et al., 2000; Levadoux-Martin et al., 2001). The translocation of MT into the nucleus during G1/S phase in tumour cells suggests that MT facilitates cell proliferation by donating zinc ions to various transcription factors. The stabilization and binding of transcription factors to DNA depend entirely on zinc binding (Ostrakhovitch et al. 2007). In this way MT may control activity of various genes, including the p53 tumour suppressor protein in cells. In *in vitro* studies the transfer of zinc ions from MT to transcription factors was demonstrated (Langmade et al., 2000). The factors involve mainly protein factors with zinc fingers domains in their structures, such as estrogen receptors and MTF-1. Binding of zinc ions by MT was found to be a reversible process: in certain conditions MT may remove zinc from other protein molecules, in this way modulating their biological activity (Davis et al., 2000; Ogra et al., 2001).

1.3 Role of MT in a neoplastic process

Recent investigations confirmed that increased synthesis of MT occurs in neoplastic cells of various origin (Dziegiel, 2004). Investigators have focused on the significance of MT in the process of carcinogenesis and tumour progression but also on the involvement of the proteins in development of tumour chemoresistance as well as the possible role of MT expression as a prognostic and predictive factor. Results of several investigations suggest that the role of MT expression in tumour cells may be linked to the processes of proliferation and apoptosis (Jayasurya et al., 2000; Bay et al., 2001; Shimoda et al., 2003). MT functions as a donor of zinc ions for transcription factors and enzymes involved in the processes of DNA and protein synthesis. This is confirmed not only by elevated MT levels in hyperplasia but also by MT translocation from cytoplasm to cell nucleus during DNA synthesis (S phase) (Woo et al., 1996; Jasani & Schmid, 1997). In neoplastic tissues, the level of MT was shown to be proportionally elevated with the concentration of zinc ions (Jayasurya et al., 2000; Florianczyk et al., 2006). Similar results have been shown in *in vitro* investigations, showing that interaction between MT and p53 protein seems to be highly significant for tumour development, due to regulation of zinc ion homeostasis by MT (Meplan et al., 2000; Ostrakhovitch et al., 2006). p53 protein represents a transcription factor with a DNA-binding domain, stabilized by zinc ions. In normal conditions it inhibits proliferation of cells with a damaged DNA and directs cells toward apoptosis. MT molecules were found to be able to remove zinc ions from p53 protein, what results in its inactivity (Rainwater et al., 1995; Meplan et al., 2000). Inactivation of p53 protein in neoplastic cells results in their excessive proliferation and in inhibition of apoptotic processes. It is suggested that an increased synthesis of MT in tumour cells promotes interaction of MT with p53 protein, resulting in an uncontrolled proliferation (Fan et al., 2002; Ostrakhovitch et al., 2007). The results were confirmed by positive correlation between expression of MT and proliferation antigens, Ki-67 and PCNA. Such a relationship was demonstrated in several tumours, such as breast cancer, cancers of ovary, kidney, and also in tumours of lungs and upper respiratory pathways (Jayasurya et al., 2000; Jin et al., 2001; Hengstler et al., 2001; Harpole et al., 2001; Mitropoulos et al., 2005). Therefore, expression of MT may be of prognostic significance in certain types of tumours. Several reports investigated the relationship between MT expression and other clinicopathological characteristics of various malignancies. In certain tumours, e.g. in colorectal carcinoma overexpression of MT was found more often in cases of tumours of a higher grade of malignancy (Dziegiel et al., 2003). An elevated level of MT was found to correlate with an abbreviated duration of survival and a shorter disease free survival in some tumour types, what may suggest usefulness of MT as a prognostic factor (Dziegiel, 2004). However, some reports did not confirm the prognostic role of MT expression, what does not permit at present to unequivocally specify prognostic value of MT in neoplastic diseases. MT was also shown to be involved in the development of resistance of cancer cells to cytostatic agents. Chemotherapy was found to induce synthesis of MT while an elevated level of the proteins decreased therapeutic efficacy of certain oncostatic proteins (Cherian et al., 2003). In several investigations it was demonstrated using experimental animals with engrafted tumour cells treated with drugs commonly used in anti-neoplastic therapy, including cisplatin, bleomycin, cyclophosphamide, that synthesis of MT in neoplastic cells increased markedly. In parallel, other drugs, such as mitomycin C, 5-fluorouracil did not alter MT expression level. Animals with engrafted tumour cells with zinc-induced MT, were shown to have significantly higher rate of chemoresitance of tumour cells to cisplatin as compared to the untreated cells. The experiments showed that MT may be responsible for both primary and acquired chemoresistance of neoplastic cells (Florianczyk, 1999; Chun et al., 2004). Mechanism of the cytoprotective MT activity during chemotherapy seems to be related to an anti-oxidative properties of MT. Some anti-neoplastic drugs act by inducing oxidative stress in tumour cells (including anthracyclines, e.g.. doxorubicin, daunorubicin), what results in their damage. MT protect cells from oxidative damage, decreasing therefore the therapeutic efficacy of cytostatic drugs (Cherian et al., 2003). In turn, affinity of MT to metal ions provides grounds for inactivation of alkylating drugs containing heavy metals (e.g. cisplatin, carboplatin). Due to MT direct interaction with the chemotherapeutic agents or their metabolites, MT may protect neoplastic cells from the cytotoxic effects (Shimoda et al., 2003; Theocharis et al., 2004). This hypothesis is confirmed by studies conducted on human malignancies (e.g. ovarian cancer, testicular cancer, colorectal cancer, breast cancer and squamocellular oesophageal cancer), showed that insensitivity of the tumours to chemotherapy was related to their MT over-expression (Yamamoto et al., 1999; Vazquez-Ramirez et al., 2000; Dziegiel et al., 2003; Surowiak et al., 2005; Surowiak et al., 2007). In view of the above, some authors include MT, in parallel to multi-drug resistance proteins (*MDR)*, to significant factors responsible for the lack of therapeutic efficacy of some cytostatic agents (Theocharis et al., 2004). Similar observations were shown regarding resistance of tumour cells to radiotherapy, which is known to generate high amounts of free radicals in tumour cells. MT, playing the function of an intracellular antioxidant inactivate reactive oxygen species, therefore protecting the tumour cells from radiotherapy induced damage, resulting in treatment failure (Cai et al., 1999; Theocharis et al., 2004). Although the role of MT in the process of carcinogenesis, proliferation and resistance of tumour cells to chemo- and radiotherapy still requires further research, MT may be considered as an additional prognostic and predictive marker in some tumour types.

2. Metallothionein in oral cancer

As overexpression of MT-1 and MT-2 was found in many malignant tumours, the studies conducted on cancers of the oral cavity concerning MT expression focused mainly on the expression of these two isoforms in oral squamous cell carcinoma (OSCC), tonque squamous cell carcinoma and tumours of the salivary glands.

2.1 Metallothionein expression in normal and dysplastic oral mucosa and oral squamous cell carcinoma

OSCC is the most frequently diagnosed oral cancer accounting for more than 95% of malignancies originating from the oral cavity with almost 25 000 new cases diagnosed annually in the US (Siegel et al., 2011). Oral leukoplakia (OL) is a premalignant and potentially malignanant lesion of the oral mucosa and proceeds OSCC in some cases (Hunt et al. 2011). On the basis of the amount of dysplastic cells and the thickness of dysplastic epithelium, this lesion is graded as mild, moderate or severe (Barnes et al., 2005). Until now, in tissues of the oral mucosa and its lesions, only isoforms of the MT-1 and MT-2 family were investigated concerning their expression. In normal oral mucosa MT-1/2 expression is restricted only to basal and parabasal cells with a mosaic cytoplasmic-nuclear expression pattern, whereas in dysplastic lesions additional foci in the spinous layer were noted (Sundelin et al., 1997; Johann et al., 2008; Pontes et al., 2009). MT-1/2 expression intensity was positively correlated with severity of dysplasia of oral leukoplakia, with the lowest MT-1/2 expression found in mild dysplastic lesions and the highest in severe dysplasia (Pontes et al., 2009). Likewise in normal and dysplastic mucosa, cancer cells of OSCC exhibited an cytoplasmic-nuclear pattern of MT-1/2 expression (Szelachowska et al., 2008; Pontes et al., 2009). In OSCC, cancer cells expressing MT-1/2 were found at the centre and the periphery of tumour islands, but interestingly in cases when keratin pearls were present, MT-1/2 expression was restricted to basal and parabasal cells (Pontes et al., 2009, Szelachowska et al, 2009).

2.1.1 Role of metallothioneins in the pathogenesis of oral squamous cell carcinoma

Three major risk factors of OSCC development are long term tobacco smoking, alcohol and areca-quid (also known as betel nut) consumption (Shiu et al, 2004). Two components of tobacco: nicotine and 4-(methylnitorosamino)-1-(3-pyridyl)-1-butanone were shown to activate Akt kinase in human airway epithelial cells (West et al., 2003; Shiu et al., 2004; West et al., 2004). Recent studies reported, that MT-1/2 expression correlated positively with phosphorylated Akt (p-Akt) expression and levels of both these proteins were significantly elevated in OSCC in comparison to normal or dysplastic oral mucosa regardless of its severity grade (Sundelin et al., 1997; Johann et al., 2008; Pontes et al., 2009). Akt/PKB (protein kinase B) is a serine/threonine kinase comprised of three isoforms and acts as a downstream target of phosphatidylinositol-3 kinase (PI3K) and is thus involved in many vital cellular pathways and is frequently activated in different human cancers (Carnero 2010; Fayard et al, 2010; Freudlsperger et al., 2011; Grabinski et al., 2011;). Its activation, similarly to MT-1/2 expression, in human cancers was associated with inhibition of apoptosis and promotion of cell proliferation (Diehl et al., 1998; Brunet et al., 1999). Epidemiological studies have also shown, that patients with head and neck cancer and OSCC frequently suffer from zinc deficiency (Doerr et al., 1997; Kleier et al., 1998). These results were also confirmed by a number of *in vivo* studies using an lingual-esophageal carcinogenesis model in mouse and rats (Fong et al., 2005; Fong et al., 2006, Liu et al., 2005). These studies have shown that deficit of zinc in diet induces MT-1 expression, along with other markers related to carcinogenesis e.g. cyclin-B2, carbonic anhydrase II and keratin 14. Moreover, zinc diet restriction potentiated the growth of lingual and esophageal tumours in p53 deficient mice, which were characterized by significantly augmented cell proliferation, keratin 14, COX-2 and MT-1 expression as compared to mice with normal p53 expression level (Liu et al., 2005; Fong et al., 2006). Zinc replenishment in the diet resulted in subsequent reduction of cell proliferation and expression of keratin 14, COX-2 and MT-I (Liu et al., 2005). These experimental results confirm the observations stemming from IHC studies on human specimens, because the carcinogenesis model clearly showed subsequent rise of MT-1 expression correlating with the noted histopathological hyperplasia-dysplasia-carcinoma model (Fong et al., 2006). Nonetheless, little is known about the interaction and possible regulation of MT-1 and MT-2 expression in dysplasia and OSCC cases.

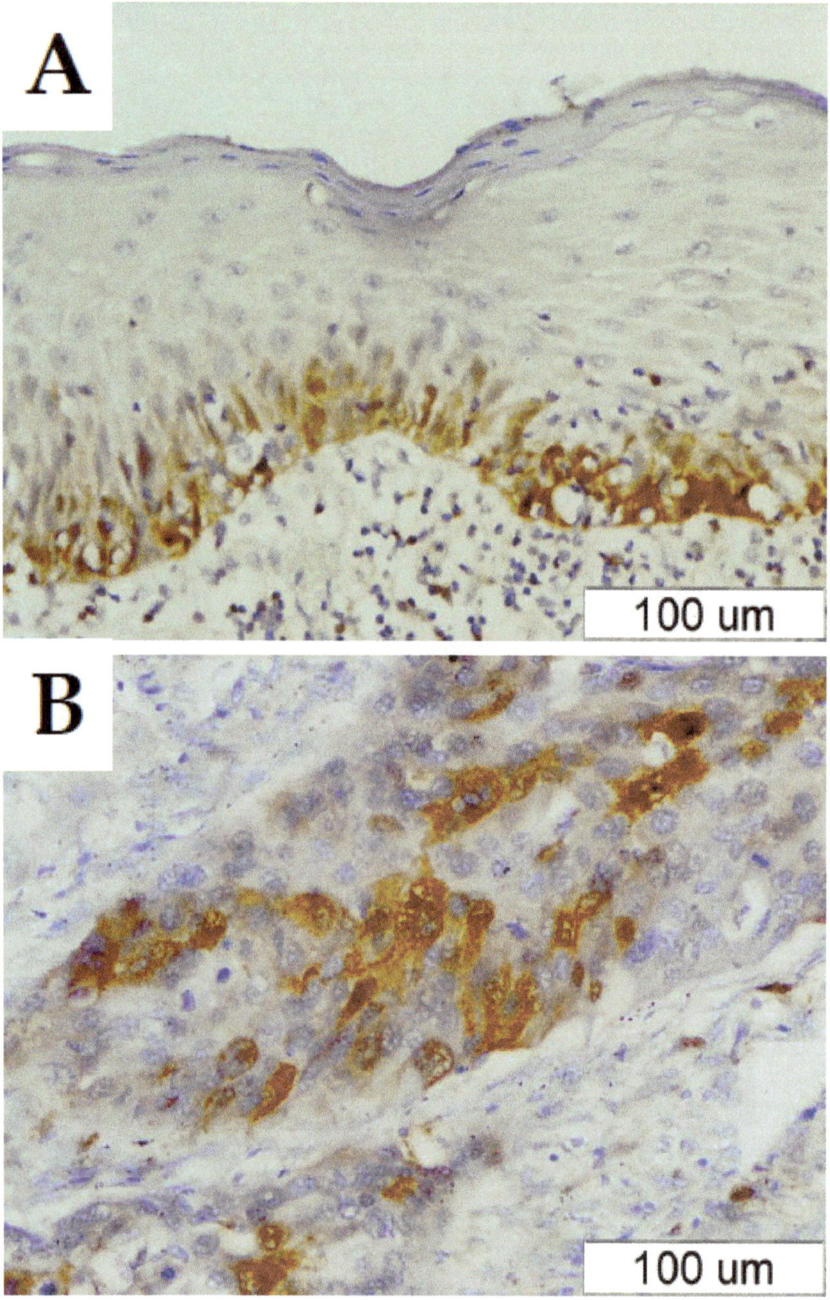

Fig. 1. MT-1/2 expression in basal layer of squamous stratified epithelium with additional foci in the upper parts of oral mucosa (A). Nuclear-cytoplasmic MT-1/2 expression in advanced OSCC (B).

2.1.1.1 Areca nuts, copper ions and reactive oxygen species (ROS)

Areca nuts chewing was shown to be associated with increased risk of OSCC development and progression (Shiu et al., 2004; Merchant et al., 2000). It is estimated that around 200-400 million people, regardless of gender consume areca nuts (Gupta and Warnakulasuriya, 2002). Moreover, almost 80% of OSCC related deaths in Taiwan are associated with areca quid consumption habit (Kwan, 1976; Lee et al., 2008). It was shown, that patients with simultaneous smoking and areca nut chewing habits are characterized be even greater risk of OSCC development, than patients consuming either of these products separately (Ko et al., 1995). The study of Lee et al. showed an upregulated expression of MT-1 in OSCC originating from patients with long-term areca nut consumption (Lee et al., 2008). Areca nuts contain high levels of copper, a metal which is bound by metallotthioneins, and is the source of ROS during chewing (Trivedy et al., 1997; Nair et al., 1992; Chen et al., 2002). This compounds were shown to be responsible for generation of OSCC in areca quid consumers (Warnakulasuriya et al., 2002). The *in vitro* experiments conducted on an oral epithelial cell line GNM originating from a patient with T2N2aM0 gingival carcinoma demonstrated an increase in MT-1 mRNA expression upon arecoline treatment in a dose dependent manner (Lee et al., 2008). Treatment of this carcinoma cell line with benzo[a]pyren (BaP) alone or in combination with arecoline resulted in an increased expression of MT-1 mRNA in GNM cells. The highest MT-1 mRNA expression was seen in the cells treated with both compounds simultaneously. Addition of a glutathione precursor, N-acetyl-L-cyteine, to the cells treated with arecoline reduced the levels of arecoline induced MT-1 mRNA levels. Nonetheless, the results of the *in vitro* experiments are in accordance with the results of the epidemiological studies conducted on Taiwan population, showing an enhanced incidence of OSCC development in patients with simultaneous areca quid and cigarette consumption (Ko et al., 1995, Lin et al., 2011). Moreover, this results also underlie the results of studies showing upregulated expression in response to reactive oxygen species (Iqbal et al., 2003; Reinecke et al., 2006). As areca nuts contain also high amounts of copper ions, high MT-1/2 expression in OSCC originating from areca nut chewers may be partially explained by its interaction with this metal ion. To note, studies have shown, that MT-1/2 expression levels is related to zinc and copper ion content in tumour cells, what points to another mechanism of MT-1/2 upregulated expression in OSCC cells originating from areca-quid consumers (Jayasurya et al., 2000; Florianczyk et al., 2006).

2.1.1.2 Cancer cell proliferation

Few studies compared the proliferative activity of OSCC tumour cells with expression levels of MT-1/2 (Cardoso et al., 2002; Szelachowska et al., 2008; Szelachowska et al., 2009). None of the studies performed on OSCC cases succeeded in noting a positive correlation between MT-1/2 expression and expression of proliferation markers. The study of Cardoso et al. found no correlation between the expression of MT-1/2 and Ki-67 antigen (Cardoso et al., 2002). Similar results were obtained in both studies performed by Szelachowska et al. on a subset of patients with OSCC (Szelachowska et al. 2008; Szelachowska et al., 2009). In the first study no correlation with Ki-67 and MCM-2 protein expression was found, when the MT-1/2 nuclear and cytoplasmic expression was analyzed separately (Szelachowska et al. 2008). Similarly, no correlations were found in the second study performed on 39 patients with OSCC between MT-1/2 expression intensity and cancer cell proliferation measured by the Ki-67 and MCM-2 expression levels (Szelachowska et al., 2009). MT-1/2 expression seems not to exert pro-mitotic effects in OSCC, which was observed in other tumour types, including the squamous cell carcinoma of the head and neck (Jayasurya et al., 2000; Dziegiel et al., 2005; Szajereka et al., 2008).

2.1.1.3 p53

Recent study performed on 100 cases of OSCC disclosed a positive correlation between the expression of MT-1/2 and p53 protein. Moreover, cases characterized by a positive nuclear MT-1/2 immunostaining yielded higher p53 expression levels (Cardoso et al., 2009). This underlies the earlier observed role of MT-1/2 in regulation of p53 expression by influencing zinc ion cell homeostasis (Rainwater et al., 1995; Meplan et al., 2000; Ostrakhovitch et al., 2006; Pastuszewski et al., 2007).

2.1.1.4 Invasiveness

Numerous studies showed the involvement of laminin in progression of different malignancies, including these of the oral cavity (Ono et al., 1999; Patarroyo et al., 2002; Stolzfus et al., 2004; Lyons and Jones, 2007). Until now, only one study analyzed the impact of MT-1/2 expression levels on the expression of invasiveness related markers in OSCC. In this immunohistochemical study a positive correlation was disclosed between the expression of MT-1/2 and laminin-5 (Szelachowska et al., 2009). Lamin in normal conditions is expressed in the epithelial basement membrane and its expression increases with severity of the dysplasia and may regulate cell motility (Kainulainen et al., 1997; Décline & Roussel, 2001; Décline et al., 2003, Lyons and Jones, 2007). This might explain the higher expression of MT-1/2 in tumours with the presence of lymph node metastases in comparison to tumours without lymph node involvement (Szelachowska et al., 2009).

2.1.1.5 Chemoresistance

As metallothionein isoforms were suggested to play a role in cancer cells chemoresistance, Nakano et al. studied the impact of cisplatin treatment of human tongue squamous cell carcinomas on MT expression (Nakano et al., 2003). These cells expressed the MT-1, MT-2 and MT-4 isoforms, whereas no expression of MT-3 was noted. The subsequent treatment of the cells with cisplatin resulted in a significant increase of expression of only the MT-1 and MT-2 isoforms in cisplatin-resistant cells (Nakano et al., 2003). Role of MT-1/2 in OSCC chemoresistance was also issued in the work of Muramutsu et al., but no difference in MT-1/2 expression levels between the treated and untreated patients was noted (Muramutsu et al., 2000).

2.1.2 Clinical implications of MT expression in OSCC

Until now six studies (Table 1) investigated the impact of MT expression regarding patients clinicopathological characteristics (Muramatsu et al., 2000; Cardoso et al., 2002; Lee et al., 2008; Szelachowska et al., 2008; Cardoso et al., 2009; Szelachowska et al., 2009). All those studies were performed on archival paraffin blocks from patients whose cancers originated mainly from oral mucosa, but in some cases specimens from cancers of the mobile part of the tongue were included (Szelachowska et al., 2008; Szelachowska et al., 2009). In case of only one study three additional tumours from the maxilla region were investigated (Muramutsu et al., 2000). Except one study of Lee et al., a primary antibody directed against MT-1/2 isoforms was used. None of the mentioned studies showed correlations with primary tumour size, grade of tumour differentiation and proliferation markers (Ki-67 and MCM-2). In three studies, a positive correlation was noted between lymph node involvement and the intensity of MT expression (Lee et al., 2008; Szelachowska et al., 2008; Szelachowska et al., 2009). Studies which analyzed the impact of metallothionein expression on patients outcome, showed that elevated MT-1/2 expression in patients with OSCC was generally an unfavourable prognostic marker (Cardoso et al., 2002; Szelachowska et al., 2008; Cardoso et al., 2009). In the study of Cardoso et. al., MT-1/2 cell positivity (cytoplasmic-nuclear staining) was counted and enrolled in the survival analysis. Univariate analysis, as well as multivariate analysis showed that MT-1/2 overexpression was an unfavorable prognostic factor in the studied patient cohort (Cardoso et al., 2002).

Publication	**Muramatsu et al., 2000**	**Cardoso et al., 2002**	**Lee et al., 2008**	**Szelachowska et al., 2008**	**Szelachowska et al., 2009**	**Cardoso et al., 2009**
Patients	28 OSCC and NPC; 3 cancers of the maxilla region	60 OSCC	*34 OSCC	50 OSCC	39 OSCC	100 OSCC
MT isoform	MT-1/2	MT-1/2	MT-1	MT-1/2	MT-1/2	MT-1/2
pT	-	-	-	-	-	NA
pN	-	-	+	+ cytoplasm	+	NA
Grade of malignancy (differentiation)	NA	-	-	-	-	-
Clinical stage	NA	-	-	not analyzed	not analyzed	-
Survival	NA	poor prognosis	NA	*poor prognosis	not analyzed	*poor prognosis
Proliferation	(-) Ki-67	(-) Ki-67	NA	(-) Ki-67, (-) MCM-2	(-) Ki-67, (-) MCM-2	-
Other markers	NA	NA	NA	NA	(+) Laminin-5	(+) p53
Notes			*Areca quid consumers	*shorter DFS and DSS in patients with high MT-1/2 expression; lack of significant impact on SFLR and OS		*combined high expression of MT-1/2 and p53 on OS

Abbreviations: SFLR - survival free of locoregional relapse; DFS - disease free survival; OS - overall survival; DSS - disease specific survival; NA - not analyzed

Table 1. Summary of studies on MT expression with regard to patients clinicpathological characteristics. (-) represents lack of correlation or relationship between the analyzed variables, whereas (+) represents positive correlations.

A more detailed analysis of MT-1/2 expression on patients outcome was performed in the study of Szelachowska et al., where cytoplasmatic and nuclear MT-1/2 expressions were analyzed separately (Szelachowska et al., 2008). For the nuclear evaluation, cells showing positive reaction were counted, whereas, for the evaluation of cytoplasmatic reaction an immunoreactive score (IRS) of Remmele and Stegner based on evaluation of number of positive cells and the intensity of colour reaction took advantage (Remmele & Stegner, 1986). The authors noted a significant correlation between the cytoplasmatic and nuclear MT-1/2 expression, but none of the evaluated types of the reaction correlated with tumour size, grade of malignancy or expression of both proliferation markers (Ki-67 and MCM-2). Interestingly, only in cases with lymph node involvement, a significant increase in MT-1/2 expression was noted when compared to cases without lymph node involvement (Szelachowska et al. 2008). Also differences regarding patients survival differed among the both analyzed expression patterns. The univariate analysis showed that cases characterized by high cytoplasmatic MT-1/2 expression had a significantly shorter disease specific survival (DSS) and disease free survival (DFS), whereas cases with high nuclear MT-1/2 expression had a significantly shorter DFS and tended to have also a shorter DSS, but this trend did not reach statistical significance. No impact of MT-1/2 expression in the cytoplasm or nucleus affected significantly patients overall survival (Szelachowska et al., 2008). In another study of Cardoso et al., no influence on patients survival was observed, when MT-1/2 expression was analyzed alone. Interestingly, a combined analysis of this protein with p53 expression, showed that high expression of both these markers predicted poor outcome of patients with OSCC (Cardoso et al, 2009). Differences in the studies concerning lymph node involvement and patients survival, may by caused be heterogenous origin of specimens used in the study (Szelachowska et al., 2008; Szelachowska et al., 2009) In summary, the above mentioned studies highlight and underlie the potential role of MT-1/2 expression in the development and tumour progression of OSCC.

2.2 Metallothionein expression in normal salivary gland and its lesions

MT were shown to be expressed in normal salivary glands as well as in benign and malignant tumours mainly in cells resembling the phenotype of myoepithelial cells (Sunardhi-Widyaputra et al., 1995; Gao et al., 1997; Hecht et al., 2002; Ogawa, 2003; Alves et al., 2007). As in the case of OSCC, the majority of studies concerning the role of MT expression in salivary glands were based on immunohistochemistry (Sunardhi-Widyaputra et al., 1995; Gao et al., 1997; Ogawa, 2003; Alves et al., 2007).

2.2.1 Role of MT in salivary gland development

MT seem to be involved in salivary gland development as shown in the studies of Hecht et al. (Hecht et al., 2002). It was found that MT is mainly the only upregulated family of genes, when human salivary gland (HSG) cells, derived from a human submandibular tumour, were cultured on a laminin-1 gel in different conditions. In gel cultures lamin-1 stimulates HSG cells to form acinar-like structures within 24-48 hours, whereas in the absence of laminin-1 in culture conditions results in a monolayer growth type. Also in microgravity culture conditions laminin-1 affects HSG cells growth by facilitating acini formation (Hoffman et al., 1998). It was seen that under laminin-1 culture conditions mRNA expression of three members of the MT family was significantly upregulated: MT-1F, MT-1B and MT-2. Subsequent immunostaining of these cells revealed a higher cytoplasmic

MT-1/2 expression in comparison to HSG cells cultured in the absence of laminin-1. An overexpression of MT-1F in HSG cells did not affect cell proliferation as compared to native and control mock-transfected cells, but MT-overexpressing cells were characterized by an augmented growth after addition of low concentrations of zinc and copper to the medium (Hecht et al., 2002). MT-overexpressing cells grew in aggregates, were larger and had more pronounced adhesive properties than the parental cells. Moreover, MT-overexpressing cells formed acini-like structures larger and faster. Despite the strong impact on cellular differentiation, MT-overexpression did not affect amylase expression or mucin production. Interestingly, when these cells were injected s.c. to nude mice, tumours formed by MT-overexpressing HSG cells were significantly smaller and more differentiated than the tumours formed by the parental cells (Hecht et al., 2002). Although, no differences in cell proliferation were observed *in vitro*, tumours originating from MT-overexpressing cells seemed to have more mitotic cells in the tumour mass (Hecht et al., 2002).

2.2.2 MT expression in normal salivary gland tissues and neoplasias

Normal salivary glands and its tumours exert a broad expression of MT-1/2 in myoepithelial cells (Sunardhi-Widyaputra et al., 1995; Gao et al., 1997; Ogawa, 2003; Alves et al., 2007, Prasad et al., 2008). In the study of Sunardhi-Widyaputra et al., performed on 21 benign and 4 malignant lesions of salivary glands, MT expression was compared with parathyroid hormone-related peptide (PTHrP) expression. In benign changes (pleomorphic adenoma, Warthin's tumour), both these proteins were coexpresed. In myoepthelioma majority of the cells expressed MT, while few have shown PTHrP reactivity. In oncocytoma, peripheries of oncotytic islands showed MT expression, while only few oncotytic PTHrP positive cells were noted. In cases of mucoepidermoid carcinomas MT and PTHrP expression was the most heterogenous. MT positivity was seen in epithelial cells and PTHrP in cyst-like structures and squamous cells (Sunardhi-Widyaputra et al., 1995). Similar results regarding MT expression were noted by Gao et al. in myoepitheliomas and myoepithelial carcinomas (Gao et al., 1997). Although these studies did not quantified MT expression, they clearly showed that MT expression may vary in regard to tumour degree of differentiation with the most heterogenous expression in the most dedifferentieted and immature tumours (Sunardhi-Widyaputra et al., 1995; Gao et al., 1997). The results of these studies are also supported by the findings of Ogawa, which demonstrated MT expression in a subset of myoepithelial cells during salivary gland development (Ogawa, 2003). MT expression in myoepithelial cells of adenoid cystic carcinomas and polymporphous low-grade adenocarcinomas was also studied as a potential marker of differentiation of these two malignancies as they may pose problems in the pathological examination (Prasad et al., 2008). This study showed, that diffuse MT expression in combination with smooth muscle acitin, calponin and smooth muscle myosin heavy chain was strongly predictive for adenoid cystic carcinoma (Prasad et al., 2008). MT expression in adenoid cystic carcinomas varied according to histological subtype (Alves et al., 2008). The most pronounced MT-1/2 staining was seen in solid and cribiform as compared to tubular subtypes of this tumour. This results support the results stemming from studies conducted on other malignanancies, showing that elevated MT-1/2 expression is linked to patients poor clinical outcome (Dziegiel, 2004). High expression of MT-1/2 in solid and low in tubular subtypes, may partially explain their distinct clinical outcome (Nascimento et al., 1986; Perez et al., 2006; Alves et al., 2008).

3. Conclusion

MT expression in OSCC seems to be of importance for the development and progression of these cancer type. Although the results of the clinical studies were not concordant (due to small sample size, heterogenous patient cohort) it is worth to mention that some of them noted a relationship between high MT expression and cancer cell metastasis and associated MT overexpression with poor patients outcome. Despite the few reports concerning MT expression in salivary glands and its lesions, one might consider MT as an interesting point of future research, mainly due to the impact of MT-1F expression on salivary tumour cells differentiation and growth. Nonetheless, further studies are needed to better characterize the role of MT expression on OSCC and tumours of the salivary glands.

4. Acknowledgment

This work was supported by the scientific grant of Wroclaw Medical University, No. ST-442.

5. References

Alves SM, Cardoso SV, de Fátima Bernardes V, Machado VC, Mesquita RA, Vieira do Carmo MA & Ferreira Aguiar MC. (2007). Metallothionein immunostaining in adenoid cystic carcinomas of the salivary glands. *Oral Oncology*, (March 2007), Vol.43, No.3, pp.252-256, ISSN: 1368-8375.

Andrews GK. (2000). Regulation of metallothionein gene expression by oxidative stress and metal ions. *Biochemical Pharmacology*, (January 2000), Vol.59, No.1, pp.95-104, ISSN 0006-2952.

Barnes L, Eveson JW, Reichert PA & Sidransky D. (2005). *Pathology and Genetics of Head and Neck Tumours*. IARC Press Lyon, ISBN 92 832 24 175, France.

Bay BH, Jin R & Jaysurya A. (2001). Analysis of Metallothionein Expression in Human Cancers. *Acta Histochemica et Cytochemica*, (September 2001), Vol.34, No.3, pp.171-176, ISSN 0044-5991.

Brunet A, Bonni A, Zigmond MJ, Lin MZ, Juo P, Hu LS, Anderson MJ, Arden KC, Blenis J & Greenberg ME. (1999). Akt promotes cell survival by phosphorylating and inhibiting a Forkhead transcription factor. *Cell*, (March 1999), Vol.96, No.6, pp.857-868, ISSN 0092-8674.

Cai L, Satoh M, Tohyama C & Cherian MG. (1999). Metallothionein in radiation exposure: its induction and protective role. *Toxicology*, (February 1999), Vol. 132, No. 2-3, pp. 85-98, ISSN 0300-483X.

Cardoso SV, Barbosa HM, Candellori IM, Loyola AM & Aguiar MC. (2002). Prognostic impact of metallothionein on oral squamous cell carcinoma. *Virchows Archives*, (April 2002), Vol.441, No.2, pp.174-178, ISSN:0174-7398.

Cardoso SV, Silveira-Júnior JB, De Carvalho Machado V, De-Paula AM, Loyola AM & De Aguiar MC. (2009). Expression of metallothionein and p53 antigens are correlated in oral squamous cell carcinoma. *Anticancer Research*, (April 2009), Vol.29, No.4, pp.1189-1193, ISSN 0250-7005.

Carnero A. (2010). The PKB/AKT pathway in cancer. *Current Pharmaceutical Design*, (January 2010), Vol.16, No.1, pp.34-44, ISSN 1381-6128.

Chen CL, Chi CW & Liu TY. (2002). Hydroxyl radical formation and oxidative DNA damage induced by areca quid in vivo. *Journal of Toxicology and Environmental Health Part A*, (February 2002), Vol.65, No.3-4, pp.327-336, ISSN 1528-7394.

Cherian MG & Apostolova MD. (2000). Nuclear localization of metallothionein during cell proliferation and differentiation. *Cellular and Molecular Biology (Noisy-le-grand)*, (March 2000), Vol.46, No.2, pp.347-356, ISSN 0145-5680.

Cherian MG & Kang YJ. (2006). Metallothionein and liver cell regeneration. *Experimental and Biological Medicine (Maywood, N.J.)*, (February 2006), Vol.231, No.2, pp.138-144, ISSN 1535-3699.

Cherian MG, Jayasurya A & Bay BH. (2003). Metallothioneins in human tumors and potential roles in carcinogenesis. *Mutation Research*, (December 2003), Vol.533, No.1-2, pp.201-209, ISSN 0027-5107.

Chun JH, Kim HK, Kim E, Kim IH, Kim JH, Chang HJ, Choi IJ, Lim HS, Kim IJ, Kang HC, Park JH, Bae JM & Park JG. (2004). Increased expression of metallothionein is associated with irinotecan resistance in gastric cancer. *Cancer Research*, (July 2004), Vol.64, No.14, pp.4703-4706, ISSN 0008-5472.

Coyle P, Philcox JC, Carey LC & Rofe AM. (2002). Metallothionein: the multipurpose protein. *Cellular and Molecular Life Sciences: CMLS*, (April 2002), Vol.59, No.4, pp.627-647, ISSN 1420-682X.

da Cruz Perez DE, de Abreu Alves F, Nobuko Nishimoto I, de Almeida OP & Kowalski LP. (2006). Prognostic factors in head and neck adenoid cystic carcinoma. *Oral Oncology*, (February 2006), Vol.42, No.2, pp.139-146, ISSN 1368-8375.

Davis SR & Cousins RJ. (2000). Metallothionein expression in animals: a physiological perspective on function. *The Journal of Nutrition*, (May 2000), Vol.130, No.5, pp.1085-1088, ISSN 0022-3166.

Décline F & Rousselle P. (2001). Keratinocyte migration requires alpha2beta1 integrin-mediated interaction with the laminin 5 gamma2 chain. J Cell Sci, (February 2001), Vol.114, No.4, pp.811-823, ISSN 0021-9533.

Décline F, Okamoto O, Mallein-Gerin F, Helbert B, Bernaud J, Rigal D & Rousselle P. (2003). Keratinocyte motility induced by TGF-beta1 is accompanied by dramatic changes in cellular interactions with laminin 5. *Cell Motility and the Cytoskeleton*, (January 2003), Vol. 54, No.1, pp.64-80, ISSN 0886-1544.

Diehl JA, Cheng M, Roussel MF & Sherr CJ. (1998). Glycogen synthase kinase-3beta regulates cyclin D1 proteolysis and subcellular localization. *Genes and Development*, (November 1998), Vol.12, No.22, pp.3499-3511, ISSN 0890-9369.

Doerr TD, Prasad AS, Marks SC, Beck FW, Shamsa FH, Penny HS & Mathog RH. (1997). Zinc deficiency in head and neck cancer patients. *Journal of the American College of Nutrition*, (October 1997), Vol.16, No.5, pp.418-422, ISSN 0731-5724.

Dziegiel P, Forgacz J, Suder E, Surowiak P, Kornafel J & Zabel M. (2003). Prognostic significance of metallothionein expression in correlation with Ki-67 expression in adenocarcinomas of large intestine. *Histology Histopathology*, (April 2003), Vol. 18, No.2, pp.401-407, ISSN 0213-3911.

Dziegiel P, Salwa-Zurawska W, Zurawski J, Wojnar A & Zabel M. (2005). Prognostic significance of augmented metallothionein (MT) expression correlated with Ki-67 antigen expression in selected soft tissue sarcomas. *Histology Histopathology*, (January 2005), Vol.20, No.1, pp. 83-89, ISSN 0213-3911.

Dziegiel P. (2004). Expression of metallothioneins in tumor cells. *Polish Journal of Pathology,* (2004), Vol.55, No.1, pp.3-12, ISSN 1233-9687.

Fan LZ & Cherian MG. (2002). Potential role of p53 on metallothionein induction in human epithelial breast cancer cells. *British Journal of Cancer,* (October 2002), Vol.87, No.9, pp.1019-1026, ISSN 0007-0920.

Fayard E, Xue G, Parcellier A, Bozulic L & Hemmings BA. (2010). Protein kinase B (PKB/Akt), a key mediator of the PI3K signaling pathway. *Current Topics in Microbiology and Immunology,* (2010), Vol. 346, pp.31-56, ISSN 0070-217X.

Florianczyk B. (1998). Metallothioneins in rats exposed to cadmium. *Roczniki Akademii Medycznej w Bialymstoku (1995),* (1998); Vol.43, pp.309-313, ISSN 0067-6489.

Florianczyk B. (2003). Copper and metallothioneins in cancer cells. *Annales Universitatis Mariae Curie Sklodowska. Sectio D: Medicina,* (2003), Vol.58, No.2, pp.390-393, ISSN 0066-2240.

Fong LY, Jiang Y & Farber JL. (2006). Zinc deficiency potentiates induction and progression of lingual and esophageal tumors in p53-deficient mice. *Carcinogenesis,* (July 2006), Vol.27, No. 7, pp.1489-1496, ISSN 0143-3334.

Fong LY, Zhang L, Jiang Y & Farber JL. (2005). Dietary zinc modulation of COX-2 expression and lingual and esophageal carcinogenesis in rats. *Journal of National Cancer Institute,* (January 2005), Vol.97, No.1, pp.40-50, ISSN 0027-8874.

Freudlsperger C, Burnett JR, Friedman JA, Kannabiran VR, Chen Z & Van Waes C. (2011). EGFR-PI3K-AKT-mTOR signaling in head and neck squamous cell carcinomas: attractive targets for molecular-oriented therapy. *Expert Opinion on Therapeutic Targets,* (January 2011), Vol.15, No.1, pp.63-74, ISSN 1472-8222.

Gao Y, Han Z & Liu X. (1997). Metallothionein expression and its significance in salivary gland tumors. Zhonghua Kou Qiang Yi Xue Za Zhi, (1997), Vol.32, No.5, pp.282-284, ISSN 1002-0098.

Ghoshal K, Majumder S, Zhu Q, Hunzeker J, Datta J, Shah M, Sheridan JF & Jacob ST. (2001). Influenza virus infection induces metallothionein gene expression in the mouse liver and lung by overlapping but distinct molecular mechanisms. *Molecular and Cellular Biology,* (December 2001), Vol.21, No.24, pp.8301-8317, ISSN 0270-7306.

Grabinski N, Bartkowiak K, Grupp K, Brandt B, Pantel K & Jücker M. (2011). Distinct functional roles of Akt isoforms for proliferation, survival, migration and EGF-mediated signalling in lung cancer derived disseminated tumor cells. *Cellular Signaling,* (July 2011), ISSN 0898-6568.

Gupta PC & Warnakulasuriya S. (2002). Global epidemiology of areca nut usage. *Addiction Biology,* (January 2002), Vol.7, No.1, pp.77-83, ISSN 1355-6215.

Haq F, Mahoney M & Koropatnick J. (2003). Signaling events for metallothionein induction. Mutation Research, (December 2003), Vol.533, No.1-2, pp.211-226, ISSN 0027-5107.

Harpole DH Jr, Moore MB, Herndon JE 2nd, Aloia T, D'Amico TA, Sporn T, Parr A, Linoila I & Allegra C. (2001). The prognostic value of molecular marker analysis in patients treated with trimodality therapy for esophageal cancer. *Clinical Cancer Research,* (March 2001), Vol.7, No.3, pp.562-569, ISSN 1078-0432.

Hecht D, Jung D, Prabhu VV, Munson PJ, Hoffman MP & Kleinman HK. (2002). Metallothionein promotes laminin-1-induced acinar differentiation in vitro and reduces tumor growth in vivo. *Cancer Research,* (September 2002), Vol.62, No.18, pp.5370-5374, ISSN 0008-5472.

Hengstler JG, Pilch H, Schmidt M, Dahlenburg H, Sagemüller J, Schiffer I, Oesch F, Knapstein PG, Kaina B & Tanner B. (2001). Metallothionein expression in ovarian cancer in relation to histopathological parameters and molecular markers of prognosis. *International Journal of Cancer*, (March 2001), Vol.95, No.2, pp.121-127; ISSN 0020-7136.

Hernández J, Carrasco J, Belloso E, Giralt M, Bluethmann H, Kee Lee D, Andrews GK & Hidalgo J. (2000). Metallothionein induction by restraint stress: role of glucocorticoids and IL-6. *Cytokine*, (June 2000), Vol.12, No.6, pp.791-796, ISSN 1043-4666.

Hidalgo J, Aschner M, Zatta P & Vasák M. (2001). Roles of the metallothionein family of proteins in the central nervous system. *Brain Research Bulletin*, (May 2001), Vol.55, No.2, pp.133-145, ISSN 0361-9230.

Hoffman MP, Nomizu M, Roque E, Lee S, Jung DW, Yamada Y & Kleinman HK. (1998). Laminin-1 and laminin-2 G-domain synthetic peptides bind syndecan-1 and are involved in acinar formation of a human submandibular gland cell line. *The Journal of Biological Chemistry*, (October 1998), Vol. 273, No.44, pp.28633-28641. Erratum in: *The Journal of Biological Chemistry*, (April 1999), Vol.274, No.18, p.12950, ISSN 1819-155X.

Hunt JL. (2011). An update on molecular diagnostics of squamous and salivary gland tumors of the head and neck. *Archives of Pathology and Laboratory Medicine*, (May 2011), Vol.135, No.5, pp.602-609, ISSN 0003-9985.

Ioachim E, Assimakopoulos D, Peschos D, Zissi A, Skevas A & Agnantis NJ. (1999). Immunohistochemical expression of metallothionein in benign premalignant and malignant epithelium of the larynx: correlation with p53 and proliferative cell nuclear antigen. *Pathological Research and Practice*, (1999), Vol.195, No.12, pp.809-814, ISSN 0344-0338.

Iqbal M, Noor R, Mizuno R & Okada S. (2003). Protective role of zinc-metallothionein (Zn-MT) in iron nitrilotriacetate (Fe-NTA)-induced renal oxidative damage. *Redox Report: Communications in Free Radicals Research*, (2003), Vol.8, No.3, pp.163-167, ISSN 1351-0002.

Jasani B & Schmid KW. (1997). Significance of metallothionein overexpression in human tumours. *Histopathology*, (September 1997), Vol.31, pp.211-214, ISSN 1365-2559.

Jayasurya A, Bay BH, Yap WM & Tan NG. (2000). Correlation of metallothionein expression with apoptosis in nasopharyngeal carcinoma. *British Journal of Cancer*, (March 2000), Vol.82, No.6, pp.1198-1203, ISSN 0007-0920.

Jayasurya A, Bay BH, Yap WM, Tan NG & Tan BK. (2000). Proliferative potential in nasopharyngeal carcinoma: correlations with metallothionein expression and tissue zinc levels. *Carcinogenesis*, (October 2000) Vol.21, No.10, pp.1809-1812, ISSN 0143-3334.

Jin R, Bay BH, Chow VT & Tan PH. (2001). Metallothionein 1F mRNA expression correlates with histological grade in breast carcinoma. Breast Cancer Research and Treatment, (April 2001), Vol.66, No.3, pp.265-272, ISSN 0167-6806.

Johann AC, da Silveira-Júnior JB, Souto GR, Horta MC, Aguiar MC & Mesquita RA. (2008) Metallothionein immunoexpression in oral leukoplakia. *Medicina Oral, Patologia Oral y Cirugia Bucal*, (March 2008), Mar 1;Vol.13, No.3, pp.156-160, ISSN 1698-4447.

Kainulainen T, Autio-Harmainen H, Oikarinen A, Salo S, Tryggvason K & Salo T. (1997). Altered distribution and synthesis of laminin-5 (kalinin) in oral lichen planus, epithelial dysplasias and squamous cell carcinomas. *British Journal of Dermatology*, (March 1997), Vol.136, No.3, pp.331-336, ISSN 0007-0963.

Kleier C, Werkmeister R & Joos U. (1998). Zinc and vitamin A deficiency in diseases of the mouth mucosa. *Mund-, Kiefer- und Gesichtschirurgie: MKG*, (November 1998), Vol.2, No.6, pp.320-325, ISSN 1434-3940.

Ko YC, Huang YL, Lee CH, Chen MJ, Lin LM & Tsai CC. (1995). Betel quid chewing, cigarette smoking and alcohol consumption related to oral cancer in Taiwan. *Journal of Oral Pathology and Medicine*, (November 1995) Vol.24, No.10, pp.450-453, ISSN 0904-2512.

Koizumi S, Suzuki K, Ogra Y, Yamada H & Otsuka F. (1999). Transcriptional activity and regulatory protein binding of metal-responsive elements of the human metallothionein-IIA gene. *European Journal of Biochemistry*, (February 1999), Vol. 259, No.3, pp.635-642, ISSN 0014-2956.

Kwan HW. (1976). A statistical study on oral carcinomas in Taiwan with emphasis on the relationship with betel nut chewing: a preliminary report. *Taiwan Yi Xue Hui Za Zhi*, (September 1976), Vol.75, No.9, pp,497-505, ISSN 0371-7682.

Langmade SJ, Ravindra R, Daniels PJ & Andrews GK. (2000). The transcription factor MTF-1 mediates metal regulation of the mouse ZnT1 gene. *Journal of Biological Chemistry*, (November 2000), Vol.275, No.44, pp.34803-34809, ISSN 0021-9258.

Lee SS, Yang SF, Ho YC, Tsai CH & Chang YC. (2008). The upregulation of metallothionein-1 expression in areca quid chewing-associated oral squamous cell carcinomas. *Oral Oncology*, (February 2008), Vol.44, No.2, pp.180-186, ISSN 1368-8375.

Levadoux-Martin M, Hesketh JE, Beattie JH, Wallace HM. Influence of metallothionein-1 localization on its function. *The Biochemical Journal*, (April 2001), Vol.355, No.2, pp.473-479; ISSN 0264-6021.

Lichtlen P, Wang Y, Belser T, Georgiev O, Certa U, Sack R & Schaffner W. (2001). Target gene search for the metal-responsive transcription factor MTF-1. *Nucleic Acids Research*, (April 2001), Vol.29, No.7, pp.1514-1523, ISSN 0305-1048.

Lin WJ, Jiang RS, Wu SH, Chen FJ & Liu SA. (2011). Smoking, alcohol, and betel quid and oral cancer: a prospective cohort study. *Journal of Oncology*, (2011), ISSN 1687-8450.

Liu CG, Zhang L, Jiang Y, Chatterjee D, Croce CM, Huebner K & Fong LY. (2005). Modulation of gene expression in precancerous rat esophagus by dietary zinc deficit and replenishment. *Cancer Research*, (September 2005), Vol.65, No.17, pp.7790-7799, ISSN 0008-5472.

Lyons AJ & Jones J. (2007). Cell adhesion molecules, the extracellular matrix and oral squamous carcinoma. *International Journal of Oral and Maxillofacial Surgery*, (August 2007), Vol.36, No.8, pp.671-679, ISSN 0901-5027.

Margoshes M & Vallee B. (1957). A cadmium protein form equine kidney cortex. *Journal of American Chemistry Society*, (September 1957), Vol.79, No.17, pp.4813-4814, ISSN 1520-5126.

Méplan C, Richard MJ & Hainaut P. (2000). Metalloregulation of the tumor suppressor protein p53: zinc mediates the renaturation of p53 after exposure to metal chelators in vitro and in intact cells. *Oncogene*, (November 2000), Vol.19, No.46, pp. 5227-5236, ISSN 0950-9232.

Merchant A, Husain SS, Hosain M, Fikree FF, Pitiphat W, Siddiqui AR, Hayder SJ, Haider SM, Ikram M, Chuang SK & Saeed SA. (2000). Paan without tobacco: an independent risk factor for oral cancer. *International Journal of Cancer*, (April 2000), Vol.86, No.1, pp.128-131, ISSN 0020-7136.

Mididoddi S, McGuirt JP, Sens MA, Todd JH & Sens DA. (1996). Isoform-specific expression of metallothionein mRNA in the developing and adult human kidney. *Toxicolgy Letters*, (April 1996), Vol.85, No.1, pp.17-27; ISSN 0378-4274, ISSN online 1879-3169.

Mitropoulos D, Kyroudi-Voulgari A, Theocharis S, Serafetinides E, Moraitis E, Zervas A & Kittas C. (2005). Prognostic significance of metallothionein expression in renal cell carcinoma. *World Journal of Surgical Oncology*, (January 2005), Vol.3, No.1, pp.5, ISSN 1477-7819.

Murata M, Gong P, Suzuki K & Koizumi S. (1999). Differential metal response and regulation of human heavy metal-inducible genes. *Journal of Cellullar Physiology*, (July 1999), Vol.180, No.1, pp.105-113, ISSN 1097-4652.

Nair UJ, Obe G, Friesen M, Goldberg MT & Bartsch H. (1992). Role of lime in the generation of reactive oxygen species from betel-quid ingredients. *Environmental Health Perspectives*, (November 1992), Vol.98, pp.203-205, ISSN 0091-6765.

Nakano M, Sogawa CA, Sogawa N, Mishima K, Yamachika E, Mizukawa N, Fukunaga J, Kawamoto T, Sawaki K, Sugahara T & Furuta H. (2003). Expression pattern of cisplatin-induced metallothionein isoforms in squamous cell carcinoma. *Anticancer Research*, (January-February 2003), Vol.23, No.1A, pp.299-303, ISSN 0250-7005.

Nascimento AG, Amaral AL, Prado LA, Kligerman J & Silveira TR. (1986). Adenoid cystic carcinoma of salivary glands. A study of 61 cases with clinicopathologic correlation. *Cancer*, (January 1986), Vol.57, No.2, pp.312-329, ISSN 0008-543X.

Nguyen T, Sherratt PJ & Pickett CB. (2003). Regulatory mechanisms controlling gene expression mediated by the antioxidant response element. *Annual Review of Pharmacology and Toxicology* (January 2002), Vol.43, pp.233-260, ISSN 0362-1642.

Ogawa Y. (2003). Immunocytochemistry of myoepithelial cells in the salivary glands. *Progress in Histochemistry and Cytochemistry*, (2003) Vol.38, No.4, pp.343-426, ISSN 0079-6336.

Ogra Y, Suzuki K, Gong P, Otsuka F & Koizumi S. (2001). Negative regulatory role of Sp1 in metal responsive element-mediated transcriptional activation. *The Journal of Biological Chemistry*, (May 2001), Vol.276, No.19, pp.16534-16539, ISSN 0021-9258.

Ono Y, Nakanishi Y, Ino Y, Niki T, Yamada T, Yoshimura K, Saikawa M, Nakajima T & Hirohashi S. (1999). Clinocopathologic significance of laminin-5 gamma2 chain expression in squamous cell carcinoma of the tongue: immunohistochemical analysis of 67 lesions. *Cancer*, (June 1999), Vol.85 No.11, pp.2315-2321, ISSN 0008-543X.

Ostrakhovitch EA, Olsson PE, Jiang S & Cherian MG. (2006). Interaction of metallothionein with tumor suppressor p53 protein. *FEBS Letters*, (February 2006), Vol.580, No. 5, pp.1235-1258, ISSN 0014-5793.

Otsuka F, Okugaito I, Ohsawa M, Iwamatsu A, Suzuki K & Koizumi S. (2000). Novel responses of ZRF, a variant of human MTF-1, to in vivo treatment with heavy metals. *Biochimica et Biophysica Acta*, (July 2000), Vol.1492, No.2-3, pp.330-340, ISSN 0167-4781.

Palmiter RD, Findley SD, Whitmore TE & Durnam DM. (1992). MT-III, a brain-specific member of the metallothionein gene family. *Proceedings of National Academy of Sciences of the United States of America*, (July 1992), Vol.89, No.14, pp.6333-6337, ISSN 0027-8424.

Palmiter RD. (1998). The elusive function of metallothioneins. *Proceedings of National Academy of Sciences of the United States of America*, (July 1998), Vol.95, No.15, pp.8428-8430, ISSN 0027-8424.

Pastuszewski W, Dziegiel P, Krecicki T, Podhorska-Okolow M, Ciesielska U, Gorzynska E & Zabel M. (2007). Prognostic significance of metallothionein, p53 protein and Ki-67 antigen expression in laryngeal cancer. *Anticancer Research*, (January-February 2007), Vol.27, No.1A, pp.335-342, ISSN 0250-7005.

Patarroyo M, Tryggvason K & Virtanen I. (2002). Laminin isoforms in tumor invasion, angiogenesis and metastasis. *Seminars in Cancer Biology*, (June 2002), Vol.12, No.3, pp.197-207, ISSN 1044-579X.

Pontes HA, de Aquino Xavier FC, da Silva TS, Fonseca FP, Paiva HB, Pontes FS & dos Santos Pinto D Jr. (2009). Metallothionein and p-Akt proteins in oral dysplasia and in oral squamous cell carcinoma: an immunohistochemical study. *Journal of Oral Pathology and Medicine*, (September 2009), Vol.38, No.8, pp. 644-650, ISSN 0904-2512.

Prasad ML, Barbacioru CC, Rawal YB, Husein O & Wen P. (2008). Hierarchical cluster analysis of myoepithelial/basal cell markers in adenoid cystic carcinoma and polymorphous low-grade adenocarcinoma. *Modern Pathology*, (February 2008), Vol.21, No.2, pp.105-114, ISSN 0893-3952.

Quaife CJ, Findley SD, Erickson JC, Froelick GJ, Kelly EJ, Zambrowicz BP & Palmiter RD. (1994). Induction of a new metallothionein isoform (MT-IV) occurs during differentiation of stratified squamous epithelia. *Biochemistry*, (June 1994), Vol.33, No.23, pp.7250-7259, ISSN 0006-2960.

Rainwater R, Parks D, Anderson ME, Tegtmeyer P & Mann K. (1995). Role of cysteine residues in regulation of p53 function. *Molecular Cell Biology*, (July 1995), Vol.15, No.7, pp.3892-3903, ISSN 0270-7306.

Rainwater R, Parks D, Anderson ME, Tegtmeyer P & Mann K. (1995). Role of cysteine residues in regulation of p53 function. *Molecular and Cellular Biology*, (July 1995), Vol.15, No.7, pp.3892-3903, ISSN 0270-7306.

Reinecke F, Levanets O, Olivier Y, Louw R, Semete B, Grobler A, Hidalgo J, Smeitink J, Olckers A & Van der Westhuizen FH. (2006). Metallothionein isoform 2A expression is inducible and protects against ROS-mediated cell death in rotenone-treated HeLa cells. *Biochemistry Journal*, (April 2006), Vol.395, No.2, pp.405-415, ISSN 0264-6021.

Remmele W & Stegner HE. (1987). Recommendation for uniform definition of an immunoreactive score (IRS) for immunohistochemical estrogen receptor detection (ER-ICA) in breast cancer tissue. *Pathologe*, (May 1987), Vol.8, No.3, pp.138-140, ISSN 0172-8113.

Samson SL & Gedamu L. (1998). Molecular analyses of metallothionein gene regulation. *Progress in Nucleic Acid Research and Molecular Biology*, (1998), Vol.59, pp.257-288; ISSN 0079-6603.

Saydam N, Adams TK, Steiner F, Schaffner W & Freedman JH. (2002). Regulation of metallothionein transcription by the metal-responsive transcription factor MTF-1:

identification of signal transduction cascades that control metal-inducible transcription. *Journal of Biological Chemistry*, (June 2002), Vol.277, No.23, pp. 20438-20445, ISSN 0021-9258.

Shimoda R, Achanzar WE, Qu W, Nagamine T, Takagi H, Mori M & Waalkes MP. (2003). Metallothionein is a potential negative regulator of apoptosis. *Toxicological Sciences*, (June 2003), Vol.73, No.2, pp.294-300, ISSN 1096-6080.

Shiu MN & Chen TH. (2004). Impact of betel quid, tobacco and alcohol on three-stage disease natural history of oral leukoplakia and cancer: implication for prevention of oral cancer. *European Journal of Cancer Prevention*, (February 2004), Vol.13, No.1, pp.39-45, ISSN 0959-8278.

Siegel R, Ward E, Brawley O & Jemal A. (2011). Cancer statistics, 2011: The impact of eliminating socioeconomic and racial disparities on premature cancer deaths. *CA: a Cancer Journal for Clinicians*, Vol.61, No.4, (July-August 2011), pp. 212-236, ISSN 0007-9235.

Stoltzfus P, Högmo A, Lindholm J, Aspenblad U, Auer G & Munck-Wikland E. (2004). The gamma2 chain of laminin-5 as an indicator of increased risk for recurrence in T1 stage tongue cancer. *Anticancer Research*, (September-October 2004), Vol.24, No.5B, pp.3109-3114, ISSN 0250-7005.

Sunardhi-Widyaputra S, van den Oord JJ, Van Houdt K, De Ley M & Van Damme B. (1995). Identification of Metallothionein- and parathyroid hormone-related peptide (PTHrP)-positive cells in salivary gland tumours. *Pathology Research and Practice*, (November 1995), Vol.191, No.11, pp.1092-1098, ISSN 0344-0338.

Sundelin K, Jadner M, Norberg-Spaak L, Davidsson A & Hellquist HB. (1997). Metallothionein and Fas (CD95) are expressed in squamous cell carcinoma of the tongue. *European Journal of Cancer*, (October 1997), Vol.33, No.11, pp.1860-1864, ISSN 0959-8049.

Surowiak P, Materna V, Kaplenko I, Spaczyński M, Dietel M, Lage H & Zabel M. (2005) Augmented expression of metallothionein and glutathione S-transferase pi as unfavourable prognostic factors in cisplatin-treated ovarian cancer patients. *Virchows Archives*, (September 2005), Vol.447, No.3, pp.626-633, ISSN 0945-6317.

Surowiak P, Materna V, Maciejczyk A, Pudełko M, Markwitz E, Spaczyński M, Dietel M, Zabel M & Lage H. (2007). Nuclear metallothionein expression correlates with cisplatin resistance of ovarian cancer cells and poor clinical outcome. *Virchows Archives*, (March 2007) Vol.450, No.3, pp.279-285, ISSN 0945-6317.

Szajerka A, Dziegiel P, Szajerka T, Zabel M, Winowski J & Grzebieniak Z. (2008). Immunohistochemical evaluation of metallothionein, Mcm-2 and Ki-67 antigen expression in tumors of the adrenal cortex. *Anticancer Research*, (September-October 2008), Vol.28, No.5B, pp.2959-2265, ISSN 0250-7005.

Szelachowska J, Dziegiel P, Jelen-Krzeszewska J, Jelen M, Tarkowski R, Spytkowska B, Matkowski R & Kornafel J. (2009). Correlation of metallothionein expression with clinical progression of cancer in the oral cavity. *Anticancer Research*, (February 2009), Vol.29, No.2, pp.589-595, ISSN 0250-7005.

Szelachowska J, Dziegiel P, Jelen-Krzeszewska J, Jelen M, Tarkowski R, Wlodarska I, Spytkowska B, Gisterek I, Matkowski R & Kornafel J. (2008). Prognostic significance of nuclear and cytoplasmic expression of metallothioneins as related to proliferative activity in squamous cell carcinomas of oral cavity. *Histology Histopathology*, (July 2008), Vol.23, No.7, pp.843-551, ISSN 0213-3911.

Theocharis SE, Margeli AP, Klijanienko JT & Kouraklis GP. (2004). Metallothionein expression in human neoplasia. *Histopathology*, (August 2004), Vol.45, No.2, pp.103-118, ISSN 0309-0167.

Trivedy C, Baldwin D, Warnakulasuriya S, Johnson N & Peters T. (1997). Copper content in Areca catechu (betel nut) products and oral submucous fibrosis. *Lancet*. (May 1997), Vol.349, No.9063, p.1447, ISSN 0140-6736.

Vasák M & Hasler DW. (2000). Metallothioneins: new functional and structural insights. *Current Opinion in Chemical Biology*, (April 2000), Vol.4, No.2, pp.177-183, ISSN 1367-5931.

Vasák M. (2005). Advances in metallothionein structure and functions. Journal of Trace Elements in Medicine and Biology, (2005), Vol.19, No.1, pp.13-17, ISSN 0946-672X.

Vázquez-Ramírez FJ, González-Cámpora JJ, Hevia-Alvarez E, Fernández-Santos JM, Ríos-Martín JJ, Otal-Salaverri C & González-Cámpora R. (2000). P-glycoprotein, metallothionein and NM23 protein expressions in breast carcinoma. *Pathology, Research and Practice*, (2000), Vol.196, No.8, pp. 553-559, ISSN 0344-0338.

West KA, Brognard J, Clark AS, Linnoila IR, Yang X, Swain SM, Harris C, Belinsky S & Dennis PA. (2003). Rapid Akt activation by nicotine and a tobacco carcinogen modulates the phenotype of normal human airway epithelial cells. *Journal of Clin Investigation*, (January 2003), Vol.111, No.1, pp.81-90, ISSN 0021-9738.

West KA, Linnoila IR, Brognard J, Belinsky S, Harris C & Dennis PA. (2004). Tobacco carcinogen-induced cellular transformation increases Akt activation in vitro and in vivo. *Chest*, (May 2004) Vol.125, No.5, pp.101-102, ISSN 0012-3692.

Woo ES, Kondo Y, Watkins SC, Hoyt DG & Lazo JS. (1996). Nucleophilic distribution of metallothionein in human tumor cells. *Experimental Cell Research*, (May 1996), Vol.224., No.2, pp.365-371, ISSN 0014-4827.

Yamamoto M, Tsujinaka T, Shiozaki H, Doki Y, Tamura S, Inoue M, Hirao M & Monden M. (1999). Metallothionein expression correlates with the pathological response of patients with esophageal cancer undergoing preoperative chemoradiation therapy. *Oncology*, (1999), Vol.56, No.4, pp.332-337, ISSN 0030-2414.

Zalups RK, Fraser J & Koropatnick J. (1995). Enhanced transcription of metallothionein genes in rat kidney: effect of uninephrectomy and compensatory renal growth. *American Journal of Physiology*, (April 1995), Vol.268, No.4 Pt 2, pp.F643-F650, ISSN 1931-857X.

Zangger K, Shen G, Oz G, Otvos JD & Armitage IM. (2001). Oxidative dimerization in metallothionein is a result of intermolecular disulphide bonds between cysteines in the alpha-domain. *Biochemical Journal*, (October 2001), Vol.359, No.2, pp.353-360, ISSN 0264-6021.

20

Epithelial-Mesenchymal Interactions in Oral Cancer Metastasis

Silvana Papagerakis[1,*] and Giuseppe Pannone[2]
[1]Department of Otolaryngology, Head and Neck Surgery, Laboratory of Oral, Head and Neck Cancer Invasion and Metastasis, Medical School, University of Michigan Ann Arbor, UM Comprehensive Cancer Center, Ann Arbor, MI
[2]Department of Surgical Sciences, Section of Anatomic Pathology and Cytopathology, University of Foggia, Foggia,
[1]USA
[2]Italy

1. Introduction

Squamous cell carcinoma of the oral cavity is one of the most prevalent tumors of the head and neck region. Despite an ever-expanding fund of knowledge regarding the etiology and pathophysiology of malignant neoplasms, oral squamous cell carcinoma (OSCC) continues to be a disfiguring and deadly disease. For patients with squamous cell carcinoma of the oral cavity or oropharynx, the 5-year survival is a dismal 56%, which has remained relatively unchanged in recent years (Davis et al., 2010). This poor prognosis reflects the fact that most patients present with advanced-stage disease, often making a complete cure a seemingly unattainable goal. In fact, just 46% of oral cavity and 16% of oropharyngeal cancers are diagnosed when there is only local disease (Davis et al., 2010). Despite recent improvements in therapeutic approaches, treatment failure takes the form of local and regional recurrences, but as disease control in these areas improves OSCC treatment failures more commonly occur as distant metastasis. Metastatic behavior is critical to survival, since patients with oral carcinomas that have distant disease have a five-year survival rate that is three times less than that of patients with spread to lymph nodes (Singh and Shah, 2003).

OSCC displays a wide range of metastatic behavior that cannot be predicted by tumor size, standard histology, or even individual gene or protein expression/activity (Singh and Shah, 2003). Despite the clinically obvious heterogeneity of OSCC, there are currently no means of predicting individual tumor behavior (Myers, 2010). Even small primary tumors of the oral cavity have a propensity to metastasize to cervical nodes, mandating that the majority of patients, even those with no clinical or radiographic evidence of nodal metastases, undergo some form of neck treatment either for staging or therapeutic purposes. Accurate prediction of metastasis in OSCC would have an immediate clinical impact through avoidance of unnecessary treatment of patients at low risk with appropriate direction of resources toward aggressive treatment of patients at high risk of having metastatic disease. Additionally,

* Corresponding Author

elucidation of key pathways and molecular mechanisms in tumor metastasis may direct therapeutic investigation and intervention.

Loss of epithelial morphology and acquisition of mesenchymal characteristics, termed the epithelial-to-mesenchymal transition (EMT), are typical for carcinoma cells during tumor progression and correlate with the local invasiveness and metastatic potential of the tumor (Birchmeier et al., 1996; Hollier et al., 2009). Cancer metastasis follows a sequential series of events, and many of the critical steps are distinctly similar to EMT-like transformations that occur during normal embryonic development. Recently, it was proposed that carcinoma cells, especially in metastatic sites, could acquire the mesenchymal-to-epithelial reverting transition (MErT) in order to adapt the microenvironments (Baum et al., 2008). This chapter explores the current status of investigations into the EMT/MErT transformations during the OSCC progression and the potential of these studies to positively impact the clinical management of OSCC in the future. The promise of using biomarker-based treatment decisions has yet to be fully realized given our limited understanding of the biology of metastatic spread in OSCC.

EMT describes a process in which epithelial cells undergo alterations in cellular architecture (lose of their characteristic epithelial polarity), adhesion (disassemble of cell-cell junctions), morphology (assuming a fibroblastoid mesenchymal morphology) and acquisition of migratory and invasive capabilities (Iwatsuki et al., 2010; Maeda et al., 2005; Thiery, 2002; Wells et al., 2008). EMT has been postulated as a versatile mechanism which facilitates cellular repositioning and redeployment during embryonic development, tissue reconstruction after injury, carcinogenesis, and tumor metastasis (Boyer et al., 2000; Roussos et al., 2010). In this context, EMT, a process first appreciated by developmental biologists, is attracting increasing attention from oncologists. Tumors are often viewed as corrupt forms of normal developmental processes (Thiery et al., 2009). Indeed, genes that are important in embryonic development are frequently found to be culprits in cancer. Conversely, genes discovered for their oncogenic role are often found to be key players in embryogenesis (Yang et al., 2008). This trend applies to the steps that initiate tumor formation. It also applies to the cross-talk with the inflammation (Lopez-Novoa and Nieto, 2009; Yadav et al., 2011) as well as to the steps that mediate tumor progression, including local invasion, intravasation into circulation and, most devastatingly, metastatic development through the establishment of secondary growths at sites distant from the primary tumor (Iwatsuki et al., 2010; Kalluri and Weinberg, 2009). There is good evidence that EMT gives rise to the dissemination of single carcinoma cells from the sites of the primary tumors (Wellner et al., 2009; Wu and Yang, 2011). More generally, it has been postulated that EMT might be involved in the dedifferentiation program that leads to malignant carcinoma. Some authors highlight the concept of altered differentiation program leading to the loss of type-specific epithelial differentiation markers and/or expression of typical mesenchymal-type proteins (Thiery, 2002). The typical example is a dedifferentiated epithelial cancer showing loss of cytokeratins and acquisition of mesenchymal markers such as Snail1, vimentin and/or fibronectin. Among many others, commonly used molecular markers for EMT include increased expression of N-cadherin and vimentin, nuclear localization of β-catenin, and increased production of the transcription factors such as Snail1 (Snail), Snail2 (Slug), Twist, EF1/ZEB1, SIP1/ZEB2, and/or E47 that inhibit E-cadherin production. Phenotypic markers for an EMT include an increased capacity for migration and three-dimensional invasion, as well as resistance to anoikis/apoptosis. Recent research conducted in embryonic model system and in normal and transformed cell lines has identified several signal-transduction pathways for EMT, and has examined the roles of a number of growth factors in inducing EMT (Said and Williams, 2011). Recent studies have focused on better understanding the role of cancer stem cells in EMT as it relates to tumor progression in general (Alison et al., 2010; Fuxe et al., 2010; Martin and Cano, 2010; Raimondi et al., 2011; Takahashi et al., 2010) and to oral, head and neck cancer in particular (Chen et al., 2011; Davis et al., 2010; Lo et al., 2011). In this review, only few of the most important EMT players are discussed with respect to other critical mediators and within most common pathways that promote the phenotypic transformation. It is important to note that individual players do not work in isolation - there is extensive crosstalk between pathways, and the effect of a given inducer on EMT seems to be contextual.

Deregulation of several other pathways has been implicated in EMT (Boyer et al., 2000). To name only few, transforming growth factor-β (TGF-β), epidermal growth factor (EGF) family members, fibroblast growth factors (FGF), hepatocyte growth factor (HGF), and insulin-like growth factor (IGF) have all been shown to induce EMT in an autocrine or paracrine manner (Baum et al., 2008). TGF-β was the first EMT inducer described in normal mammary epithelial cells by signaling through its receptor serine-threonine kinase complex (Fuxe et al., 2010). It remains the main and the best-characterized inducer of EMT phenotype in a variety of biological and patho-physiological conditions. TGF-β has an important tumor suppressor function at the early stage of tumorigenesis by inducing apoptosis and cell cycle arrest. However, it acts as a positive modulator of tumor progression in the late phase of tumorigenesis. This tumor promotional function of TGF-β, which is consistent with its EMT-induction activity, plays an important role in tumor progression including invasion and metastasis (Fuxe et al., 2010). Recent evidence indicates that the underlying mechanism of the prognostic value of Smad (2 and 6) for overall survival in OSCC patients is the aberrant TGF-β signaling (Mangone et al., 2010). Disruption in TGF-β induced Smad signaling occur during induced hamster buccal-pouch squamous cell carcinogenesis (Chen et al., 2011). Furthermore, the inhibition of TGF-β pathway in normal human oral keratinocytes leads to suppression of Bmi1-mediated cell senescence (Kim et al., 2010). TGF-β also seems to play an important role in the bone invasion by OSCC cells (Goda et al., 2010) as well as in the metastatic dissemination of salivary adenoid cystic carcinoma (Dong et al., 2011). Being a major inducer of EMT, TGF-β is able to regulate the activation of other signaling pathways besides establishing a hierarchical gene network. TGF-β-mediated signaling during EMT involves both gene expression-dependent and -independent pathways (Said and Williams, 2011). TGF-β cooperates with Wnt, Hedgehog, Notch and Ras signaling pathways to induce complete EMT. EMT signaling pathways have many common endpoints and E-cadherin is a central target (Thiery and Sleeman, 2006).

Loss of E-cadherin: E-cadherin is emerging as one of the caretakers of the epithelial phenotype with critical roles in adherens junctions and desmosomes (Garrod et al., 1996; Papagerakis et al., 2009). Our groups have devoted a large number of studies on the cadherin/catenin mediated adhesion in oral carcinogenesis (Lo Muzio et al., 2005; Lo Muzio et al., 2004; Lo Muzio et al., 2002; Lo Muzio et al., 1999; Pannone et al., 1998; Papagerakis et al., 2011; Papagerakis et al., 2004; Papagerakis et al., 2009) Among the mechanisms largely associated with the metastatic conversion of epithelial cells and the EMT, the loss of E-cadherin-mediated cell adhesion is prominent; overall there is a trend towards a loss of E-cadherin during carcinoma progression including the OSCC (Huber et al., 2011). E-cadherin production is maintain in most differentiated tumors including carcinomas of the head and neck, but there seems to be an inverse correlation between E-cadherin levels and patient survival (Hirohashi, 1998; Kaur et al., 2009; Nguyen et al., 2011). In most cases, down-regulation of E-cadherin during OSCC carcinoma progression occurs by epigenetic mechanisms, including transcriptional repression and promoter hypermethylation (Kudo et al., 2004). Occasionally, the E-cadherin gene is mutated leading to the absence or to the expression of a non-functional protein (Berx et al., 1995; Yoshimura et al., 1996), however no mutations have been reported in OSCC. In vitro, there is a direct correlation between the lack of E-cadherin production and loss of epithelial phenotype (Behrens et al., 1989). Acquisition of the mesenchymal phenotype has been also associated with invasive behavior in vitro in three-dimensional collagen gels and hearts explants (Chen and Obrink, 1991) and the partial or complete reversal of the invasive mesenchymal phenotype was observed if E-cadherin is constitutively produced (Behrens et al., 1991; Kim et al., 2000; Vleminckx et al., 1991). Recently, it was proposed that carcinoma cells, especially in metastatic sites, could acquire the mesenchymal-to-epithelial reverting transition (MErT) in order to adapt the microenvironments and re-expression of E-cadherin be a critical indicator of MErT (Baum et al., 2008; Wells et al., 2008). Among E-cadherin repressors counts Snail, considered a "master gene" in the conversion from the epithelial to fibroblastic state, and a closely related member of the same family, Slug, both detected at sites of EMT in vertebrates (Nieto et al., 1994). Carcinoma cell lines that lack E-cadherin produce significant amounts of Snail, and the transfection of E-cadherin-positive lines with Snail results in the induction of EMT and the expression of mesenchymal markers (Batlle et al., 2000; Cano et al., 2000). There seems to be a causal link between the production of these transcriptional repressors and the down-regulation of E-cadherin during tumor progression. Snail expression was inversely correlated with E-cadherin expression in a number of cancers including OSCC (Batlle et al., 2000; Cano et al., 2000; Takkunen et al., 2006; Yokoyama et al., 2001). Transcriptional repressors of the E-cadherin gene are activated downstream in these pathways, leading to the loss of the epithelial phenotype. Given that in most advanced human tumors including OSCC, the loss of E-cadherin might be incomplete, with foci of E-cadherin-positive carcinoma cells mingling with negative areas, along with E-cadherin detection in metastatic tumors, it may suggest that rather than a single-gene control it could be more likely a general mechanism that is associated with the dedifferentiation program in which E-cadherin is lost. It is important to note that the immunohistological detection of E-cadherin within the positive tumoral foci is not necessarily indicative of a normal function of the protein; additional investigations are required to asses its functionality even in the presence of an apparent normal cellular distribution. In vivo evidence of EMT in tumors can be difficult to obtain due to the transient nature of the EMT process and may require combined immunohistochemical staining for several EMT markers. The loss of E-cadherin in normal epithelial cells and more importantly in carcinoma cells might deregulate cell growth, suggesting that in addition to contributing to the maintenance of the differentiation program, E-cadherin might also regulate cell proliferation, via activation of the Fos oncogene (Eger et al., 2000; Reichmann et al., 1992) or by altering the ß-catenin transcriptional activity through the Wnt signaling pathway (Gottardi et al., 2001; Stockinger et al., 2001).

Cadherin switching: Aberrant N-cadherin expression and E-cadherin/N-cadherin switching (EN-Switch) have been involved in EMT. They represent an independent prognostic marker in cancer progression; this concept has been well documented in gastric, prostate and oral carcinomas (Gravdal et al., 2007; Kim et al., 2009; Liu et al., 2010). Furthermore, some studies demonstrate that cadherin switching is necessary for increased motility but it is not required for the morphological changes that accompany EMT (Maeda et al., 2005) therefore, immunohistochemical detection should be performed in order to detect EN-Switch and the consequent EMT in oral cancer.

Wnt signaling: Our groups have a particular interest in WNT/ ß-catenin pathway (Lo Muzio et al., 2002; Pannone et al., 2010; Papagerakis et al., 2011). Dysregulation of the Wnt pathway via ß-catenin is a frequent event in EMT involved in the pathogenesis of several human cancers. In OSCC its roles still remain unclear. Although it is evident that constitutive activation of the Wnt / ß-catenin is frequently observed in oral cancer progression, only infrequent mutations have been found in genes encoding various components of this pathway that are commonly mutated in other cancers (adenomatous polyposis coli APC, (Kok et al., 2002); Axin, (Iwai et al., 2005; Rui et al., 2007); no ß-catenin mutations have been reported in OSCC, (Lo Muzio et al., 2005). This suggests activation of this pathway by multiple mechanisms. Furthermore, the interaction between epithelial tumor cells and the different components of the surrounding microenvironment can locally affect the intracellular level of Wnt/ß-catenin signaling components and differentially trigger tumor cell stemness, EMT, invasive behavior, and metastasis (Myers, 2010).

β-catenin: has a dual role in the EMT; it enhances cell–cell adhesion when bound to cadherin complexes in adherens junctions and also functions as a transcriptional co-activator upon entry into the nucleus. When the WNT pathway is in resting state, cytoplasmic ß-catenin is phosphorylated by glycogen synthase kinase (GSK)3-ß and actively degraded by a multiprotein destruction complex that also includes casein kinase 1, APC and Axin. Thus, the levels of free ß-catenin are kept bellow the threshold where aberrant transcriptional activity will occur. In response to Wnt ligand binding to its specific receptor, the destruction complex is inactivated by inhibiting the activity of GSK3-ß which results in dephosphorylation and stabilization of ß-catenin, enabling it to accumulate within the nucleus, where it interacts with T-cell factor 4 /lymphocyte enhancer factor (TCF4/LEF) transcription factors to activate the transcription of Wnt target genes (Behrens et al., 1996; van de Wetering et al., 1997). It has been demonstrated that a number of genes targeted by nuclear ß-catenin LEF/TCF pathway plays a significant role in EMT (Table 1). Repression of E-cadherin by Snail, Twist, or other repressors leads indirectly to expression of vimentin and other mesenchymal gene products, partly because of β-catenin/TCF–Lef1 activation. TGF-β is known to activate this canonical Wnt pathway; TGF-β and Wnt pathway can independently or cooperatively regulate LEF/TCF target genes (Huber et al., 2005). TGF-β also directly activates the TCF–Lef1 transcription complex through tyrosine phosphorylation of SMAD-2. It has been reported that Smad-2/4 repressed E-cadherin transcription through TCF–Lef1 (Masszi et al., 2004; Nawshad et al., 2005). Loss of membranous ß-catenin and E-cadherin associated with EMT have been shown to correlate with metastatic formation and poor prognosis in multiple solid tumors and is a common feature of OSCC (Kudo et al., 2004; Odajima et al., 2005; Tanaka et al., 2003; Wang and Ma, 2007; Williams et al., 1998). Several studies have demonstrated that cytoplasmic and nuclear localization of β-catenin is correlated with tumor progression, invasion and metastatic potential of OSCC (Ishida et al., 2007; Lo Muzio et al., 1999; Odajima et al., 2005; Yu et al., 2005). Cytoplasmic/nuclear β-catenin expression has also been found to significantly correlate with EGFR expression in OSCC (Odajima et al., 2005). In addition to the change in subcellular localization, phosphorylation of β-catenin may also be associated with OSCC progression and EMT (Tamura et al., 2003). It has been shown that tyrosine phosphorylation of β-catenin by EGFR is associated with the perturbation of E-cadherin - mediated cell adhesion and EMT acquisition and leads to increased cell motility that are requisite for metastatic dissemination (Hirohashi, 1998; Thiery, 2003). Furthermore, some authors have uncovered a new EMT pathway via p68 to nuclear ß-catenin (Yang et al., 2006). Given that EGF and TGF-β also induce p68 tyrosine phosphorylation, the nuclear ß-catenin is not simply a consequence of E-cadherin down-regulation during EMT, because phosphorylated p68 promotes ß-catenin nuclear localization regardless of whether E-cadherin is depleted or expressed. P68/ß-catenin axis may represent a common output for several signaling pathways. These pathways offer additional routes to nuclear ß-catenin signaling that are parallel to the Wnt pathway, which does not involve p68. The ability of β-catenin to enhance cadherin-dependent adhesion depends on β-catenin binding to α-catenin and on α-catenin binding to the cadherin (Chu et al., 2004). Phosphorylation of β-catenin residue Y142 prevents α-catenin interaction and enhances the binding of β-catenin to BCL9-2, which is the vertebrate homologue of the Drosophila melanogaster legless gene (Brembeck et al., 2006; Brembeck et al., 2004). Interaction of β-catenin with BCL9-2 enhances nuclear accumulation of both proteins simultaneously decreasing cadherin-mediated adhesion and activating catenin target gene transcription. Ectopic BCL9-2 expression is sufficient to induce EMT in cultured cells, and siRNA-mediated BCL9-2 inactivation drives the reverse mesenchymal–epithelial transition. Birchmeier reported that Y142 can be phosphorylated by the Met tyrosine kinase, indicating the existence of an EMT activation pathway where Met induces β-catenin nuclear translocation by enhancing BCL9-2 interaction (Heuberger and Birchmeier, 2010). This pathway satisfactorily links these two well known EMT regulators.

Akt pathway: Recently, activation of the Akt axis is emerging as a central feature of EMT. The Akt family of kinases is a downstream effector of phosphatidylinositol 3-kinase (PI3K) and is frequently activated in human epithelial cancers, including OSCC (Nakayama et al., 2001; Testa and Bellacosa, 2001). Akt activation in OSCC was linked to aggressive clinical behavior and the loss of histological features of epithelial differentiation (Lim et al., 2005). Akt-induced EMT involves down-regulation of E-cadherin, which appears to result from up-regulation of the transcription repressor Snail. Accordingly, inhibition of Akt activity induced down-regulation of EMT-related transcription factor Snail. Akt activity is induced by ligand stimulation of growth factor receptors such as the insulin-like growth factor-I receptor (IGF-IR) and the EGFRs (Hong et al., 2009; Hynes and Lane, 2005). It has been demonstrated that OSCC cells engineered to express constitutively active Akt underwent EMT, characterized by down-regulation of epithelial markers (desmoplakin, E-cadherin, β-catenin) and up-regulation of the mesenchymal marker vimentin, and exhibited enhanced tumor invasion (Grille et al., 2003). In contrast, the inhibition of Akt activity was able to restore epithelial characteristics, deplete mesenchymal features and reduce the migratory ability. This indicates that the inhibition of Akt activity could induce the MErT in OSCC cells and that the gain of epithelial characteristic might be an earlier or more prominent event in the MErT of the OSCC than the loss of mesenchymal one (Hong et al., 2009).

Name	Function	References
TNF-alpha	proinflammatory cytokine	Cawthorn WP et al *Cell Death Differ.* 2007
Osteopontin	extracellular matrix protein	Phlilip S et al *J Biol Chem.* 2005
Cyclin-D1 CCND1	Oncogene involved in cell proliferation	Cao J et al *World J Gastroenterol* 2006
c-myc	proto-oncogene involved in cellular proliferation	Cao J et al *World J Gastroenterol* 2006
Splicing Factor-1		
(SF-1)	regulates beta-cat gene transactivation and premessenger RNA splicing activities	Shitashige M et al *Gastroentetology* 2007
Notch1	transmembrane receptor that determines cell fate after its translocation to the nucleus where it activates gene transcription	Balint K et al *J Clin Invest.* 2005
Brn2	cell lineage-restricted genes	Larue L, Delmas V *Front Biosci.* 2006
Mitf-M	melanocyte-specific gene, with critical role in cell survival, proliferation and differentiation	Larue L, Delmas V *Front Biosci.* 2006
Dct	melanocyte-specific gene involved in melanoma proliferation	Larue L, Delmas V *Front Biosci.* 2006
MCP-1/CCL2	CC-chemokine implicated in tumour progression events such as angiogenesis or tumour associated macrophage (TAM) infiltration	Mestdagt M et al *Int J Cancer*, 2006
MYCBP	(myc binding protein)	Jung HC, Kim K *Life Sci.* 2005
MMP-7	Matrix Metalloproteinase Metastasis	Monaghan H.et al. *Histopathology.* 2007
CX43 (Connexin 43),	gap junctional protein	Husoy T et al. *Carcinogenesis.* 2003
PPAR-delta	peroxisome proliferator-activated receptor	Gupta RA et al *Proc Natl Acad Sci U S A.* 2000
ITF2 initiation transcription factor 2	transcription factor	Zhai Y et al. *Am J Pathol.* 2002
Survivin	Inhibition of apoptosis	Kim PJ et al. *Lancet* 2003
VEGF	Vascular endothelial growth factor	Calviello G et al *Carcinogenesis.* 2006
MT1-MMP	Membrane Type1-Matrix Metalloproteinase	Calviello G et al *Carcinogenesis.* 2006

Table 1.

C-met and tyrosine kinase receptors: The c-Met pathway has been implicated in the EMT during oral carcinogenesis; activating mutations have been found in metastatic head and neck carcinomas, but not in the corresponding primary tumors (Di Renzo et al., 2000).The activation of several other tyrosine kinase receptors, including fibroblast growth factor (FGF), insulin-like growth factor (IGF) and the ERBB family has been found to induce EMT in vivo and in vitro (Valles et al., 1990). Although the Met receptor-mediated signaling results in cell scattering, it has not been made clear whether Met signaling also has a more permanent effect on the expression or localization of some of the effectors of EMT, such as E-cadherin and β-catenin. Recent work suggests that Met also regulates intracellular localization of β-catenin (Heuberger and Birchmeier, 2010).

Twist: The basic helix-loop-helix transcription factor Twist, a master regulator of embryonic morphogenesis essential for initiating mesoderm development during gastrulation, was recently added to the growing list of developmental genes with a key role in E-cadherin repression and EMT induction, as well as metastasis (Kang and Massague, 2004; Martin and Cano, 2010). However, there have been very few reports on the relationship of Twist with the EMT in oral cancer cells. Hong et al (2009) reported that inhibition of Akt activity induced down-regulation of EMT-related Twist in OSCC cells. It has been recently reported that Twist directly regulates the stemness factor Bmi1, and that both proteins are required for the induction of EMT and stemness in head and neck squamous cell carcinoma (Yang et al., 2010). Twist is also induced by hypoxia showing a link between tumor microenvironment and the expression of EMT promoting transcription factors (Yang and Wu, 2008). Twist over-expression correlates with aggressive phenotypes and poor outcome in HNSCC (Yang et al., 2008). Twist can be up-regulated by Wnt signaling (Howe et al., 2003) and can bind and repress the E-cadherin promoter (Vesuna et al., 2008) in epithelial cells. Twist confers metastatic properties to breast tumor cells and stem-like properties in epithelial cells (Mani et al.; Morel et al., 2008; Yang et al., 2004).

Accumulating evidence demonstrates that tumor cells undergoing EMT acquire the capacity to migrate, invade the stroma and metastasize. EMT also involves other inducers such as matrix metalloproteinases (MMPs) and urokinase plasminogen activator which like growth factors, may be secreted by either the tumor cells themselves or by the surrounding tumor stromal cells. These molecules degrade the components of basal lamina leading to invasion of the migrating cancer cells into reactive stroma and subsequently lymphatic vessels and systemic circulation (Said and Williams, 2011). EMT cells also acquire stem cells characteristics suggesting crosstalk between EMT and pathways involved in promoting cellular stemness and that EMT might provide cells with both migratory and stem cells properties. Brabletz and colleagues proposed first the idea that disseminating cancer stem cells (CSC) represent the origin of metastasis (Brabletz et al., 2005). The experimental evidence to support this idea was provided by Weinberg and colleagues, by showing that cells induced to undergo EMT (by Twist/Snail/TFG-β) acquired a $CD44^{high}/Cd24^{low}$ signature, similar to a small sub-population of breast cancer stem cells that previously had been isolated and identified to have a unique ability to form tumors in xenograft models (Al-Hajj et al., 2003; Mani et al., 2008). Furthermore, EMT cells exhibited many properties of stem cells (mammospheres formation, ability to differentiate into cells of different lineages and to reconstitute a heterogenous tumor, (Mani et al., 2008). Another study reported that cells induced to undergo EMT by Ras-MAPK activation also displayed stem-like properties and a $CD44^{high}/CD24^{low}$ signature (Morel et al., 2008). Colleagues at the University of

Michigan first demonstrated that a CD44+ population of cells possesses the properties of CSC in head and neck cancer (Prince et al., 2007), followed by other reports on head and neck cancer stem cells using other markers in addition to CD44 (Clay et al., 2010; Krishnamurthy et al., 2010; Krishnamurthy and Nor, 2011). In our recent study, we reported increased motility of CD44^{high} CSC from head and neck cancer which is characteristic of cells undergoing EMT, and this may explain why, in our study, head and neck CSCs formed lung lesions in vivo, while non-CSCs did not (Davis et al., 2010). In fact, Takahashi et al. showed that, in EMT induced by tumor necrosis factor, the interaction between CD44 and hyaluronan indeed mediated cell-cell dissociation, actin remodeling, and, as a result, enhanced motility (Takahashi et al., 2010). These findings, in conjunction with our own, suggest that cell motility and the ability to undergo EMT are some of the most important characteristics of a metastatic cell, and it appears that CSCs may have those capabilities. Cancer stem cells seems to localize at the invasive fronts of the head and neck squamous cell carcinomas in the proximity of the blood vessels (Krishnamurthy and Nor, 2011) Future studies focused on better understanding the role of CSCs in EMT as it relates to oral, head and neck carcinomas are needed. In addition, further purification of the stemlike cell population in HNSCC is necessary to clarify what metastatic characteristics are indeed unique to these cells. Our laboratories are currently investigating these underlying mechanisms. Such knowledge would allow clinicians to exploit this particular set of attributes to target cancer cells that keep a tumor growing and allow it to spread. Furthermore, a better understanding of the EMT/MErT transformations during the OSCC progression will positively impact the clinical management of OSCC in the future.

2. References

Al-Hajj, M., M.S. Wicha, A. Benito-Hernandez, S.J. Morrison, and M.F. Clarke. 2003. Prospective identification of tumorigenic breast cancer cells. *Proc Natl Acad Sci U S A*. 100:3983-8.

Alison, M.R., S.M. Lim, and L.J. Nicholson. 2010. Cancer stem cells: problems for therapy? *J Pathol*. 223:147-61.

Batlle, E., E. Sancho, C. Franci, D. Dominguez, M. Monfar, J. Baulida, and A. Garcia De Herreros. 2000. The transcription factor snail is a repressor of E-cadherin gene expression in epithelial tumour cells. *Nat Cell Biol*. 2:84-9.

Baum, B., J. Settleman, and M.P. Quinlan. 2008. Transitions between epithelial and mesenchymal states in development and disease. *Semin Cell Dev Biol*. 19:294-308.

Behrens, J., M.M. Mareel, F.M. Van Roy, and W. Birchmeier. 1989. Dissecting tumor cell invasion: epithelial cells acquire invasive properties after the loss of uvomorulin-mediated cell-cell adhesion. *J Cell Biol*. 108:2435-47.

Behrens, J., J.P. von Kries, M. Kuhl, L. Bruhn, D. Wedlich, R. Grosschedl, and W. Birchmeier. 1996. Functional interaction of beta-catenin with the transcription factor LEF-1. *Nature*. 382:638-42.

Behrens, J., K.M. Weidner, U.H. Frixen, J.H. Schipper, M. Sachs, N. Arakaki, Y. Daikuhara, and W. Birchmeier. 1991. The role of E-cadherin and scatter factor in tumor invasion and cell motility. *EXS*. 59:109-26.

Berx, G., A.M. Cleton-Jansen, F. Nollet, W.J. de Leeuw, M. van de Vijver, C. Cornelisse, and F. van Roy. 1995. E-cadherin is a tumour/invasion suppressor gene mutated in human lobular breast cancers. *EMBO J*. 14:6107-15.

Birchmeier, C., W. Birchmeier, and B. Brand-Saberi. 1996. Epithelial-mesenchymal transitions in cancer progression. *Acta Anat (Basel)*. 156:217-26.

Boyer, B., A.M. Valles, and N. Edme. 2000. Induction and regulation of epithelial-mesenchymal transitions. *Biochem Pharmacol*. 60:1091-9.

Brabletz, T., A. Jung, S. Spaderna, F. Hlubek, and T. Kirchner. 2005. Opinion: migrating cancer stem cells - an integrated concept of malignant tumour progression. *Nat Rev Cancer*. 5:744-9.

Brembeck, F.H., M. Rosario, and W. Birchmeier. 2006. Balancing cell adhesion and Wnt signaling, the key role of beta-catenin. *Curr Opin Genet Dev*. 16:51-9.

Brembeck, F.H., T. Schwarz-Romond, J. Bakkers, S. Wilhelm, M. Hammerschmidt, and W. Birchmeier. 2004. Essential role of BCL9-2 in the switch between beta-catenin's adhesive and transcriptional functions. *Genes Dev*. 18:2225-30.

Cano, A., M.A. Perez-Moreno, I. Rodrigo, A. Locascio, M.J. Blanco, M.G. del Barrio, F. Portillo, and M.A. Nieto. 2000. The transcription factor snail controls epithelial-mesenchymal transitions by repressing E-cadherin expression. *Nat Cell Biol*. 2:76-83.

Chen, W.C., and B. Obrink. 1991. Cell-cell contacts mediated by E-cadherin (uvomorulin) restrict invasive behavior of L-cells. *J Cell Biol*. 114:319-27.

Chen, Y.K., S.H. Yang, A.H. Huang, S.S. Hsue, and L.M. Lin. 2011. Aberrant expression in multiple components of the transforming growth factor-beta1-induced Smad signaling pathway during 7,12-dimethylbenz[a]anthracene-induced hamster buccal-pouch squamous-cell carcinogenesis. *Oral Oncol*. 47:262-7.

Chu, E.Y., J. Hens, T. Andl, A. Kairo, T.P. Yamaguchi, C. Brisken, A. Glick, J.J. Wysolmerski, and S.E. Millar. 2004. Canonical WNT signaling promotes mammary placode development and is essential for initiation of mammary gland morphogenesis. *Development*. 131:4819-29.

Clay, M.R., M. Tabor, J.H. Owen, T.E. Carey, C.R. Bradford, G.T. Wolf, M.S. Wicha, and M.E. Prince. 2010. Single-marker identification of head and neck squamous cell carcinoma cancer stem cells with aldehyde dehydrogenase. *Head Neck*. 32:1195-201.

Davis, S.J., V. Divi, J.H. Owen, C.R. Bradford, T.E. Carey, S. Papagerakis, and M.E. Prince. 2010. Metastatic potential of cancer stem cells in head and neck squamous cell carcinoma. *Arch Otolaryngol Head Neck Surg*. 136:1260-6.

Di Renzo, M.F., M. Olivero, T. Martone, A. Maffe, P. Maggiora, A.D. Stefani, G. Valente, S. Giordano, G. Cortesina, and P.M. Comoglio. 2000. Somatic mutations of the MET oncogene are selected during metastatic spread of human HNSC carcinomas. *Oncogene*. 19:1547-55.

Dong, L., Y.X. Wang, S.L. Li, G.Y. Yu, Y.H. Gan, D. Li, and C.Y. Wang. 2011. TGF-beta1 promotes migration and invasion of salivary adenoid cystic carcinoma. *J Dent Res*. 90:804-9.

Eger, A., A. Stockinger, B. Schaffhauser, H. Beug, and R. Foisner. 2000. Epithelial mesenchymal transition by c-Fos estrogen receptor activation involves nuclear translocation of beta-catenin and upregulation of beta-catenin/lymphoid enhancer binding factor-1 transcriptional activity. *J Cell Biol*. 148:173-88.

Fuxe, J., T. Vincent, and A. Garcia de Herreros. 2010. Transcriptional crosstalk between TGF-beta and stem cell pathways in tumor cell invasion: role of EMT promoting Smad complexes. *Cell Cycle*. 9:2363-74.

Garrod, D., M. Chidgey, and A. North. 1996. Desmosomes: differentiation, development, dynamics and disease. *Curr Opin Cell Biol.* 8:670-8.

Goda, T., T. Shimo, Y. Yoshihama, N.M. Hassan, S. Ibaragi, N. Kurio, T. Okui, T. Honami, K. Kishimoto, and A. Sasaki. 2010. Bone destruction by invading oral squamous carcinoma cells mediated by the transforming growth factor-beta signalling pathway. *Anticancer Res.* 30:2615-23.

Gottardi, C.J., E. Wong, and B.M. Gumbiner. 2001. E-cadherin suppresses cellular transformation by inhibiting beta-catenin signaling in an adhesion-independent manner. *J Cell Biol.* 153:1049-60.

Gravdal, K., O.J. Halvorsen, S.A. Haukaas, and L.A. Akslen. 2007. A switch from E-cadherin to N-cadherin expression indicates epithelial to mesenchymal transition and is of strong and independent importance for the progress of prostate cancer. *Clin Cancer Res.* 13:7003-11.

Grille, S.J., A. Bellacosa, J. Upson, A.J. Klein-Szanto, F. van Roy, W. Lee-Kwon, M. Donowitz, P.N. Tsichlis, and L. Larue. 2003. The protein kinase Akt induces epithelial mesenchymal transition and promotes enhanced motility and invasiveness of squamous cell carcinoma lines. *Cancer Res.* 63:2172-8.

Heuberger, J., and W. Birchmeier. 2010. Interplay of cadherin-mediated cell adhesion and canonical Wnt signaling. *Cold Spring Harb Perspect Biol.* 2:a002915.

Hirohashi, S. 1998. Inactivation of the E-cadherin-mediated cell adhesion system in human cancers. *Am J Pathol.* 153:333-9.

Hollier, B.G., K. Evans, and S.A. Mani. 2009. The epithelial-to-mesenchymal transition and cancer stem cells: a coalition against cancer therapies. *J Mammary Gland Biol Neoplasia.* 14:29-43.

Hong, K.O., J.H. Kim, J.S. Hong, H.J. Yoon, J.I. Lee, S.P. Hong, and S.D. Hong. 2009. Inhibition of Akt activity induces the mesenchymal-to-epithelial reverting transition with restoring E-cadherin expression in KB and KOSCC-25B oral squamous cell carcinoma cells. *J Exp Clin Cancer Res.* 28:28.

Howe, L.R., O. Watanabe, J. Leonard, and A.M. Brown. 2003. Twist is up-regulated in response to Wnt1 and inhibits mouse mammary cell differentiation. *Cancer Res.* 63:1906-13.

Huber, G.F., L. Zullig, A. Soltermann, M. Roessle, N. Graf, S.K. Haerle, G. Studer, W. Jochum, H. Moch, and S.J. Stoeckli. 2011. Down regulation of E-Cadherin (ECAD) - a predictor for occult metastatic disease in sentinel node biopsy of early squamous cell carcinomas of the oral cavity and oropharynx. *BMC Cancer.* 11:217:1-8.

Huber, M.A., N. Kraut, and H. Beug. 2005. Molecular requirements for epithelial-mesenchymal transition during tumor progression. *Curr Opin Cell Biol.* 17:548-58.

Hynes, N.E., and H.A. Lane. 2005. ERBB receptors and cancer: the complexity of targeted inhibitors. *Nat Rev Cancer.* 5:341-54.

Ishida, K., S. Ito, N. Wada, H. Deguchi, T. Hata, M. Hosoda, and T. Nohno. 2007. Nuclear localization of beta-catenin involved in precancerous change in oral leukoplakia. *Mol Cancer.* 6:62.

Iwai, S., W. Katagiri, C. Kong, S. Amekawa, M. Nakazawa, and Y. Yura. 2005. Mutations of the APC, beta-catenin, and axin 1 genes and cytoplasmic accumulation of beta-catenin in oral squamous cell carcinoma. *J Cancer Res Clin Oncol.* 131:773-82.

Iwatsuki, M., K. Mimori, T. Yokobori, H. Ishi, T. Beppu, S. Nakamori, H. Baba, and M. Mori. 2010. Epithelial-mesenchymal transition in cancer development and its clinical significance. *Cancer Sci*. 101:293-9.

Kalluri, R., and R.A. Weinberg. 2009. The basics of epithelial-mesenchymal transition. *J Clin Invest*. 119:1420-8.

Kang, Y., and J. Massague. 2004. Epithelial-mesenchymal transitions: twist in development and metastasis. *Cell*. 118:277-9.

Kaur, G., S. Carnelio, N. Rao, and L. Rao. 2009. Expression of E-cadherin in primary oral squamous cell carcinoma and metastatic lymph nodes: an immunohistochemical study. *Indian J Dent Res*. 20:71-6.

Kim, J.B., S. Islam, Y.J. Kim, R.S. Prudoff, K.M. Sass, M.J. Wheelock, and K.R. Johnson. 2000. N-Cadherin extracellular repeat 4 mediates epithelial to mesenchymal transition and increased motility. *J Cell Biol*. 151:1193-206.

Kim, M.A., H.S. Lee, H.E. Lee, J.H. Kim, H.K. Yang, and W.H. Kim. 2009. Prognostic importance of epithelial-mesenchymal transition-related protein expression in gastric carcinoma. *Histopathology*. 54:442-51.

Kim, R.H., M.B. Lieberman, R. Lee, K.H. Shin, S. Mehrazarin, J.E. Oh, N.H. Park, and M.K. Kang. 2010. Bmi-1 extends the life span of normal human oral keratinocytes by inhibiting the TGF-beta signaling. *Exp Cell Res*. 316:2600-8.

Kok, S.H., J.J. Lee, H.C. Hsu, C.P. Chiang, Y.S. Kuo, and M.Y. Kuo. 2002. Mutations of the adenomatous polyposis coli gene in areca quid and tobacco-associated oral squamous cell carcinomas in Taiwan. *J Oral Pathol Med*. 31:395-401.

Krishnamurthy, S., Z. Dong, D. Vodopyanov, A. Imai, J.I. Helman, M.E. Prince, M.S. Wicha, and J.E. Nor. 2010. Endothelial cell-initiated signaling promotes the survival and self-renewal of cancer stem cells. *Cancer Res*. 70:9969-78.

Krishnamurthy, S., and J.E. Nor. 2011. Head and Neck Cancer Stem Cells. *J Dent Res*.

Kudo, Y., S. Kitajima, I. Ogawa, M. Hiraoka, S. Sargolzaei, M.R. Keikhaee, S. Sato, M. Miyauchi, and T. Takata. 2004. Invasion and metastasis of oral cancer cells require methylation of E-cadherin and/or degradation of membranous beta-catenin. *Clin Cancer Res*. 10:5455-63.

Lim, J., J.H. Kim, J.Y. Paeng, M.J. Kim, S.D. Hong, J.I. Lee, and S.P. Hong. 2005. Prognostic value of activated Akt expression in oral squamous cell carcinoma. *J Clin Pathol*. 58:1199-205.

Liu, L.K., X.Y. Jiang, X.X. Zhou, D.M. Wang, X.L. Song, and H.B. Jiang. 2010. Upregulation of vimentin and aberrant expression of E-cadherin/beta-catenin complex in oral squamous cell carcinomas: correlation with the clinicopathological features and patient outcome. *Mod Pathol*. 23:213-24.

Lo, J.F., C.C. Yu, S.H. Chiou, C.Y. Huang, C.I. Jan, S.C. Lin, C.J. Liu, W.Y. Hu, and Y.H. Yu. 2011. The epithelial-mesenchymal transition mediator S100A4 maintains cancer-initiating cells in head and neck cancers. *Cancer Res*. 71:1912-23.

Lo Muzio, L., G. Goteri, R. Capretti, C. Rubini, A. Vinella, R. Fumarulo, F. Bianchi, F. Mastrangelo, E. Porfiri, and M.A. Mariggio. 2005. Beta-catenin gene analysis in oral squamous cell carcinoma. *Int J Immunopathol Pharmacol*. 18:33-8.

Lo Muzio, L., G. Pannone, M.D. Mignogna, S. Staibano, M.A. Mariggio, C. Rubini, M. Procaccini, M. Dolci, P. Bufo, G. De Rosa, and A. Piattelli. 2004. P-cadherin expression predicts clinical outcome in oral squamous cell carcinomas. *Histol Histopathol.* 19:1089-99.

Lo Muzio, L., G. Pannone, S. Staibano, M.D. Mignogna, M. Grieco, P. Ramires, A.M. Romito, G. De Rosa, and A. Piattelli. 2002. WNT-1 expression in basal cell carcinoma of head and neck. An immunohistochemical and confocal study with regard to the intracellular distribution of beta-catenin. *Anticancer Res.* 22:565-76.

Lo Muzio, L., S. Staibano, G. Pannone, M. Grieco, M.D. Mignogna, A. Cerrato, N.F. Testa, and G. De Rosa. 1999. Beta- and gamma-catenin expression in oral squamous cell carcinomas. *Anticancer Res.* 19:3817-26.

Lopez-Novoa, J.M., and M.A. Nieto. 2009. Inflammation and EMT: an alliance towards organ fibrosis and cancer progression. *EMBO Mol Med.* 1:303-14.

Maeda, M., K.R. Johnson, and M.J. Wheelock. 2005. Cadherin switching: essential for behavioral but not morphological changes during an epithelium-to-mesenchyme transition. *J Cell Sci.* 118:873-87.

Mangone, F.R., F. Walder, S. Maistro, F.S. Pasini, C.N. Lehn, M.B. Carvalho, M.M. Brentani, I. Snitcovsky, and M.H. Federico. 2010. Smad2 and Smad6 as predictors of overall survival in oral squamous cell carcinoma patients. *Mol Cancer.* 9:106.

Mani, P., A. Jarrell, J. Myers, and R. Atit. Visualizing canonical Wnt signaling during mouse craniofacial development. *Dev Dyn.* 239:354-63.

Mani, S.A., W. Guo, M.J. Liao, E.N. Eaton, A. Ayyanan, A.Y. Zhou, M. Brooks, F. Reinhard, C.C. Zhang, M. Shipitsin, L.L. Campbell, K. Polyak, C. Brisken, J. Yang, and R.A. Weinberg. 2008. The epithelial-mesenchymal transition generates cells with properties of stem cells. *Cell.* 133:704-15.

Martin, A., and A. Cano. 2010. Tumorigenesis: Twist1 links EMT to self-renewal. *Nat Cell Biol.* 12:924-5.

Masszi, A., L. Fan, L. Rosivall, C.A. McCulloch, O.D. Rotstein, I. Mucsi, and A. Kapus. 2004. Integrity of cell-cell contacts is a critical regulator of TGF-beta 1-induced epithelial-to-myofibroblast transition: role for beta-catenin. *Am J Pathol.* 165:1955-67.

Morel, A.P., M. Lievre, C. Thomas, G. Hinkal, S. Ansieau, and A. Puisieux. 2008. Generation of breast cancer stem cells through epithelial-mesenchymal transition. *PLoS One.* 3:e2888.

Myers, J. 2010. Oral Cancer Metastasis Springer Science+Business Media, LLC, New York, NY

Nakayama, H., T. Ikebe, M. Beppu, and K. Shirasuna. 2001. High expression levels of nuclear factor kappaB, IkappaB kinase alpha and Akt kinase in squamous cell carcinoma of the oral cavity. *Cancer.* 92:3037-44.

Nawshad, A., D. Lagamba, A. Polad, and E.D. Hay. 2005. Transforming growth factor-beta signaling during epithelial-mesenchymal transformation: implications for embryogenesis and tumor metastasis. *Cells Tissues Organs.* 179:11-23.

Nguyen, P.T., Y. Kudo, M. Yoshida, N. Kamata, I. Ogawa, and T. Takata. 2011. N-cadherin expression is involved in malignant behavior of head and neck cancer in relation to epithelial-mesenchymal transition. *Histol Histopathol.* 26:147-56.

Nieto, M.A., M.G. Sargent, D.G. Wilkinson, and J. Cooke. 1994. Control of cell behavior during vertebrate development by Slug, a zinc finger gene. *Science.* 264:835-9.

Odajima, T., Y. Sasaki, N. Tanaka, Y. Kato-Mori, H. Asanuma, T. Ikeda, M. Satoh, H. Hiratsuka, T. Tokino, and N. Sawada. 2005. Abnormal beta-catenin expression in oral cancer with no gene mutation: correlation with expression of cyclin D1 and epidermal growth factor receptor, Ki-67 labeling index, and clinicopathological features. *Hum Pathol.* 36:234-41.

Pannone, G., P. Bufo, A. Santoro, R. Franco, G. Aquino, F. Longo, G. Botti, R. Serpico, B. Cafarelli, A. Abbruzzese, M. Caraglia, S. Papagerakis, and L. Lo Muzio. 2010. WNT pathway in oral cancer: epigenetic inactivation of WNT-inhibitors. *Oncol Rep.* 24:1035-41.

Pannone, G., L. Lo Muzio, P. Bucci, M. Canfora, L. Santacroce, T. Bucci, and S. Staibano. 1998. [Physiopathology of beta and gamma catenin expression in the oral epithelium]. *Minerva Stomatol.* 47:583-8.

Papagerakis, P., G. Pannone, A.-H. Shabana, J. Depondt, A. Santoro, K. Ghirtis, A. Berdal, and S. Papagerakis. 2011. Aberrant ß-catenin and LEF1 expression may predict the clinical outcome for patients with oropharyngeal cancer (*under review*).

Papagerakis, S., A.H. Shabana, J. Depondt, L. Pibouin, C. Blin-Wakkach, and A. Berdal. 2004. Altered plakoglobin expression at mRNA and protein levels correlates with clinical outcome in patients with oropharynx squamous carcinomas. *Hum Pathol.* 35:75-85.

Papagerakis, S., A.H. Shabana, B.H. Pollock, P. Papagerakis, J. Depondt, and A. Berdal. 2009. Altered desmoplakin expression at transcriptional and protein levels provides prognostic information in human oropharyngeal cancer. *Hum Pathol.* 40:1320-9.

Prince, M.E., R. Sivanandan, A. Kaczorowski, G.T. Wolf, M.J. Kaplan, P. Dalerba, I.L. Weissman, M.F. Clarke, and L.E. Ailles. 2007. Identification of a subpopulation of cells with cancer stem cell properties in head and neck squamous cell carcinoma. *Proc Natl Acad Sci U S A.* 104:973-8.

Raimondi, C., A. Gradilone, G. Naso, B. Vincenzi, A. Petracca, C. Nicolazzo, A. Palazzo, R. Saltarelli, F. Spremberg, E. Cortesi, and P. Gazzaniga. 2011. Epithelial-mesenchymal transition and stemness features in circulating tumor cells from breast cancer patients. *Breast Cancer Res Treat.*

Reichmann, E., H. Schwarz, E.M. Deiner, I. Leitner, M. Eilers, J. Berger, M. Busslinger, and H. Beug. 1992. Activation of an inducible c-FosER fusion protein causes loss of epithelial polarity and triggers epithelial-fibroblastoid cell conversion. *Cell.* 71:1103-16.

Roussos, E.T., Z. Keckesova, J.D. Haley, D.M. Epstein, R.A. Weinberg, and J.S. Condeelis. 2010. AACR special conference on epithelial-mesenchymal transition and cancer progression and treatment. *Cancer Res.* 70:7360-4.

Rui, Y., Z. Xu, B. Xiong, Y. Cao, S. Lin, M. Zhang, S.C. Chan, W. Luo, Y. Han, Z. Lu, Z. Ye, H.M. Zhou, J. Han, A. Meng, and S.C. Lin. 2007. A beta-catenin-independent dorsalization pathway activated by Axin/JNK signaling and antagonized by aida. *Dev Cell.* 13:268-82.

Said, N.A., and E.D. Williams. 2011. Growth factors in induction of epithelial-mesenchymal transition and metastasis. *Cells Tissues Organs.* 193:85-97.

Singh, B., and J.P. Shah. 2003. Oral cancer. *In* Complications and their management. J.P. Shah, N.W. Johnson, and J.G. Batsakis, editors, London: Martin Dunitz. 367-72

Stockinger, A., A. Eger, J. Wolf, H. Beug, and R. Foisner. 2001. E-cadherin regulates cell growth by modulating proliferation-dependent beta-catenin transcriptional activity. *J Cell Biol.* 154:1185-96.

Takahashi, E., O. Nagano, T. Ishimoto, T. Yae, Y. Suzuki, T. Shinoda, S. Nakamura, S. Niwa, S. Ikeda, H. Koga, H. Tanihara, and H. Saya. 2010. Tumor necrosis factor-alpha regulates transforming growth factor-beta-dependent epithelial-mesenchymal transition by promoting hyaluronan-CD44-moesin interaction. *J Biol Chem.* 285:4060-73.

Takkunen, M., R. Grenman, M. Hukkanen, M. Korhonen, A. Garcia de Herreros, and I. Virtanen. 2006. Snail-dependent and -independent epithelial-mesenchymal transition in oral squamous carcinoma cells. *J Histochem Cytochem.* 54:1263-75.

Tamura, I., T. Sakaki, B. Chaqour, P.S. Howard, T. Ikeo, and E.J. Macarak. 2003. Correlation of P-cadherin and beta-catenin expression and phosphorylation with carcinogenesis in rat tongue cancer induced with 4-nitroquinoline 1-oxide. *Oral Oncol.* 39:506-14.

Tanaka, N., T. Odajima, K. Ogi, T. Ikeda, and M. Satoh. 2003. Expression of E-cadherin, alpha-catenin, and beta-catenin in the process of lymph node metastasis in oral squamous cell carcinoma. *Br J Cancer.* 89:557-63.

Testa, J.R., and A. Bellacosa. 2001. AKT plays a central role in tumorigenesis. *Proc Natl Acad Sci U S A.* 98:10983-5.

Thiery, J.P. 2002. Epithelial-mesenchymal transitions in tumour progression. *Nat Rev Cancer.* 2:442-54.

Thiery, J.P. 2003. Epithelial-mesenchymal transitions in development and pathologies. *Curr Opin Cell Biol.* 15:740-6.

Thiery, J.P., H. Acloque, R.Y. Huang, and M.A. Nieto. 2009. Epithelial-mesenchymal transitions in development and disease. *Cell.* 139:871-90.

Thiery, J.P., and J.P. Sleeman. 2006. Complex networks orchestrate epithelial-mesenchymal transitions. *Nat Rev Mol Cell Biol.* 7:131-42.

Valles, A.M., B. Boyer, J. Badet, G.C. Tucker, D. Barritault, and J.P. Thiery. 1990. Acidic fibroblast growth factor is a modulator of epithelial plasticity in a rat bladder carcinoma cell line. *Proc Natl Acad Sci U S A.* 87:1124-8.

van de Wetering, M., R. Cavallo, D. Dooijes, M. van Beest, J. van Es, J. Loureiro, A. Ypma, D. Hursh, T. Jones, A. Bejsovec, M. Peifer, M. Mortin, and H. Clevers. 1997. Armadillo coactivates transcription driven by the product of the Drosophila segment polarity gene dTCF. *Cell.* 88:789-99.

Vesuna, F., P. van Diest, J.H. Chen, and V. Raman. 2008. Twist is a transcriptional repressor of E-cadherin gene expression in breast cancer. *Biochem Biophys Res Commun.* 367:235-41.

Vleminckx, K., L. Vakaet, Jr., M. Mareel, W. Fiers, and F. van Roy. 1991. Genetic manipulation of E-cadherin expression by epithelial tumor cells reveals an invasion suppressor role. *Cell.* 66:107-19.

Wang, Z., and Q. Ma. 2007. Beta-catenin is a promising key factor in the SDF-1/CXCR4 axis on metastasis of pancreatic cancer. *Med Hypotheses.* 69:816-20.

Wellner, U., J. Schubert, U.C. Burk, O. Schmalhofer, F. Zhu, A. Sonntag, B. Waldvogel, C. Vannier, D. Darling, A. zur Hausen, V.G. Brunton, J. Morton, O. Sansom, J. Schuler, M.P. Stemmler, C. Herzberger, U. Hopt, T. Keck, S. Brabletz, and T. Brabletz. 2009. The EMT-activator ZEB1 promotes tumorigenicity by repressing stemness-inhibiting microRNAs. *Nat Cell Biol.* 11:1487-95.

Wells, A., C. Yates, and C.R. Shepard. 2008. E-cadherin as an indicator of mesenchymal to epithelial reverting transitions during the metastatic seeding of disseminated carcinomas. *Clin Exp Metastasis*. 25:621-8.

Williams, H.K., D.S. Sanders, J.A. Jankowski, G. Landini, and A.M. Brown. 1998. Expression of cadherins and catenins in oral epithelial dysplasia and squamous cell carcinoma. *J Oral Pathol Med*. 27:308-17.

Wu, K.J., and M.H. Yang. 2011. Epithelial-mesenchymal transition and cancer stemness: the Twist1-Bmi1 connection. *Biosci Rep*. 31:449-55.

Yadav, A., B. Kumar, J. Datta, T. Teknos, and P. Kumar. 2011. IL-6 promotes head and neck tumor metastasis by inducing epithelial-mesenchymal transition via the JAK-STAT3-SNAIL signaling pathway. *AACR 102nd annual meeting, 2011.*

Yang, J., S.A. Mani, J.L. Donaher, S. Ramaswamy, R.A. Itzykson, C. Come, P. Savagner, I. Gitelman, A. Richardson, and R.A. Weinberg. 2004. Twist, a master regulator of morphogenesis, plays an essential role in tumor metastasis. *Cell*. 117:927-39.

Yang, L., C. Lin, and Z.R. Liu. 2006. P68 RNA helicase mediates PDGF-induced epithelial mesenchymal transition by displacing Axin from beta-catenin. *Cell*. 127:139-55.

Yang, M.H., D.S. Hsu, H.W. Wang, H.J. Wang, H.Y. Lan, W.H. Yang, C.H. Huang, S.Y. Kao, C.H. Tzeng, S.K. Tai, S.Y. Chang, O.K. Lee, and K.J. Wu. 2010. Bmi1 is essential in Twist1-induced epithelial-mesenchymal transition. *Nat Cell Biol*. 12:982-92.

Yang, M.H., and K.J. Wu. 2008. TWIST activation by hypoxia inducible factor-1 (HIF-1): implications in metastasis and development. *Cell Cycle*. 7:2090-6.

Yang, M.H., M.Z. Wu, S.H. Chiou, P.M. Chen, S.Y. Chang, C.J. Liu, S.C. Teng, and K.J. Wu. 2008. Direct regulation of TWIST by HIF-1alpha promotes metastasis. *Nat Cell Biol*. 10:295-305.

Yokoyama, K., N. Kamata, E. Hayashi, T. Hoteiya, N. Ueda, R. Fujimoto, and M. Nagayama. 2001. Reverse correlation of E-cadherin and snail expression in oral squamous cell carcinoma cells in vitro. *Oral Oncol*. 37:65-71.

Yoshimura, M., Y. Ihara, Y. Matsuzawa, and N. Taniguchi. 1996. Aberrant glycosylation of E-cadherin enhances cell-cell binding to suppress metastasis. *J Biol Chem*. 271:13811-5.

Yu, Z., P.M. Weinberger, E. Provost, B.G. Haffty, C. Sasaki, J. Joe, R.L. Camp, D.L. Rimm, and A. Psyrri. 2005. beta-Catenin functions mainly as an adhesion molecule in patients with squamous cell cancer of the head and neck. *Clin Cancer Res*. 11:2471-7.

Permissions

The contributors of this book come from diverse backgrounds, making this book a truly international effort. This book will bring forth new frontiers with its revolutionizing research information and detailed analysis of the nascent developments around the world.

We would like to thank Kalu U. E. Ogbureke, for lending his expertise to make the book truly unique. He has played a crucial role in the development of this book. Without his invaluable contribution this book wouldn't have been possible. He has made vital efforts to compile up to date information on the varied aspects of this subject to make this book a valuable addition to the collection of many professionals and students.

This book was conceptualized with the vision of imparting up-to-date information and advanced data in this field. To ensure the same, a matchless editorial board was set up. Every individual on the board went through rigorous rounds of assessment to prove their worth. After which they invested a large part of their time researching and compiling the most relevant data for our readers. Conferences and sessions were held from time to time between the editorial board and the contributing authors to present the data in the most comprehensible form. The editorial team has worked tirelessly to provide valuable and valid information to help people across the globe.

Every chapter published in this book has been scrutinized by our experts. Their significance has been extensively debated. The topics covered herein carry significant findings which will fuel the growth of the discipline. They may even be implemented as practical applications or may be referred to as a beginning point for another development. Chapters in this book were first published by InTech; hereby published with permission under the Creative Commons Attribution License or equivalent.

The editorial board has been involved in producing this book since its inception. They have spent rigorous hours researching and exploring the diverse topics which have resulted in the successful publishing of this book. They have passed on their knowledge of decades through this book. To expedite this challenging task, the publisher supported the team at every step. A small team of assistant editors was also appointed to further simplify the editing procedure and attain best results for the readers.

Our editorial team has been hand-picked from every corner of the world. Their multi-ethnicity adds dynamic inputs to the discussions which result in innovative outcomes. These outcomes are then further discussed with the researchers and contributors who give their valuable feedback and opinion regarding the same. The feedback is then collaborated with the researches and they are edited in a comprehensive manner to aid the understanding of the subject.

Apart from the editorial board, the designing team has also invested a significant amount of their time in understanding the subject and creating the most relevant covers. They scrutinized every image to scout for the most suitable representation of the subject and create an appropriate cover for the book.

The publishing team has been involved in this book since its early stages. They were actively engaged in every process, be it collecting the data, connecting with the contributors or procuring relevant information. The team has been an ardent support to the editorial, designing and production team. Their endless efforts to recruit the best for this project, has resulted in the accomplishment of this book. They are a veteran in the field of academics and their pool of knowledge is as vast as their experience in printing. Their expertise and guidance has proved useful at every step. Their uncompromising quality standards have made this book an exceptional effort. Their encouragement from time to time has been an inspiration for everyone.

The publisher and the editorial board hope that this book will prove to be a valuable piece of knowledge for researchers, students, practitioners and scholars across the globe.

List of Contributors

Kalu U. E. Ogbureke
Department of Oral Biology, College of Dental Medicine, Georgia Health Sciences University, Augusta, Georgia, USA

Christopher Bingham
Department of Periodontology, College of Dental Medicine, Georgia Health Sciences University, Augusta, Georgia, USA

Raghu Radhakrishnan, Bijayata Shrestha and Dipshikha Bajracharya
Department of Oral Pathology, Manipal College of Dental Sciences, Manipal University, India

Nicolás Bolesina, Fabián L. Femopase, Silvia A. López de Blanc, Rosana A. Morelatto and María Alicia Olmos
Universidad Nacional de Córdoba, Córdoba, Argentina

C. S. Farah, P. J. Ford, K. Allen and A. Vu
The University of Queensland, School of Dentistry, Brisbane, Australia
The University of Queensland, UQ Centre for Clinical Research, Herston, Australia

M. J. McCullough
The University of Melbourne, Melbourne Dental School, Melbourne, Australia

Shih-An Liu
National Yang-Ming University, Taichung Veterans General Hospital, Taiwan, ROC

Chi-Ting Chiang
Green Energy and Environment Research Laboratories, Industrial Technology Research Institute, Taiwan, ROC

Tsun-Kuo Chang
Department of Bioenvironmental Systems Engineering, National Taiwan University, Taiwan, ROC

Ie-Bin Lian
Graduate Institute of Statistics and Information Science, National Changhua University of Education, Taiwan

Che-Chun Su
Department of Internal Medicine, Changhua Christian Hospital, Taiwan, ROC

Yang Kuo-Tsai
Department of Oral and Maxillofacial Surgery, Changhua Christian Hospital, Taiwan, ROC

Yaw-Huei Hwang
Department of Public Health, National Taiwan University, Taiwan, ROC

Michael J. McCullough and Gareema Prasad
The University of Melbourne, Melbourne Dental School, Melbourne, Australia

Sarah Zhao and Camile S. Farah
The University of Queensland, School of Dentistry, Brisbane, Australia
The University of Queensland, UQ Centre for Clinical Research, Herston, Australia

Nur Mohammad Monsur Hassan
Department of Oral and Maxillofacial Surgery, Division of Oncological Science, Okayama University Graduate School of Medicine, Dentistry and Pharmaceutical Sciences, Okayama, Japan
Division of Cancer-Related Genes, Institute for Genetic Medicine, Hokkaido University, Sapporo, Japan

Akira Sasaki
Department of Oral and Maxillofacial Surgery, Division of Oncological Science, Okayama University Graduate School of Medicine, Dentistry and Pharmaceutical Sciences, Okayama, Japan

Mitsuhiro Tada, Jun-ichi Hamada and Tetsuya Moriuchi
Division of Cancer-Related Genes, Institute for Genetic Medicine, Hokkaido University, Sapporo, Japan

Nobuo Inoue and Haruhiko Kashiwazaki
Department of Geriatric Stomatology, Hokkaido University Graduate School of Dental Medicine, Sapporo, Japan

Masanobu Shindoh
Department of Oral Pathology, Hokkaido University Graduate School of Dental Medicine, Sapporo, Japan

Yutaka Yamazaki
Department of Oral Diagnosis and Oral Medicine, Division of Oral Health Science, Hokkaido University Graduate School of Dental Medicine, Sapporo, Japan

Yuichi Ashikaga
Department of Oral and Maxillofacial Surgery, Division of Oral Health Science, Hokkaido University Graduate School of Dental Medicine, Sapporo, Japan

Pegah Mosannen Mozafari, Zahra Delavarian and Nooshin Mohtasham
Oral and Maxillofacial Diseases Research Center, Mashhad Dental Faculty, Mashhad University of Medical Sciences, Mashhad, Iran

S. Gokul
YMT Dental College and Hospital, India

Pablo Varela Centelles, Juan Manuel Seoane-Romero, Iria Gómez, Pedro Diz-Dios, Nilce Santos de Melo and Juan Seoane
University of Santiago de Compostela, Spain
University of Brasilia, Brazil

Mônica Lúcia Rodrigues, Hugo Fontan Köhler and Luiz Paulo Kowalski
Department of Head and Neck Surgery and Otolaryngology, A. C. Camargo Hospital, Brazil

Kiyoto Shiga, Katsunori Katagiri, Ayako Nakanome, Takenori Ogawa and Toshimitsu Kobayashi
Department of Otolaryngology-Head and Neck Surgery, Tohoku University Hospital, Japan

Carlos Campi, Livia Escovich, Liliana Racca, Amelia Racca, Carlos Cotorruelo and Claudia Biondi
National University of Rosario, Argentina

Masumi Tsuda and Yusuke Ohba
Laboratory of Pathophysiology and Signal Transduction, Hokkaido University Graduate School of Medicine, Japan

G. Pannone and P. Bufo
Department of Surgical Sciences, Section of Pathological Anatomy and Cytopathology, University of Foggia, Foggia, Italy

A. Santoro
Department of Surgical Sciences, Section of Pathological Anatomy and Cytopathology, University of Foggia, Foggia, Italy
Department of Surgical Sciences, Institute of Pathological Anatomy, University of Bari, Bari, Italy

R. Serpico and A. Guida
Department of Oral Pathology, Orthodontics and Oral Surgery, Second University of Napoli, Napoli, Italy

L. Lo Muzio
Department of Surgical Sciences, Section of Oral Pathology, University of Foggia, Foggia, Italy

S. Papagerakis
Department of Otolaryngology - Head and Neck Surgery and Oncology, Medical School University of Michigan Ann Arbor, Ann Arbor, MI, USA

Takashi Muramatsu
Oral Health Science Center hrc8, Tokyo Dental College, Chiba, Japan
Department of Pathology, Tokyo Dental College, Chiba, Japan
Department of Clinical Pathophysiology, Tokyo Dental College, Chiba, Japan

Walter Giaretti
Biophysics and Cytometry Section, Department of Diagnostic Oncology, National Institute for Cancer Research, Genoa, Italy

Dziegiel Piotr, Pula Bartosz and Podhorska-Okolow Marzena
Department of Histology and Embryology, Wroclaw Medical University, Poland

Silvana Papagerakis
Department of Otolaryngology, Head and Neck Surgery, Laboratory of Oral, Head and Neck Cancer Invasion and Metastasis, Medical School, University of Michigan Ann Arbor, UM Comprehensive Cancer Center, Ann Arbor, MI, USA

Giuseppe Pannone
Department of Surgical Sciences, Section of Anatomic Pathology and Cytopathology, University of Foggia, Foggia, Italy